COGNITIVE-BEHAVIORAL STRATEGIES IN CRISIS INTERVENTION

Cognitive-Behavioral Strategies in *Crisis Intervention*

THIRD EDITION

EDITED BY

Frank M. Dattilio
Arthur Freeman

Foreword by AARON T. BECK

THE GUILFORD PRESS
New York   London

© 2007 The Guilford Press
A Division of Guilford Publications, Inc.
72 Spring Street, New York, NY 10012
www.guilford.com

Printed in the United States of America

This book is printed on acid-free paper.

Last digit is print number: 9 8 7 6 5 4 3 2 1

The authors have checked with sources believed to be reliable in their efforts to provide
information that is complete and generally in accord with the standards of practice that are
accepted at the time of publication. However, in view of the possibility of human error or
changes in medical sciences, neither the authors, nor the editor and publisher, nor any other
party who has been involved in the preparation or publication of this work warrants that the
information contained herein is in every respect accurate or complete, and they are not
responsible for any errors or omissions or the results obtained from the use of such
information. Readers are encouraged to confirm the information contained in this book with
other sources.

Library of Congress Cataloging-in-Publication Data

Cognitive-behavioral strategies in crisis intervention / edited by Frank M. Dattilio, Arthur
Freeman ; foreword by Aaron T. Beck.—3rd ed.
    p. ; cm.
    Includes bibliographical references and index.
    ISBN-10: 1-59385-487-0   ISBN-13: 978-1-59385-487-4 (cloth: alk. paper)
    1. Cognitive therapy.   2. Crisis intervention (Mental health services)   I. Dattilio, Frank M.
II. Freeman, Arthur, 1942–
    [DNLM: 1. Crisis Intervention—methods. 2. Cognitive Therapy. 3. Mental Disorders—
therapy. WM 401 C676 2007]
    RC480.6.C63 2007
    616.89′142—dc22

                                                              2007011928

About the Editors

Frank M. Dattilio, PhD, ABPP, maintains a dual faculty position in psychiatry at both Harvard Medical School and the University of Pennsylvania School of Medicine. He is a clinical psychologist and is listed in the National Register of Health Service Providers in Psychology. He is also a diplomate in behavioral psychology and clinical psychology of the American Board of Professional Psychology; a founding fellow of the Academy of Cognitive Therapy; and a visiting professor at several major universities throughout the world. Dr. Dattilio trained in behavior therapy in the Department of Psychiatry at Temple University School of Medicine under the direct supervision of the late Joseph Wolpe; he completed a postdoctoral fellowship at the Center for Cognitive Therapy, University of Pennsylvania School of Medicine, under Aaron T. Beck. He has more than 200 professional publications to his credit in the areas of anxiety disorders, behavioral problems, and marital and family discord. He has also presented extensively on cognitive-behavioral therapy throughout the United States, Canada, Africa, Europe, South America, New Zealand, Australia, Cuba, the West Indies, and Mexico. Dr. Dattilio's works have been translated into 22 languages and are used as required reading worldwide. Among his many publications are *Cognitive Therapy with Couples, Comprehensive Casebook of Cognitive Therapy, Cognitive Therapy with Children and Adolescents: A Casebook for Clinical Practice, Case Studies in Couple and Family Therapy: Systemic and Cognitive Perspectives, The Family Therapy Treatment Planner, Relationship Dysfunction: A Practitioner's Guide to Comparative Treatments,* and *Panic Disorder: Assessment and Treatment through a Wide-Angle Lens.* He is on the boards of several professional journals, including *The New England Journal of Medicine,* and has received a number of professional awards for outstanding achievement in the fields of psychology, psychiatry, and medicine.

Arthur Freeman, EdD, ABPP, is Visiting Professor in the Department of Psychology at Governors State University, University Park, Illinois, and Director of Training at Sheridan Shores Care and Rehabilitation, Chicago. Dr. Freeman completed a postdoctoral fellowship at the Center for Cognitive Therapy, University of Pennsylvania School of Medicine, under Aaron T. Beck and also studied with Albert Ellis in New York. In addition to over 40 book chapters, reviews, and journal articles, he has published 20 professional books, including *Cognitive Therapy of Personality Disorders* (with Aaron T. Beck), *Clinical Applications of Cognitive Therapy* (with James Pretzer, Barbara Fleming, and Karen M. Simon), and *Comprehensive Casebook of Cognitive Therapy* (with Frank M. Dattilio), and two popular books, *Woulda, Coulda, Shoulda: Overcoming Mistakes and Missed Opportunities* and *The 10 Dumbest Mistakes Smart People Make, and How to Overcome Them* (both with Rose DeWolf). His work has been translated into almost a dozen languages. Dr. Freeman serves on the editorial boards of several U.S. and international journals. He is a diplomate in behavioral psychology and clinical psychology of the American Board of Professional Psychology and a fellow of the American Psychological Association, the American Psychological Society, the Academy of Clinical Psychology, and the Pennsylvania Psychological Association. He is past president of the Association for Advancement of Behavior Therapy. Dr. Freeman has been a visiting professor of psychiatry and psychology at the Universities of Umeå and Göteborg (Sweden), the University of Catania (Italy), and the Shanghai Second Medical University (China). He has lectured in more than 22 countries.

Contributors

Emily Becker-Weidman, BA, is a student in the doctoral program in clinical psychology at Northwestern University Feinberg School of Medicine. After graduating from the University or Pennsylvania, she worked at the Beck Institute for Cognitive Therapy and Research as a research assistant, executive assistant to the director, and education coordinator.

Frank M. Dattilio (see "About the Editors").

Elizabeth A. Davis, MD, is an instructor in the Massachusetts General Hospital Department of Psychiatry, Harvard Medical School, Boston, and has an outpatient practice at the Massachusetts Mental Health Center. She is boarded in internal medicine after completing her primary care training at the Cambridge Hospital, Cambridge, Massachusetts. She also completed a fellowship in psychosomatic medicine in 2003 in the Department of Psychiatry at the Cambridge Hospital.

Esther Deblinger, PhD, is a licensed clinical psychologist and professor at the University of Medicine and Dentistry of New Jersey–School of Osteopathic Medicine. She is cofounder and codirector of the New Jersey Child Abuse Research Education and Service (CARES) Institute, which is a member center of the National Child Traumatic Stress Network (NCTSN). Dr. Deblinger has conducted extensive clinical research examining the mental health impact of child abuse and the treatment of posttraumatic stress disorder and other abuse-related difficulties. She has authored numerous scientific articles and book chapters and published four professional books.

Helen M. DeVries, PhD, is professor and director of the doctoral program in clinical psychology at Wheaton College. She completed postdoctoral training in geropsychology at Stanford University School of Medicine and the VA Palo Alto Health Care System and in neuropsychology at the Medical College of Virginia, Department of Rehabilitation Medicine. Her teaching and research interests are in clinical geropsychology and midlife and late-life family coping.

Norman B. Epstein, PhD, is professor of family studies and director of the marriage and family therapy program at the University of Maryland, College Park. He is a fellow of the American Psychological Association and a clinical member and approved supervisor of the American Association for Marriage and Family Therapy. He has published over 80 journal articles and book chapters as well as four books, including the 2002 text *Enhanced*

Cognitive-Behavioral Therapy for Couples: A Contextual Approach (coauthored with Donald H. Baucom). Throughout his career, he has maintained a part-time clinical practice with individuals, couples, and families.

Arthur Freeman (see "About the Editors").

Sharon Morgillo Freeman, PhD, is president-elect of NAADAC, the Association for Addiction Professionals, and serves on the board of directors of the International Association for Cognitive Psychotherapy. She is associate faculty at Indiana–Purdue University, Fort Wayne, Indiana, and a board-certified advanced-practice clinical nurse specialist. In addition, she is director of the Center for Brief Therapy in Fort Wayne, Indiana. Dr. Freeman has lectured nationally and internationally on the problems of substance misuse and addiction issues and the use of cognitive therapy with chronic pain problems, mood disorders, psychopharmacology, personality disorders, and trauma.

Gina M. Fusco, PsyD, a licensed psychologist and graduate of the Philadelphia College of Osteopathic Medicine, is the executive clinical director for the Northeastern Region of Alternative Behavioral Services. She has designed, developed, and implemented residential and continuum-of-care services for high-risk adolescents; provided clinical oversight to crisis intervention and high-risk programs; and provided trauma-focused evaluation and crisis services. Her publications include books on borderline personality disorder and numerous textbook chapters on crisis intervention, borderline personality disorder, and cognitive-behavioral therapy.

Tamar Galai-Gat, MA, is a clinical and medical psychologist specializing in trauma and crisis work and has extensive experience as a clinical psychologist specializing in adolescent and adult counseling. Ms. Galai-Gat has trained both in the United States and in Israel. She is the author of a number of professional articles in the field of psychotrauma and is the founder and director of Metiv, the first and only walk-in crisis center in Israel. Metiv is a unit of the Israel Center for the Treatment of Psychotrauma, Herzog Hospital. In her capacity as director of Metiv, Ms. Galai-Gat has developed and implemented a unique model of crisis intervention. She has also been instrumental in the creation of programs for first responders (firefighters, police, and paramedics) in the Jerusalem area.

Robert M. Goisman, MD, is associate professor of psychiatry at Harvard Medical School and director of medical student education at the Massachusetts Mental Health Center in Boston. Dr. Goisman was one of the first psychiatrists in the United States to practice and teach cognitive-behavioral therapy. His areas of interest include anxiety disorders, social skills training, and psychosocial rehabilitation, and he has won awards for his teaching and clinical work from Harvard Medical School, the Massachusetts Psychiatric Society, and the American Psychiatric Association.

Wayne A. Gordon, PhD, is the Jack Nash Professor of Rehabilitation Medicine, associate director of the Department of Rehabilitation Medicine, and chief of the Rehabilitation Psychology and Neuropsychology Services in the Department of Rehabilitation Medicine, Mount Sinai School of Medicine, New York City. Dr. Gordon is a diplomate in clinical neuropsychology and a fellow in the Academy of Behavioral Medicine Research. He has published more than 100 articles and book chapters. Dr. Gordon is the project director of two grants funded by the National Institute on Disability and Rehabilitation Research focusing on the effects of traumatic brain injury, and he received a recognition award in 1996 from the New York State Department of Health for his visionary work in the field.

L. Kevin Hamberger, PhD, is a professor of family and community medicine at the Medical College of Wisconsin. Since the mid-1980s, he has conducted research and treatment in the area of intimate partner violence, working with both perpetrators and survivors. He has published over 85 journal articles and book chapters and 6 books and guest-edited several journal special issues devoted to intimate partner violence. He is presently the co-chair of the Wisconsin Governor's Council on Domestic Abuse.

Anne Hope Heflin, PhD, is an associate professor of clinical psychology at the American School of Professional Psychology of Argosy University, Washington, DC, campus. Her research and clinical interests have focused on the evaluation and treatment of children and adolescents, particularly those who have been exposed to trauma such as child sexual abuse. She coauthored the book *Treating Sexually Abused Children and Their Nonoffending Parents: A Cognitive Behavioral Approach* and has published a variety of articles and chapters on children's mental health issues.

Mary R. Hibbard, PhD, is a professor of rehabilitation medicine and psychiatry at the Mount Sinai School of Medicine, New York City. She holds a diplomate in rehabilitation psychology and membership in the American Board of Rehabilitation Psychology and is a fellow and the current secretary of Division 22 (Rehabilitation Psychology) of the American Psychological Association. Dr. Hibbard is the director of research for the New York TBI Model System Program, director of training for the Research and Training Center on TBI Interventions, and project director for an Advanced Rehabilitation Research Training Program. She has published more than 60 articles and book chapters in the field of clinical neuropsychology, rehabilitation psychology, traumatic brain injury, and stroke. She has received several awards, including the Ted Weiss Advocacy Award for her advocacy work for individuals with traumatic brain injury.

Stevan E. Hobfoll, PhD, is Distinguished Professor of Psychology at Kent State University and director of their Applied Psychology Center and the Summa–Kent State University Center for the Treatment and Study of Traumatic Stress. He is also a fellow of the Center for National Security Studies at the University of Haifa, Israel. Formerly an officer in the Israeli Defense Forces, Dr. Hobfoll remains involved with the problem of stress in Israel. He was co-chair of the American Psychological Association (APA) Commission on Stress and War during Operation Desert Storm, helping plan for the prevention of prolonged distress among military personnel and their families; a member of the task force on bioterrorism; and a member of the APA Task Force on Resilience in Response to Terrorism. Dr. Hobfoll has authored and edited 11 books, including *Traumatic Stress, The Ecology of Stress*, and *Stress, Culture, and Community*. In addition, he has authored over 160 journal articles, book chapters, and technical reports and has been a frequent workshop leader on stress, war, and terrorism.

Amy Holtzworth-Munroe, PhD, is a professor of psychology at Indiana University, Bloomington. She has conducted research on the problem of relationship aggression since the mid-1980s, recently focusing on the study of subtypes of male batterers. Dr. Holtzworth-Monroe has published more than 50 journal articles and book chapters and serves on various journal editorial boards and grant review panels in the area of domestic violence. She has led batterer intervention groups and worked with a local domestic violence task force to set up batterer programs.

Dawn M. Johnson, PhD, is an assistant professor and clinic coordinator of the Summa–Kent State University Center for the Treatment and Study of Traumatic Stress in Akron, Ohio. She is currently in her fourth year of support from a career development award where she is developing and evaluating the initial efficacy of a shelter-based treatment for battered women with posttraumatic stress disorder. Chapter 17 in this volume, illustrating Dr. Johnson's work with women who are currently under ongoing threat, was used in part as a model for treatment of victims of terrorism and mass casualty.

Philip C. Kendall, PhD, is the Laura H. Carnell Professor of Psychology and director of the Child and Adolescent Anxiety Disorders Clinic at Temple University. He is an internationally recognized expert on clinical child and adolescent psychology and clinical psychological research. As author/coauthor of over 300 research publications and books, Dr. Kendall's work has advanced our understanding of the nature of psychological disorders of youth (e.g., anxiety) and the outcomes associated with psychological treatments (e.g., cognitive-behavioral therapy). Dr. Kendall has been editor of the *Journal of Consulting and Clinical Psychology* and is past president of Division 53 (Clinical Child and Adolescent Psychology) of the American Psychological Association and the Association for Behavioral and Cognitive Therapies.

Samuel Knapp, EdD, is the director of professional affairs of the Pennsylvania Psychological Association. His primary area of research is in professional ethics, but he also has interests in religion and psychology and multiculturalism.

Lynne M. Kothera, PhD, is a senior psychologist in the Department of Rehabilitation Medicine, Mount Sinai Medical Center, New York City. She is the codirector of training for an American Psychological Association-accredited predoctoral internship program within the Department of Rehabilitation Medicine. Dr. Kothera has completed a 2-year fellowship in clinical neuropsychology at the Institute of Living, Hartford, Connecticut, and postdoctoral training in psychoanalysis and psychotherapy at New York University.

Lata K. McGinn, PhD, is associate professor of psychology at the Ferkauf Graduate School of Psychology, Yeshiva University/Albert Einstein College of Medicine, and director of the Doctoral Clinical Program and the Cognitive Behavior Training Program. Dr. McGinn specializes in cognitive-behavioral therapy of anxiety and depression and has authored numerous publications, including a book on the treatment of obsessive–compulsive disorder. Dr. McGinn is a founding fellow of the Academy of Cognitive Therapy (ACT) and is on the executive board of the International Association for Cognitive Psychotherapy. She also served on the ACT Trauma Taskforce developed to address the needs of individuals suffering from the aftermath of the World Trade Center attack.

Joop J. Meijers, PhD, a clinical psychologist and psychotherapist, is chair of the Department of Clinical Child and Educational Psychology at the School of Education of the Hebrew University in Jerusalem. He is also chair of the Israeli Association for Cognitive-Behavior Therapy. Dr. Meijers teaches and supervises students in cognitive-behavioral therapy (CBT). His main research interests include problem-solving therapy with conduct-disordered children, and intrusive thoughts and CBT for children with obsessive–compulsive disorder. In addition to his academic assignment, Dr. Meijers has a private practice in CBT.

Laurence Miller, PhD, is a psychologist specializing in clinical, forensic, and law enforcement psychology, as well as corporate consulting and management training. Dr. Miller is the police psychologist for the West Palm Beach Police Department and consults with other local, regional, and national law enforcement agencies. He is a certified trainer by the International Critical Incident Stress Foundation and is a member of the Psychological Services Section of the International Association of Chiefs of Police. Dr. Miller is an instructor at the Criminal Justice Institute of Palm Beach County and is on the adjunct faculty of Florida Atlantic University. He conducts continuing education workshops and training seminars around the United States and is the author of numerous publications pertaining to the brain, behavior, health, law, criminal justice, and crisis management. His most recent book is *Practical Police Psychology: Stress Management and Crisis Intervention for Law Enforcement.*

Elizabeth Muran, PhD, completed graduate and postdoctoral training in cognitive-behavioral therapy. She has authored and presented professional papers on posttraumatic stress disorder. She is currently in independent practice in New York City.

Suzann M. Ogland-Hand, PhD, is a geriatric consultant and supervising geropsychologist with the Pine Rest Christian Mental Health Services in Grand Rapids, Michigan, and an adjunct assistant professor in the Department of Psychiatry at Michigan State University.

Mark A. Reinecke, PhD, professor of psychiatry and behavioral sciences and chief of the Division of Psychology at Northwestern University's Feinberg School of Medicine, is a distinguished fellow and former president of the Academy of Cognitive Therapy and a diplomate of the American Board of Professional Psychology in clinical psychology and clinical child and adolescent psychology. His research and clinical interests include vulnerability for depression and suicide, empirically supported treatments of childhood depression and anxiety, and cognitive mediation of adjustment to chronic illness. Dr. Reinecke serves on the editorial boards of several professional journals. Among his published works are *Cognitive Therapy of Suicidal Behavior, Cognitive Therapy with Children and Adolescents, Comparative Treatments of Depression, Cognitive Therapy across the Lifespan,* and *Encyclopedia of Cognitive Behavior Therapy.*

Stephen E. Schlesinger, PhD, is a licensed psychologist in private practice with offices in Chicago and Oak Park, Illinois. He is a cofounder of The Couples' Workshop, an organization that teaches couples effective relationship skills, and is an assistant professor at Northwestern University Medical School. Dr. Schlesinger's research and publications are in the areas of addictions and marital and family education and therapy.

Carrie B. Spindel, PsyD, is a clinical psychologist working with children, adolescents, adults, and families, and coordinator of the Cognitive Behavioral Consultants of Westchester, a group practice in White Plains, New York. Dr. Spindel has advanced training in cognitive and behavioral treatment of anxiety disorders, trauma, and depression, and in dialectical behavior therapy for borderline personality disorder, suicidal, and self-injurious behavior. She recently coauthored *Child Maltreatment: Advances in Psychotherapy—Evidence-Based Practice.* Dr. Spindel serves as the membership associate for the International Association for Cognitive Psychotherapy and has served on the planning committee for the International Society for the Improvement and Teaching of Dialectical Behavior Therapy conference.

Misti Storie, MS, holds a master's degree in justice, law, and society from American University and is currently the Education and Training Coordinator for NAADAC, the Association for Addiction Professionals based in Alexandria, Virginia. Among other projects, Ms. Storie has authored *The Basics of Addiction Counseling: Desk Reference and Study Guide* (9th ed.); *Campral Awareness Training,* which is used across the United States; and numerous articles concerning addiction for *NAADAC News.*

Stephen Timchack, MS, is a fourth-year doctoral student in clinical psychology at the Philadelphia College of Osteopathic Medicine. He also holds adjunct faculty appointments in the Department of Psychology at College Misericordia, where he teaches courses in developmental psychology and introductory psychology, as well as the University of Scranton's graduate program in counseling and human services, where he teaches courses on psychopathology and provides supervision to master's-level counseling students on internship. Mr. Timchack has presented locally, statewide, and nationally on topics including cognitive-behavioral therapy, applied behavior analysis, and autism/pervasive developmental disorder.

Leon VandeCreek, PhD, is professor in the School of Professional Psychology at Wright State University, Dayton, Ohio. His primary areas of interest are professional ethics and issues, including professional liability, and psychological assessment.

Jason J. Washburn, PhD, is a research assistant professor in the Department of Psychiatry and Behavioral Sciences at Northwestern University's Feinberg School of Medicine. His research and clinical interests include psychosocial treatments for children and adolescents, antisocial behavior, juvenile justice, and diversity.

Patricia J. Watson, PhD, is deputy to the director of the National Center for Posttraumatic Stress Disorder, an educational specialist for the National Center for PTSD, and an assistant professor at Dartmouth Medical School in the Department of Psychiatry. She currently collaborates with the Substance Abuse and Mental Health Services Administration and the Centers for Disease Control and Prevention and subject-matter experts to create publications for public and mental health interventions following large-scale terrorism, disaster, and pandemic flu. Dr. Watson also serves as vice president and secretary of the Mobility Without Barriers Foundation, a nonprofit organization that offers all-terrain mobility devices to disabled individuals in programs that foster increased quality of life.

Foreword

This third edition of *Cognitive-Behavioral Strategies in Crisis Intervention* comes on the heels of a number of major worldwide crises that have occurred since the second edition appeared in 2000, forever changing the way we think and feel about crisis situations. Although this third edition covers many of the topics presented in the former two editions, all the chapters have been updated with the most recent research on assessment and treatment interventions on each topic, along with a number of new chapters that address the broader spectrum of crisis intervention.

The introductory chapter by the editors provides an overview of crisis intervention and the need for short-term effective treatments. The remaining chapters highlight the clinical syndromes that are commonly encountered in outpatient settings, such as panic disorder, cluster B disorders, suicide/depression, substance abuse, rape trauma, child sexual abuse, divorce, and problems with couples, families, and older adults.

A comprehensive chapter on neurological problems and medical patients as well as one on ethical and legal issues address areas that are of particular concern to today's mental health practitioners. There are also several new additions to the book that cover timely topics, such as dealing with victims of terrorist attacks. Special chapters on anger and aggression in children and adolescents and dealing with acute and chronic pain have been added, along with a revised section on large-scale disasters and an innovative chapter on crisis intervention for law enforcement and mental health professionals.

Because crises and natural disasters occur throughout the world on a daily basis, the need for effective strategies in crisis intervention has become more essential than ever, especially in light of the rapid growth of our world's population and the increasing conflicts between nations.

The editors, both former students of mine, have become leaders in the world of cognitive therapy. Frank Dattilio and Art Freeman have once again compiled a powerful text, prepared by some of the finest experts in the field of cognitive therapy and applied to a comprehensive range of crisis situations.

The text's quality is the result of an excellent selection of authors with a background rich in clinical experience and empirical research. In addition, each chapter has been strategically organized to provide the reader with a thorough overview of the application of cognitive therapy to a broad variety of settings. Drs. Dattilio and Freeman are highly respected worldwide as authors and educators of cognitive therapy. Combined, their works have been translated into more than 30 languages and are used as primary teaching references. In fact, the earlier editions of the text have been used by mental health experts working in countries that have been the heaviest victims of terroristic attacks and natural disasters.

This third edition of *Cognitive-Behavioral Strategies in Crisis Intervention* provides the most up-to-date information on cutting-edge interventions. This compendium of interventions will prove invaluable to clinicians who wish to sharpen their skills in the area of crisis work. This text is a necessity for the front-line practitioner and will clearly serve as a resource for continued research in the field.

AARON T. BECK, MD
University Professor of Psychiatry
University of Pennsylvania School of Medicine

Preface

We are both pleased and honored that, since 1994, the first two editions of this crisis intervention book have been translated into several languages and have been used by clinicians and training programs worldwide. This clearly says something about the unique contribution that the text has to offer. It is with great pride that we go forward in 2007 with the third edition of this text.

Crisis intervention continues to be an important and crucial area of the mental health delivery system. Despite the increased need for improved strategies for crisis intervention, the literature in cognitive-behavioral therapy is sparse but continues to grow as world crises also continue to grow. It is our hope that this third edition will improve the professional literature on the application of cognitive-behavioral interventions. As with the first two editions, this edition of the book has been designed for both active crisis workers, who come in contact daily with crisis situations in outpatient and outreach programs, as well as private practitioners, who will undoubtedly encounter crisis situations in their work. Regardless of the setting, the techniques and strategies discussed in each chapter are short term and time effective.

The chapters selected for this text were carefully designed to address the spectrum of situations found among crisis settings. Although it is impossible to include every type of crisis imaginable, we have attempted to focus the chapters on a representative sampling of the most common themes encountered, particularly those suggested to us by many of the readers of the first two editions.

Cognitive-behavioral techniques as they stand are practical to use with many of the disorders found in crisis settings. In addition, they are well adapted to short-term or brief therapy, and they are compatible with many other modalities of treatment.

It is for these reasons that this text will serve both students and seasoned practitioners and researchers who are working in the field of crisis intervention.

FRANK M. DATTILIO
ARTHUR FREEMAN

Acknowledgments

We consider ourselves fortunate to have a group of contributors who are not only seasoned writers but excellent clinicians as well. Many of the contributors are colleagues with whom we have worked with on previous texts or in actual clinical practice. So, to them we extend our hearty thanks. It has been an honor and a pleasure to work with them.

Our information and our inspiration as editors and writers are also attributed to our teacher and mentor, Aaron T. Beck, to whom we owe much of what we know on the topic of cognitive therapy. His research and literary work sparked our own resolve to put into writing what we know and to gather the expertise of our colleagues/contributors.

Such a work is not produced without an excellent support staff. We thank Ms. Carol Jaskolka for her superb word processing and organizational skills. We are also grateful to the fine editorial and production staff at The Guilford Press, in particular, Seymour Weingarten, editor-in-chief, and Jim Nageotte, with whom it is always a pleasure to work.

Finally, we thank our spouses and family members for their patience and forbearance while we were engrossed in this project.

FRANK M. DATTILIO
ARTHUR FREEMAN

Contents

PART III. CHILD AND FAMILY CRISES

PART IV. ENVIRONMENTAL AND SITUATIONAL CRISES

PART V. GENERAL ISSUES IN CRISIS WORK

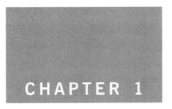

CHAPTER 1

Introduction

Frank M. Dattilio
Arthur Freeman

*E*very civilization has been subjected to crisis situations at one time or the other. From the beginning crisis events have undoubtedly plagued the human condition, be it physical illness, natural disasters, and so on. Although the magnitude and frequency of crisis situations may vary, their occurrence remains constant. What has changed, however, is the manner in which we deal with crisis situations and the degree to which they affect the human psyche. Because of the great number of crisis situations, our world is more in need of crisis intervention than ever before.

The term *crisis* generally evokes an image of any one of a number of extreme negative life events. Natural disasters, terrorist attacks, rapes, illness, loss, all by their very nature involve situations of life-threatening proportions. The pictures and experiences of the victims of these disasters strike a chord within all of us. Nowhere does this ring truer than when watching the events of September 11, 2001. However, a crisis may also relate to circumstances or experiences that threaten one's home, family, property, or sense of well-being. A psychological crisis may involve a loss or threat of a loss or a radical change in one's relationship with oneself or with some significant other (Goldenberg, 1983). For a child, it may involve a sudden relocation of home to another state and saying good-bye to friends. For an adolescent, it may be the breakup of a romantic relationship or being ostracized by one's peers. What produces, or fuels, a crisis is not simply defined by a particular situation or set of circumstances but rather by the individual's perception of the event and his/her ability (or inability) to effectively cope with that circumstance. In the same situation, different individuals deal with the potential crisis with varying degrees of competence or success. Simply stated, crisis results when stress and tension in an individual's life mount to unusual proportions and take a negative toll on them (Greenstone & Leviton, 1993).

HISTORY OF CRISIS INTERVENTION

Historically, the concept of crisis intervention dates to the Lemberger Freiwilligern Rettungsgesellschaft (Lemberg Rescue Society) organized in Vienna in the latter part of the 19th century (1883–1906). In 1906, the Anti-Suicide Department of the Salvation Army was organized in London, and the National Save-a-Life League was set up in New York City (Farberow & Schneidman, 1961). Crisis counseling was developed during World War II, when psychologists and psychiatrists who were working near the battlefield saw cases of extreme "battle fatigue" ("shell shock" in World War I; posttraumatic stress disorder in Vietnam). They found that dealing with the crisis close to the front line rather than being sent back to a rear-area hospital was very helpful for the soldiers in distress. The intervention that was used at that time took a focused approach. The goal was to return the soldier to active duty as quickly as possible.

With the opening of the Suicide Prevention Center in Los Angeles in the early 1950s, a basic model for the modern crisis center was established and, soon after, similar suicide prevention centers and general crisis intervention hotlines began to spring up around the country. In large part, they emerged in answer to the general climate of social concern and awareness of the late 1950s and 1960s. This became particularly pronounced with the enactment of then President John F. Kennedy's Community Mental Health Centers Act of 1963, in which crisis units played a major role (Dattilio, 1984). With the innovation of the suicide prevention hotline, crisis intervention hotlines began to diversify and specify their focus. This came about because suicide intervention centers were asked to help people deal with all types of crisis. Out of this developed teen hotlines, drug abuse hotlines, rape hotlines, and hotlines for the elderly. The telephone began to be used as a means of keeping in contact and following up with patients discharged from psychiatric facilities. Poison control hotlines were developed, community rumor control hotlines, homework hotlines, and general community service hotlines appeared to help callers with problems such as garbage removal or pest control, low standard of housing, voter registration, pollution, and many others.

Currently there are more than 1,400 grass-roots crisis centers and crisis units affiliated with the American Association of Suicidology or local community mental health centers. There are also more than 11,000 victim assistance programs, rape crisis, and child sexual abuse intervention programs as well as 1,250 battered women's shelters and hotlines. Roberts and Camasso (1994) estimate that each year as many as 4.3 million documented calls come into crisis hotlines. Roberts (2005) further projects that if we were to take this figure and broaden it to include all natural and local 24-hour crisis lines, including those for crime victims, survivors of terrorist attacks, battered women, sexual assault victims, troubled employees, adolescent runaways, and child abuse victims as well as the crisis intervention units at mental health centers, the total estimate would be approximately 35–45 million crisis callers per year (p. 11). This does not include the thousands of crisis services available through community hospital emergency rooms or psychiatric emergency service centers.

CRISIS THEORY

Crisis intervention, based on crisis theory, is one of the most widely used types of brief treatment employed by mental health professionals working in community settings (Ell, 1996). Burgess and Roberts (2005) and Burgess and Holstrom (1974) posit that crisis results when homeostasis is disrupted; that is, when the individual's balance—however precarious or firm it might be—is thrown off and the individual is no longer able to cope with the situation effectively. The result would be that the individual would then manifest a number of symptoms that become the clinical markers for the crisis response, often necessitating some crisis intervention. In general, crisis intervention is aimed at a psychological resolution of an immediate crisis in an individual's life and restoring him/her to at least the precrisis level of functioning (Aguilera, 1990). Rosenbaum and Calhoun (1977) regard a crisis as involving some precipitating event that is time limited and disrupts the individual's usual coping and problem-solving capabilities. Slaiku (1990) offers a definition that synthesizes the definitions of crisis as "a temporary state of upset and disorganization, characterized chiefly by an individual's inability to cope with a particular situation using customary methods of problem-solving, and by the potential for a radically positive or negative outcome" (p. 15). This definition focuses on several specific areas. The first part of the definition addresses the "temporary" nature of crisis situations. For most individuals, crises are immediate, transient, and temporary. For other individuals, however, the temporary nature of crisis may lead to years of upset. Their life crises may become part of a posttraumatic stress that is long term and chronic. Other individuals have a predisposition to view certain stimuli as dangerous and thereby damaging. They may see many circumstances as crisis laden. For these individuals, there is no one crisis but a series of "brushfires" that continue to strain their coping ability throughout life.

The second part of the definition addresses the individual's response of being upset. The term *upset* can be broadened to include the most common responses to crisis, those of anxiety and depression. In more severe reactions, the individual may also be disorganized. This disorganization may involve confusion and decreased problem-solving ability. In its severest form, it might include brief reactive psychoses. The disorganization may be cognitive (e.g., mental confusion), behavioral (e.g., acting in random or uncharacteristic ways), or emotional (e.g., being emotionally labile). The individual's inability to cope, the focus of the next part of the definition, revolves more specifically around the issue of problem-solving ability. If an individual's balance is disrupted and some form of anxiety results, the individual's cognitive flexibility decreases, problem solving suffers, and avoidance or denial may be used as a coping strategy. By using the common or traditional techniques for personal coping, many individuals find themselves overwhelmed. Their customary methods of problem solving are not adequate to the present task requirements (Roberts, 2000).

The final part of the definition involves the potential for rather weighty consequences. Loss of health, property, or loved ones and death are well within the definition of weighty consequences that could lead to radically positive or negative outcomes. Negative outcomes would include loss of self-esteem, loss of esteem of others, or, in cultural contexts, loss of "face." Slaiku (1990) suggests the possibility that the crisis situation could also lead to powerful positive outcomes, including the opportunity for new experiences, starting over, or gaining new skills, behaviors, and even insights, including the appreciation of our human vulnerability to life's perils.

A classic example is evident in two of the more recent crises that occurred in the United States: the events of 9/11 and Hurricane Katrina. Both of these events produced weighty consequences, including loss of life, health, property, not to mention an increased vulnerability to life's perils. In fact, the events of 9/11 alone represented the largest loss of life of U.S. citizens in one day in our history (Roberts, 2005).

Americans did learn a powerful lesson from both of these events—that one must be prepared for life-threatening events at anytime, and that, as human beings, we are, by nature, always vulnerable.

Usually, when individuals are in a crisis situation and their present resources are not adequate to the task, they call on little-used reserves of personal fortitude and spirit to carry them through. They may also call on little-used or infrequently practiced skills to help them prevail. Or, if they have the added advantage of a family or social network on which they might rely for assistance, support, or encouragement, they use that network as an expanded resource. In addition, they may search for or create temporary systems of support to assist them through the crisis period. With an extensive repertoire of coping strategies and the techniques to implement the strategies, a supportive family system, good friends, or a therapist on whom to call, potential life crises can be more easily weathered.

Why a particular situation or event is moved to a level of a crisis at one time and not another is a central issue underlying the treatment of the individual who ends up in crisis. The strategies and techniques for intervening in crisis situations are the focus of this volume. Our goal in this chapter is to provide a theoretical and conceptual basis as well as a rationale for a cognitive-behavioral format for the delivery of crisis intervention services.

DISCUSSION

Erikson's (1950) psychosocial theory of development was formulated as a "crisis theory" based on the concept that crises are not necessarily negative life occurrences that injure or destroy the individual but, rather, serve as points of growth. This growth can add to individuals' strength, provide them with a coping repertoire, and help them to succeed in every area of life. Erikson further believed that the lack of resolution of these crises could lead to a poor coping style. This theory would obviously be opposed by some victims of a crisis in the short term. Most individuals who are the victims of disaster or terrorist attacks fail to see Erikson's crisis concept. It is a concept that is only likely to be accepted years after the crisis event has occurred.

Erikson's model states that throughout his/her lifetime, an individual encounters a number of predictable life crises (Erikson identified eight). By the nature and degree of resolution or nonresolution of these crises, the individual grows and develops in a particular direction. This growth and development lead to the conceptualization of an idiosyncratic life view and its attendant behaviors, cognitions, and emotions. Individually, and in combination, the eight crises subsume virtually every possible life schema. Overall, the resolution or nonresolution of the life crises determines the development of the individual's personal, family, cultural, gender, and age-related schema (Freeman, 1993). This schema then becomes a template for that individual's behavior. Erikson views the initial resolution of these crises as amenable to change throughout life, inasmuch as all eight crises are concurrent rather than sequential (aging, death, illness, etc.). A particular crisis may be more prevalent at a particular point in life (i.e., crises do not start and end during a particular developmental period). This fact then presents a much more optimistic view for ongoing crisis resolution. If an individual has not managed to successfully cope with a particular crisis or resolve it in a positive manner, he/she has other opportunities to resolve it throughout life.

By understanding the particular types of behaviors that emerge from the resolution or nonresolution of these life crises, the therapist can understand the individual's coping style and strategies. This understanding of the individual's schema sets the stage for tailoring interventions more effectively to help individuals and families resolve or cope with present life crises. The first major therapeutic task is discerning and manifesting a particular schema that will then allow therapists to work with their patients to examine the schema, the advantages and disadvantages of maintaining it, and methods for disputing and/or altering it. This schematic focus is central to the cognitive-behavioral approach to crisis intervention.

SCHEMATA

Schemata are hypothesized structures that guide and organize the processing of information and the understanding of life experience. Beck (1967, 1976) has suggested that schemata are the cognitive substrate that generates the various cognitive distortions often observed in patients. These schemata serve to increase or decrease the individual's vulnerability to various situations. These schemata or basic rules of life begin to form as a force in cognition and behavior from the earliest points in life and are well ingrained by the middle childhood years. They involve the accumulation of the individual's learning and experience within the family group; religious group; ethnic, gender, or regional subgroup; and broader society. The particular extent or effect that a given schema has on an individual's life depends on (1) how strongly that schema is held; (2) how essential the individual sees that schema to his/her safety, well-being, or existence; (3) the individual's previous learning vis-à-vis the importance and essential nature of a particular schema; (4) how early a particular schema was internalized; and (5) how powerfully, and by whom, the schema was reinforced.

Schemata can be active or dormant, with the more active schemata serving as the rules that govern day-to-day behavior. The dormant schemata are called into play to control behavior in times of stress. The schemata may be either compelling or noncompelling. The more compelling the schemata, the more likely it is that the individual or family will respond to the schemata.

Schemata are in a constant state of change and evolution. Environmental data and experience are only taken in by individuals as they can use them in terms of their own subjective experience. The self-schemata then become selective as the individual may ignore environmental stimuli. There is an active and evolutionary process by which all perceptions and cognitive structures are applied to new functions (*assimilation*) while new cognitive structures are developed to serve old functions in new situations (*accommodation*). Some individuals persist in utilizing old structures without fitting them to the new circumstances in which they are involved—they use them *in toto* without measuring fit or appropriateness. They may further fail to accommodate or build new structures.

Schemata are cognitive structures that can be described in great detail. We can also deduce them from behavior or automatic thoughts. The behavioral component involves the manner in which the belief system governs the individual's responses to a particular stimulus or set of stimuli. In seeking to alter a particular schema that has endured for a long time, the professional must help the individual deal with the belief from as many different perspectives as possible. A pure cognitive strategy would leave the behavioral and affective untouched. The pure affective strategy is similarly limited, and, of course, the strict behavioral approach is limited by its disregard for cognitive–affective elements. In many cases we find that an individual's particular schemata are consensually validated.

The cognitive-behavioral approach initially involves an intrapsychic focus on the individual's automatic thoughts and schemata. This part of the therapeutic work deals with the individual's belief systems; assumptions about self, world, experience, and the future; and general perceptions. A second focus of the therapy is interpersonal and deals with the individual's style of relating to others.

The third focus of the therapy is external, and it involves changing behaviors to affect a more productive coping style. This external focus involves learning new behaviors/responses, trying the new behaviors, evaluating the result of the new behaviors, and developing and using available resources.

The particular attributes of cognitive therapy make it ideal for crisis intervention work. The eight specific attributes involve the *activity* of the model. This part of the model invites the patient to be an active part of the therapy, helping to restore a sense of control over his/her life.

The *directiveness* of the model is important because it encourages the therapist to be active and direct in guiding the therapy. The therapist's job is more than restatement and reformulation. The therapist shares hypotheses; utilizes guided discovery;

encourages the patient; serves as a resource person; and is a case manager and, in certain cases, an advocate for the patient.

The *structure of the therapy* calls for the establishment of a discrete problem list that helps both patient and therapist clarify where the therapy is going and evaluate how the therapy is progressing. This structure is essential for the patient in crisis and commensurate with most models of crisis intervention (Greenstone & Leviton, 1993; Roberts, 2005).

The content and the direction of the therapy are established early in the collaboration. Having established and agreed on a problem list and focus for therapy, the therapist and patient structure the individual sessions through agenda setting and homework.

Agenda setting provides for maximum success in the minimal time often available to the therapy. Rather than having the therapy session wander and meander, the therapist can work with the patient to set an agenda for the session, which helps to focus the therapy work and makes better use of time, energy, and available skills. Agenda setting at the beginning of the session allows both patient and therapist to place issues of concern on the agenda for the day. Accomplishing the items on the agenda requires that the therapist be skilled at setting priorities and pacing the session, taking into account the needs of the patient. This is a skill refined through practice and experience. However, even seasoned therapists may feel tense and anxious and exhibit a loss of effectiveness when they are first learning how to pace a session that is built around a collaborative agenda. This is only a natural part of adjusting to the patients' needs and establishing a footing in treatment.

The *short-term nature of the therapy* is a fourth element in crisis intervention. Research protocols for testing the efficacy of cognitive therapy generally involve 12 to 20 sessions over a period of no more than 20 weeks, whereas the treatment of a crisis situation may need to be more rapid but not necessarily limited to 20 weeks. For certain patients the length of therapy may be 6 sessions; for other patients, 50 sessions. The length of the therapy and the frequency and length of the sessions are all negotiable. There is also some discussion in the professional literature about the pros and cons of early-intervention techniques (Brom & Kleber, 1989; Foa, Hearst-Ikeda, & Perry, 1995; Schützwohl, 2000). This aspect is something that therapists need to consider seriously in regard to the effectiveness of any intervention.

In addition to the aforementioned, the problems being addressed, the skills of the patient and the therapist, the time available for therapy, and financial resources all have the potential to dictate the parameters of treatment.

Another issue is the development of *collaboration*. The therapist and patient must work together as a team. This concept has long been the backbone of cognitive-behavioral therapy (Beck, Rush, Shaw, & Emery, 1979). The collaboration is not always 50:50 but may, with the crisis patient, be 70:30 or 90:10, with the therapist providing most of the energy or work within the session or in the therapy more generally. The more stressed the patient is, the less energy he/she may have available to use during the course of therapy. The therapeutic focus would be to help such patients make maximum use of their energy and build greater energy resources.

A sixth issue is that the cognitive therapy model is a *dynamic* model of therapy. The dynamic cognitive approach to therapy promotes rapid self-disclosure of individual cognitions in order to increase understanding through enhanced knowledge and an understanding of thoughts, beliefs, and attitudes. Early schemata develop and are modified within the family group. Cognitive therapy with families can provide a context for observing these schemata in operation 'see Dattilio, 1993, 1998, 2005, Chapter 13, this volume; Teichman, 1992).

Also, cognitive therapy is a *psychoeducational* model of therapy. It is a skill-building or coping model of therapy as opposed to a cure model. Patients in cognitive therapy ideally gain skills to cope more effectively with their own thoughts and behaviors that may be dysfunctional. Rather than cure, the cognitive therapist helps the patient to acquire a range of coping strategies for present and future exigencies of life.

Finally, the cognitive therapy model is a *social/interpersonal* model. We do not exist in social vacuums. The relationships of the individual to his/her significant others, friends, and work colleagues are all schematically based and are essential foci for the therapy. If the individual is isolated, there may be great gaps in his/her resource network.

Clearly, if one does not have external resources and few internal resources on which to rely, a crisis will result. In some cases individuals have what objectively appears to be a wealth of support, but the support is not accepted by the individual or is perceived by the hopeless individual as not sufficient or available. In Edward Arlington Robinson's poem *Richard Cory*, Cory was seen to have everything. He was wealthy, handsome, well dressed, and sophisticated. Despite all these apparent resources however, "one calm summer night, [Richard Cory] went home and put a bullet through his head."

Highlighting the importance of understanding the individual's schemata, available resources, and belief in those resources, we can look at the Social Readjustment Scale (Holmes & Rahe, 1967). In this scale, the death of a spouse is rated number 1. It is seen as the most powerful stressor and the standard against which all other life stressors are measured. The death of a close family member is rated as 5 on the scale, and the death of a friend as 7. If the spouse was much loved, it is easily understandable as to why it is perceived as a situation of the highest stress. In the case of an embittered and estranged couple, the death of a spouse may be a solution to long-term stress, bringing with it relief and even financial security. Or, in the case of a loved spouse with a terminal illness and intractable pain, the eventual death of that spouse, family member, or friend may be prayed for out of love and caring. The eventual death may be a great relief because of the peace and surcease the death will bring to the terminally ill individual. In such cases, then, the rating level on the Social Readjustment Scale would be lower.

Slaiku (1990) states, "Short-term, time-limited therapy is the treatment of choice in crisis situations" (p. 98). In this respect, the active, directive, goal-oriented, structured, collaborative, and problem-solving nature of cognitive therapy makes it the ideal crisis intervention treatment model. The immediate goals of cognitive-behavioral strategies in crisis intervention are threefold: (1) the evaluation and assessment of the immediacy of the crisis situation, (2) an assessment of the individual's coping repertoire to deal with the crisis, and (3) the generation of options of thought, perception, and behavior. Some individuals have a skill deficit in problem solving. This requires the direct teaching of better problem-solving skills. Other individuals have the problem-solving strategies and techniques available but see their ability as far less than it is. A more behavioral approach is necessary in the former situation, whereas a more cognitive approach is called for in the latter situation.

Using Slaiku's (1990) definition described earlier, there are several possible points of intervention. The initial point of intervention is the recognition that the situation that brings on the upset and disorganization is *temporary*. This implies that by seeing the situation with a long-term focus it may be possible to "wait it out." For example, panic patients have difficulty seeing the long view because the immediacy of the physiological symptoms and the misinterpretation of danger draws their focus to the "here and now" (see Dattilio & Kendall, Chapter 3, this volume). The idea of waiting out the bodily response and not responding by running is somehow viewed by the panic patient as impossible. Working with the patient to develop the long-term view may help to decrease the crisis perception. The perception of immediate danger and the need to avoid it cause panic patients to act in self-defeating ways in the ideal interest of saving their life.

A second point of intervention involves the *upset*. Clearly, if the situation were not as upsetting, there would be no crisis. The upset is caused by a perception that can be questioned or challenged. For example, a businessman reported being in crisis over the economic downturn and the possible loss of his business. He reported that every time he thought of losing his business he would then extend the thought to losing everything. He would picture losing his home, his car, his wife, his children, his self-respect, and the respect of others. He would, in his view, be living on a hot-air vent in the street, housed in a large cardboard carton. His upset came not simply from the reality of his business difficulties but rather from his catastrophic style of thinking.

The third point of intervention relates to the *disorganization*. If the individual's thoughts, actions, and emotions are confused and disorganized, the clear therapeutic strategy is to offer some structure and a format for problem solving. The therapist must recognize that confusion and disorganization are common themes for virtually all psychological problems. Patients' complaints that they "need to get their life/head/marriage together" are quite common. For patients seeing themselves in crisis, this collection of parts or pieces may be more emergent. The cognitive therapy model is especially helpful with the disorganized patient. For example, a woman who was date raped saw her only avenue of action being to flee her job and school program. She was overwhelmed by the thoughts, images, and feelings related to the rape. She was further confused by the contradictory advice and information offered by others, which was compounded by legal issues and threats. She described her reaction as running off in 10 directions simultaneously. No direction gave her answers or peace.

Each of us uses a fairly limited repertoire of techniques for coping with life. Our day-to-day life is rather familiar and comfortable. We can expect certain consequences when we act in particular ways. If, for example, an individual begins her morning commute at 6:30 A.M., she will likely experience little traffic. If, however, she leaves at 8:00 A.M., she may be in the middle of the heaviest commuter traffic. She then knows that she has to leave earlier to avoid the "crisis" of the morning rush. If she lives in an area that experiences heavy winter snow, she considers driving in snow to be part of the risk or price to pay for living in that area. Ideally, she has coped by having snow tires, sand in the trunk, a shovel, cold-weather gear, a blanket, and flares. If there is snow in an area that is not prepared for it, even a coating of snow becomes a crisis of major proportions.

A final point of intervention is to help the individual *reduce the potential for a radical outcome*. If the outcome were uncomfortable rather than catastrophic, the crisis potential would be significantly reduced.

ASSESSMENT

As in any other circumstance, assessment is crucial during crisis situations, particularly because the given situation may be critical at the time and require an almost immediate response. What makes assessment difficult is that it must be conducted almost three times as quickly as in the normal course of treatment and, in some cases, under difficult circumstances. When a crisis situation presents itself with little or no opportunity to implement formal assessment inventories or questionnaires, a paradigm is recommended for quick structured interviewing. Greenstone and Leviton (1993) recommend adhering to the following steps:

1. *Immediacy.* Intervention usually begins at the moment the intervener encounters the individual in crisis. The intervener must immediately attempt to size up the situation, alleviate anxiety, prevent further disorientation, and ensure that sufferers do not harm themselves or cause harm to others.

2. *Taking control.* Here it is important for the intervener to be clear about what and whom he/she is attempting to control. The purpose of assuming control is not to conquer or overwhelm the victim but to help reorder the chaos that exists in the sufferer's world at the moment of the crisis. The one conducting the crisis intervention provides the needed structure until the victim(s) is able to regain control. Consequently, it is important to enter the crisis scene cautiously.

Approaching the crisis situation slowly and carefully can prevent unnecessary grief and give the professional time to mentally absorb what he/she is encountering. It is important for the professional intervening to make every attempt to remain stable, supportive, and able to establish a structured environment. This may involve using personal presence, including strength control, and making every effort to have a calming effect on the crisis situation and exercising some emotional control over the victim. Research usually indicates that victims respond to structure and those who represent it, if they sense genuineness and sincerity by the professional doing the interview.

3. *Assessment.* Intervening usually involves making a quick, on-the-spot evaluation. This means attempting to understand how and why the individual got into a cri-

sis situation at this particular time and which specific problem is of immediate concern. Assessment also involves the use of management and identifying any variables that would hinder the problem management process.

The bottom line consists of how the intervener can be most effective in the least amount of time. Consequently, lengthy histories are forfeited in favor of focusing on the assessment of the present crisis and the events that occurred within the immediate hours surrounding the crisis—more specifically, pinpointing the precipitating events.

A number of inventories have been designed for use in crisis situations, although, unfortunately, there is a surprising lack of standardized instruments with strong psychometric properties available to mental health practitioners engaged in crisis work.

One assessment measure that has been designed to provide a rapid assessment for measuring perceived psychological trauma and perceived problems in coping efficacy is the Crisis State Assessment Scale (Lewis, 2002). This scale is still in the process of validation, but it offers constructs mentioned earlier and is used to predict or indicate the magnitude of a crisis state. This assessment measure may be helpful initially in order to aid in the direction of future treatment.

Another inventory is the modified version of the Structured Clinical Interview Schedule for DSM-IV, which is known as the Upjohn version (SCID-UP-R). This is an abridged version of the Structured Clinical Interview Schedule that allows the intervener to provide a more expedient method of assessment in crisis situations (Spitzer & Williams, 1986). In addition, there are other scales such as the American Academy of Crisis Interveners Lethality Scale (Greenstone & Leviton, 1993, pp. 19–20). This scale allows an individual to quickly assess criteria in a crisis situation by summing up the scores and matching the total with the criteria.

4. *Decide how to handle the situation after the assessment*. This essentially involves using the material that was gathered during the assessment stage and deciding on an avenue for intervention. It may also involve exploring the possible options available to the individual in crisis and either handling the situation at the moment or referring it out as needed.

The reader is referred to the individual chapters of this book for more detail on various assessment tools for particular crisis situations.

TREATMENT

Obviously, models of brief psychotherapy have been the treatment of choice in crisis settings. There are several models of brief psychotherapy; however, they all have the common goal of removing and alleviating specific symptoms in a timely fashion. The intervention may lead to some personality reconstruction, but this is not considered a primary goal (Aguilera, 1990).

The focused cognitive therapy approach to crisis intervention has five stages: The first stage is the development of a relationship with the patient and a building of rapport. This also follows in line with the cognitive model's notion of collaboration. The patient must feel comfortable enough to allow a free flow of information about the crisis in which he/she is currently involved. The therapist's behavior is instrumental in developing this rapport. The therapist has to be able to convey a nonjudgmental attitude to the patient and a feeling of interest and concern in the patient's problem. In a more serious crisis, levels of trust tend to develop more easily; thus the patient may have already assumed a certain level of trust in meeting with the therapist. Therefore, to some degree rapport will not be as difficult to develop. However, in a less serious crisis, rapport is an especially important aspect of the counseling relationship because it may be more difficult to develop.

The second stage is the initial evaluation of the severity of the crisis situation. Such an evaluation allows the therapist to get some idea of the immediate physical danger to the patient. It might also offer some idea as to the type of schemata held by the person with whom the therapist is dealing. The therapist must determine which course of action to take. Finally, the therapist must assist the patient in identifying the specific problem he/she is experiencing. Often patients' confusion and disorganization render them unable to define their problem. The therapist must make every effort to help individuals focus on the specific areas creating problems as opposed to attempting to deal with the vagaries of "depression", "anxiety," or "communication problems." It is important, however, not to focus on one specific problem too early in the contact because there is a chance the therapist could be overlooking other significant problems. Developing a problem list ensures a more specific focus within the broader context.

Once the problem is established, the third stage involves helping the patient assess and mobilize his/her strengths and resources. This may be in the form of identifying friends in the immediate vicinity who could help as well as various internal strengths and resources the person in crisis is likely to overlook. It is extremely useful to have the cognitive and behavioral resources menu handy and available.

In the fourth stage the therapist and patient must work jointly to develop a positive plan of action (collaboration and problem solving). An essential aspect of this collaboration includes eliciting the patient's commitment to the plan of action. At this point, the technique of problem solving is especially applicable. If the nature of the crisis is such that problem solving is not an appropriate mechanism, the last stage becomes necessary. A resource that may be called into play at this point is the therapist as advocate for the patient. In such cases, the therapist may need to become more demonstrative in aiding the patient in making a decision.

The fifth stage involves testing ideas and new behaviors. How well the new coping techniques work can be evaluated and the strategies revised accordingly.

CRISIS PATIENTS

The therapist who deals with patients in crisis is under a special pressure. Burnout occurs rather frequently. There is often no place for therapists to vent their own frustrations and upset, which may create a perception of crisis for the therapist. The notion of "therapist heal thyself" is easier said than done. Crisis workers may need peer supervision or some outlet for the pressure of working with patients in crisis. The reader is referred to Miller (Chapter 4, this volume) on traumatized psychotherapists for a more elaborate discussion of this topic.

The crisis intervention work often represents the only link that individuals in crisis believe they have. Even when there is not a life-or-death outcome, the patient's perception is often that in some vague way his/her very existence is being threatened. When the individual is experiencing a peak in his/her emotional distress, the therapeutic environment can be seen as the only tie, however tenuous, to survival. For the patient accustomed to the idea of receiving help, the decision to seek professional help is less frightening. Too often, patients do not seek help until the problems have reached crisis proportions. For more dependent patients, help seeking may in fact be overdeveloped as a coping strategy (Beck, Freeman, & Associates, 1990). Such patients see every problem as a potential crisis; therefore, they frequently seek help and need support. Conversely, the more autonomous patient may avoid seeking help, fearing ridicule or criticism on the part of the therapist.

Given the need for rather rapid conceptualization and intervention, we divide crisis patients into the following five general categories.

1. *The adolescent style.* Such patients may or may not be chronologically adolescent. They are generally experiencing some major life changes having to do with self-image. They are extremely reluctant to show any signs that might suggest dependency, vulnerability, weakness, or lack of self-confidence. For this reason, any request for help may be perceived by these patients as very threatening to their self-image. Typical schemata for these individuals revolve around issues of loss, dependence, and fear.

2. *The isolate.* Such individuals are typically distressed to the point of lacking all motivation to make social contact. Their crises revolve around social interactions or the lack of social involvement. Their main problems include their frequent lack of social skills, fear of rejection, passivity, and apathy. Their schemata often dictate that unless they receive absolute guarantees of recognition or support, they will refuse to become socially involved.

3. *The desperate individual.* Such patients exemplify for many what crisis intervention is all about. They experience some sudden psychological shock and are in desperate need of some type of immediate help. This shock may come from an environmental disaster or a psychological loss. As a result of this shock, the desperate individual has most likely lost contact with reality or this contact is extremely shaky. The therapist may represent his/her final link to reality. Often, the mere sound of a caring, concerned voice is enough to begin to bring this patient back from a state of despair. For example, a therapist reported meeting with a woman patient who was in crisis. He extended the session to double its time to help her move away from her determination of suicide. At some point in the session the patient asked for a cigarette. The therapist's office partner smoked and kept a pack of cigarettes in the desk drawer. He offered one to the patient and he smoked one also even though he had not smoked cigarettes in many years. When he believed that the patient was able to weather the cri-

sis, he ended the session and set another appointment time for the following day. When the patient came in the next day, she was calmer and less confused. When the therapist asked her about her reaction to the previous day's session, she replied, "I don't remember anything that we talked about. All I remember is that you gave me a cigarette."

4. *The one-shot crisis contact.* Such individuals are typically relatively normal and emotionally stable. Although the crises experienced by such people vary, there are specific reasons they call for therapy. They come to therapy to get help to deal with the specific crisis situation. They perceive themselves as mainly seeking someone to help them through some current situation. For this reason, a brief cognitive approach is especially well suited. This individual is simply looking for some immediate advice or someone to act as a sounding board to advise him/her on alternatives to the plans of action the individual may have already developed.

5. *The chronic patient.* Such patients seek therapy for another in a long history of brushfires. Therapy means that they will be able to call at any time and that whenever they call they will be able to find someone to listen to them and help them through the crisis of the day. We are reminded of the Confucian idea that if we give a person a fish he can eat for a day, but if we teach him to fish, he can feed himself. For this type of patient, long histories of therapeutic contact have taught them that they do not need to learn to cope. They can come to therapy and have the therapist do their coping for them.

The use of cognitive therapy techniques in crisis intervention offers advantages both to patients in their ability to receive help and to therapists in their ability to offer help. The patient often feels powerless to change his/her circumstances or unmotivated to problem-solve and reason a solution. By working collaboratively and actively to identify cognitive distortions and automatic thoughts and to suggest alternatives, the therapist can provide such patients with some hope for resolving their seemingly insoluble difficulties.

Cognitive-behavioral therapy is attractive "because most of the concepts of cognitive and behavior therapy are consistent with commonly shared notions of human nature, the neophyte therapist can readily assimilate them" (Beck, 1976, p. 318). The theories of cognitive-behavioral therapy are easily delineated, and, most important, the link between theory and practice is clear. By virtue of its ease of learning, cognitive and behavior therapy techniques also make crisis intervention work much more satisfying for the therapist.

ISSUES IN CRISIS INTERVENTION

Confidentiality

The issue of confidentiality is a sensitive one; knowing when to maintain confidentiality and when it is essential to break confidentiality is a very important issue (see VandeCreek & Knapp, Chapter 21, this volume, for an expanded discussion). Although confidentiality relies in large part on therapist judgment and accurate assessment of the severity of the situation, there is a general set of ethical standards. A life-threatening situation is one in which the patient is in danger of bodily injury or death. Once the therapist has established that there is a life-threatening situation, the therapist is no longer ethically bound to confidentiality and may have to exercise certain options. For example, if there is a crisis or emergency (e.g., homicide or suicide) the therapist may need to involve the police or insist that the patient offer the name of the spouse, friend, roommate, parent, or significant other who can be an available resource if assistance is necessary. The individual in crisis can enlist the support of these resources throughout the treatment process.

Cognitive Functioning

We use the term *cognitive functioning* to include intelligence, ability to comprehend and process information, and ability to understand both practical and abstract concepts of crisis, illness, injury, and health. The disorganization of the patient at the point of crisis may thus alter the therapeutic approach.

If, for example, patients or family members do not have a sufficient fund of knowledge to understand the nature of the present trauma, care must be taken to ensure that explanations are made in the simplest terms. Jargon, complex medical explanations, shorthand descriptions, or abstract concepts may be acknowledged as understood but really leave the patient and family puzzled by the events, treatment, and sequelae of the trauma (or treatment).

If the family is non-English-speaking, it is essential that explanations be offered in their primary language and within the context of their cultural values. Trauma service interpreters must be trained in addressing the practical and emotional needs of the patients and families and be able to translate the psychological concepts of the therapist into clear and digestible understanding (Dattilio, 1999).

Case Example

Ramon, age 6, was struck by a car while playing in the street. He was rushed to the hospital and was in treatment in the trauma unit. He was conscious but had several lacerations causing a great deal of bleeding. His mother, who had accompanied him in the ambulance, was distraught. She spoke Spanish and was demanding explanations of what was happening to her son. Would he live? Would he be able to walk again? While her questions were understood, it was difficult to explain the nature of the treatment and the necessary periods of observation and care. In addition to being upset, this woman was uneducated and unsophisticated. A Spanish-speaking nurse was unable to communicate to her the problems and the treatment, but a Spanish-speaking 8-year-old girl in the waiting room offered her services to the interpreter. The girl understood both Spanish and English, and when the treatment was explained to her she could both frame and phrase it in terms the mother could understand and thus the crisis diminished.

Mourning

Any loss has the effect of reducing one's ability to cope. The sequelae of an emergency may be the permanent loss of a family member through death or the temporary loss of a family member who is hospitalized. In addition, the result of the crisis might be the loss of a cognitive faculty, physical skill or ability, body parts, or intellectual or physical prowess.

The therapist must recognize and deal directly with losses, both real and imagined. In some cases family members may refuse to recognize the loss. The therapist must walk the line between maintaining hope and facing reality, encouraging the search for treatment options while evaluating the potential for success, and preparing for the worst while hoping for the best.

The mourning process must be identified for the patient. Patients must be helped to accept that any loss must be mourned and that the mourning process is normal, natural, and necessary. Often, follow-up treatment is especially important because the initial loss and mourning will be followed by another mourning process that might begin long after the immediate crisis. There is, in many cases, a "sleeper effect" in which the full effect of the loss does not become clear until the patient or significant other is gone.

Case Example

Alexander, age 62, was brought into the trauma unit by ambulance because he had suffered a stroke at home. Sara, his wife of 41 years, had called 911, and she stayed with him in the trauma unit. At first it was not clear whether Alexander would survive. When he was examined and stabilized, the doctors discovered that he had suffered a massive stroke that had affected both motor and language areas.

Alexander had been physically active since his retirement; he and Sara played golf, weather permitting, throughout the year. Alexander also jogged daily. Sara kept repeating, "He'll be running again soon. You'll see. He's never been sick." When the doctors pointed out that Alexander would need a long recuperative period, physical therapy, and probably speech and language therapy, Sara continued to repeat her mantra about his rapid recovery. The goal of the crisis intervention was to help Sara to build a positive outlook while taking into account the reality of the damage to her husband. If she were to maintain unrealistic expectations, refuse to mourn the loss of the man she had known for 43 years, or make demands of Alexander that he could not meet, serious interpersonal and intrapsychic conflicts would ensue.

Premorbid Personality, Lifestyle, and Interests

The particular interpersonal style, life choices, or intrapsychic conflicts can often provide a context for understanding the patient's or spouse's reaction to the crisis. In many cases the dependent individual reacts to the trauma by seeking help, reassurance, or comfort. The more autonomous individual may be resistant to help, refuse treatment, and generally avoid therapy with statements such as "I'll be OK," "Just leave me (us) alone," "I (we) can do it myself (ourselves)." In other cases, the premorbid personality style may not be a good predictor of the emotional reaction to the trauma. For example, under stress the "strong, silent type" becomes helpless and dependent whereas the weak and helpless individual shows an internal strength and fortitude that may carry an entire family throughout the crisis. This can be explained by the existence of dormant schemata (Freeman, 1993; Freeman & Leaf, 1989) that become active under the stress of the trauma. When the stress of the trauma is removed, however, the individual may return to his/her previous style of functioning.

Case Example

Sal was a 51-year-old male. He was driving on a rain-slick highway when he was hit by a tractor–trailer from behind. He suffered severe head injuries and his survival was uncertain. The family was concerned for his wife, Alice; they felt she would be unable to survive his death. "She needs him. She cannot take care of herself. She has serious health problems." Sal did eventually die as a result of the accident, but it was Alice who was clearly the support for the rest of the family. In the wake of Sal's death she seemed to rise to the occasion, supporting the children and other relatives. The weakness and deference she had displayed throughout her entire life was put aside so that she could care for others. On follow-up she maintained her strength for several weeks. However, she soon suffered a "nervous breakdown" and was seen for inpatient psychiatric treatment. She became depressed, helpless, and dependent, requesting the help of the nursing staff with almost all of her activities of daily living.

Discrepancy between Actual and Perceived Difficulty in Coping

As much as possible, it is important to make clear the discrepancy between actual and predicted problems for effective coping. It is essential for the patient to be realistic in terms of expectations for coping, recovery, and survival.

Case Example

Al, a 39-year-old construction worker, was injured in the collapse of a structure while working on a home construction site. He was rushed to the hospital by a community ambulance team after having his back, neck, and head stabilized and supported. He reported no feeling in the lower extremities on admission. After receiving a phone call with the news, his wife rushed to the trauma unit along with her mother and three children (ages 2, 3, and 5). Despite assurances that tests and radiological studies showed no damage and a good prognosis for complete recovery, Al, his wife, and his mother-in-law were negative and pessimistic about his ever walking again. The family perceived Al as being a quadriplegic—unable to work, confined to a wheelchair, unable to care for or feed himself, and ultimately dying. Even though some sensation returned to Al's legs rather quickly, their view was that the crisis was only beginning.

Reinforce Even Small Therapeutic Gains

A frequent concomitant of crisis is depression. The negative view of self ("I am unable to cope"), the world, and experience ("It's unfair; why has this happened to me?") and the negative view of the future ("I will always be this way; I will die") are the progenitors of depressive affect (Beck et al., 1979; Freeman, Pretzer, Fleming, & Simon, 1990). The patient's awareness of depressive symptomatology moderates the therapeutic strategy to identify the areas of greatest difficulty and focus rather quickly on these issues. Any small gain or improvement in dealing with the crisis must be identified and reinforced. Such reinforcement can lift the patient's mood. It is necessary to socialize patients to the cognitive model and help them to begin identifying automatic thoughts and schemata.

Case Example

Marla came for therapy as a result of her loss of a relationship. When Marla's fiancé told her that he no longer wanted to marry her, Marla reacted by trying to kill herself. She was in the hospital for several days as a result of a drug overdose. She had ingested a lethal amount of medication but was found when the police broke into her apartment after receiving a call from Marla's mother. Prior to the overdose, Marla had not been going to work and voiced hopelessness regarding a recovery. She saw only dark, bleak, and empty days ahead of her. The only solution was death.

As Marla became better equipped to view the crisis of the breakup in perspective, she was helped to challenge some of her depressogenic thoughts (e.g., "I will never find anyone who will love me this much," "My love will never be returned," "I will never have children," and "I have no worth"). As she challenged these thoughts, Marla's level of depression decreased and she was less suicidal.

The next step was to go beyond the immediate crisis and help "inoculate" Marla from responding in the same way to future losses.

Emphasize the Collaborative Therapeutic Relationship

The therapist must be seen as a warm, supportive, competent, reasonable individual and must work toward building and maintaining the working alliance. Given the nature of crises the relationship must be built immediately. Empathy is the most important element; when patient is in crisis, sympathy is likely to have a negative effect on the overall therapeutic work. There are probably many other people in the patient's world who offer sympathy. The patient needs someone who can enter his/her internal reality and then offer support and strategies for effective coping.

Case Example

Mary had lost her family in a house fire. She felt profound guilt for not having died along with her children and her husband. Neighbors offered their condolences, her minister made several visits to the hospital to express his sorrow and sympathy, and she received sympathy cards from her children's schoolmates. Nothing seemed to help her. After Mary expressed her anger over yet another sympathy card, her sister asked, "What do you want from these people? They are trying their best to let you know how they feel." Mary's response was that everyone was expressing how they felt and no one seemed to try to understand how she felt.

Barriers to Patient Empowerment

Empowerment is essential in treating patients in crisis. Patients must be helped to recognize their right and ability to be empowered. The goal of empowerment may be limited by the manner in which it is presented, by its implementation, or by misunderstanding the idea or model.

By definition, empowerment implies that one person or agency gives, offers, provides, or allows another person or agency to have or assume power. This definition assumes that the power giver has it within his/her purview to give or allow power. It further implies that the receiver is willing to assume the proffered power. The power may be related to work or taking charge of one's life or one's surroundings. Given the admirable goal, demonstrated potential, and egalitarian focus, empowerment may be doomed to fail for a variety of reasons. The ability to facilitate change in oneself and/ or one's family group is critical to the development of empowerment. Too often self-change is impeded by repetitive, stylistic errors in personal information processing. Simply put, we can make errors in judgment, computation, reasoning, or perception. There are many examples of individuals who are smart, educated, talented, perceptive, and competent but who continue to repeat the same mistakes and find themselves in sequential crises. Their mistake-making style becomes idiosyncratic and may cause them difficulties at work, at home, in relationships, or within themselves. It is important to help individuals to identify their particular schematic style and then to develop strategies to overcome impediments to change. Impediments to change include lack of practice in new behavior, environmental stressors interfering with change, personal ideas about ability to change oneself or family, personal ideas about consequence of change to self or group, group or family ideas about the need to avoid change, secondary gain from maintaining status quo in spite of cost, lack of motivation, rigidity, and vague or unrealistic goals. In therapy, if the goals are not agreed on, patient frustration will result.

Threshold and Vulnerability

The ability to cope with a stressor and whether the same stressors precipitate a crisis depend on the individual's threshold for response. In different situations, the individual's threshold will be very different. A surgeon working in a critical care setting is able to deal with medical emergencies with competence and skill. Once past the doors of the operating room, he/she may be unable to cope with the normal exigencies of life.

If we picture coping ability on a scale of 0–100, we can literally map an individual's normal threshold for coping. If, for example, the normal stress of life is 60 and one's threshold is 75, there is a cushion of 15 to accommodate extraordinary stress. If, due to higher than normal stress, the stress of life increases to 80, the individual would be overwhelmed and in difficulty. If, however, the stressors of life remain the same but one's threshold decreases, the individual will likewise be overwhelmed.

Vulnerability factors lower one's threshold. These are circumstances, situations, or deficits that have the effect of decreasing the patient's ability to cope effectively with life stressors or to see available options.

The following list gives examples of such factors (Freeman & Simon, 1989):

1. *Acute illness.* This may span the range from a severe and debilitating illness to more transient illnesses such as headaches, viral infections, and so on.
2. *Chronic illness.* When the health problem is chronic, there can be an acute exacerbation of suicidal thinking.
3. *Deterioration of health.* There may be a loss of activity due to aging.
4. *Hunger.* During times of food deprivation, the individual is often more vulnerable to a variety of stimuli. Recent studies have linked a depressive diagnosis to those with an eating disorder.
5. *Anger.* When individuals are angry, they can lose appropriate problem-solving ability. They may also lose impulse control or overrespond to stimuli that they are usually able to ignore.
6. *Fatigue.* In a similar fashion, fatigue decreases both problem-solving strategies and impulse control.
7. *Loneliness.* When individuals see themselves as isolated, leaving this unhappy world may seem to be a reasonable option.
8. *Major life loss.* Following the loss of a significant other through death, divorce, or separation, individuals often see themselves as having reduced options. They lose interest in what happens to them.
9. *Poor problem-solving ability.* Certain individuals may have impaired problem-solving ability. This deficit may not be obvious until the individual is placed in situations of great stress. The ability to deal with minor problems is a poor indicator of the individual's ability to deal with a crisis.
10. *Substance abuse.* The abuse of many substances can cause two types of problems: acute, in which the patient's judgment is compromised during periods of intoxication, and more chronic, in which judgment may be impaired more generally. Such problems increase suicidality.
11. *Chronic pain.* Chronic pain may cause the individual to view suicide as a method for ending the pain.
12. *Poor impulse control.* Certain patients have poor impulse control because of organic (hyperactivity) or functional problems. Patients with bipolar illness, borderline, antisocial, or histrionic personality disorders may all have impulse control deficits.
13. *New life circumstances.* Changing jobs, marital status, homes, or family status are all stressors that are vulnerability factors.

These factors can, alone or in combination, increase the patient's suicidal thinking or actions, lower threshold for anxiety stimuli, or increase the patient's vulnerability to depressogenic thoughts and situations (Freeman & Simon, 1989). The vulnerability factors can have a summation effect. That is, when several vulnerability factors operate at the same time, they may continue to lower one's threshold. For example, if an individual who has a history of effective coping (threshold = 90; life stress = 60) suddenly loses the ability to cope and ends up in crisis, the family is often surprised. They may disregard the fact that the individual has had a stroke (–10), his wife has a broken leg (–7), his son is getting divorced (–6), his daughter has lost her job (–5), his oldest grandchild is having difficulty in school (–5), and his pet dog has been hit by a car (–4). His threshold is now 54, low enough to have him respond to normal life stress as if it were a crisis. Rather than thinking in terms of the sequence of losses, families may respond by thinking that the patient has dealt with similar problems in the past so it is unclear why at this point he is having such a negative response.

Assessment of vulnerability factors may help to explain the ability to deal with crises and to predict the possibility of withdrawal, suicidal ideation, depression, or anxiety.

REFERENCES

Aguilera, D. C. (1990). *Crisis intervention: Theory and methodology.* St. Louis, MO: Mosby.

Beck, A. T. (1967). *Depression: Causes and treatment.* Philadelphia: University of Pennsylvania Press.

Beck, A. T. (1976). *Cognitive therapy and the emotional disorders.* New York: International Universities Press.

Beck, A. T., Freeman, A., & Associates. (1990). *Cognitive therapy of personality disorders.* New York: Plenum Press.

Beck, A. T., Rush, A. J., Shaw, B. F., & Emery, G. (1979). *Cognitive therapy of depression.* New York: Guilford Press.

Brom, D., & Kleber, R. J. (1989). Prevention of posttraumatic stress disorders. *Journal of Traumatic Stress, 2,* 335–351.

Burgess, A., & Holstrom, L. (1974). *Rape: Victims of crisis.* Bowie, MD: Robert J. Brady.

Burgess, A. W., & Roberts, A. R. (2005). Crisis intervention for persons diagnoses with clinical disorders based on the Stress Crisis Continuum. In A. R. Roberts (Ed.), *Crisis intervention handbook: Assessment, treatment and research* (3rd ed., pp. 120–140). New York: Oxford University Press.

Dattilio, F. M. (1984). The mental health delivery system. In M. Braswell & T. A. Seay (Eds.), *Approaches to counseling and psychotherapy* (pp. 229–237). Prospect Heights, IL: Waveland Press.

Dattilio, F. M. (1993). Cognitive therapy with couples and families. *The Family Journal, 1*(1), 51–65.

Dattilio, F. M. (Ed.). (1998). *Case studies in couple and family therapy: Systemic and cognitive perspectives.* New York: Guilford Press.

Dattilio, F. M. (1999, January/February). Cultural sensitivities in forensic psychological evaluations. *The Forensic Examiner, 8*(1&2), 26–27.

Dattillio, F. M. (2005). Restructuring family schemas: A cognitive-behavioral perspective. *Journal of Marital and Family Therapy, 31*(1), 15–30.

Ell, K. (1996). Crisis theory and social work practice. In F. Turner (Ed.), *Social work treatment* (pp. 168–190). New York: Free Press.

Erikson, E. (1950). *Childhood and society.* New York: Norton.

Farberow, N. L., & Schneidman, E. S. (Eds.). (1961). *The cry for help.* New York: McGraw-Hill.

Foa, E. B., Hearst-Ikeda, D., & Perry, K. J. (1995). Evaluation of a brief cognitive-behavioral program for the prevention of chronic PTSD in recent assault victims. *Journal of Consulting and Clinical Psychology, 63,* 948–955.

Freeman, A. (1993). A psychosocial approach for conceptualizing schematic development for cognitive therapy. In K. T. Kuhlwein & H. Rosen (Eds.), *Cognitive therapies in action: Evolving innovative practices.* San Francisco: Jossey-Bass.

Freeman, A., & Leaf, R. C. (1989). Cognitive therapy applied to personality disorders. In A. Freeman, K. M. Simon, L. E. Beutler, & H. Arkowitz (Eds.), *Comprehensive Handbook of cognitive therapy* (pp. 403–433). New York: Plenum Press.

Freeman, A., Pretzer, J., Fleming, B., & Simon, K. M. (1990). *Clinical applications of cognitive therapy.* New York: Plenum Press.

Freeman, A., & Simon, K. M. (1989). Cognitive therapy of anxiety. In A. Freeman, K. M. Simon, L. E. Beutler, & H. Arkowitz (Eds.), *Comprehensive handbook of cognitive therapy* (pp. 347–365). New York: Plenum Press.

Goldenberg, H. (1983). *Contemporary clinical psychology* (2nd ed.). Pacific Grove, CA: Brooks/Cole.

Greenstone, J. L., & Leviton, S. C. (1993). *Elements of crisis intervention.* Pacific Grove, CA: Brooks/Cole.

Holmes, T. H., & Rahe, R. H. (1967). The social readjustment rating scale. *Journal of Psychosomatic Research, 11,* 213–218.

Lewis, S. J. (2002). A Crisis State Assessment Scale: Development and validation of a new instrument. *Dissertation Abstract International Section A; Humanities and social sciences, 62*(11-A), 3935.

Roberts, A. L. (1990). An overview of crisis theory and crisis intervention. In A. L. Roberts (Ed.), *Crisis intervention handbook* (pp. 3–16). Belmont, CA: Wadsworth.

Roberts, A. L. (2000). An overview of crisis theory and crisis intervention. In A. L. Roberts (Ed.), *Crisis intervention handbook: Assessment, treatment and research* (2nd ed., pp. 3–36). New York: Oxford University Press.

Roberts, A. (2005). Bridging the past and present to the future of crisis intervention and crisis management. In A. Roberts (Ed.), *Crisis intervention handbook* (3rd ed., pp. 3–34). New York: Oxford University Press.

Roberts, A. R., & Camasso, M. (1994). Staff turnover at crisis intervention units and programs: A national survey. *Crisis Intervention and Time Limited Treatment, 1*(1), 1–9.

Rosenbaum, A., & Calhoun, J. F. (1977). The use of the telephone hotline in crisis intervention: A review. *Journal of Community Psychology, 5,* 325–330.

Schützwohl, M. (2000). Frühintervention nacht traumatisierenden erfahrugen: Ein überblick über mapnahmen und deren wirksamkeit. *Fortschritte der Neurologie Psychiatric, 68*(9), 423–430.

Slaiku, K. A. (1990). *Crisis intervention* (2nd ed.). Boston: Allyn & Bacon.

Spitzer, R. L., & Williams, J. B. W. (1986). *Structured clinical interview for DSM-III-R, Upjohn version* (SCID-UP-R). New York: New York State Psychiatric Institute, Biometrics Research.

Teichman, Y. (1992). Family treatment with an acting out adolescent. In A. Freeman & F. M. Dattilio (Eds.), *Comprehensive casebook of cognitive therapy* (pp. 331–346). New York: Plenum Press.

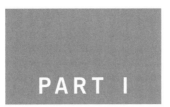

PART I

Psychological Crises

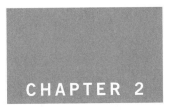

CHAPTER 2

Depression and Suicide

Mark A. Reinecke
Jason J. Washburn
Emily Becker-Weidman

> How small a thought it takes to fill someone's whole life! Just as a man can spend his life traveling around the same little country and think there is nothing outside it! You see everything in strange perspective (or projection): the country that you keep traveling around strikes you as enormously big; the surrounding countries all look like narrow border regions. If you want to go down deep you do not need to travel far; indeed, you don't have to leave your most immediate and familiar surroundings.
>
> —WITTGENSTEIN (1946/1980, p. 50)

When Ludwig Wittgenstein wrote this in 1946 he was commenting not on thought and language but on the ways in which focusing on a specific philosophical issue can lead to a misperception of the larger world. One can come to view everything from the perspective of the thought (which, from an external point of view may appear relatively small and unimportant). One becomes focused on it. Traveling deeper and deeper, one becomes fixated on the issue and the outer world becomes a narrow borderland.

His point was well taken. Our experience of ourselves and our world is guided by our inner language and the issues we identify as important. As a small thought may fill a life with meaning, value, and richness, so too can it end it. "I just can't take it anymore and there's nothing I can do, I might as well be dead." Simple statements such as these are frightening, both for individuals who feel that there is no solution for their problems other than their own destruction and for the therapist who must address them. Suicide is, by its very nature, a crisis. Decisions about patients who are considering suicide, or who have made a suicide attempt, must be made rapidly. There is little room for error. Suicidality can, as such, represent a crisis for the therapist as well as for the patient.

Slaikeu (1990) defined a crisis as "a temporary state of upset and disorganization, characterized chiefly by an individual's inability to cope with a particular situation using customary methods of problem solving, and by the potential for a radically positive or negative outcome" (p. 15). The four components of a crisis—its transient nature, the accompanying state of disorganization and distress, the failure of customary solutions or problem-solving skills, and the opportunity for reintegration and a positive outcome—apply both to our understanding of suicidality and to its treatment. Suicidal crises are, in most cases, time limited. Although suicidal thoughts may persist for extended periods of time, the intense and highly charged "urge to act," as well as the internal sense of being unable to control or resist the impulses, often subsides after a relatively short period. With support and strategic interventions, the accompanying feelings of distress can be alleviated. New problem-solving skills can be developed such that there is an opportunity for a positive outcome. With preparation and the refinement of coping skills, future crises can be averted.

The goal of this chapter is threefold: (1) to review the recent literature on factors associated with suicidal risk; (2) to provide clinicians with useful tools and recommendations for managing suicidal crises; and (3) to provide guidelines for treating suicidal patients. The latter objectives, crisis management and longer-term treatment, can be viewed as separate but related processes. The primary goal in managing a suicidal crisis is to protect patients from themselves—to ensure their survival. Protection can be accomplished in several ways—through hospitalization, with medications, through intensive outpatient therapy, by alleviating stressors or problems that may have precipitated the crisis, and by developing a more supportive and secure environment. Treatment of suicidal patients involves identification and resolution of factors that have contributed to their suicidality. It is not sufficient simply to alleviate the stressors that have contributed to the current suicidal episode. Other problems or stressors may arise in the future. Rather, the goal of treatment is to identify factors that lead individuals to consider suicide a viable alternative and to develop other strategies for coping with the problems and stresses of life. This is a longer-term goal and is typically accomplished once the patient has been stabilized and the immediate crisis has passed.

Crisis situations are varied and highly personal, and they tend to fluctuate over time. Thus, it would be difficult to prepare a list of specific "rules" for their management. Rather, an attempt is made here to draw on contemporary cognitive-behavioral theory for guidelines that can be used in a flexible, creative manner. Suicidality among children and adolescents is an increasingly important problem; however, a review of the literature is beyond the scope of this chapter (see Brent, 2001; Commission on Adolescent Suicide Prevention, 2005; Freeman & Reinecke, 1993; Gould, Greenberg, Velting, & Shaffer, 2003; Piacentini, Rotheram-Borus, & Cantwell, 1995; Spirito, Overholser, & Vinnick, 1995; Trautman, 1995; Weersing & Brent, 2003, for thoughtful discussions of cognitive-behavioral approaches for assessing and treating suicidal youth).

COGNITIVE MODELS OF DEPRESSION AND SUICIDE

At their most basic level, cognitive models of psychopathology are based on the assumption that transactional relationships exist between how individuals think and how they subsequently feel and behave. Individuals' assumptions, schemata, memories, beliefs, goals, attributions, expectations, wishes, plans, inferences, and perceptual biases all influence how they respond, both behaviorally and emotionally, to events in their world. These cognitive processes are adaptive, selective, and automatic. Emotional and behavioral problems, including suicidality, are seen as stemming from distorted or maladaptive mental representations and thought processes that were learned at an earlier point in time.

Clinically, the therapist's objective is to assist the patient to identify these maladaptive cognitive processes and dysfunctional beliefs, and to encourage the development of more adaptive or functional beliefs and coping skills. Although the emphasis is on understanding and changing beliefs, expectations, assumptions, and schemata, cognitive therapy acknowledges the importance of attending to social, environmental, biological, emotional, and behavioral factors that may be contributing to the patient's distress.

Both research and clinical observation suggest a strong link between depression and suicidality. Psychological autopsies of completed suicides show that many had a mental disorder at the time of death, and nearly all had depressive symptoms (Bertolote, Fleischmann, De Leo, & Wasserman, 2004; Cheng, 1995; Henriksson et al., 1993; Lönnqvist, 2000). The lifetime incidence of suicide among clinically depressed persons is likely between 4 and 8% (Bostwick & Pankratz, 2000; Brodaty, Luscombe, Peisah, Anstey, & Andrews, 2001; Inskip, Harris, & Barraclough, 1998; Simon & Von Korff, 1998). Although virtually all psychiatric disorders increase risk for suicide (Harris & Barraclough, 1997), patients with a major affective disorder are at a particular risk (Bostwick & Pankratz, 2000). Why might this be?

Research initiated by Aaron Beck in the early 1960s (1967, 1973, 1976) suggests that depressed individuals experience a range of negativistic thoughts about themselves, their world or experience, and their future. They tend to view themselves as flawed in important ways and believe that others are rejecting or unsupportive. As a consequence, they tend to believe that they do not possess the resources to resolve their difficulties and view their future as hopeless. In an attempt to preserve what resources they retain, they become passive or withdrawn and tend to seek reassurance from others. Their depressed affect biases their memory—such that they selectively recall other instances of failure in their past (Bower, 1981)—as well as their perceptions of current events (Beck, Rush, Shaw, & Emery, 1979). The dark lens of negativistic beliefs leads depressed individuals to perceive that they lack control over important events in their life, leading them to feel helpless (Abramson, Metalsky, & Alloy, 1989). Recent prospective studies indicate that cognitive factors may increase individual's vulnerability to both depression and suicide (Abela & Brozina, 2004; Hankin, Fraley, & Abela, 2005; Hunt & Forand, 2005; Robinson & Alloy, 2003; Scher, Ingram, & Segal, 2005).

Depressed individuals tend to pay attention to the immediate (rather than the delayed) consequences of their behavior and may make inappropriate attributions about their responsibility for negative events. Depressed individuals tend not to reward themselves for their successes, are less responsive to rewards, and can become highly self-punitive when they fail to meet their standards or goals (Henriques & Davidson, 2000; Rehm, 1977). They tend to view themselves in negative ways and demonstrate high levels of discrepancy between how they view themselves and how they feel they "ought" to be.

Given these beliefs, expectations, self-appraisals and attributions, highly depressed individuals can become suicidal. They feel that their current predicament is intolerable and believe there is no hope for it to change. As a consequence, suicide becomes a viable solution. They believe that their attempt will communicate their distress to others and so may effect a change in the environment, or that it will provide them with a sense of relief from their problems. Moreover, many suicidal patients experience intense feelings of psychic anxiety, agitation, and turmoil (Fawcett et al., 1990), leading them to seek an immediate solution to their distress. As Shneidman (1985) cogently observed, "The common stimulus in suicide is unendurable psychological pain" (p. 124), and the "common purpose is to seek a solution" (p. 129). Cognitive therapy is directed toward alleviating specific cognitive biases and distortions, developing behavioral skills, reducing environmental stress, developing supports, and assisting patients to communicate their concerns to others more clearly and adaptively.

Suicide, from this perspective, is a state of mind. It is there we must go if we are to understand and address it. In addition to the cognitive distortions often associated with feelings of depression and anxiety, several cognitive distortions appear to contribute to the risk of suicide. Most prominent among these is "tunnel vision" or "constriction" (Shneidman, 1985)—the inability to see alternative courses of action and outcomes— and "dichotomous thinking." Studies suggest that suicidal individuals tend to categorize events or experiences into polar extremes. They rigidly adopt an absolutist, black-or-white perspective and experience difficulty acknowledging nuances, subtleties, or relativistic alternatives (Neuringer, 1968; Neuringer & Lettieri, 1971; Wetzel, 1976). Moreover, suicidal individuals appear to manifest increased levels of irrational or dysfunctional beliefs (Prezant & Neimeyer, 1988) and behave in an impulsive manner (Ellis & Ratliff, 1986; Linehan, Camper, Chiles, Strosahl, & Shearin, 1987; Schotte & Clum, 1987; Tarter, Kirisci, Reynolds, & Mezzich, 2004). Recent work indicates that they may also experience deficits in "positive future thinking" (Conaghan & Davidson, 2002; Lavender & Watkins, 2004; MacLeod & Salaminiou, 2001). The cognitive model posits that an individual's beliefs are heavily influenced by his/her social experiences, and that dysfunctional attitudes develop in a social context. Depressed and suicidal patients tend to withdraw from others and report feeling that their families are not cohesive or supportive. These social difficulties serve to exacerbate their feelings of alienation and provide further evidence for their beliefs that others are rejecting.

A number of studies indicate that suicidal individuals may demonstrate deficits in social problem solving (Chang, 1998; D'Zurilla, Chang, Nottingham, & Faccini,

1998; Linehan et al., 1987; Rudd, Rajab, & Dahm, 1994; Schotte & Clum, 1987; Pollock & Williams, 2004). It has been postulated that these difficulties may interact with hopelessness and stressful life events in placing individuals at risk for suicidal thoughts and behavior (Bonner & Rich, 1988). Suicidal thoughts and behavior may result from a failure to obtain a satisfactory solution to persistent psychological discomfort and pain (Schneidman, 1985). Specific deficits have been observed in problem-solving orientation, confidence in being able to solve problems, generating alternative solutions, and use of "active" problem-solving strategies (Bonner & Rich, 1988; Clum & Febbraro, 1994; Jollant et al., 2005; Linehan et al., 1987; Schotte & Clum, 1987). Although it is not clear that problem-solving deficits are a stable predictor of suicidal behavior (Schotte, Cools & Payvar, 1990), they may play a role in the treatment process (Joiner, Voelz, & Rudd, 2001; Lerner & Clum, 1990; Reinecke, 2006; Salkovskis, Atha, & Storer, 1990).

THE ROLE OF HOPELESSNESS

An extensive body of research suggests that hopelessness is an important predictor and mediator of suicide among adults. Hopelessness, which may be defined as a general set of negative expectancies about oneself and the future, appears to be both a concomitant of depression and a predictor of suicidal behavior (Beck, 1967, 1986; Dyer & Kreitman, 1984; Weishaar & Beck, 1992). Hopelessness has been found, for example, to be a more powerful predictor of suicidal intent than is depression among suicidal ideators (Beck, Steer, Beck, & Newman, 1993; Nekanda-Trepka, Bishop, & Blackburn, 1983; Wetzel, Margulies, Davis, & Karam, 1980) and nonreferred adults (Cole, 1988; Joiner & Rudd, 1996). It has been found to predict eventual suicide among individuals diagnosed with major affective disorders (Chioqueta & Stiles, 2003; Coryell & Young, 2005), schizophrenia (Drake & Cotton, 1986), and alcohol abuse (Beck, Weissman, & Kovacs, 1976). Moreover, it appears to discriminate suicidal from nonsuicidal patients with equivalent levels of depression (Ellis & Ratliff, 1986; Heisel, Flett, & Hewill, 2003). Hopelessness appears to be a strong predictor of suicide among patients who have made a prior suicide attempt (Beck, Kovacs, & Weissman, 1975; Beck et al., 1976; Dyer & Kreitman, 1984; Kovacs, Beck, & Weissman, 1975; Petrie & Chamberlain, 1983; Weissman, Beck, & Kovacs, 1979; Wetzel, 1976; Brinkman-Sull, Overholser, & Silverman, 2000; Spirito, Valeri, Boergers, & Donaldson, 2003). Finally, longitudinal studies suggest that hopelessness may be a useful long-term predictor of completed suicide (Beck, Steer, Kovacs, & Garrison, 1985; Beck, Brown, & Steer, 1989; Fawcett et al., 1990; Wen-Hung, Gallo, & Eaton, 2004).

Taken together, these findings are impressive and compelling. They suggest that hopelessness may be a useful long-term predictor of suicidal risk among adults, and that feelings of pessimism may be an important target for therapy (Freeman & Reinecke, 1993). In a prospective study of 1958 outpatients, for example, hopelessness was found to be strongly associated with eventual suicide (Beck, Brown,

Berchick, Stewart, & Steer, 1990). Given the large sample employed, the authors were able to use statistical techniques derived from signal detection theory to determine optimum cutoff scores for both the Beck Depression Inventory (BDI) and the Beck Hopelessness Scale (HS) for predicting suicide. Employing receiver operating characteristic curves, they found that a cutoff score of 9 or above on the HS and 23 or above on the BDI yielded an accurate prediction of suicidal risk. Although the BDI had greater specificity, the HS had superior sensitivity in predicting ultimate suicide. The authors suggest that these findings indicate that hopelessness "is more directly related than is depression alone to suicidal intent" (Beck et al., 1990, p. 193). These findings are congruent with those of an earlier prospective study of 165 adults who had been hospitalized due to suicidal ideations (Beck et al., 1985). Of the 11 patients who committed suicide over a 10-year follow-up period, 10 (90%) had HS scores greater than 9. Only one patient who ultimately committed suicide received a hopelessness score below 10. Similar results have been found in prospective studies of psychiatric outpatients. In a study of 2,174 adults, Beck (1986) found that a cutoff score of 10 correctly identified 9 of 10 eventual suicides, yielding a false negative rate of 10%. Of concern, however, was the fact that 1,137 of the 2,164 patients who did not commit suicide (52.5%) also received HS scores of 10 or above. The specificity rate for this cutoff score, then, was 47.5%—unacceptably high for most clinical practices. Beck observed that a more stringent criterion—a cutoff score of 17 or above—identifies a "high-risk group" whose rate of eventual suicide is 15 times greater than that of other outpatients.

Recent work suggests that there may be both state and trait components to scores on the HS (Young et al., 1996). In a study of 316 adults, they found that patients manifest a relatively stable, "trait" level of hopelessness when they are not depressed, as well as an incremental, "state-dependent" increase in pessimism which accompanies the depressive episode. Patients' baseline or trait level of hopelessness predicted future suicide attempts, whereas the incremental increase and total score did not. It appears, then, that patients who maintain a chronic, pessimistic outlook may be at higher long-term risk for suicidal gestures and attempts than are patients who do not. They suggest that it may be useful to assess "how pessimistic this is patient when not depressed, and how much more hopeless do he/she becomes during the depressive episode. MacLeod, Pankhania, Lee, and Mitchell (1997) find that suicidal patients anticipated fewer positive events than controls but not more negative experiences. Suicidal patients are significantly more pessimistic than controls, and there is no difference between depressed and nondepressed suicidal patients. Taken together, these findings indicate that hopelessness might best be viewed as a predictor of suicidal potential rather than a predictor of a specific behavior at a specific point in time. It can be used, in conjunction with other clinical information, in estimating suicidal risk.

It is worth acknowledging that although hopelessness appears to be a strong predictor of suicidal risk among adults, equivocal findings have been reported (Kennedy & Reinecke, 1998; Dieserud, Roysamb, Braverman, Dalgard, & Ekeberg, 2003). Robust relationships between hopelessness and suicidality are most often found among patients with a history of suicidal gestures and among more severely depressed inpatients and outpatients. Research with the elderly (Uncapher, Gallagher-Thompson, Osgood, & Bongar, 1998), adolescents (Rotheram-Borus & Trautman, 1988), prison inmates (Ivanoff & Jang, 1991), and college students (Konick & Gutierrez, 2005), however, are less consistent. Taken together, these findings highlight the importance of considering depression and hopelessness simultaneously when assessing and treating suicidal adults, and of viewing hopelessness within the context of a broader range of cognitive, social, and psychiatric risk factors.

TOWARD AN INTEGRATED MODEL OF RISK

A number of psychiatric, social, environmental, and cognitive factors are associated with severity of suicidal thoughts. They may serve as predictors of suicidal risk. Although studies have tended to examine these variables in isolation, recent work based on diathesis–stress models of psychopathology suggests that these factors may interact in contributing to vulnerability for suicide. In an early attempt to evaluate an integrative model, Rudd (1990) found that stressful life events were a significant predictor of both depression and hopelessness, which, in turn, mediated the relationship between negative life events and severity of suicidal thoughts. Significant relationships were also observed between perceived social support, life events, and suicidality. In a similar manner, Clum and Febbraro (1994) found that stressful life events, social support, and social problem-solving skills interacted in predicting severity of suicidality in a sample of 59 chronically suicidal college students. This was congruent with observations by Yang and Clum (1994), who found that social support and problem-solving skills may mediate relationships between stressful life events and suicidal ideations among young adults. Attributional style has also been found to interact with stressful life events in predicting levels of depression, hopelessness, and suicidality among college students (Joiner & Rudd, 1995).

It has been more than 20 years since Ellis (1986) suggested that the pattern of cognitive deficits observed among suicidal patients may distinguish them from other individuals, and that these differences may warrant developing distinct treatment programs for suicidal patients. It appears that the cognitive characteristics of suicidal patients he described—problem-solving deficits, cognitive rigidity, cognitive distortions, a view of suicide as a viable solution, anxious agitation, and hopelessness—may interact with stressful life events, behavioral impulsivity, and the availability of social supports in placing individuals at risk. Although the specific relationships between these factors are not yet known, the general outlines of an integrated model of vulnerability and treatment are beginning to emerge. Individuals function in a dynamic social world; our models must address all the variables associated with suicide risk, the relationships among variables, and their environmental contexts. The model proposed by Rudd, Joiner, and Rajab (2001) meets these model criteria. It suggests that specific predisposing vulnerabilities interact with internal or external stressors and a person's cognitive organization, behavioral and motivational system, physiological system, and affect in leading to suicidal ideation and behavior.

SOCIAL AND PSYCHIATRIC RISK FACTORS

A number of social and psychiatric factors have also been identified that place a person at risk for suicide. Suicidality does not represent a singular entity but reflects a continuum from ideation to attempt to completed suicide. Research suggests that meaningful differences exist between individuals who think about suicide (ideators) and those who attempt or complete the act. These three groups—ideators, attempters, and completers—are, in important ways, independent and distinct. It is worth keeping in mind, then, that different factors may be associated with risk for each of these groups. We often tacitly assume that research with ideators and attempters will inform our understanding of individuals who ultimately commit suicide. Unfortunately, this is not always the case. Moreover, differences appear to exist within each of these groups with regard to the individual's level of intent, lethality of means, the presence of mitigating circumstances, and the availability of deterrents. Thus, it is essential that one adopt an idiographic approach to assessing suicidality.

Finally, it is important to define what is meant by a risk factor or predictor. Risk factors may be thought of as experiences, events, or propensities that make a particular outcome—in this case, an attempted or completed suicide—more likely. They may play a causal role in the development of the crisis—that is, they may be necessary and/or sufficient for the person to become suicidal—or they may simply be contributory. That is, they increase the likelihood of a suicide attempt but are neither necessary nor sufficient for the act to occur. Causal factors may also be proximal or distal. That is, they may have occurred immediately before the outset of the suicidal crisis (e.g., an executive who is fired for embezzlement then borrows a gun to commit suicide) or further in the patient's past. Both prospective and retrospective studies suggest, for example, that stressful life events (including work or legal problems, humiliating social events, the recent loss of a loved one, and changes of residence) are associated with an increased risk of suicide (Hagnell & Rorsman, 1980). It is also known that the loss of a parent during childhood increases the risk of suicide years later (Adam, Bouckoms, & Streiner, 1982; Goldney, 1981; Roy, 1984). These findings are important in that negative early experiences—including family psychopathology, negative peer relationships, abuse and neglect, family instability, and a chaotic home environment—appear to be associated with both cognitive markers of vulnerability and later suicidal behavior (Gibb et al., 2001; Yang & Clum, 2000).

Factors that are predictive of suicide in the short term differ from those that are associated with risk over longer periods. Research has shown a large range of variables are associated with suicide, including family structure (marital status, parenthood, spousal qualities), economic factors (employment and income), demographic factors (age, sex, race), health status, history of suicide attempts, and psychiatric illness (Qin, Agerbo, & Mortensen, 2005). A recent review of the literature identified long-term risk factors in the prediction of inpatient suicide. Standard or long-term factors included in traditional risk profiles include previous suicide attempts (acts and gestures), suicidal thoughts, hopelessness, being male, previous admissions to inpatient units, and duration of hospitalization (Cassells, Paterson, Dowding, & Morrison, 2005).

Several scales have been developed to assess suicide risk among individuals who have made a suicide attempt. In a provocative study of individuals who attempted suicide by overdose, Buglass and Horton (1974) identified six factors associated with an increased risk of further suicide attempts:

1. Problems with the use of alcohol.
2. Sociopathic personality disorder.
3. Previous inpatient psychiatric treatment.
4. Previous outpatient psychiatric treatment.
5. Previous suicide attempts resulting in hospital admission.
6. Not living with a relative.

The probability of an additional suicide attempt during a 1-year follow-up period ranged from 5% for individuals who received a score of 0 to approximately 45% for those who scored 5 or 6. This scale was cross-validated by Garzotto, Siani, Zimmerman-Tansella, and Tansella (1976) and Siani, Garzotto, Zimmerman-Tansella, and Tansella (1979). Once again, psychiatric and social factors (in this case, social isolation) were found to be strong predictors of suicidal behavior. Motto, Heilbron, and Juster (1985) developed an empirical suicide risk scale for adults hospitalized due to a depressive or suicidal state. The authors studied 2,753 subjects prospectively regarding 101 psychosocial variables. The risk scale is composed of 15 items that were identified through statistical analysis and validation procedures as significant predictors of suicide in a 2-year follow-up. In another prospective study of 929 clinically depressed patients, Fawcett et al. (1987), found that hopelessness, anhedonia, and mood cycling predicted completed suicide during the 12 months after a suicide attempt.

A statistical model for identifying repeat suicide attempters, developed by Corcoran et al. (1997) includes only data available to nonclinical hospital personnel and not information about psychiatric diagnosis or use of treatment services. A number of demographic and sociological variables serve as potential predictors, such as age, gender, marital status, level of education, previous suicide attempt, method of suicide attempt, drug or alcohol use at time of attempt, past or present substance abuse, history of harm due to alcohol, and any change in domestic situation around the time of the attempt. This model predicted 96% of repeaters and 86% of nonrepeaters.

Taken together, these studies suggest that a number of variables—including demographic, social, environmental, behavioral, psychiatric, and psychological factors—are associated with risk of suicide (Buerk, Kurz, & Moeller, 1985). When faced with a suicidal crisis, each of these domains should be assessed. Caution should be taken, however, when employing scales in that the limited reliability of individual items may reduce the utility of the scales for predicting suicide attempts in some populations (Spirito, Brown, Overholser, & Fritz, 1991).

As noted, individuals with a diagnosable psychiatric disorder are at an increased risk of attempting suicide (Prigerson, Desai, Lui-Mares, & Roseheck, 2003; Bertole, Fleischmann, De Leo, & Wasserman, 2003). The risk is greatest among individuals with depression, bipolar disorder, schizophrenia, an eating disorder, substance abuse, or a personality disorder (Chioqueta & Stiles, 2003; MacKinnon et al., 2005; Warman, Forman, Henriques, Brown, & Beck, 2004; Meltzer, 2003; Herzog et al., 2000; Preuss et al., 2002; Gorwood, 2001; Borges, Walters, & Kessler, 2000; Verona, Patrick, & Joiner, 2001; Yen et al., 2003; Caldwell & Gottesman, 1990). Discrepant findings have been reported for panic disorder (Beck, Steer, Sanderson, & Skeie, 1991; Friedman, Jones, Chernen, & Barlow, 1992). Recent studies suggest that depressive disorders but not anxiety disorders constitute a risk for suicide (Chioqueta & Stiles, 2003; Placidi et al., 2000; Warshaw, Dolan, & Keller, 2000). Other studies report that panic disorder is associated with higher risk for suicide (Fawcett et al., 1990; MacKinnon et al., 2005; Khan, Leventhal, Khan, & Brown, 2002). Noyes (1991) proposes that suicide risk in patients with panic disorder is not triggered by panic attacks but by other stressors, such as interpersonal loss. It is clear that anxiety plays an important role in suicidal behavior. Two prospective studies by Fawcett, Busch, Jacobs, Kravitz, and Fogg (1997) observes some form of anxiety (panic attacks, psychic anxiety, ruminations, or agitation) in almost all depressed patients who later committed suicide. The authors highlight the importance of differentiating between acute and persistent suicide risk. With this in mind, a careful diagnostic assessment is recommended as part of an evaluation of suicide risk.

Current findings suggest that there may be a relationship between certain personality traits and suicidal ideation. Results show that Neuroticism is positively related to suicidal thoughts in nonclinical samples (Lester, 1987; Mehryar, Hekmat, & Khajavi, 1977). These findings are supported in a more recent study using undergraduates, where high scores on the Neuroticism scale of the NEO Personality Inventory—Revised (NEO PI-R) are correlated with higher incidence of suicidal ideation (Velting, 1999). Chioqueta and Stiles (2005) also find that suicidal ideation is positively predicted by Neuroticism but none of the other personality traits in the five-factor model. The relationship between comprehensive measures of personality and suicidality warrants further investigation. Identification of personality factors that create a vulnerability for suicide ideation may be an important tool for clinicians and intervention efforts.

Recent research with a nonpsychiatric sample of young adults suggests that many chronically suicidal individuals have a history of childhood psychiatric problems, and that severity of suicidal ideations among adults may be associated with early psychopathology (Clum & Weaver, 1997). These findings are both complex and intriguing. They suggest that developmental continuities may exist in vulnerability for chronic suicidality and that an assessment of early psychopathology may play a role in a comprehensive evaluation of suicidal risk.

Our goal as clinicians is to identify individuals who are at risk for making a suicide attempt in the immediate future (within hours or days). Predictors of imminent risk appear to differ, however, from predictors of long-term risk. Moreover, although demographic, social, psychiatric, and psychological factors are useful in identifying groups of individuals who are at an increased risk of suicide, they have not been found useful in predicting the behavior of individuals. Given the relatively low incidence of completed suicide in the general population (and even among a number of high-risk groups), rating scales based on demographic, social, and psychological characteristics are accompanied by unacceptably high false-positive and false-negative rates. Suicide risk for an individual appears to be more strongly related to clinical and proximate risk factors than to demographic characteristics. As Lester (1974) observed, scales based on demographic variables tend, by their very nature, to overlook individual differences. This is not meant to minimize the value of these studies or the usefulness of these scales. In practice risk scales, such as those described, and clinical ratings complement one another. Together, they form the foundation of a comprehensive and sensitive evaluation of suicidal risk. Suicide risk scales might best be used as a guide, and information derived from them should be integrated with the results of clinical interviews and a review of the patient's history in estimating current risk. Inasmuch as the likelihood of making a successful suicide attempt is greater during the months after an initial nonfatal attempt, clinicians working with suicidal patients should be particularly attentive immediately following their attempt or their discharge from the hospital.

SUBTYPES OF MOTIVATION FOR SUICIDE

Freeman and Reinecke (1993) described four groups of suicidal patients: (1) hopeless suicide, (2) psychotic suicide, (3) rational suicide, and (4) histrionic or impulsive suicide. The hopeless subtype refers to individuals who believe that their predicament is intolerable and that there is no hope that the situation will improve. They become highly pessimistic and view suicide as a reasonable solution to their problems. Quite often, these individuals are motivated by a desire for relief from their difficulties and consider suicide "adaptive." Although they are often ambivalent about ending their lives, their pervasive sense of personal helplessness presses them toward action. While suicidal patients often feel other emotions—including anger or rage, guilt, shame, fear, isolation, and loneliness—their feelings of hopelessness and impotence, their belief that they cannot effect a change, are what lead them to death. Clinical experience suggests that hopeless individuals do envision a future, but it is worse than their current state. They believe that their suffering will continue, that the canyon into which they have fallen is bottomless, and that suicide is their only solution.

The second group, psychotic suicides, includes patients who experience command hallucinations or delusions (Caldwell & Gottesman, 1990; Gardner & Cowdry, 1985; Roy, Mazonson, & Pickar, 1984). Although suicide is the leading cause of premature death among individuals with a history of schizophrenia, research does not consistently support the belief that delusional patients attempt suicide in response to command hallucinations (Nathan & Rousch, 1984). Rather, schizophrenic individuals often attempt suicide during periods of relative lucidity. It is the chronicity of the illness and the inexorable recurrence of psychotic episodes that place the individuals at risk for suicide. As they become aware of their deteriorating condition and lose confidence in the effectiveness of their treatment, feelings of pessimism develop and suicide risk increases.

Rational suicides constitute a third subgroup of patients. Most often, these individuals suffer from a terminal illness or a progressive disease and view suicide as a reasonable course of action. Like "hopeless" patients, these individuals are typically motivated by a desire for relief from their illness or by a desire to avoid pain or hardship stemming from their deteriorating condition. Only a small percentage of suicidal patients, about 2%, are terminally ill at the time of their attempt. Of these, the majority also manifest an acute mental disorder, such as depression. As such, it is unclear that these attempts are "rational" in the traditional sense of the term.

Histrionic or manipulative individuals constitute a fourth subgroup of suicidal patients. They are motivated not by a desire for relief but by a desire for stimulation or excitement. They do not tend, as a group, to feel particularly hopeless or pessimistic. Rather, often they are motivated by a desire for attention or revenge—they want to "make someone pay" for a perceived wrong. Although their attempts are often impulsive and may be seen by others as "attention seeking," they should not be overlooked or their significance minimized.

It should be acknowledged that there is some overlap between these alternatives, and that other conceptual schemes for understanding suicidal behavior have been proposed (Arensman & Kerkhof, 1996; Reynolds & Berman, 1995). Typologies such as this can be a clinically useful tool for rapidly assessing suicidal motivation and for developing a treatment plan. Of particular interest is the fact that of the four subtypes, in all but one (the histrionic–manipulative) suicide is mediated by feelings of pessimism or hopelessness. This typology is consistent with the results of a study of 200 adults hospitalized after making a suicide attempt (Kovacs et al., 1975). Of these patients, 111 (56%) reported that they attempted suicide as a means of gaining a sense of relief from their problems, whereas 13% had attempted suicide "for the sole purpose of taking a chance on effecting some change in others or in the environment" (p. 365).

This conceptual scheme is similar in many ways to one proposed by Beck, Rush, et al. (1979). They also suggested that suicidal individuals may be differentiated with regard to their motivation for considering suicide. They proposed that some individuals are motivated by a "desire for escape or surcease," whereas others are motivated by a "desire to communicate" their concerns to others. They, suggested that those who are motivated by a desire for escape may be more hopeless or pessimistic than those motivated by a desire to express their concerns to others. An assessment of a patient's motivation for considering suicide is clinically important in that treatment goals may differ for each of the groups. Feelings of pessimism might, for example, be a reasonable target for the hopeless or rational individual, whereas appropriate communication and regulation of anger might be the focus of treatment for the histrionic–manipulative patient.

ASSESSMENT

Although suicidal risk should regularly be assessed when working with depressed individuals, there are two situations in which a more formal evaluation is needed—when patients express suicidal thoughts and after they have made a suicidal gesture or attempt (Williams & Wells, 1989; Yufit & Bongar, 1992). Given the range of factors that are associated with risk of completed suicide, a comprehensive evaluation includes a diagnostic and developmental interview, an assessment of suicide risk indicators, completion of objective rating scales, and a more extended assessment of risk and protective factors.

Clinical Interviews

Assessing suicidal risk typically begins with clinical interviews of the patient and family members. As we have seen, factors have been identified that are associated with an increased risk of suicide. As a consequence, a number of issues should be addressed in a clinical interview. These include an assessment of the patient's

- Current mood (including feelings of anxiety, hopelessness, and agitation)
- Motivation for attempting suicide
- Degree of intent to die
- History of impulsive behavior
- Adaptive and maladaptive coping strategies
- Family and community supports
- Cognitive flexibility
- Deterrents (including their nature, durability and strength)
- Ability to envision alternative future scenarios
- Attitudes toward death

It also is important to determine whether the patient manifests a specific psychiatric disorder. In addition to unipolar and bipolar affective disorders, the clinician will want to inquire about the patients lifetime history of alcohol or substance abuse, psychosis, externalizing behavior problems (such as conduct disorder or antisocial personality), anxiety (including panic disorder, posttraumatic stress disorder, obsessive–compulsive disorder, and generalized anxiety disorder), and personality disorder.

Similar recommendations were made by Motto (1989), who observed that factors associated with suicidal risk can be assessed by directly asking patients about their recent experiences. Empathic, sensitive questioning can be useful in identifying factors contributing to the suicidal crisis. Recommended questions include the following:

1. Do the patients experience periods of feeling depressed or despondent about their life?
2. How long do these periods last? How frequent are they? How severe? Are their associated symptoms of depression?
3. Do they feel hopeless, discouraged, or self-critical?
4. Are there suicidal ideations? What is their nature?
5. How are these feelings managed?
6. What supports are available?

If patients express suicidal thoughts, it is essential to determine their specific reasons or motives for considering suicide. The strength of their desire to attempt suicide as well as the development of a specific plan should be assessed. Have they developed a specific plan? What is their understanding of the lethality of their plan? Do they have the means and opportunity to kill themselves? Have they made a suicide attempt before? Further questioning might focus on the availability of effective deterrents to making an attempt. Do they have reasons for wanting to live? How strong or important are these reasons? The evaluation would continue with a discussion of stresses and supports they perceive and an assessment of their typical approach to solving problems. It would conclude with a review of their medical and psychiatric history and an evaluation of their current mood. Particular attention would be given to assessing their current levels of depression, hopelessness, anxiety, and anger.

Rating Scales

Assessing suicidal risk can be a complex endeavor. Standardized rating scales can be quite useful in this regard and are a valuable adjunct to a clinical interview (Reinecke & Franklin-Scott, 2005). Many of the measures available are concise and easy to administer and have proven clinical utility. In addition to providing a quantitative index of the patient's mood and suicidality, the specific items endorsed can provide the clinician with important insights into areas that are most problematic. Although many of these scales have received extensive empirical support, it is worth keeping in mind that they are face valid. Thus, they are subject to distortion should patients wish to minimize or exaggerate their current distress. Corroborating evidence should be sought, as a consequence, from the patient's family or friends.

Among the most useful measures for assessing suicidality is the Scale for Suicidal Ideation (SSI; Beck, Kovacs, & Weissman, 1979). The scale contains 19 items, which are rated by a clinician on a scale of 0 (least severe) to 3 (most severe). Total scores are derived for both the current episode and a time in the patient's past when he/she "felt the worst." The scale is administered as a semistructured interview and yields a quantitative estimate of the intensity of the patient's suicidal thoughts and impulses. The assessment of suicide ideation at its worst point is of particular interest as recent work suggests that this may identify a subgroup of patients at relatively high risk for eventual suicide (Beck, Brown, Steer, Dahlsgaard, & Grisham, 1999). A modified version of this scale, the Modified Scale for Suicidal Ideation (MSSI; Miller, Norman, Bishop, & Dow, 1986; Clum & Yang, 1995), is also available. Both scales are useful qualitatively as well in that they provide information about the patient's motivations for considering suicide and deterrents that are available.

The Suicide Intent Scale (SIS; Beck, Schuyler, & Herman, 1974) is a 15-item questionnaire assessing the intensity of an attempter's wish to die at the time of his/her attempt. This information may be a useful predictor of long-term risk. The authors suggest that suicidal intent—the seriousness of the wish to end one's life—is one of several components of suicidal risk. Other factors include the availability of means, the presence of deterrents or "protective individuals," and knowledge about the lethality of the method selected. Suicidal intent is conceptualized as reflecting a balance between the wish to die and life-protective wishes, and it is believed to be based on the estimates made by patients about the probability that their attempt will be successful. Suicidal intent or risk may be viewed, then, as a continuum. As Beck, Rush, et al. (1979) observed, "At one extreme is an absolute intention to kill oneself and at the other extreme is an intention to go on living" (p. 210). One's position on this continuum is not static but varies in accord with one's perceptions and beliefs. Suicidal intent is conceptually independent from the lethality of an attempt. This is clinically important in that individuals may possess a high degree of suicidal intent yet may make an ineffective, nonlethal attempt (e.g., they might take a relatively small number of aspirin). The SIS includes items about the suicidal gesture, as well questions about the patients' thoughts and feelings at the time of their attempt. Items include the following:

1. How isolated was the person at the time of the attempt?
2. Was the attempt timed so that an intervention by someone else was likely or unlikely?
3. Did the individual take precautions against discovery?
4. Did the individual seek help during or after the attempt?
5. Did the individual make any final acts in anticipation of death?
6. Was the attempt planned?
7. Did the individual write a suicide note?
8. Did the individual communicate his/her intent to others?
9. Was the purpose of the attempt to manipulate the environment or to provide the individual with relief from problems?
10. Did the individual expect to die?
11. How certain was the individual that his/her means were "lethal"?
12. Did the individual consider the attempt to be "serious"?
13. Did the individual believe that the attempt was "reversible" if he/she received medical attention?
14. Was the attempt premeditated or impulsive?

The Lethality of Suicide Attempt Rating Scale (LSARS; Smith, Conroy, & Ehler, 1984) is another useful measure for estimating the lethality of an attempt. It differs from the SIS in that it does not incorporate judgments about patients' intent, premeditation, or understanding of the lethality of their attempt. As a result, it is less susceptible to biases in reporting by the patient. Rather, a clinician estimates the degree of lethality of the attempt on an 11-point (0–10) scale, using a table of risk variables and a set of nine well-defined anchor points as a guide.

Other measures of suicidal risk include the Los Angeles Suicide Prevention Scale/Suicidal Death Prediction Scale (LASPC/SDPS; Lettieri, 1974), the SAD Persons scale (SP; Patterson, Dohn, Bird, & Patterson, 1983), the Suicidal Ideation Questionnaire (SIQ; Reynolds, 1987), the Suicide Risk Assessment Scale (SRAS; Motto et al., 1985), the Scale for Assessing Suicidal Risk (SASR; Tuckman & Youngman, 1968), the Suicide Probability Scale (SPS; Cull & Gill, 1982), the Suicide Risk Measure (Plutchik, van Praag, Conte, & Picard, 1989), the Short Risk Scale (SRS; Pallis,

Barraciough, Levey, Jenkins, & Sainsbury, 1982), Intent Scale (Pierce, 1977), and the Index of Potential Suicide (IPS; Zung, 1974).

The Reasons for Living Inventory (RLI; Linehan, Goodstein, Nielsen, & Chiles, 1983; Linehan, 1985) is an interesting and valuable instrument in that it does not assess suicidal ideations. Rather, it is a 48-item self-report scale that taps feelings and beliefs about not attempting suicide. The scale is useful in identifying deterrents that may be meaningful for patients as well as their strength. As such, it can assist in identifying targets for clinical intervention.

Among the most valuable measures currently available for assessing pessimism is the Beck HS (Beck, Weissman, Lester, & Trexler, 1974). As noted, hopelessness or pessimism is a strong predictor of suicidal risk among adults and stands as an important target for therapy.

The BDI (Beck, Ward, Mendelson, Mock, & Erbaugh, 1961) is a 21-item self-report scale assessing depressive attitudes, feelings, and symptoms. It is the most widely used depression rating scale in the world, and has become "the standard in its class" (Rabkin & Klein, 1987, p. 64) and "a touchstone against which to compare assessments derived from other measures" (Steer, Beck, & Garrison, 1986, p. 123). Items are scored from 0 (not at all) to 3 (severe) and are summed to yield a total score. Concerns about the BDI's content validity motivated development of a second edition, the Beck Depression Inventory–II (BDI-II; Beck, Steer, & Brown, 1996). Twenty-three item changes were made in the recent edition. Two items moved location; four items concerning weight loss, body image, work difficulty, and somatic preoccupation were replaced with four new items related to agitation, worthlessness, concentration, and loss of energy; and wording was altered for 17 other items. The number of items and scoring system remain the same, but recommended cutoff scores on the BDI-II are higher. The psychometric characteristics of the BDI-II are comparable to those reported for the BDI, and the two instruments are highly correlated (.93). Differences between the scales do not seem to pose a problem for clinical or research interpretation (Beck et al., 1996). Scores on the BDI and the BDI-II, are highly correlated with suicidal intent and measures of self-esteem, pessimism, and anxiety.

As noted, recent research suggests that anxious patients, particularly those with a history of recurrent panic attacks, may be at an increased risk of suicide. Moreover, depressed and suicidal patients are often highly anxious and agitated. With this in mind, it is often helpful to assess levels of anxiety among depressed or suicidal patients. Several questionnaires have been developed during recent years that are useful in this regard. They include the Beck Anxiety Inventory, the Zung Anxiety Scale, and the State–Trait Anxiety Scale.

The Dysfunctional Attitude Scale (DAS; Weissman & Beck, 1978) is a 100-item self-report scale for measuring assumptions and beliefs thought to reflect the content of personal schemas. Significant associations have been found between dysfunctional attitudes, depression, and suicide. Ranieri et al. (1987) find that DAS scores are correlated with suicidal ideation among inpatients even after controlling for level of depression and hopelessness. Beck, Steer, and Brown (1993), however, do not find a significant correlation between dysfunction attitudes and suicidal ideation for psychiatric outpatients. The DAS appears to be a reliable and valid measure of depressive cognitions. The notion that it may be associated with long-term vulnerability for suicide is interesting and deserves further consideration. The DAS can provide useful clinical information about schema and beliefs associated with suicidality (Reinecke & Franklin-Scott, 2005).

INTERVENTIONS

As Bongar (1991) observed in his discussion of outpatient management of suicidal crises:

> If the clinician becomes preoccupied with the issue and threat of a patient's suicide, it can divert the clinician from the primary task of attending to more disposition-based treatment-therapeutics that are solidly grounded in an understanding of the power of a sound therapeutic alliance and on a well-formulated treatment plan. . . . (p. 104)

Quite true. Effective treatment of suicidality, like other clinical problems, begins with the establishment of a trusting therapeutic collaboration and the development of a clear, simple, and parsimonious conceptualization and treatment plan.

Beck, Rush, et al. (1979) described a series of steps in working with suicidal individuals. After assessing suicidal risk and gaining an understanding of the patient's motives for considering suicide, the therapist's first goal is to "step into his world and view it through the patient's lens" (p. 212). A phenomenological stance is an integral part of the cognitive model (Freeman & Reinecke, 1995) and forms a foundation for understanding and addressing the patient's most pressing concerns. Empathizing with patients' despair, understanding their motives for considering their own destruction, and acknowledging their belief that there are no other alternatives can provide them with a sense of being understood and accepted.

As Freeman and Reinecke (1993) noted, it can be helpful to acknowledge that "suicide is an option, things are bad for you, and death is something that might be considered" (p. 61). As one suicidal patient said:

> "You're the first person who ever really understood that. Everybody else just tries to talk me out of it, or tells me things could be worse . . . God, that would be something."

This acknowledgment would be followed by a discussion of other available alternatives and the development of a list of concrete steps that might be taken. In addition to enhancing rapport, this approach may reduce manipulative gains some patients seek through suicidal threats. Patients may be reassured by the therapist's candor in discussing their most terrifying thoughts and concerns. Suicidal persons typically view death as a reasonable solution to their predicament. In fact, they may view it as the *only* solution available. A therapeutic goal is to enhance their sense of hope by demonstrating that although suicide remains an option, it is not their only option. Moreover, it is not their best option.

The goal of crisis management is simple—to preserve the patient's life. This is achieved by restoring the patient's hope, developing effective deterrents, alleviating stressors, and providing support. When faced with a suicidal crisis, therapists adopt an active, problem-oriented stance. In contrast to traditional psychotherapy, minimal emphasis is placed on the interpretation of the therapeutic relationship or an examination of developmental events. As noted, impaired problem solving and cognitive distortions often contribute to the suicidal crisis. The therapist attempts to serve, then, as a supportive "rational guide"—an external ego, if you will, to supplant the patient's limited cognitive resources. Whereas suicidal patients typically see few alternatives, the therapist actively assists in developing solutions. When patients report feeling that their problems are numerous and overwhelming, the therapist breaks them into smaller units that can be attacked individually. When patients engage in maladaptive attempts to cope (such as using alcohol or drugs), the therapist works to develop more effective coping skills.

Suicidal patients frequently feel isolated from others and believe there is no one to whom they can reliably turn for support. Therapist availability, thus, is essential. Regular sessions should be scheduled as frequently as necessary, and patients might be given a card with emergency telephone numbers that they can call day or night. This might include the therapist's pager or home telephone number, an emergency room or crisis center number, and a backup therapist's telephone number. The provision of reliable and unwavering support is often quite reassuring to suicidal patients. The therapeutic message that someone will be reliably available to ensure their security is paramount. A calm, active therapeutic stance is employed to demonstrate that problems are endurable and solutions can be developed.

Family or friends, if available, might be recruited to assist with crisis management. They might be asked, for example, to accompany the patient home, or to allow the patient to stay with them until the next therapy session. The objectives are to ensure the patient's safety and provide the patient with an experience that is inconsistent with his/her belief that others are uncaring or unsupportive. If conflicts at home have contributed to the crisis (which is not uncommon), these would be directly addressed. As Fremouw, de Perczel, and Ellis (1990) stated, "A therapist's assistance in defining problems, articulating feelings, communicating wishes, and engineering solutions can prove invaluable in helping resolve stressful interpersonal conflicts" (pp. 104–105).

If a patient has a means for attempting suicide, it should be removed. Guns should be locked and removed and the patient's access to knives, prescription medications, poisons, and the like should be strictly monitored.

Given the role of hopelessness in suicidality, an immediate goal is to address the source of the patient's sense of pessimism and demoralization. This goal should be accomplished in the first session, during subsequent sessions, and throughout the follow-up period, through cognitive and behavioral exercises or assignments and by the therapist's modeling of effective problem solving and optimism in the face of difficult problems. If the patient feels he/she will be unable to resist the impulse to attempt suicide until the next therapy session, or the patient will be returning to a stressful, conflict-laden home, hospitalization should be considered. Hospitalization protects the patient and provides the therapist with the opportunity to complete a more thorough assessment of factors contributing to the crisis. Medication trials can be initiated and patients can participate in intensive individual and group psychotherapy (Davis & Schrodt, 1992).

Once the crisis has passed, longer-term treatment can begin. The issues and concerns that contributed to the emergency can be addressed. Strategic cognitive therapy of depression and anxiety can be initiated (Beck, Rush, et. al., 1979), with the goal of providing the patient with more effective cognitive and behavioral tools for coping with life's problems. Goals of therapy might include developing stable and supportive interpersonal relationships and learning more effective or adaptive ways of communicating one's concerns to others. Social skills training and marital or family therapy might prove useful in this regard (Epstein, Schlesinger, & Dryden, 1988).

Attempts also might be made to address problems with alcohol or substance abuse (Beck, Wright, & Newman, 1992). Given their important role in suicide, therapy might be directed toward reducing behavioral impulsivity, developing a positive attitude toward addressing life problems, and promoting flexible problem solving (Lerner & Clum, 1990). Patients are encouraged to recognize their ability to influence events in their life, and their belief that suicide is a viable solution is directly disputed. An objective is to enhance the patients' sense of control and personal effectiveness. As patients become better able to generate solutions that might be pursued in lieu of a suicide attempt, the link between thought and impulsive action is broken. Patients' reasons for living and dying are openly discussed, and patients are encouraged to envision alternative, positive future scenarios. As Markus and Nurius (1986) observed, an individual's beliefs, goals, and expectations for the future—the individual's sense of a "possible self"—have important behavioral and emotional implications. These beliefs and expectations affect not only an individual's motivation but also his/her self-concept. Direct attempts are made to identify and alleviate depressogenic beliefs and cognitive distortions. The focus is on changing dysfunctional schemata and interpersonal behavioral patterns (Linehan, 1987; Young, 1991).

As can be seen, cognitive therapy of suicidal patients is multidimensional and acknowledges the importance of behavioral, affective, social, and environmental factors in suicide. Cognitive interventions include rational responding, thought monitoring, cognitive distraction, guided imagery, thought stopping, self-instruction, scaling, guided association, reattribution, and examination of idiosyncratic meanings. Behavioral interventions are directed primarily toward developing coping skills, and they include activity scheduling, assertiveness or relaxation training, graded task assignments, mastery and pleasure ratings, behavioral rehearsal, *in vivo* exposure, and bibliotherapy. These and other techniques have been discussed at length by Beck, Rush, et al. (1979), Freeman and Reinecke (1995), McMullin (1986), and Reinecke and Didie (2005).

No-suicide contracts are commonly employed in work with suicidal patients and may, in fact, be viewed as "standard practice" in some settings. Unfortunately, there is relatively little empirical support for their effectiveness in reducing suicidal gestures and attempts among acutely suicidal patients (Busch, Fawcett, & Jacbos, 2003; Lee & Bartlett, 2005; Weis, 2001). The possibility exists, then, that they serve as much to alleviate the clinician's anxiety as to reduce the patients' distress. There are some situations in which the use of this approach may be contraindicated (Mahrer & Bongar, 1993) or increase risk (Drew, 2001; Reid, 2005). Although we regularly use no-suicide contracts or agreements in our clinical work, they are not a substitute for sensitive, ongoing assessment of suicidal risk or a systematic program of treatment.

Efficacy of Cognitive Therapy

The question remains: Is cognitive therapy clinically useful in reducing suicidal behavior? Whereas a substantial body of research indicates that cognitive-behavioral therapy can be effective for treating clinically depressed adults, few controlled studies have focused specifically on the prevention of suicidal behavior. Although research on the treatment of suicidal patients is limited, recent findings have been promising.

In an early study, Patsiokas and Clum (1985) examined the effectiveness of three forms of treatment—cognitive-restructuring, problem-solving training, and nondirective therapy—for reducing suicidal ideations in a sample of 15 psychiatric inpatients admitted after having made suicide attempts. Results indicated that all three treatments were effective in reducing the intensity of patients' suicidal thoughts. Lerner and Clum (1990) reported that social problem-solving therapy was more effective than supportive psychotherapy in reducing depression, hopelessness, and loneliness among suicidal young adults, and that these gains were maintained at 3-month follow-up. This approach was not significantly better, however, at reducing suicidal ideations. Social problem-solving training was, however, found to be effective in reducing suicidality in a study of 39 patients who had attempted to poison themselves. McLeavey, Daly, Ludgate, and Murray (1994) reported that interpersonal problem-solving training was effective in reducing levels of hopelessness, enhancing self-perception, improving social problem-solving skills, and improving patients' perceived ability to cope with ongoing problems. As important, patients in this condition reportedly made fewer suicidal gestures during a 1-year follow-up period than did patients in a control treatment condition. More recently, Wingate, Van Order, Joiner, Williams, and Rudd (2005) demonstrated that problem-solving treatment of suicidal behavior may be more effective when it is used to compensate for problem-solving deficits than when it is used to capitalize on existing problem-solving strengths.

Brown et al. (2005) recently published results of a randomized controlled trial of cognitive therapy with 120 adults who attempted suicide. Compared to enhanced usual care, participants in the cognitive therapy group were 50% less likely to reattempt suicide at the 18-month follow-up assessment. Cognitive therapy also resulted in significantly lower severity of self-reported depression than the enhanced usual care group at the 6-, 12-, and 18-month follow-up assessments. Although cognitive therapy was superior to enhanced usual care for reducing incidents of reattempts and severity of depression, no significant difference between rates of suicide ideation was reported.

Dialectical behavior therapy (DBT), a form of cognitive-behavioral therapy, has shown efficacy in reducing suicidality among patients diagnosed with borderline personality disorder (BPD) (Bohus et al., 2000; Linehan, 1993, 1999; Linehan, Armstrong, Suarez, Allmon, & Heard, 1991; Linehan, Heard, & Armstrong, 1993; Low, Jones, Duggan, Power, & MacLeod, 2001; Verheul et al., 2003). In a study of 39 women with BPD who had a history of suicidal gestures, for example, a combination of intensive individual and group cognitive-behavioral therapy (DBT) was contrasted with community treatment. During the initial 6 months of the follow-up period, patients who had received DBT reportedly made fewer suicidal gestures, were less angry, and demonstrated better social adjustment than those in the control condition. Moreover, during the subsequent 6 months they had fewer inpatient days and better interviewer-rated social adjustment.

These findings are consistent with other controlled studies (Evans et al., 1999; Salkovskis et al., 1990), and with the results of a meta-analytic review of randomized controlled trials of interventions for suicide attempters (van der Sande, Buskens, Allart, van der Graaf, & van Engeland, 1997). Yet, not all studies of cognitive-behavioral treatments have shown efficacy in reducing self-harm or suicide attempts. For example, a large, multicenter evaluation of a brief form of cognitive-behavioral therapy in England found no significant difference in rates of deliberate self-harm from treatment as usual (Tyrer et al., 2003).

Taken together, most findings indicate that cognitive-behavioral therapy may be more effective than community-based "treatment as usual" in reducing the frequency of suicidal gestures and in improving psychosocial adjustment of patients with a history of suicide attempts. Are these gains maintained over time? It is difficult to know. Results thus far are generally positive, but the long-term stability of gains observed has not been examined. Moreover, it is not clear whether the gains observed are clinically meaningful, or what factors discriminate those patients who are best able to benefit from these interventions. Given the limited number of studies completed, however, additional research is required before we can have confidence in the effectiveness of these approaches for treating suicidal patients.

CASE STUDY

Presenting Problems

G.L. was 41 years old at the time of her referral to our clinic. She had recently been discharged from an inpatient psychiatric treatment program and was experiencing recurrent, subjectively severe feelings of depression, anxiety, and anger. She was completing her doctorate in history and worked part time as a college instructor. Although G.L. had been raised in a devout Jewish home, she and her husband were atheists. G.L. had been divorced twice and now lived with her husband of 16 years and their three teenage children.

Presenting concerns included feelings of irritability, fear, anxiety, and depression. Although G.L. reportedly had lost 30 pounds during the past 3 months, medical tests revealed no physical basis for her loss of appetite or weight. She was, nonetheless, quite concerned that she might have a serious physical illness. She had been diagnosed with breast cancer approximately 8 months before, and the treatment had been successful. A node of cancerous cells reportedly was quite small and was excised completely. As there was no evidence of metastasis, radiation treatments and chemotherapy were not recommended. G.L.'s brother- in-law had, however, died of cancer several years before, leading her to suspect that she might be vulnerable to a physical illness. G.L. was highly sensitive to bodily sensations and reported experiencing a range of vague somatic problems. G.L. reported that she had felt depressed "all of her life," and that these feelings had become progressively more severe during the past 5 years. This worsening of her condition coincided with the beginning of her doctoral studies. She stated that she felt "frustrated about being alive" and commented that "everything I touch is destroyed." When asked to elaborate, she stated, "I mess up people's lives, I'm not fun, I make people miserable, and I can't stand myself." As a consequence, she observed that she "doesn't like to be alone; but I'm not able to be with others either." G.L. reported that she experienced a "lack of joy and fulfillment in life" and that this was "just the way I am." She recalled having struggled with feelings of guilt since her childhood, and remarked that she felt she "needed to be believed . . . and validated by others." G.L.'s specific symptoms, then, included the following:

Affective: dysphoria, irritability, guilt, anxiety, anger, fear, worrying, anhedonia, hopelessness, helplessness.

Cognitive: ruminations about past mistakes, depersonalization, feelings of unreality, low self-esteem, confusion, suicidal ideations, impaired concentration and memory.

Physiological: fatigue, decreased libido, loss of appetite, severe weight loss, nausea, insomnia, nightmares, early-morning awakening, dry mouth.

Behavioral: severe psychomotor retardation, agitation, hand wringing, frequent crying, social avoidance, angry outbursts, restlessness, yelling at children.

G.L. stated that these difficulties were worse just prior to taking exams, and she reported fearing that she was "going to fail." She reportedly became depressed and anxious prior to appointments with physicians or psychologists and when she was away from her children. She became quite fearful at those times and said that she experienced images of her children being killed in an accident. G.L. also became depressed while on vacations with her family. She stated that she "always had difficulty with unstructured time" and was fearful that she would "ruin it for everyone else." A structured diagnostic interview revealed that G.L. met the criteria in the fourth edition of *Diagnostic and Statistical Manual for Mental Disorders* (DSM-IV; American Psychiatric Association, 1994) for major depression—recurrent, dysthymia, and generalized anxiety disorder. These difficulties were superimposed on a range of borderline and dependent traits. The latter observation was of some concern given recent research suggesting that BPD may be associated with an increased risk of both attempted and completed suicide (Kjellander, Bongar, & King, 1998).

Assessment

A clinical interview, including the SSI, was completed to assess G.L.'s current level of suicidal risk. She stated that she had "no wish to live" and felt a "strong desire to die"—she simply "felt like being dead." Her thoughts of suicide were frequent and persistent. Although she stated that she was "ambivalent" about attempting suicide, she had no sense of control over these impulses. G.L. was deterred from attempting suicide by thoughts of the effects of her death on her family and a fear of pain or serious injury if she failed. She later acknowledged feeling, however, that she was a "bad mother and wife," and that her family would soon forget her if she were dead. She was motivated to consider attempting suicide by a desire for relief from her problems. Although G.L. had considered writing a suicide note, she had not developed a plan and did not have a lethal means available for attempting suicide. Moreover, she did not feel she would be able to carry out an attempt and had a supportive and caring family. She was able to agree not to make a suicide attempt prior to our next therapy session and was comfortable making this promise. With these considerations in mind, and given the fact that there was no history of prior suicidal gestures or attempts, rehospitalization was not indicated.

G.L. reported that there were no acute stressors or problems in her life. As her husband was a successful attorney, finances were not a concern. Although she characterized her graduate program as "difficult," she noted that she had earned A's in all her courses. Her children reportedly were polite and well mannered and were doing reasonably well in school. G.L. remarked, however, that she had few close friends and so felt isolated and estranged. Although she had numerous acquaintances and friendly neighbors, she felt she did not have anyone she could confide in. As a consequence, G.L. felt isolated and alienated. She stated that her husband was supportive, but she characterized her marriage as "living with a saint"—a situation she resented. She remarked that her husband was rarely critical of her, and that given her recent behavior was "either a saint or the biggest masochist in the world."

G.L.'s responses on a battery of objective rating scales were consistent with the results of the clinical interview and suggested that she was highly depressed, anxious, and pessimistic and was moderately suicidal. Her self-esteem was low, and she acknowledged being fearful of many situations. G.L.'s responses on the Young–Brown Schema Questionnaire (Young, 1991) revealed that she believed that others would not be able to provide emotional support or protection for her and that she was vulnerable to harm or illness. She viewed herself as incompetent and unable to handle day-to-day problems without support and felt that she was fundamentally flawed and unlovable. G.L. acknowledged that she had very high standards for herself, and that she felt she could never meet them. As a consequence, she continually felt discouraged and dissatisfied. Table 2.1 presents a summary of G.L.'s scores on the self-report questionnaires and clinician rating scales.

As noted, G.L. was highly depressed, anxious, agitated, and pessimistic at the time of her referral. Of particular concern was the fact that she was experiencing mod-

TABLE 2.1. Summary of Objective Rating Scales

	Scale	Score	Level
Depression	BDI	55	Severe
	CES-D	54	Severe
	Hamilton (HRSD)	52	Severe
Anxiety	BAI	38	Severe
	Zung	30	Severe
	Hamilton (HARS)	38	Severe
Hopelessness	HS	20	Severe
Suicidality	SSI		
	Current	19	Moderate
	Past	15	Moderate

Note. BAI, Beck Anxiety Inventory; CES-D, Center for Epidemiological Studies Depression Scale; HARS, Hamilton Anxiety Rating Scale; HRSD, Hamilton Rating Scale for Depression.

erately severe suicidal thoughts and demonstrated a number of significant cognitive distortions. Table 2.2 presents a summary of her suicide risk indicators.

Summary of Developmental and Medical History

When asked what may have led her to become so depressed, G.L. remarked, "I blame my mother. . . . I wasn't meant to be born." She recounted that she was the youngest of two children (her sister was approximately 15 years older) and that her mother was 45 years old when she became pregnant. Her mother reportedly had several abortions during the preceding years and had "attempted to miscarry me by throwing herself down a ladder." G.L. stated that her mother "never forgave me for being born," and she recalled her mother admonishing her to act appropriately or she would be "abandoned on a street corner . . . or in the park." Although G.L. was quiet, polite, and studious during her childhood, she recalled her mother berating her as "a bad child" and "an idiot." She described her mother as "angry and tense" and characterized her relationship with her mother as "frightening." These experiences may have contributed to G.L.'s belief that people are rejecting and unpredictable and that she was fundamentally unlovable, defective, and vulnerable. They are consistent, as well, with the possibility that she manifested an insecure attachment with her mother, and that this may have contributed to the development of her negativistic beliefs.

G.L. described her father in somewhat different terms. Her father was employed as a watchmaker and worked in a small jewelry shop attached to their house. G.L. characterized her father as a "political and social activist" and noted that he was "full of life when he was away from home." She described her relationship with him as "distant" and recalled him stating that "life at home doesn't exist . . . one should always be working for society." She recalled feeling that he was unresponsive to her

TABLE 2.2. Summary of Risk Indicators

Indicator	Interpretation
Daily functioning	Moderately good Cares for children; well respected at work Frustrated, angry at children
Lifestyle	Stable, but engages in no enjoyable activities; few social activities
Supports	Caring husband and family; few close friends; tends to withdraw
Stressors	Moderate stress at work; good performance, but avoids tasks
Coping	Adequate resources available; intelligent; motivated; good sense of humor
Psychiatric history	Extensive psychotherapy and medications Cooperative with treatment, but poor response No prior suicide attempts
Family history of suicide	None
Medical history	Breast cancer (in remission) Chronic fatigue and somatic complaints
Recent losses	None
Depression	Severe
Anxiety	Severe
Pessimism	Severe
Positive future thinking	Negligible; severe
Anger/irritability	Moderate
Impulsivity	Low
Alcohol/drug use	None
Suicidal ideations	Moderate to severe
Prior suicide attempts	None
Problem solving	Poor; negative problem orientation
Cognitive distortions	Severe
Constriction/dichotomizing	Severe
Self-focused attention	Severe
Ruminative style	Severe

concerns during her childhood, and noted that "no one was allowed to become upset at home . . . that was a sign you were self-centered." G.L.'s father is now almost 90 years old and lives several thousand miles away. Although she frequently sends him money, G.L. feels guilty that she is not able to be more supportive. She visits her father every several years but describes these visits as "tense."

G.L. lived at home until she was 18 years old, when she married. She stated that she was "never separated" from either of her parents during her childhood, and that she was frightened of being left alone. As she stated, "Even now I can't tolerate being separated from my family." As noted, G.L. has been married three times. She said that she divorced her first two husbands "just because," and remarked that "I think I get afraid they will leave me because I'm horrible, so I quit before they fire me." She continued by observing, "I never had a good reason for believing they'd leave me . . . I'm just too afraid."

G.L. reported that her parents had emigrated from Poland, and that many of her relatives were killed in the Holocaust. In addition, many of G.L.'s relatives and friends were arrested, tortured, and killed during military coups in South America during the 1970s. These experiences contributed to her belief that "individuals have no value in society" and to her feelings of guilt.

G.L. had participated in individual and family therapy for approximately 5 years but did not find the interventions helpful. In addition, she has received trials of numerous medications, including imipramine, nortriptyline, trazodone, phenelzine sulfate (Nardil), fluoxetine hydrochloride (Prozac), lorazepam (Ativan), diazepam, chlorpromazine hydrochloride (Thorazine), and lithium. The medications were ineffective, however, and were discontinued due to aversive side effects. The fact that she had not benefited from prior therapy is of concern given observations that unfavorable response to treatment may be a predictor of completed suicide (Dahlsgaard, Beck, & Brown, 1998).

Cognitive Conceptualization

Several cognitive-behavioral models of depression have been proposed during recent years, each emphasizing a specific facet of clinical depression (Ingram, Miranda, & Segal, 1998). Cognitive theorists and researchers have noted the importance of cognitive errors, distortions and negativistic beliefs (Beck, Rush, et al., 1979), impaired problem solving and self-reinforcement (Fuchs & Rehm, 1977; Rehm, 1977), depressogenic schemata (Beck, Rush, et al., 1979; Guidano & Liotti, 1983; Segal, 1988), reduced social reinforcement (Lewinsohn, 1975), attributional style (Abramson, Metalsky, & Alloy, 1989; Alloy, Abramson, Metalsky, & Hartlage, 1988; Barnett & Gotlib, 1988); helplessness, reduced perceptions of control over important outcomes (Seligman, 1975), hopelessness (Weishaar & Beck, 1992), and behavioral activity (Freeman, Pretzer, Fleming, & Simon, 1990) in depression.

G.L. demonstrated features of many of these models. A range of cognitive distortions was readily apparent as she described herself and her relationships with others, and she appeared to maintain highly negative views of herself, the world, and her future. She believed that she was essentially unlovable, that others were unsupportive and rejecting, and that she lacked the attributes or abilities necessary to succeed. Moreover, she actively avoided social activities and behaved in ways that might elicit rejection from her friends and family. G.L. demonstrated little "social interest" or empathy for others. Rather, she tended to ruminate about her concerns and experienced difficulty identifying possible solutions. As a consequence, she felt both hopeless and helpless. G.L. avoided challenging tasks and engaged in few activities that would provide her with a sense of competence or pleasure. She maintained high standards for her personal performance (both as a mother and a graduate student) and was highly self-critical when she did not meet these standards. She gave herself little credit for her successes ("Anyone can get a PhD . . . it's easy," she noted) and believed that she ultimately would be punished if she allowed herself to feel happy. These beliefs, expectations, attributions, behavioral skills deficits, and difficulties in problem solving became the focus of treatment. A cognitive-behavioral conceptualization of G.L.'s difficulties includes the following components:

Behavioral coping strategies: avoidance; withdrawal; excessive reassurance seeking.

Cognitive processes: dichotomizing; personalization; magnification/minification; selective abstraction; should statements; self-focused attention; ruminative style; dependent/sociotropic stance.

Automatic thoughts: "I'll never be as good as others; they don't care . . . they won't want to see me again; I destroy everything I touch; I'm a horrible, castrating person; I'll be punished for feeling happy; there's no one who can help; all people care about is money . . . people have no value; I can't function . . . I'll never be as capable as I should be; something bad is going to happen . . . I just know it; life isn't worth living; I can't manage on my own; I'm too old to get a job."

Assumptions: "If I stay with my family, I can feel secure; one should never be happy—the letdown afterward is worse."

Schemata: "I'm defective and unlovable; people are uncaring and rejecting; the world is a dangerous place."

Problem solving: negative problem orientation; she is capable of solving problems rationally, but does not anticipate that her efforts will be effective.

Treatment

The first goal of crisis intervention is to ensure the patient's immediate safety. With that in mind, a comprehensive review of G.L.'s concerns and a systematic assessment of suicide risk factors were completed. Given G.L.'s poor response to psychodynamic therapy in the past, as well as her tendency to magnify and personalize problems, it was felt that insight-oriented approaches or anxiety-provoking interventions could further disorganize her and might exacerbate the suicidal risk. With this in mind, the initial focus of therapy was on addressing the sources of her feelings of hopelessness and on providing her with cognitive and behavioral skills for managing her feelings of depression.

At the outset of the first treatment session, G.L. noted that it was "normal to feel afraid and scared" and that she did not believe that therapy would be effective. As she stated, "This treatment won't work . . . it never works." Given her limited improvement over the years, there may have been some support for this belief. These thoughts—that it was normal to feel afraid and that treatment would not work—were particularly important in that if they were true, they would undermine G.L.'s motivation for participating in cognitive therapy. Our first interventions, then, were straightforward—demonstrating the relationship between her thoughts and current mood and examining evidence for and against these beliefs. G.L. readily recognized that she felt "despondent . . . and paralyzed" when she thought about therapy in these terms and acknowledged that many people did not feel anxious or depressed—it was not "normal" for others. She noted, however, that if her mood improved, others would "expect more of her." As she stated, "I'm hiding behind my depression." Her comment raised the possibility that there were secondary gains from her problems—an issue that would be addressed later in treatment. G.L. reported that she was worried about an upcoming exam, and that she had not been studying due to a fear of failing the test. She agreed that a behavioral homework assignment might be helpful and made plans to study for the test for 1 hour that night. Although this assignment was, admittedly, small and would have little effect on her grade, it served her well in that it demonstrated that she could return to work on her degree. Not surprisingly, she passed the test.

G.L. continued to believe that it was impossible to consciously influence one's mood. She felt that moods "were hormonal" and regularly commented on how her feelings of depression had worsened "for no real reason." She experienced difficulty identifying automatic thoughts and was unable to recall times when she had not felt depressed. The latter difficulty may have been related to the effects of her dysphoria on her ability to recall mood-incongruent events (Bower, 1981) or to an actual paucity of enjoyable experiences during recent years. With this in mind, G.L. was asked to recall her early childhood. She began smiling, and described images of playing with her relatives. "It was wonderful," she stated, "I was happy, I felt human . . . that was the way it should be." G.L.'s mood had improved, if only for a few moments, in response to a conscious intervention. Our clinical goal had been met; G.L. learned that she did have the capacity to influence her feelings of depression.

A goal in crisis intervention is to actively help the patient to respond to the specific negativistic perceptions or beliefs that contributed to the crisis. This process is quite selective. The objective is to identify and resolve only those beliefs that are exacerbating or maintaining the crisis. This involves several steps: (1) identifying and labeling the negative emotion; (2) identifying thoughts or events that triggered this feeling; (3) identifying automatic thoughts that are maintaining this emotional state (e.g., "What is going through your mind that leads you to feel this way?"); (4) having the patient recognize the central importance of this perception or belief; (5) collecting evidence that is inconsistent with this belief; (6) identifying the most persuasive evidence against the belief or perception; (7) developing an alternative, more adaptive, conceptualization of the triggering event; (8) assisting patients to see how their mood would shift if they were to accept this alternative viewpoint; and (9) developing a behavioral plan for using this information to cope with the situation. It is often helpful to provide patients with more adaptive and objective "coping statements" and to help them to decatastrophize the situation by pointing out that it is, in fact, possible to endure the problem. G.L. noted, for example, that she "couldn't tolerate" her feelings of depression any longer. When asked how long she had felt this way she remarked "all my life." When it was pointed out that it seemed she had been able to tolerate these feelings for quite some time, she smiled and responded, "Sure, I just don't like it . . . I wish it would end, but I don't know what to do . . . just tell me what to do."

The emphasis in crisis intervention is on resolving current problems rather than addressing past losses or failures. In working with G.L., our focus was on two particularly malignant beliefs—that "nobody really cares" and "I'm not able to function." She came to see that there were a number of people in her life (including her husband, children, friends, and therapist) who were concerned about her well-being, and that she had, in fact, done quite well in her studies and as a teacher. G.L. was asked to read a number of books and articles on cognitive therapy during the next several weeks and to think about how they might apply to her concerns. She read *Coping with Depression* (Beck & Greenberg, 1978), a pamphlet describing cognitive and behavioral tools for managing depression, but found it "simplistic." She next read *Reinventing Your Life* (Young & Klosko, 1993), a book on the development and treatment of maladaptive beliefs, and "Possible Selves" (Markus & Nurius, 1986), a review article on the role of expectations and goals in human behavior. G.L. found these readings interesting and useful. Moreover, they demonstrated that she was, in fact, able to assimilate and remember fairly complex material—something she had felt unable to do in class. Although there are risks in providing patients with readings that have been prepared for a professional audience, it is important to select articles that meet the patient's specific needs. Flexibility in developing homework assignments and selecting readings for bibliotherapy is essential. In this case, the readings not only served a didactic function (teaching G.L. about cognitive therapy and its procedures) but also provided G.L. with an experience that was inconsistent with a central belief—that she was unable to function academically.

Subsequent sessions focused on identifying and changing negativistic assumptions and schemata. The downward-arrow procedure (Beck, Rush, et. al., 1979) was introduced to identify depressogenic assumptions. We began, for example, with the thought "I can't do my dissertation." When asked, "What comes to mind when you think of that?", she remarked, "I won't move forward." The remainder of the downward arrow is presented below.

"I can't do my dissertation. I won't move forward."
"I'll never finish my degree."

"Everything I start is unfinished."

"My mother told me I couldn't finish things. I can't help others."

"I'm a terrible person."

"I'll never support myself. I'll wind up in the streets."

"I have to depend on others. What if they die? I'll be a burden."

G.L. recognized a number of themes in her statements, including the beliefs that "I'm incapable" and "people will abandon me." As noted, these were long-standing beliefs and seem to have stemmed from early experiences with her mother. At this point, G.L. became angry at the therapist and remarked, "Are you married? . . . I don't know how anyone could stand to be with you." When asked what had gone through her mind at that point, she remarked tersely, "I'm the biggest failure." She reportedly experienced an image of her mother sitting near her admonishing her that she was "making a fool of herself" and that she should "shut up and go to the corner." She stated that she heard the voice of her mother telling her that her participation in therapy was "proof that she'd failed" and that she had "failed because she wasn't strong." G.L. became quite agitated at the outset of the following therapy session. She reported feeling that the therapist would "test her" and that she would be "thrown out" if she did not "do therapy right." Upon questioning, she noted that there was nothing the therapist had done or said to suggest that she might "fail therapy," and that these thoughts and feelings were internally generated. The therapeutic relationship, then, served as evidence that was inconsistent with her belief that she would ultimately be abandoned. This theme reemerged several weeks later when she asked for assistance in processing an insurance claim. She reported that she had received a denial of coverage, which served as proof that "people have no value" and "I'm just another policy to you . . . I don't matter." Once again, a patient reappraisal of the event led her to conclude that the therapist was concerned for her well-being and that "maybe not everyone will abandon you." Interventions directed toward activating tacit beliefs can be quite powerful and should be undertaken only after the initial crisis has passed and a strong therapeutic rapport has developed.

G.L.'s feelings of anger toward her husband and children were examined during subsequent sessions. The beliefs that she had "damaged the children beyond repair" and that she "had become just like her mother" were discussed at length, as were her feelings of anxiety when apart from her family. She acknowledged that it was necessary for her teenage children to become more independent, but she resented their increasing autonomy. As she stated, "I do a lot for them . . . kids ask more and more, then they leave you . . . they abandon you." Upon examination, she noted that her children were not "abandoning her," and that her belief that "I have nothing except my children" was both untrue and maladaptive. Behavioral interventions, including relaxation training and scheduling of pleasurable activities, were introduced. G.L. was also asked to resume work on her dissertation—an activity that she felt would provide her with a sense of accomplishment. She began by reading a short research article but experienced a great deal of difficulty understanding it. The experience was taken as further evidence of her "defectiveness." A behavioral experiment was developed to assess the validity of this belief. G.L. asked a colleague to review the article and to share his thoughts with her. He reportedly felt the article was "an awful piece . . . poorly written," leading G.L. to recognize that her difficulties nay have stemmed, at least in part, from the quality of the article.

After 10 weeks of therapy, G.L. reported, with some surprise, that her mood was "reasonably good" and that she was "feeling better" about her classes and teaching. Her scores on each of the objective rating scales had improved dramatically and she reportedly felt less isolated, defective, and dependent on others. As she stated, "Life isn't always horrible." Although the suicidal crisis had passed and important therapeutic gains had been made, much work remained to be accomplished. G.L. continued to feel emotionally depleted and pessimistic about her future. Moreover, her anxiety about separation from her family was not fully resolved. She still feared abandonment and experienced difficulty separating from her children. These became the focus of her ongoing therapy.

CONCLUSION

This chapter reviewed the assessment and management of suicidality among depressed adults. In concluding, several general statements can be made. First, the general outline of an integrated model of suicidality is beginning to emerge. Studies indicate that a number of cognitive, social, environmental and psychiatric factors are associated with an increased risk of suicidal thoughts and gestures. These variables can serve as targets of intervention in a comprehensive treatment program. The specific manner in which these variables interact over time in contributing to vulnerability to suicide, however, is not yet known.

Second, the prediction of suicidal behavior remains a daunting clinical task. Although progress has been made in understanding the social, psychiatric, cognitive, and emotional concomitants of suicidal ideations, the astute reader will note that prediction of suicidal behavior for individual patients remains an imprecise endeavor. Additional research into the clinical prediction of suicidal ideations and behavior is warranted.

The primary goal in addressing a suicidal crisis is, of course, to ensure the patient's safety. This is accomplished by alleviating environmental pressures or stresses, recruiting the support of others, and helping the patient to cope with immediate problems. Attention is directed only toward those perceptions, beliefs, attributions, or expectations that are contributing to the crisis. Other maladaptive cognitions are not addressed at that time. After the crisis has been resolved, the therapeutic focus can shift to identifying and changing ancillary maladaptive beliefs as well as dysfunctional schemata or assumptions that contributed to the suicidal crisis. The goals of therapy are to identify the cognitive, behavioral, and social factors that placed the patient at risk and to provide the patient with alternative ways of coping with problems that arise. While cognitive and behavioral techniques are useful, the importance of a trusting, reliable, and supportive therapeutic relationship should not be minimized. Clinicians should be aware of their beliefs or expectations and sensitive to the ways that these can influence the course of therapy. Negative biases—including thoughts that a patient "looks untreatable" or is "just being manipulative"—can affect both the tone of the therapeutic relationship and the nature of the interventions that are made. As when examining the validity or utility of a patient's beliefs, it is often helpful to examine the evidence for and against the therapist's perceptions, whether there is a more reasonable interpretation, and how one's behavior is affected by it (Rudd & Joiner, 1997).

Although the results of recent controlled outcome studies are promising, it is not clear, at this point, that psychotherapy can reliably reduce the frequency and severity of suicidal ideations, reduce the risk of suicide attempts among ideators, or prevent further attempts by individuals with a history of suicidal behavior. Nonetheless, cognitive models of depression and suicide have empirical support, and interventions derived from them can be clinically useful. In the absence of evidence for the effectiveness of specific interventions, clinicians would do well to adopt a broad view and use a range of cognitive and behavioral techniques when working with acutely suicidal patients.

It has been 12 years since the first edition of this book was published, and the question naturally comes to mind, "What have we learned during the interim?" Unfortunately, the prevention and treatment of suicide remain significant clinical and social concerns. Although suicide has increasingly come to be viewed as an important public health problem, there have been no substantive or paradigmatic changes in our understanding of vulnerability or treatment. Suicide remains a leading cause of death in many countries, including the United States, and our clinical practices are not appreciably different than those in 1995. That said, research completed over the past 10 years indicates that (1) dialectical behavior therapy and cognitive-behavioral therapy *may* be effective in reducing suicidal behavior, at least for some individuals; (2) psychic anxiety and agitation may serve as short-term predictors of risk; and (3) medications, including lithium and fluoxetine, can be useful in reducing suicidal ideations and behavior. Beyond this, however, progress has been limited. Much work remains to be done.

Working with acutely suicidal patients can be both challenging and stressful. With this in mind, regular consultation with colleagues can be quite helpful. Consultation is viewed by some, in fact, as an essential component of effective care and risk management (Bongar, 1993; Linehan, 1993). It can provide clinicians with a sense of support as well as practical recommendations. Therapists can have confidence in that cognitive models have proven useful for conceptualizing depression and suicidality. The interventions derived from the model are clinically powerful. Cognitive and behavioral interventions can be of value in alleviating suicidal patients' feelings of depression, pessimism, anxiety, and anger. They are useful in reducing impulsivity, enhancing social relationships, and improving their ability to cope with reality-based problems. For the acutely suicidal patient, then, there is hope.

REFERENCES

Abela, J. R. Z., & Brozina, K. (2004). The use of negative events to prime cognitive vulnerability to depression. *Cognitive Therapy and Research, 28,* 209–227.

Abramson, L., Metalsky, G., & Alloy, L. (1989). Hopelessness depression: A theory-based subtype of depression. *Psychological Review, 96*(2), 358–372.

Adam, K., Bouckoms, A., & Streiner, D. (1982). Parental loss and family stability in attempted suicide. *Archives of General Psychiatry, 39,* 1081–1085.

Alloy, L., Abramson, L., Metalsky, G., & Hartlage, S. (1988). The hopelessness theory of depression: Attributional aspects. *British Journal of Clinical Psychology, 27,* 5–21.

American Psychiatric Association. (1994). *Diagnostic and statistical manual of mental disorders* (4th ed.). Washington, DC: Author.

Arensman, E., & Kerkhof, A. (1996). Classification of attempted suicide: A review of empirical studies, 1963–1993. *Suicide and Life-Threatening Behavior, 26*(1), 46–67.

Barnett, P., & Gotlib, I. (1988). Psychosocial functioning in depression: Distinguishing among antecedents, concomitants, and consequences. *Psychological Bulletin, 104,* 97–126.

Beck, A. (1967). *Depression: Clinical, experimental, and theoretical aspects.* New York: Harper & Row.

Beck, A. (1973). *The diagnosis and management of depression.* Philadelphia: University of Pennsylvania Press.

Beck, A. (1976). *Cognitive therapy and the emotional disorders.* New York: International Universities Press.

Beck, A. (1986). Hopelessness as a predictor of eventual suicide. *Annals of the New York Academy of Science, 487,* 90–96.

Beck, A., Brown, G., Berchick, R., Stewart, B., & Steer, R. (1990). Relationship between hopelessness and ultimate suicide: A replication with psychiatric outpatients. *American Journal of Psychiatry, 147,* 190–195.

Beck, A., Brown, G., & Steer, R. (1989). Prediction of eventual suicide in psychiatric inpatients by clinical ratings of hopelessness. *Journal of Consulting and Clinical Psychology, 57,* 309–310.

Beck, A., Brown, G., Steer, R., Dahlsgaard, K., & Grisham, J. (1999). Suicide ideation at its worst point: A predictor of eventual suicide in psychiatric outpatients. *Suicide and Life-Threatening Behavior, 29*(1), 1–9.

Beck, A., & Greenberg, R. (1978). *Coping with depression.* Unpublished manuscript, University of Pennsylvania, Philadelphia.

Beck, A., Kovacs, M., & Weissman, A. (1975). Hopelessness and suicidal behavior: An overview. *Journal of the American Medical Association, 234,* 1146–1149.

Beck, A., Kovacs, M., & Weissman, A. (1979). Assessment of suicidal intention: The scale for suicidal ideation. *Journal of Consulting and Clinical Psychology, 47,* 343–352.

Beck, A., Rush, A., Shaw, B., & Emery, G. (1979). *Cognitive therapy of depression.* New York: Guilford Press.

Beck, A., Schuyler, D., & Herman, 1. (1974). Development of suicidal intent scales. In A. Beck, H. Resnick, & D. Lettieri (Eds.), *The prediction of suicide* (pp. 45–56). Philadelphia: Charles Press.

Beck, A., Steer, R., Beck, J., & Newman, C. (1993). Hopelessness, depression, and suicidal ideation, and clinical diagnosis of depression. *Suicide and Life-Threatening Behavior, 23,* 139–145.

Beck, A., Steer, R., & Brown, G. (1993). Dysfunctional attitudes and suicidal ideation in psychiatric outpatients. *Suicide and Life-Threatening Behavior, 23,* 11–20.

Beck, A., Steer, R., & Brown, G. (1996). *Manual for Beck Depression Inventory–II.* San Antonio, TX: Psychological Corporation.

Beck, A., Steer, R., Kovacs, M., & Garrison, B. (1985). Hopelessness and eventual suicide: A 10-

year prospective study of patients hospitalized with suicidal ideation. *American Journal of Psychiatry, 142*, 559–563.

Beck, A., Steer, R., Sanderson, W., & Skeie, T. (1991). Panic disorder and suicidal ideation and behavior: Discrepant findings in psychiatric out-patients. *American Journal of Psychiatry, 148*(9), 1195–1199.

Beck, A., Ward, C., Mendelson, M., Mock, J., & Erbaugh, J. (1961). An inventory for measuring depression. *Archives of General Psychiatry, 4*, 561–571.

Beck, A., Weissman, A., & Kovacs, M. (1976). Alcoholism, hopelessness, and suicidal behavior. *Journal of Studies on Alcohol, 37*, 66–77.

Beck, A., Weissman, A., Lester, D., & Trexler, L. (1974). The measurement of pessimism: The Hopelessness Scale. *Journal of Consulting and Clinical Psychology, 42*, 861–865.

Beck, A., Wright, F., & Newman, C. (1992). Cocaine abuse. In A. Freeman & F. Dattilio (Eds.), *Comprehensive casebook of cognitive therapy* (pp. 185–192). New York: Plenum Press.

Bertole, J., Fleischmann, A., De Leo, D., & Wasserman, D. (2003). Suicide and mental disorders: Do we know enough? *British Journal of Psychiatry, 183*, 382–383.

Bertolote, J. M., Fleischmann, A., De Leo, D., & Wasserman, D. (2004). Psychiatric diagnoses and suicide: Revisiting the evidence. *Crisis: The Journal of Crisis Intervention and Suicide Prevention, 25*, 147–155.

Bohus, M., Haaf, B., Stiglmayr, C., Pohl, U., Bohme, R., & Linehan, M. (2000). Evaluation of inpatient dialectical-behavioral therapy for borderline personality disorder—A prospective study. *Behaviour Research and Therapy, 38*, 875–887.

Bongar, B. (1991). *The suicidal patient: Clinical and legal standards of care.* Washington, DC: American Psychological Association.

Bongar, B. (1993). Consultation and the suicidal patient. *Suicide and Life-Threatening Behavior, 23*(4), 299–306.

Bonner, R., & Rich, A. (1988). Negative life stress, social problem-solving, self-appraisal, and hopelessness: Implications for suicide research. *Cognitive Therapy and Research, 12*(6), 549–556.

Borges, G., Walters, E., & Kessler, R. (2000). Associations of substance use, abuse, and dependence with subsequent suicidal behaviour. *American Journal of Epidemiology, 151*, 781–789.

Bostwick, J. M., & Pankratz, V. S. (2000). Affective disorders and suicide risk: A reexamination. *American Journal of Psychiatry, 157*, 1925–1932.

Bower, G. (1981). Mood and memory. *American Psychologist, 36*, 129–148.

Brent, D. A. (2001). Assessment and treatment of the youthful suicidal patient. In H. Hendin & J. J. Mann (Eds.), *The clinical science of suicide prevention* (pp. 106–131). New York: New York Academy of Sciences.

Brinkman-Sull, D., Overholser, J., & Silverman, E. (2000). Risk of future suicide attempts in adolescent psychiatric inpatients at 18-month follow-up. *Suicide and Life-Threatening Behavior, 30*, 327–340.

Brodaty, H., Luscombe, G., Peisah, C., Anstey, K., & Andrews, G. (2001). A 25-year longitudinal, comparison study of the outcome of depression. *Psychological Medicine, 31*, 1347–1359.

Brown, G. K., Have, T. T., Henriques, G. R., Xie, S. X., Hollander, J. E., & Beck, A. T. (2005). Cognitive therapy for the prevention of suicide attempts: A randomized controlled trial. *Journal of the American Medical Association, 294*, 563–570.

Buerk, F., Kurz, A., & Moeller, H. (1985). Suicide risk scales: Do they help to predict suicidal behaviour? *European Archives of Psychiatry and Neurological Sciences, 235*(3), 153–157.

Buglass, D., & Horton, J. (1974). A scale for predicting subsequent suicidal behaviour. *British Journal of Psychiatry, 124*, 573–578.

Busch, K. A., Fawcett, J., & Jacobs, D. G. (2003). Clinical correlates of inpatient suicide. *Journal of Clinical Psychiatry, 64*(1), 14–19.

Caldwell, C., & Gottesman, I. (1990). Schizophrenics kill themselves too: A review of risk factors for suicide. *Schizophrenia Bulletin, 16*(4), 571–589.

Cassells, C., Paterson, B., Dowding, D., & Morrison, R. (2005). Long- and short-term risk factors in the prediction of inpatient suicide: Review of the literature. *Crisis, 26,* 53–63.

Chang, E. C. (1998). Cultural differences, perfectionism, and suicidal risk in a college population: Does social problem solving still matter? *Cognitive Therapy and Research, 22,* 237–254.

Cheng, A. T. (1995). Mental illness and suicide: A case-control study in East Taiwan. *Archives of General Psychiatry, 52,* 594–603.

Chioqueta, A., & Stiles, T. (2003). Suicide risk in outpatients with specific mood and anxiety disorders. *Crisis: The Journal of Crisis Intervention and Suicide Prevention, 24,* 105–112.

Chioqueta, A., & Stiles, T. (2005). Personality traits and the development of depression, hopelessness, and suicide ideation. *Personality and Individual Differences, 38,* 1283–1291.

Clum, G., & Febbraro, G. (1994). Stress, social support, and problem-solving appraisal/skills: Prediction of suicide severity within a college sample. *Journal of Psychopathology and Behavioral Assessment, 16*(1), 69–83.

Clum, G., & Weaver, T. (1997). Diagnostic morbidity and its relationship to severity of ideation for a nonpsychiatric sample of chronic and severe suicide ideators. *Journal of Psychopathology and Behavioral Assessment, 19*(3), 191–206.

Clum, G., & Yang, B. (1995). Additional support for the reliability and validity of the Modified Scale for Suicide Ideation. *Psychological Assessment, 7*(1), 122–125.

Cole, D. (1988). Hopelessness, social desirability, depression, and parasuicide in two college student samples. *Journal of Consulting and Clinical Psychology, 56,* 131–136.

Commission on Adolescent Suicide Prevention. (2005). Youth suicide. In D. L. Evans, E. B. Foa, R. E. Gur, H. Hendin, C. P. O'Brien, M. E. P. Seligman, et al. (Eds.), *Treating and preventing adolescent mental health disorders* (pp. 433–493). New York: Oxford University Press.

Conaghan, S., & Davidson, K. M. (2002). Hopelessness and the anticipation of positive and negative future experiences in older parasuicidal adults. *British Journal of Clinical Psychology, 41,* 233–242.

Corcoran, P., Kelleher, M., Keeley, H., Byrne, S., Burke, U., & Williamson, E. (1997). A statistical model for identifying repeaters of parasuicide. *Archives of Suicide Research, 3,* 65–74.

Coryell, W., & Young, E. (2005). Clinical predictors of suicide in primary major depressive disorder. *Journal of Clinical Psychiatry, 66,* 412–417.

Cull, J., & Gill, W. (1982). *Suicide Probability Scale.* Los Angeles: Western Psychological Services.

Dahlsgaard, K., Beck, A., & Brown, G. (1998). Inadequate response to therapy as a predictor of suicide. *Suicide and Life-Threatening Behavior, 28*(2), 197–204.

Davis, M., & Schrodt, G. (1992). Inpatient treatment. In A. Freeman & F. Dattilio (Eds.), *Comprehensive casebook of cognitive therapy* (pp. 293–301). New York: Plenum Press.

Dean, R., Miskimins, W., DeCook, R., Wilson, L., & Maley, R. (1967). Prediction of suicide in a psychiatric hospital. *Journal of Clinical Psychology, 23,* 296–301.

Dieserud, G., Roysamb, E., Braverman, M., Dalgard, O., & Ekeberg, O. (2003). Predicating repetition of suicide attempt: A prospective study of 50 suicide attempters. *Archives of Suicide Research, 7,* 1–15.

Drake, R., & Cotton, P. (1986). Depression, hopelessness, and suicide in chronic schizophrenia. *British Journal of Psychiatry, 148,* 554–559.

Drew, B. L. (2001). Self-harm behavior and no-suicide contracting in psychiatric inpatient settings. *Archives of Psychiatric Nursing, 15,* 99–106.

Dyer, J., & Kreitman, N. (1984). Hopelessness, depression, and suicidal intent in parasuicide. *British Journal of Psychiatry, 144,* 127–133.

D'Zurilla, T. J., Chang, E. C., Nottingham, E. J. I. V., & Faccini, L. (1998). Social problem-solving deficits and hopelessness, depression, and suicidal risk in college students and psychiatric inpatients. *Journal of Clinical Psychology, 54*, 1091–1107.

Ellis, T. (1986). Toward a cognitive therapy for suicidal individuals. *Professional Psychology—Research and Practice, 17*(2), 125–130.

Ellis, T., & Ratliff, K. (1986). Cognitive characteristics of suicidal and nonsuicidal psychiatric patients. *Cognitive Therapy and Research, 1*, 625–634.

Epstein, N., Schlesinger, S., & Dryden, W. (1988). *Cognitive-behavioral therapy with families.* New York: Bruner/Mazel.

Evans, K., Tyrer, P., Catalan, J., Schmidt, U., Davidson, K., Dent, J., et al. (1999). Manual-assisted cognitive-behaviour therapy (MACT): A randomized controlled trial of a brief intervention with bibliotherapy in the treatment of recurrent deliberate self-harm. *Psychological Medicine, 29*(1), 19–25.

Fawcett, J., Busch, K., Jacobs, D., Kravitz, H., & Fogg, L. (1997). Suicide: A four-pathway clinical–biochemical model. *Annals of the New York Academy of Sciences, 836*, 288–301.

Fawcett, J., Scheftner, W., Clark, D., Hedeker, D., Gibbons, R., & Coryell, W. (1987). Clinical predictors of suicide in patients with major affective disorders: A controlled prospective study. *American Journal of Psychiatry, 144*, 35–40.

Fawcett, J., Scheftner, W., Fogg, L., Clark, D., Young, M., Hedeker, D., et al. (1990). Time-related predictors of suicide in major affective disorder. *American Journal of Psychiatry, 147*(9), 1189–1194.

Freeman, A., Pretzer, J., Fleming, B., & Simon, K. (1990). *Clinical applications of cognitive therapy.* New York: Plenum Press.

Freeman, A., & Reinecke, M. (1993). *Cognitive therapy of suicidal behavior.* New York: Springer.

Freeman, A., & Reinecke, M. (1995). Cognitive therapy. In A. Gurman & S. Messer (Eds.), *Essential psychotherapies: Theory and practice* (pp. 182–225). New York: Guilford Press.

Fremouw, W., de Perczel, M., & Ellis, T. (1990). *Suicide risk: Assessment and response guidelines.* New York: Pergamon Press.

Friedman, S., Jones, J., Chernen, L., & Barlow, D. (1992). Suicidal ideation and suicide attempts among patients with panic disorder: A survey of two outpatient clinics. *American Journal of Psychiatry, 149*(5), 680–685.

Fuchs, C., & Rehm, L. (1977). A self-control behavior program for depression. *Journal of Consulting and Clinical Psychology, 45*, 206–215.

Gardner, D. L., & Cowdry, R. W. (1985). Suicidal and parasuicidal behavior in borderline personality disorder. *Psychiatric Clinics of North America, 8*, 389–403.

Garzotto, N., Siani, R., Zimmerman-Tansella, C., & Tansella, M. (1976). Cross-validation of a predictive scale for subsequent suicidal behaviour in an Italian sample. *British Journal of Psychiatry, 128*, 137–140.

Gibb, B., Alloy, L., Abramson, L., Rose, D., Whitehouse, W., & Hogan, M. (2001). Childhood maltreatment and college students' current suicidal ideation: A test of the hopelessness theory. *Suicide and Life-Threatening Behavior, 31*, 405–415.

Goldney, R. (1981). Parental loss and reported childhood stress in young women who attempt suicide. *Acta Psychiatrica Scandinavica, 64*, 34–59.

Gorwood, P. (2001). Biological markers for suicidal behavior in alcohol dependence. *Journal of European Psychiatry, 16*, 410–417.

Gould, M. S., Greenberg, T., Velting, D. M., & Shaffer, D. (2003). Youth suicide risk and preventive interventions: A review of the past 10 years. *Journal of the American Academy of Child and Adolescent Psychiatry, 42*, 386–405.

Guidano, V., & Liotti, G. (1983). *Cognitive processes and emotional disorders: A structural approach to psychotherapy.* New York: Guilford Press.

Hagnell, O., & Rorsman, B. (1980). Suicide in the Lundby study: A controlled prospective investigation of stressful life events. *Neuropsychobiology, 6*, 319–332.

Hankin, B. L., Fraley, R. C., & Abela, J. R. Z. (2005). Daily depression and cognitions about stress: Evidence for a traitlike depressogenic cognitive style and the prediction of depressive symptoms in a prospective Daily diary study. *Journal of Personality and Social Psychology, 88*, 673–685.

Harris, E. C., & Barraclough, B. (1997). Suicide as an outcome for mental disorders: A meta-analysis. *British Journal of Psychiatry, 170*, 205–228.

Heisel, M., Flett, G., & Hewitt, P. (2003). Social hopelessness and college student suicide ideation. *Archives of Suicide Research, 7*, 221–235.

Henriksson, M. M., Aro, H. M., Marttunen, M. J., Heikkinen, M. E., & Isometsa, E. T. (1993). Mental disorders and comorbidity in suicide. *American Journal of Psychiatry, 150*, 935–940.

Henriques, J. B., & Davidson, R. J. (2000). Decreased responsiveness to reward in depression. *Cognition and Emotion, 14*, 711–724.

Herzog, D. B., Greenwood, D. N., Dorer, D. J., Flores, A. T., Ekeblad, E. R., Richards, A., et al. (2000). Mortality in eating disorders: A descriptive study. *International Journal of Eating Disorders, 28*, 20–26.

Hunt, M., & Forand, N. R. (2005). Cognitive vulnerability to depression in never depressed subjects. *Cognition and Emotion, 19*, 763–770.

Ingram, R., Miranda, J., & Segal, Z. (1998). *Cognitive vulnerability to depression.* New York: Guilford Press.

Inskip, H. M., Harris, E. C., & Barraclough, B. (1998). Lifetime risk of suicide for affective disorder, alcoholism and schizophrenia. *British Journal of Psychiatry, 172*, 35–37.

Ivanoff, A., & Jang, S. (1991). The role of hopelessness and social desirability in predicting suicidal behavior: A study of prison inmates. *Journal of Consulting and Clinical Psychology, 59*(3), 394–399.

Joiner, T., & Rudd, M. (1995). Negative attributional style for interpersonal events and the occurrence of severe interpersonal disruptions as predictors of self-reported suicidal ideation. *Suicide and Life-Threatening Behavior, 25*(2), 297–304.

Joiner, T., & Rudd, M.(1996). Disentangling the interrelations between hopelessness, loneliness, and suicidal ideation. *Suicide and Life-Threatening Behavior, 26*(1), 19–26.

Joiner, T. E., Jr., Voelz, Z. R., & Rudd, M. D. (2001). For suicidal young adults with comorbid depressive and anxiety disorders, problem-solving treatment may be better than treatment as usual. *Professional Psychology: Research and Practice, 32*, 278–282.

Jollant, F., Bellivier, F., Leboyer, M., Astruc, B., Torres, S., Verdier, R., et al. (2005). Impaired decision making in suicide attempters. *American Journal of Psychiatry, 162*(2), 304–310.

Kennedy, J., & Reinecke, M. (1998). *Hopelessness and suicide among adults: A review and meta-analysis.* Paper presented at the 10th annual convention of the American Psychological Society, Washington, DC.

Khan, A., Leventhal, R., Khan, S., & Brown, W. (2002). Suicide risk in patients with anxiety disorders: A metaanalysis of the FDA database. *Journal of Affective Disorders, 68*, 183–190.

Kjellander, C., Bongar, B., & King, A. (1998). Suicidality in borderline personality disorder. *Crisis, 19*(3), 125–135.

Konick, L., & Gutierrez, P. (2005). Testing a model of suicide ideation in college students. *Suicide and Life-Threatening Behavior, 35*, 181–192.

Kovacs, M., Beck, A., & Weissman, A. (1975). Hopelessness: An indicator of suicidal risk. *Suicide, 5*, 98–103.

Lavender, A., & Watkins, E. (2004). Rumination and future thinking in depression. *British Journal of Clinical Psychology, 43*, 129–142.

Lee, J. B., & Bartlett, M. L. (2005). Suicide prevention: Critical elements for managing suicidal clients and counselor liability without the use of a no-suicide contract. *Death Studies, 29*, 847–865.

Lerner, M., & Clum, G. (1990). Treatment of suicide ideators: A problem-solving approach. *Behavior Therapy, 21*(4), 403–411.

Lester, D. (1974). Demographic versus clinical prediction of suicidal behaviors: A look at some issues. In A. Beck, H. Resnik, & D. Lettieri (Eds.), *The prediction of suicide* (pp. 71–84). Philadelphia: Charles Press.

Lester, D. (1987). Suicidal preoccupation and dysthymia in college students, *Psychological Reports, 61,* 762.

Lettieri, D. (1974). Research issues in developing prediction scales. In C. Neuringer (Ed.), *Psychological assessment of suicidal risk.* Springfield, IL: Thomas.

Lewinsohn, P. (1975). The behavioral study and treatment of depression. In M. Hersen, R. Eisler, & P. Miller (Eds.), *Progress in behavior modification* (Vol. 1, pp. 19–64). New York: Academic Press.

Linehan, M. M. (1985). The reasons for living inventory. In P. Keller & L. Ritt (Eds.), *Innovations in clinical practice: A sourcebook* (pp. 321–330). Sarasota, FL: Professional Resource Exchange.

Linehan, M. M. (1987). Dialectical behavior therapy: A cognitive-behavioral approach to parasuicide. *Journal of Personality Disorders, 1,* 328–333.

Linehan, M. M. (1993). *Cognitive-behavioral treatment of borderline personality disorder.* New York: Guilford Press.

Linehan, M. M. (1999). Standard protocol for assessing and treating suicidal behaviors for patients in treatment. In D. Jacobs (Ed.), *The Harvard Medical School guide to suicide assessment and intervention* (pp. 146–187). San Francisco: Jossey-Bass.

Linehan, M. M., Armstrong, H. E., Suarez, A., Allmon, D., & Heard, H. L. (1991). Cognitive-behavioral treatment of chronically parasuicidal borderline patients. *Archives of General Psychiatry, 48,* 1060–1064.

Linehan, M. M., Camper, P., Chiles, J., Strosahl, K., & Shearin, E. (1987). Interpersonal problem-solving and parasuicide. *Cognitive Therapy and Research, 11*(1), 1–12.

Linehan, M. M., Goodstein, J., Nielsen, S., & Chiles, J. (1983). Reasons for staying alive when you are thinking of killing yourself: The reasons for living inventory. *Journal of Consulting and Clinical Psychology, 51,* 276–286.

Linehan, M. M., Heard, H., & Armstrong, H. (1993). Naturalistic follow-up of a behavioral treatment for chronically parasuicidal borderline patients. *Archives of General Psychiatry, 50*(12), 971–974.

Lönnqvist, J. K. (2000). Psychiatric aspects of suicidal behaviour: Depression. In K. Hawton & K. Van Heeringen (Eds.), *The international handbook of suicide and attempted suicide* (pp. 107–120). Chichester, UK: Wiley.

Low, G., Jones, D., Duggan, C., Power, M., & MacLeod, A. (2001). The treatment of deliberate self-harm in borderline personality disorder using dialectical behaviour therapy: A pilot study in a high security hospital. *Behavioural and Cognitive Psychotherapy, 29,* 85–92.

MacKinnon, D., Potash, J., McMahon, F., Simpson, S., Depaulo, J., & Zandi, P. (2005). Rapid mood switching and suicidality in familial bipolar disorder. *Bipolar Disorders, 7,* 441–448.

MacLeod, A., Pankhania, B., Lee, M., & Mitchell, D. (1997). Parasuicide, depression and the anticipation of positive and negative future experiences. *Psychological Medicine, 27,* 973–977.

MacLeod, A. K., & Salaminiou, E. (2001). Reduced positive future-thinking in depression: Cognitive and affective factors. *Cognition and Emotion, 15,* 99–107.

Mahrer, J., & Bongar, B. (1993). Assessment and management of suicide risk and the use of the no-suicide contract. In L. VandeCreek, S. Knapp, & T. L. Jackson (Eds.), *Innovations in clinical practice: A source book* (Vol. 12, pp. 277–293). Sarasota, FL: Professional Resource Press/Professional Resource Exchange.

Markus, H., & Nurius, P. (1986). Possible selves. *American Psychologist, 41,* 954–969.

McLeavey, B., Daly, R., Ludgate, J., & Murray, C. (1994). Interpersonal problem-solving skills training in the treatment of self-poisoning patients. *Suicide and Life-Threatening Behavior, 24*(4), 382–394.

McMullin, R. (1986). *Handbook of cognitive therapy techniques*. New York: Norton.

Mehryar, A., Hekmat, H., & Khajavi, A. (1977). Some personality correlated of contemplated suicide, *Psychological Reports, 40*, 1291–1294.

Meltzer, H. (2003). Reducing the risk for suicide in schizophrenia and affective disorders. *Journal of Clinical Psychiatry, 64*, 1122–1129.

Miller, I., Norman, W., Bishop, S., & Dow, M. (1986). The Modified Scale for Suicidal Ideation: Reliability and validity. *Journal of Consulting and Clinical Psychology, 54*(5), 724–725.

Motto, J. (1989). Problems in suicide risk assessment. In D. Jacobs & H. Brown (Eds.), *Suicide: Understanding and responding: Harvard Medical School perspectives on suicide* (pp. 129–142). Madison, CT: International Universities Press.

Motto, J., Heilbron, D., & Juster, R. (1985). Development of a clinical instrument to estimate suicide risk. *American Journal of Psychiatry, 142*(6), 680–686.

Nathan, R., & Rousch, A. (1984). Which patients commit suicide? American Journal of Psychiatry, *141*, 1017.

Nekanda-Trepka, C., Bishop, S., & Blackburn, I. (1983). Hopelessness and depression. *British Journal of Clinical Psychology, 22*, 49–60.

Neuringer, C. (1968). Divergencies between attitudes towards life and death among suicidal, psychosomatic, and normal hospitalized patients. *Journal of Consulting and Clinical Psychology, 32*, 59–63.

Neuringer, C., & Lettieri, D. (1971). Cognition, attitude, and affect in suicidal individuals. *Suicide and Life-Threatening Behavior, 1*, 106–124.

Noyes, R. (1991). Suicidal ideation and panic disorder: A review. *Journal of Affective Disorders, 22*, 1–11.

Pallis, D., Barraciough, B., Levey, A., Jenkins, J., & Sainsbury, P. (1982). Estimating suicide risk among attempted suicides: 1. The development of new clinical scales. *British Journal of Psychiatry, 141*, 37–44.

Patsiokas, A., & Clum, G. (1985). Effects of psychotherapeutic strategies in the treatment of suicide attempters. *Psychotherapy, 22*(2), 281–290.

Patterson, W., Dohn, H., Bird, J., & Patterson, G. (1983). Evaluation of suicide patients: The SAD Persons Scale. *Psychosomatics, 24*, 343–352.

Petrie, K., & Chamberlain, K. (1983). Hopelessness and social desirability as moderator variables in predicting suicidal behavior. *Journal of Consulting and Clinical Psychology, 51*, 485–487.

Piacentini, J., Rotheram-Borus, M., & Cantwell, C. (1995). Brief cognitive-behavioral family therapy for suicidal adolescents. In L. VandeCreek, S. Knapp, & T. L. Jackson (Eds.), *Innovations in clinical practice: A source book* (Vol. 14, pp. 151–168). Sarasota, FL: Professional Resource Press.

Pierce, D. (1977). Suicidal intent in self-injury. *Britich Journal of Psychiatry, 130*, 377–385.

Placidi, G., Oquendo, M. H., Malone, K. M., Brodsky, B., Ellis, S. P., & Mann, J. (2000). Anxiety in major depression: Relationship to suicide attempts. *American Journal of Psychiatry, 157*, 1614–1618.

Plutchik, R., van Praag, H., Conte, H., & Picard, S. (1989). Correlates of suicide and violent risk: 1. The Suicide Risk Measure. *Comprehensive Psychiatry, 30*, 296–302.

Pokorny, A. (1983). Prediction of suicide in psychiatric patients. *Archives of General Psychiatry, 40*, 249–257.

Pollock, L., & Williams, J. M. G. (2004). Problem-solving in suicide attempters. *Psychological Medicine, 34*, 163–167.

Preuss, U., Schuckit, M. A., Smith, T. L., Danko, G. P., Buckman, K., Bierut, L., et al. (2002). Comparison of 3190 alcohol-dependant individuals with and without suicide attempts. *Alcoholism, Clinical and Experimental Research, 26*, 471–477.

Prezant, D., & Neimeyer, R. (1988). Cognitive predictors of depression and suicide ideation. *Suicide and Life-Threatening Behavior, 18*(3), 259–264.

Prigerson, H., Desai, R., Lui-Mares, W., & Roseheck, R. (2003). Suicidal ideation and suicide attempts in homeless mentally ill persons. *Social Psychiatry and Psychiatric Epidemiology, 38,* 213–219.

Qin, P., Agerbo, E., & Mortensen, P. B. (2005). Factors contributing to suicide: The epidemiological evidence from large-scale registers. In K. Hawton (Ed.), *Prevention and treatment of suicidal behavior: From science to practice* (pp. 11–28). Oxford, UK: Oxford University Press.

Rabkin, J., & Klein, D. (1987). The clinical measurement of depressive disorders. In A. Marsella, R. Hirschfeld, & M. Katz (Eds.), *The measurement of depression* (pp. 30–83). New York: Guilford Press.

Ranieri, W., Steer, R., Lavrence, T., Rissmiller, D., Piper, G., & Beck, A. (1987). Relationship of depression, hopelessness, and dysfunctional attitudes to suicide ideation in psychiatric patients. *Psychological Reports, 61,* 967–975.

Rehm, L. (1977). A self-control model of depression. *Behavior Therapy, 8,* 787–804.

Reid, W. H. (2005). Contracting for safety redux. *Journal of Psychiatric Practice, 11,* 54–57.

Reinecke, M. A. (2006). Problem solving: A conceptual approach to suicidality and psychotherapy. In T. Ellis (Ed.) *Cognition and suicide: Theory, research, and therapy* (pp. 237–260). Washington, DC: American Psychological Association.

Reinecke, M. A., & Didie, E. R. (2005). Cognitive-behavioral therapy with suicidal patients. In R. I. Yufit, & D. Lester (Eds.), *Assessment, treatment, and prevention of suicidal behavior* (pp. 205–234). Hoboken, NJ: Wiley.

Reinecke, M., & Franklin-Scott, R. (2005). Assessment of suicide: Beck's Scales for Assessing Mood and Suicidality. In R. Yofit & D. Lester (Eds.), *Assessment, treatment, and prevention of suicidal behavior* (pp. 29–61). Hoboken, NJ: Wiley.

Reynolds, F., & Berman, A. (1995). An empirical typology of suicide. *Archives of Suicide Research, 1*(2), 97–109.

Reynolds, W. (1987). *Suicide Ideation Questionnaire: Professional manual.* Odessa, FL: Psychological Assessment Resources.

Robinson, M. S., & Alloy, L. B. (2003). Negative cognitive styles and stress-reactive rumination interact to predict depression: A prospective study. *Cognitive Therapy and Research, 27,* 275–292.

Rotheram-Borus, M., & Trautman, P. (1988). Hopelessness, depression, and suicidal intent among adolescent suicide attempters. *Journal of the American Academy of Child and Adolescent Psychiatry, 27*(6), 700–704.

Roy, A. (1984). Suicide in recurrent affective disorder patients. *Canadian Journal of Psychiatry, 29,* 319–322.

Roy, A., Mazonson, A., & Pickar, D. (1984). Attempted suicide in chronic schizophrenia. *British Journal of Psychiatry, 144,* 303–306.

Rudd, M. (1990). An integrative model of suicidal ideation. *Suicide and Life-Threatening Behavior, 20*(1), 16–30.

Rudd, M., & Joiner, T. (1997). Countertransference and the therapeutic relationship: A cognitive perspective. *Journal of Cognitive Psychotherapy, 11*(4), 231–250.

Rudd, M., Joiner, T., & Rajab, M. (2001). *Treating suicidal behavior: An effective, time-limited approach.* New York: Guilford Press.

Rudd, D. M., Rajab, H. M., & Dahm, F. P. (1994). Problem-solving appraisal in suicide ideators and attempters. *American Journal of Orthopsychiatry, 64*(1), 136–149.

Salkovskis, P., Atha, C., & Storer, D. (1990). Cognitive-behavioural problem solving in the treatment of patients who repeatedly attempt suicide: A controlled trial. *British Journal of Psychiatry, 157,* 871–876.

Scher, C. D., Ingram, R. E., & Segal, Z. V. (2005). Cognitive reactivity and vulnerability: Empirical evaluation of construct activation and cognitive diatheses in unipolar depression. *Clinical Psychology Review, 25,* 487–510.

Schotte, D., & Clum, G. (1987). Problem-solving skills in suicidal psychiatric patients. *Journal of Consulting and Clinical Psychology, 55*, 49–54.

Schotte, D., Cools, J., & Payvar, S. (1990). Problem-solving deficits in suicidal patients: Trait vulnerability or state phenomenon? *Journal of Consulting and Clinical Psychology, 58*(5), 562–564.

Segal, Z. (1988). Appraisal of the self-schema construct in cognitive models of depression. *Psychological Bulletin, 103*(2), 147–162.

Seligman, M. (1975). *Helplessness: On depression, development, and death.* New York: Freeman.

Shneidman, E. (1985). *The definition of suicide.* New York: Wiley-Interscience.

Siani, R., Garzotto, N., Zimmerman-Tanselia, C., & Tansella, M. (1979). Predictive scales for parasuicide repetition: Further results. *Acta Psychiatrica Scandinavica, 59*, 17–23.

Simon, G. E., & Von Korff, M. (1998). Suicide mortality among patients treated for depression in an insured population. *American Journal of Epidemiology, 147*, 155–160.

Slaikeu, K. (1990). *Crisis intervention* (2nd ed.). Boston: Allyn & Bacon.

Smith, K., Conroy, R., & Ehler, B. (1984). Lethality of suicide attempt rating scale. *Suicide and Life-Threatening Behavior, 14*(4), 215–242.

Spirito, A., Brown, L., Overholser, J., & Fritz, G. (1991). Use of the risk-rescue rating scale with adolescent suicide attempters: A cautionary note. *Death Studies, 15*(3), 269–280.

Spirito, A., Overholser, J., & Vinnick, L. (1995). Adolescent suicide attempters in general hospitals: Psychological evaluation and disposition planning. In J. Wallander & L. J. Siegel (Eds.), *Adolescent health problems: Behavioral perspectives (Advances in pediatric psychology)* (pp. 97–116). New York: Guilford Press.

Spirito, A., Valeri, S., Boergers, J., & Donaldson, D. (2003). Predictors of continued suicidal behavior in adolescents following a suicide attempt. *Journal of Clinical Child and Adolescent Psychology, 32*, 284–289.

Steer, R., Beck, A., & Garrison, B. (1986). Applications of the Beck Depression Inventory. In N. Sartorius & T. Ban (Eds.), *Assessment of depression* (pp. 123–142). New York: Springer-Verlag.

Tarter, R., Kirisci, L., Reynolds, M., & Mezzich, A. (2004). Neurobehavior disinhibition in childhood predicts suicide potential and substance use disorder by young adulthood. *Drug and Alcohol Dependence, 76*(Suppl. 7), S45–S52.

Trautman, P. (1995). Cognitive behavior therapy of adolescent suicide attempters. In J. Zimmerman & G. M. Asnis (Eds.), *Treatment approaches with suicidal adolescents* (pp. 155–173). New York: Wiley.

Tuckman, J., & Youngman, W. F. (1968). A scale for assessing suicide risk of attempted suicides. *Journal of Clinical Psychology, 24*(1), 17–19.

Tyrer, P., Thompson, S., Schmidt, U., Jones, V., Knapp, M., Davidson, K., et al. (2003). Randomized trial of brief cognitive behavior therapy versus treatment as usual in recurrent deliberate self-harm: The POPMACT Study. *Psychological Medicine, 33*(6), 969–976.

Uncapher, H., Gallagher-Thompson, D., Osgood, N., & Bongar, B. (1998). Hopelessness and suicidal ideation in older adults. *Gerontologist, 38*(1), 62–70.

van der Sande, R., Buskens, E., Allart, E., van der Graaf, Y., & van Engeland, H. (1997). Psychosocial intervention following suicide attempt: A systematic review of treatment interventions. *Acta Psychiatrica Scandinavica, 96*(1), 43–50.

Velting, D. (1999). Suicidal ideation and the five-factor model of personality, *Personality and Individual Differences, 27*, 943–952.

Verheul, R., van den Bosch, L. M. C., Koeter, M. W. J., de Ridder, M. A. J., Stijnen, T., & van den Brink, W. (2003). Dialectical behaviour therapy for women with borderline personality disorder: 12-month, randomised clinical trial in The Netherlands. *British Journal of Psychiatry, 182*, 135–140.

Verona, E., Patrick, C., & Joiner, T. (2001). Psychopathy, antisocial personality, and suicide risk. *Journal of Abnormal Psychology, 110,* 444–451.

Warman, D., Forman, E., Henriques, G., Brown, G., & Beck, A. (2004). Suicidality and psychosis: Beyond depression and hopelessness. *Suicide and Life-Threatening Behavior, 34,* 77–86.

Warshaw, M., Dolan, R., & Keller, M. (2000). Suicidal behavior in patients with current or past panic disorder: Five years of prospective data from Harvard/Brown Anxiety Research program. *American Journal of Psychiatry, 157,* 1876–1878.

Weersing, V. R., & Brent, D. A. (2003). Cognitive-behavioral therapy for adolescent depression: Comparative efficacy, mediation, moderation and effectiveness. In A. E. Kazdin & J. R. Weisz (Eds.), *Evidence-based psychotherapies for children and adolescents* (pp. 135–147). New York: Guilford Press.

Weishaar, M., & Beck, A. (1992). Hopelessness and suicide. *International Review of Psychiatry, 4,* 185–192.

Weisman, A., & Beck, A. (1978). *Development and validation of the Dysfunctional Attitude Scale: A preliminary investigation.* Paper presented at the meeting of the Association for Advancement of Behavior Therapy, Chicago.

Weissman, A., Beck, A., & Kovacs, M. (1979). Drug abuse, hopelessness, and suicidal behavior. *International Journal of Addiction, 14,* 451–464.

Weiss, A. (2001). The no-suicide contract: Possibilities and pitfalls. *American Journal of Psychotherapy, 55,* 414–419.

Wen-Hung, K., Gallo, J., & Eaton, W. (2004). Hopelessness, depression, substance disorder, and suicidality: A 13-year community-based study. *Social Psychiatry and Psychiatric Epidemiology, 39,* 497–501.

Wetzel, R. (1976). Hopelessness, depression, and suicide intent. *Archives of General Psychiatry, 33,* 1069–1073.

Wetzel, R., Margulies, T., Davis, R., & Karam, E. (1980). Hopelessness, depression, and suicide intent. *Journal of Clinical Psychiatry, 4(5),* 159–160.

Williams, J., & Wells, J. (1989). Suicidal patients. In J. Scott, J. Williams, & A. Beck (Eds.), *Cognitive therapy in clinical practice: An illustrative casebook* (pp. 206–226). London: Routledge.

Wittgenstein, L. (1980). *Culture and value.* Chicago: University of Chicago Press. (Original work published 1946)

Yang, B., & Clum, G. (1994). Life stress, social support, and problem-solving skills predictive of depressive symptoms, hopelessness, and suicide ideation in an Asian student population: A test of a model. *Suicide and Life-Threatening Behavior, 24(2),* 127–139.

Yang, B., & Clum, G. (2000). Childhood stress leads to later suicidality via its effect on cognitive functioning. *Suicide and Life-Threatening Behavior, 30,* 183–198.

Yen, S., Sheam, T., Pagano, M., Samislow, C. A., Grilo, C. M., McGlashan, T., et al. (2003). Axis I and axis II disorders as predictors of prospective suicide attempts: Findings from the collaborative longitudinal personality disorders study. *Journal of Abnormal Psychology, 112,* 375–381.

Young, J. (1991). *Cognitive therapy of personality disorders: A schema-focused approach.* Sarasota, FL: Professional Resource Exchange.

Young, M., Fogg, L., Scheftner, W., Fawcett, J., Akiskal, H., & Maser, J. (1996). Stable trait components of hopelessness: Baseline and sensitivity to depression. *Journal of Abnormal Psychology, 105(2),* 155–165.

Yufit, R., & Bongar, B. (1992). Structured clinical assessment of suicide risk in emergency room and hospital settings. In B. Bongar (Ed.), *Suicide: Guidelines for assessment, management, and treatment* (pp. 144–159). New York: Oxford University Press.

Zung, W. (1974). Index of Potential Suicide (IPS): A rating scale for suicide prevention. In A. Beck, H. Resnick, & D. Lettieri (Eds.), *The prediction of suicide* (pp. 221–249). Philadelphia: Charles Press.

SUGGESTED READINGS

Bongar, B., Berman, A., Maris, R., Silverman, M., Harris, E., & Packman, W. (Eds.). (1998). *Risk management with suicidal patients*. New York: Guilford Press.

Ellis, T. (1987). A cognitive approach to treating the suicidal client. In P. A. Keller & S. R. Heyman (Eds.), *Innovations in clinical practice: A sourcebook* (Vol. 5, pp. 93–107). Sarasota, FL: Professional Resource Exchange.

Freeman, A., & Reinecke, M. (1993). *Cognitive therapy of suicidal behavior*. New York: Springer.

Freeman, A., & White, D. (1989). The treatment of suicidal behavior. In A. Freeman, K. Simon, H. Arkowitz, & L. Beutler (Eds.), *Comprehensive handbook of cognitive therapy* (pp. 321–346). New York: Plenum Press.

Greenberger, D. (1992). The suicidal patient. In A. Freeman & F. M. Dattilio (Eds.), *Comprehensive casebook of cognitive therapy* (pp. 139–146). New York: Plenum Press.

Hawton, K. (1997). Attempted suicide. In D. M. Clark & C. Fairburn (Eds.), *Cognitive behaviour therapy: Science and practice* (pp. 285–312). Oxford, UK: Oxford University Press.

Hawton, K., & Catalan, J. (1982). *Attempted suicide: A practical guide to its nature and management*. Oxford, UK: Oxford University Press.

Overholser, J. (1995). Cognitive-behavioral treatment of depression: I. Assessment of depression and suicide risk. *Journal of Contemporary Psychotherapy, 25*(3), 185–204.

Weishaar, M., & Beck, A. (1990). The suicidal patient: How should the therapist respond? In K. Hawton & P. Cowan (Eds.), *Dilemmas and difficulties in the management of psychiatric patients* (pp. 65–76). Oxford, UK: Oxford University Press.

Williams, J., & Wells, J. (1989). Suicidal patients. In J. Scott, J. Williams, & A. Beck (Eds.), *Cognitive therapy in clinical practice: An illustrative casebook* (pp. 206–226). London: Routledge.

CHAPTER 3

Panic Disorder

Frank M. Dattilio
Philip C. Kendall

Angela, a 42-year-old emergency room nurse, was driving home from a 12-hour shift in the emergency room. She had experienced a particularly stressful shift due to several auto accidents and their victims, one of whom was a young child.

En route home, Angela began to experience what she describes as a frightening sensation. Initially, she shrugged the experience off to being "wound up from work," but after the same sensation occurred a second and third time, along with an increased heart rate, she became concerned and thought, "My God, I'm going into 'V-tac' [ventricular tachycardia]." She experienced heart palpitations with profuse sweating. It was at that point that Angela felt a hot flash radiate through her weak body like a bolt of lightning. As her symptoms intensified, she became increasingly distressed. Consequently, she turned her vehicle around and sped back to the hospital emergency room. Once there, she spoke with the physician on call who quickly hooked her up to an electrocardiogram (EKG) and ordered an arterial blood gas profile. All results were normal and Angela was informed that she had experienced a panic attack. Angela was administered alprazolam, 0.5 mg, as needed, and released to the care of her primary care physician. It was also suggested that she might want to consider seeing a mental health professional for stress management. What Angela experienced is an example a spontaneous panic attack, a condition that is not common but is also not uncommon among individuals who work in intensely stressful circumstances. She believed her symptoms were life threatening, causing her to seek immediate medical attention.

According to the *Diagnostic and Statistical Manual of Mental Disorders*, fourth edition, text revision (DSM-IV-TR; American Psychiatric Association, 2000), panic attacks are diagnosed by the presence of at least four of the following symptoms: (1) shortness of breath or suffocating sensation; (2) dizziness, unsteady feelings, or faintness; (3) palpitations or accelerated heart rate; (4) trembling or shaking; (5) sweating; (6) choking; (7) nausea or abdominal distress; (8) depersonalization or derealization—a feeling that the sufferer's body or environment, respectively, is not real; (9) numbness or tingling sensations in one or more parts of the body; (10) hot flashes or chills; (11) chest pain or discomfort; (12) fear of dying; and (13) fear of going crazy or losing self-control. A condition of these criteria involves "unexpected (uncued) panic attacks," which is required for a diagnosis of panic disorder as well as the symptoms' reaching a peak within 10 minutes (American Psychiatric Association, 2000).

Panic disorder is one of the common and disabling psychological disorders encountered in both mental health and general medical settings and for some time has continued to rank among the top 10 disorders found in psychiatric emergencies (Wayne, 1966; Goldenberg, 1983). In past studies, investigators have estimated that the 1-month prevalence of panic disorder among primary care patients was 1.4% (Von Korff et al., 1987). This appears to hold true with a slight increase to date (Dattilio & Salas-Auvert, 1999). In addition, previous statistics derived from a study assessing community-based epidemiological catchment areas estimate that in any given month 0.5% of the population will be diagnosed with panic disorder (Regier et al., 1988).

Panic is reportedly a common diagnosis among hospital emergency room patients as well as in primary care facilities (Rosenman, 1985; Dunner, 1985; Roy-Byrne, et al., 2005). This situation is in part due to the fact that heart palpitations are among the most common symptoms expressed during a panic attack (Ehlers & Breuer, 1992; Dattilio & Salas-Auvert, 2000), and panic episodes are particularly common in cardiology patients (Beitman, DeRosear, Basha, Flaker, & Corcoran, 1987). Outpatient mental health clinics also report a high frequency of complaints of panic symptoms, with estimated incidences in the general population of 1.6–2.9% among women and 0.4–1.7% among men (Crowe, Noyes, Pauls, & Slymen, 1983; Boyd, 1986).

Although the literature on crisis and crisis intervention in general is abundant (e.g., Aguilera, 1990; Kocmur & Zavasnik, 1991; Roberts, 1990), very little research has been devoted to specifically addressing crisis intervention for reports of panic and panic disorder (Aronson & Logue, 1988; Dattilio & Kendall, 1994, 2000; Diez, Gastó, & Vallejo, 1989). This situation is surprising, because it is well documented that physicians have, for the past 120 years, experienced difficulty in differentially diagnosing panic disorder from a variety of physiological disorders (DaCosta, 1871; Oppenheimer & Rothschild, 1918; Prince & Putnam, 1912; Skerrit, 1983; Westphal, 1871). Moreover, because the primary goal of crisis intervention is to reduce the patient's self-reported emotional distress (Kendall & Norton-Ford, 1982), it is not surprising that panic would appear near the top of the list of disorders targeted in crisis intervention.

The scarcity of crisis intervention literature regarding panic may be because panic attacks are often viewed as crisis manifestations of some other underlying problem. In the medical setting, for example, a physician usually focuses immediately on any chronic underlying condition suspected of precipitating the panic symptoms, such as temporal lobe epilepsy, coronary artery disease, alcohol or tranquilizer withdrawal, hyperthyroidism, pheochromocytoma, electrolyte abnormalities, or stimulant medications/decongestants (see Katon, 1992, for a more extensive list). In addition, symptoms of panic can be secondary to other mental disorders such as major affective disorders (Breir, Charney, & Heninger, 1984), personality disorder (Barlow, 2002; Beck, Freeman, & Associates, 1990) and alcohol withdrawal (Katon, 1992). For a more extensive review of this subject, the reader is referred to Dattilio and Salas-Auvert (2000).

TWO THEORIES OF PANIC

There have been several attempts to explain the etiology of panic. Psychobiologists have contributed a number of hypotheses, which include the septohippocampal theory (Gray, 1982), the locus coeruleus theory (Charney, Heninger, & Breier, 1984; Svensson, 1987), and the gamma-aminobutyric acid–benzodiazepine hypothesis (Skolnick & Paul, 1983). More recently, cholecystokinin tetrapeptide (cck-4) has been studied as a panicogenic agent (Bradwejn, Koszycki, Payeur, Bourin, & Borthwick, 1992). These theories seek to explain panic by the action of certain neurochemicals in the brain. Another possibility is that there is a specific genetic basis for inheriting a predisposition to panic disorder. Recent research on deoxyribonucleic acid (DNA) has analyzed the genetic structure of panic victims and members of their families who also reported a history of experiencing panic or related symptoms. A genetic linkage among individuals diagnosed with panic disorder has been hypothesized for some time (Knowles & Weissman, 1995; Weissman, 1993; Weismann & Merikangas, 1986). Such a linkage is most likely to be true of individuals who describe an early onset of panic (Goldstein, Wickramaratne, Horwath, & Weissman, 1997). Recently, a series of studies were undertaken to test this hypothesis (Hamilton et al., 1999; Knowles et al., 1998). In one particular study, the investigators used a family-based design to test for genetic association and linkage between panic disorder and a functional polymorphism in the promoter of the gene 5-HTT. In this study, 340 individuals in 45 families, as well as 75 haplotype relative risk "trios," were genotyped at the polymorphic locus, which consists of 44 base pair deletion/insertion. The results yielded nonsignificant differences in allele frequencies or occurrence of genotypes within the triads. Furthermore, no linkage between the 5-HTT polymorphism and panic disorder was observed in the multiplex families, using a variety of simulations for dominant and recessive models of inheritance. The results of this study suggest that the genetic basis of panic disorder may be distinct from anxiety-related traits assessed by personality inventories in normal populations (Hamilton et al., 1999).

One of the more popular theories is the sodium lactate theory, proposed as a result of the early studies by Pitts and McClure (1967). This study examined the effects of sodium lactate infusion, which induced panic attacks only in subjects who had a history of panic and not in others in the study who had no history of panic. Other studies were repeated yielding similar results (Appleby, Klein, Sachar, & Levitt, 1981; Dager, Cowley, & Dunner, 1987). On the other hand, Ley (1986), in his reexamination of the original data of the 1967 Pitts and McClure study, uncovered that the 1967 panic subjects actually experienced an increase in a sensitivity to uncomfortable symptoms. This requires a determination as to whether it was an actual chemical chain reaction that occurred or a catastrophic misinterpretation that caused the subjects in the study to experience panic.

Even more provocative are the findings from the study conducted by Margraf and Ehlers (1989), which investigated panic-disordered individuals' reactions to hyperventilation and compared them to a normal population. The influence of subjects' expectancies was tested by manipulating instructions that were presented during an exercise. Two groups (panic and normals) were informed that they were participating in a "biological panic attack test" as opposed to the others, who were told that they were involved in a "fast-paced breathing task." Apparently, the increase in panic subjects' anxiety and arousal depended on what they were told. The expectation that they were taking a panic test produced physiological reactions and self-reported elevations in both anxiety and arousal. Conversely, the manipulation of the instructions and expectations had no effect on normal subjects' responses. As a likely consequence of these biology-based theories, the treatment of choice in medical settings involves a pharmacological regimen of high-potency benzodiazepines, tricyclic antidepressants, or monoamine oxidase inhibitors (Sheehan, 1982) coupled with behavior therapy (Brown, Rakel, Well, Downs, & Akisdal, 1991).

Although the psychobiological explanation of panic has merit, it retains several drawbacks. For one, there is little evidence to prove a psychobiological etiology for panic disorder—that is, there is no sure method to test for chemical imbalances or other difficulties in the brain. In fact, additional evidence recently reviewed in Kendall and Hammen (1999) suggests that the biological model of panic disorder does not explain as much as once thought. In an interesting study at Vanderbilt University, researchers had individuals diagnosed with panic disorder inhale carbon dioxide either with or without an accompanying safe person who was chosen by the individual. The researchers hypothesized that if panic was solely biological in nature, a person's presence should have little effect on the panic episode. The results indicated that those panic-disordered individuals who were without a "safe person" reported greater distress, more catastrophic cognitions, and an increase in physiological arousal than did those who were accompanied by a "safe person." These results support the cognitive-behavioral theory of panic (Clark, Salkovskis, & Chalkley, 1985). The explosion of research relying on magnetic resonance imaging (MRI), positron emission tomography (PET) scans, and brain electrical area mapping (BEAM) studies have generated tremendous interest in psychobiological research of panic disorders. Nevertheless, the complexity of brain-related behavior continues to stall a comprehensive understanding of brain mechanisms involved in panic and anxiety. Although pharmacotherapy can expeditiously alleviate symptoms and possibly reduce the likelihood of phobic avoidance by reducing or ameliorating spontaneous panic attacks, it remains less than a cure. Pharmacotherapy provides the afflicted individual with little in the way of true coping mechanisms other than the reliance on simply taking the prescribed compound as instructed. In addition, individuals with panic disorder can be among the most difficult groups of patients to treat with medication—all pharmacological compounds have side effects and panic attack patients are often hypersensitive to bodily sensations (Katon, 1992).

Pharmacological compounds have offered the most expedient treatment in crisis settings and have long been the treatment of choice for emergency situations involving panic and acute anxiety symptoms. The medical literature still suggests, however, that the first stage of treatment in primary care and emergency settings should be to negotiate explanatory models of the illness with the patients (Katon & Kleinman, 1980) and to elicit patients' beliefs about their illness prior to the actual treatment intervention. Open-ended questions such as "What do you believe is the problem?" and "What reasons would you give for the onset of symptoms at this particular time?" are recommended (Katon, 1992).

Unfortunately, questioning can be limited to gathering some background information about the patient's relevant medical history subsequent to a blood profile and/or EKG, and medication is often dispensed without further exploration or explanation. Psychobiological theories argue that panic is essentially the result of biochemical abnormalities associated with genetic predispositions (Sheehan, 1982; Weiss & Uhde, 1990); however, more recent literature suggests that psychological theories are better supported by empirical research (Beck & Emery, with Greenberg, 1985; Dattilio & Salas-Auvert, 2000).

A cognitive-behavioral theory of panic contends that it is psychological factors rather than solely psychobiological factors that precipitate panic symptoms. Whereas the cognitive-behavioral theories do acknowledge the neurochemical components of autonomic symptoms, they place more emphasis on the perception of threat or danger whether it involves internal (bodily sensations) or external (environmental) events (Dattilio, 1986; Ottaviani & Beck, 1987; Raskin, Peeke, Dickman, & Pinsker, 1982). Specifically, the misattribution theory introduced in the literature within the last two decades proposes that specific symptoms resulting in hyperventilation elicit panic in individuals who are predisposed, genetically or psychologically, to catastrophic misattribution of internal bodily sensations (Clark, 1986; Ley, 1985). According to this theory, the most commonly occurring physical sensations during a panic attack include dizziness, vertigo, blurred vision, tachycardia, palpitations, numbness, tingling in the hands and feet, nausea and breathlessness (Clark et al., 1985; Hibbert, 1984; Kerr, Dalton, & Gliebe, 1937). Clark et al. (1985) noticed that these sensations were similar to those produced by hyperventilation.

Thus it was hypothesized that hyperventilation may play an important role in the initiation of panic attacks (Clark et al., 1985). The theory purports that some individuals increase respiration under stress. This increase causes carbon dioxide to be expelled from the lungs, triggering a decrease in the partial pressure of carbon dioxide (pCO2) in the blood with an increase of pH in the blood. Such changes in the blood's chemistry manifests uncomfortable body sensations such as the aforementioned to which the individuals respond with startle and apprehension. This increased apprehension elicits further rapid breathing, which can spiral into a full-blown panic attack. Clark et al. (1985) contend that it is either the perception of the feared stimulus itself or the induction of fear already elicited by other stimuli that contributes to the catastrophic reaction during this event that precipitates panic. Hence, teaching individuals how to avoid hyperventilation when under stress via breathing retraining is an important part of the treatment.

Although panic attacks have often been reported as occurring "spontaneously," Beck et al. (1985) have found that some particular experiences appear to activate a person's "alarm system" (p. 112) involving cognitive–affective and physiological components. In addition, the aspect of perceived control has received increasing attention in explaining outcome effects in the treatment of panic (Borden, Clum, & Salmon, 1991; Dattilio & Salas-Auvert, 1999).

ASSESSMENT AND DIAGNOSIS

A comprehensive assessment protocol for diagnosing panic is quite complex and usually involves a structured interview. Such interviews may be performed with assessment instruments such as the Structured Interview Schedule for DSM-III-R (SCID; Spitzer, Williams, & Gibbon, 1985) or the Anxiety Disorders Interview Schedule—Revised (ADIS-R; DiNardo et al., 1985). Unfortunately, such comprehensive assessment usually requires a considerable amount of time, which is not always available during crisis situations. Some abridged versions have been developed in recent studies to provide a more expedient method of assessment in crisis situations, for example, the Upjohn version of the SCID (SCID-UP-R; Spitzer & Williams, 1986; Swinson, Soulios, Cox, & Kuch, 1992).

It is recommended that, at a minimum, a brief clinical interview be conducted, including an excerpt from the panic section of the ADIS-R and screening questions that elicit the individual's medical history (particularly cardiac or seizure disorders) along with all medication currently in use. Some of the briefer diagnostic questionnaires may also help to pinpoint specific symptoms and to support information that has been obtained from the patient verbally. Such quick screening questionnaires include the Beck Anxiety Inventory (BAI; Beck, 1987), the Body Sensations Questionnaire (BSQ; Chambless, Caputo, Bright, & Gallagher, 1984), the Anxiety Sensitivity Index (ASI; Reiss, Peterson, Gursky, & McNally, 1986), and the Zung Anxiety Scale (Zung, 1975), any of which can be completed in a matter of minutes. In addition, Table 3.1 includes some of the more important questions to ask during crisis situations. There are also myriad questionnaires and inventories that have been empirically tested and are available in one text (Antony, Orsillo, & Roemer, 2001). Because much of the cognitive-behavioral literature stresses the importance of relating symptoms to the misinterpretation of interoceptive cues and catastrophic cognitions (Alford, Beck, Freeman, & Wright, 1990; Dattilio, 1986, 1987, 1990, 1992a, 1994a; Ottaviani & Beck, 1987), a formal system for linking panic symptoms to thoughts and emotional-behavioral responses is essential. A recently developed assessment technique known as the SAEB (symptoms–automatic thoughts–emotions–behavior) system is also of interest as an approach for helping panic sufferers recognize the link between their panic

TABLE 3.1. Questions for Crisis Intervention

1. Have you recently adjusted, discontinued, or changed any medications, either prescription or nonprescription?
2. Have you experienced any illness or deaths or changes in relationships, job, or financial situation in the past 6 months?
3. Have you recently experienced childbirth, surgery, or a change in menstrual pattern?
4. Has anyone in your immediate family or family of origin experienced symptoms similar to those you are experiencing now?
5. Have you recently commenced or discontinued any use of tobacco, drugs, or alcohol?
6. Do you have any history of medical disorders such as hypoglycemia, cardiac abnormalities, seizure disorder, etc.?
7. Have you experienced these types of symptoms in the past?
8. Are you currently using stimulant/diet drugs such as crank, speed, cocaine, crack, etc.?

symptoms and their catastrophic responses to their initial bodily sensations (Dattilio, 1990, 1992a, 1992b; Dattilio & Berchick, 1992). The unique design of the SAEB system allows the treating clinician to align specific catastrophic thoughts and misinterpretations of symptoms with the onset of subsequent symptoms in a quick, expedient fashion. The system thus allows the panic victim to see the connections between stages of the escalation process setting the stage for the next step, which involves the treatment intervention (see Figure 3.1).

This system is applied by having patients identify the beginning symptom of the panic episode. If the individual has experienced more than one attack, the repetitive sequence of each attack is more credible. For example, in Figure 3.1, a "spontaneous increase in heart rate" was the initial symptom experienced by Angela, the nurse depicted in the case study, at the onset of each attack. This was followed by "difficulty breathing" and subsequently by "hot flashes and sweating," and so on. Once the symptoms have been aligned, the automatic thoughts accompanying each symptom are indicated along with the associated emotion and behavior. Vectors are then drawn in order to demonstrate to the patient in a collaborative fashion how the catastrophic thought content may be in reaction to the autonomic symptoms experienced and how these thoughts contribute to the subsequent behavior and possibly to the subsequent escalation of the symptoms (Dattilio, 1990). This technique is demonstrated in detail in a videotape (Dattilio, 1994b) as well as by Dattilio and Salas-Auvert (2000).

This SAEB system sets the stage for the implementation of several cognitive-behavioral treatment strategies that are explained later in this chapter. It is useful as a quick method of assessment for tracking the cognitive, affective, behavioral, and physiological sequence of panic. Pinpointing specific triggers of panic symptoms (e.g., stress; hot, stuffy climates; excessive exercise) is also another important aspect of assessment that has been emphasized in the literature (Beck et al., 1985; Dattilio & Berchick, 1992). It is also an excellent method for teaching individuals how to differentiate symptoms of anxiety from other physiological symptoms of more severe illness (Dattilio, 2005; Dattilio & Castaldo, 2001, 2006).

SYMPTOMS

AUTOMATIC
THOUGHT

EMOTION/
BEHAVIOR

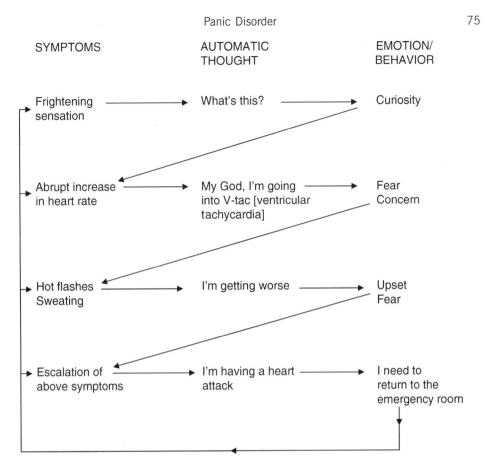

FIGURE 3.1. Angela's panic sequence.

COGNITIVE-BEHAVIORAL INTERVENTION STRATEGIES

A great deal of professional literature has focused on the use of cognitive-behavioral strategies and their effectiveness in treating panic and anxiety disorders (Beck et al., 1985; Barlow, 2002). Treatments utilizing cognitive and behavioral techniques have consistently demonstrated efficacy in the treatment of panic disorder with or without agoraphobia (Gould, Otto, & Pollack, 1995). Specifically, exposure-based treatments have been reasonably successful in reducing panic (Clark & Ehlers, 1993; Barlow, 2002), particularly when used in concert with pharmacological interventions (Zitrin, Klein, & Woerner, 1978). Cognitive-behavioral treatment focusing on panic control through education, cognitive restructuring, interoceptive exposure, and breathing retraining have been reported in some cases with success in a group format (Telch et al., 1993). More recently, didactic group approaches have been used in Scotland by White, Keenan, and Brooks (1992) to accommodate the large number of anxiety-disordered patients referred to primary care services. The therapy sessions employ a combination of cognitive-behavioral strategies and elements of traditional group therapy with a psychoeducational self-help package. The goal is to turn individuals into their own therapists, providing them with the education and skills necessary to recognize and overcome anxiety or panic.

Most recently, brief treatments of panic attacks in emergency situations have used exposure instruction with relative effectiveness (Swinson et al., 1992). In one particular study, 33 patients with panic attacks were seen in two emergency room settings. Forty percent of the patients had been diagnosed with the SCID as meeting the criteria for panic disorder with agoraphobia. Patients were randomly assigned to groups receiving either reassurance or exposure instruction. Outcome measures demonstrated significant improvement over a 6-month period for individuals of the exposure group. Individuals of the reassurance group showed no improvement on any measure and, in fact, reported increased symptomatology (Swinson et al., 1992). The specific treatment involved informing patients that the most effective way to reduce their fear was to confront the situation in which the attack occurred. Patients were advised to return to the situation as soon as possible after the interview and to wait until their anxiety decreased. Although this approach improves on the sole use of pharmacological interventions, it still falls short of providing the individual with any specific set of coping techniques, especially for dealing with future panic episodes. It also relies on extinction procedures and appears to require more time for reducing symptoms and may not always be practical depending on the circumstances in which the individual experienced the attack.

A number of additional cognitive-behavioral strategies may prove to be more satisfactory alternatives in the treatment of panic in crisis settings by providing the individual with specific coping mechanisms to apply during future episodes or attacks.

Controlled Breathing and Respiratory Feedback

Early studies on anxiety refer to the use of progressive muscle relaxation and controlled breathing as well as carbon dioxide inhalation (Wolpe, 1958). These techniques are based on the premise that a state of relaxation and a state of anxiety cannot coexist. Some view these techniques as being all that is necessary to put a stop to recurrent panic attacks (Clark et al., 1985; Lum, 1981).

The concept of controlled breathing is an offshoot of the hyperventilation hypothesis mentioned previously, which contends that individuals commonly hyperventilate prior to panicking (Hibbert, 1984). Individuals who hyperventilate tend to breathe through their mouths, taking short, shallow breaths of air or sighing frequently. Diaphragmatic breathing is one form of breathing retraining for counteracting hyperventilation. Individuals are instructed to breathe through the nose normally and to count the number of breaths while at rest, keeping the frequency to 9 to 16 times per minute. They are also told to place both hands over the abdomen while breathing, noticing the movement of the diaphragm. Individuals are instructed to practice the exercise during both panic and nonpanic periods (Clum, 1990). If, during a severe panic attack, the diaphragmatic method does not enable the individual to obtain a full breath, which is often the case, breathing into a paper bag or cupped hands may be used in order to increase the level of carbon dioxide (Dattilio, 1990). An alternative is to exhale through the mouth as much as possible and then slowly inhale through the nose, repeating the process several times. While practicing these techniques, distraction may be used to divert one's attention from the panic symptoms to enhance the positive effects of the breathing exercise.

Another technique often seen in the professional literature is "respiratory feedback." This involves actually training patients to change their breathing patterns. Unfortunately, breathing has rarely been measured objectively or through monitoring therapy results. A new breathing training method has been introduced recently that makes use of respiratory biofeedback to teach individuals to modify four respiratory characteristics: increased ventilation (respiratory rate × tidal volume), breath-to-breath irregularity in rate and depth, and chest breathing (Meuret, Wilhem, & Roth, 2004). This technique is used during the long course of treatment after the crisis intervention techniques have been initiated.

Symptom Induction and Deescalation

The cognitive-behavioral model of panic contends that individuals' misinterpretations of bodily sensations play an integral role in the escalation of panic symptoms. Consequently, such misinterpretations can be responsible for maintaining the vicious panic cycle (Argyle, 1988; Beck et al., 1985; Dattilio, 1987; Ottaviani & Beck, 1987). During this period of vulnerability, individuals tend to overestimate perceived danger and underestimate their capacity for coping (Dattilio, 1987, 1990; Greenberg, 1989).

In symptom induction, clients are presented with a therapeutic exercise whereby they are instructed to follow the therapist in taking short successive breaths of air, inhaling and exhaling, for approximately 2 to 3 minutes. This procedure reproduces the symptoms of panic by activating the autonomic nervous system and disrupting the balance of oxygen and carbon dioxide levels, sometimes causing hyperventilation as well (Dattilio, 1990). Symptom induction allows the therapist to obtain a direct report of the client's thought processes as the attack develops and to assist the client firsthand in controlling the attack through progressive breathing and thought restructuring. The goal here is to reproduce the types of symptoms that are similar to an attack and then show the client that he/she can "turn on" as well as "turn off" the attacks. Once the symptoms have been induced, the therapist records the sequence of events that occur, paying particular attention to the specific symptoms, the automatic thoughts, and the emotional reaction experienced as a result. Figure 3.1 provides an example of how to track the client's panic sequence during an attack. In response to the initial symptom, spontaneous increase in heart rate, the automatic thought is overreactive in the sense that it is assumed that "something is wrong" or that the client "could faint." It is essential that all clients who are candidates for this technique receive medical clearance prior to the exercise to ensure that the approach is not contraindicated by a preexisting medical condition. The therapist can then begin to intervene with the deescalation techniques by collaboratively focusing with the client on the initial symptoms.

In the case presented in Figure 3.1, a spontaneous increase in heart rate followed by the thought, "Something is wrong" or "I'm going to faint," translated into increased fear. By identifying the early onset of symptoms in the panic cycle, the thera-pist can aid clients in the deescalation of symptoms. This process has patients down-play the severity of the symptoms by altering their misinterpretations. For example, the individual in Figure 3.1 had developed a pattern of responding to increased heart rate by perceiving it as dangerous and a sure sign that "something is wrong." In restructuring their thoughts, clients are asked to consider an alternative response that may involve a less catastrophic implication. For instance, "Just because I have an increase in heart rate doesn't mean that this is necessarily dangerous or that something is wrong. It is perhaps just benign autonomic activity that will last for a limited time." This cognitive response is then supported by having the client log each attack and review the log for reassurance that because nothing dangerous has occurred in the past, it is unlikely to occur in the future. Clients are then taught controlled breathing in order to regulate their oxygen intake level and reduce autonomic activity. The pur-pose of this type of restructuring is to lessen the likelihood that the individual's auto-matic thoughts are fueling the subsequent increase in symptoms and emotional reaction and to persuade them that their fear ("I might faint") is unsubstantiated. This point can be affirmed with cognitive correction via factual information (e.g., in order to faint, one must experience a decrease in blood pressure; blood pressure increases with increased heart rate and anxiety). In addition, this serves to improve their per-ceived sense of bodily control, which reduces the intensity of threat and danger. This type of thought correction is followed throughout the entire panic cycle and then rein-forced by virtue of reexposure to symptoms through the use of the panic induction exercise. It is the combination of the artificial induction of symptoms (e.g., purposely increasing heart rate), as well as the reinterpretation of these symptoms (e.g., it will not hurt me), deescalation of the catastrophic thoughts (e.g., this will not last forever), and eventual reduction of symptom severity that makes the technique effective. In addition, follow-through on having clients expose themselves to real-life situations is also an important component to treatment so that the ability to generalize the tech-niques to a variety of situations can develop.

This strategy has been well received by panic sufferers, particularly after they have overcome their initial apprehension about raising their autonomic activity level. With those clients who sometimes do not benefit from the intervention (e.g., they become too overwhelmed or are unable to increase their autonomic activity level), it is recom-mended that the same technique of cognitive restructuring be used without the symp-tom induction exercise.

Paradoxical Intention

Paradoxical intention, originally developed by Frankl (1984), is similar to symptom induction in that it involves a behavioral prescription for clients to perform responses that seem incompatible with the goal for which they are seeking help. The specific dif-ference, however, is that in paradoxical intention clients are asked to exaggerate their anticipations rather than behaviorally induce the symptoms by deliberately hyper-ventilating. For example, individuals who experience panic attacks and fear that they may die suddenly or become "overwhelmed" would be instructed to "go ahead and let themselves die" or do whatever they fear they might do (Dattilio, 1987). After several attempts, they often discover that they are unable to achieve the feared response, and their anxiety then diminishes. At this point, many clients are able to perceive the absurd or irrational aspect of their apprehensions, which is strongly encouraged by the therapist. They are then instructed to repeat this same procedure in selected settings at graded levels of panic-evoking situations until they experience few or no symptoms. This approach also differs from symptom induction and deescalation in that there is no deescalation of symptoms and no instruction in the use of controlled breathing as an anxiety-reducing agent. In fact, it poses the opposite approach to the client with the reliance on the paradoxical focus itself as the trigger in reducing anxiety (Dattilio, 1987, 1994a, 1994c; Dattilio & Salas-Auvert, 2000).

Paradoxical intention has at times been rather loosely defined in the literature, particularly as it has been utilized by therapists of varying theoretical orientations who conceptualize it quite differently (Dell, 1981; Efran & Caputo, 1984; Ascher, 1984: Dowd & Trutt, 1988; Sexton, Montgomery, Goff, & Nugent, 1993). More specifically, the debate appears to center around whether or not the "intention" referred to is the patient's or the therapist's. This issue is discussed by Dowd and Trutt (1988), and the intention was clearly defined earlier by Frankl (1975) as being the patient's. Thus the technique of paradoxical intention may fall more clearly within the bounds of a cognitive intervention, because it first forces a behavioral change, which is followed by a restructuring of cognition upon reflection on the implication of the behavioral change. This point has been challenged, however, by others (Bandura, 1977) arguing that the behavioral change precedes the restructured cognition. Paradoxical intention appears antithetical to the other cognitive-behavioral treatments for panic, such as symptom induction, deescalation, and the relaxation-based techniques, mainly because it seems to provide patients with few coping techniques for anxiety. However, at times certain individuals may prove to benefit more from paradoxical treatments than others because of the extinction-based philosophy. It may be recommended for individuals who may experience relaxation-induced anxiety (Heide & Borkovec, 1983; Cohen, Barlow, & Blanchard, 1985; Lazarus & Mayne, 1990), in which many of the more traditional anxiety-reducing techniques are less effective. Side effects such as tingling, numbness, dizziness, paradoxical increases in tension, increased heart rate, and other untoward reactions have been reported with relaxation-based treatment (Borkovec & Grayson, 1980; Edinger & Jacobsen, 1982). Patients have reportedly often lost interest in progressive muscle relaxation or have repeatedly fallen asleep. Relaxation techniques may at times even evoke seizure activity or traumatic memories, which may undermine the intention of the treatment (Kiselica & Baker, 1992). Paradoxical intention would also be recommended in patients who appear resistant to techniques that involve actual symptom induction, as well as patients with a history of cardiovascular disorders. Even though paradoxical intention encourages the symptoms to worsen, there is no direct induction of symptoms (e.g., overbreathing); thus, the likelihood of cardiovascular stress is reduced. It is therefore suggested as an alternative treatment when induction is contraindicated and when an expedient intervention is required such as with crisis situations.

Symptom induction, deescalation, breathing retraining, and paradoxical intention are all nonpharmacological strategies that may be applied for amelioration of panic symptoms in emergency and crisis situations. In combination with exposure and/or pharmacological interventions, these techniques may prove to be the most efficacious (Brown et al., 1991).

Eye Movement Desensitization and Reprocessing

Shapiro and Forrest (1997) propose a method, called eye movement desensitization and reprocessing (EMDR), that has purported to have benefit in the treatment of traumatic memories and has recently been explored as a potential intervention in panic disorder.

Shapiro reports initially developing EMDR while working with some 70 people over the course of about 6 months, with refinements added over the past 10 years. As a result of her work, she reports developing a standard procedure that alleviated patients' complaints. Because the primary focus of EMDR was on reducing anxiety, this has become Shapiro's targeted population. Shapiro reported results of EMDR in the treatment of posttraumatic stress disorder (PTSD; Shapiro, 1996, 1998).

Goldstein and Feske (1994) reported on the use of EMDR in the treatment of panic disorder. They initially selected seven panic-disordered subjects who were patients at anxiety disorder clinics. The patients were treated with EMDR for memories of past and anticipated panic attacks and other anxiety-evoking memories of personal reference. Standardized report inventories and behavioral monitoring instruments were employed to measure changes with treatment. After only five sessions of EMDR, subjects reported a decrease in the frequency of panic attacks, fear of experiencing a panic attack, general anxiety, fear of body sensations, depression, and other symptom measures. These results sparked the authors' further investigation of the effectiveness of EMDR for panic.

In a subsequent study, the same authors (Feske & Goldstein, 1997) randomly assigned 43 outpatients diagnosed with panic disorder to six sessions of EMDR. A control group was assigned to the same treatment, but with the omission of the eye movement and with a waiting list. Posttest comparisons showed EMDR to be more effective in alleviating panic and panic-related symptoms than the waiting-list procedure. Compared with the same treatment without the eye movement, EMDR led to a greater improvement on two of five primary outcome measures. EMDR's advantages had dissipated 3 months after treatment. Consequently, this study fails to support the eye movement component of the treatment of panic disorder (Feske & Goldstein, 1997). Shapiro (1998) argued that Feske and Goldstein removed part of the treatment package (e.g., self-control imagery, attention to physical stimuli, and log reporting), features that may have been crucial to effectiveness. This issue is a topic of debate regarding the efficacy of eye movement (Feske & Goldstein, 1997) article.

Pharmacotherapy

Because medication is used in many crisis settings, it is important that it be addressed in this chapter. As mentioned earlier, pharmacotherapy has been the medical treatment of choice in most crisis or emergency settings involving acute anxiety or panic. This is particularly due to the quick-acting effects of many of the pharmacological agents, particularly the benzodiazepines, which act more rapidly than any other antipanic agents (Liebowitz, Fryer, & Goman, 1986). Recently, pharmacological treatment guidelines for panic disorder have changed as new treatment options have become available (Cloos, 2005). Bruce et al. (2003) examined how the use of psychotropic compounds have shifted over the course of 10 years. Treatment patterns for psycho-tropic medications have remained stable over the past decade with benzodiazepines being the most commonly prescribed compounds for panic disorder. Alprazolam is probably the most widely used benzodiazepine (Ballenger, Burrows, & Dupont, 1988). A variety of other benzodiazepines, including clonazepam, lorazepam and diazepam, also have antipanic effects when administered in significant doses (Brown et al., 1991) and as an add-on to selective serotonin reuptake inhibitors (SSRI) in the treatment of panic disorder. Benzodiazepines act rapidly and are well tolerated, but their use pres-ents clinical issues such as dependence, rebound anxiety, memory impairment, and dis-continuation syndrome (Chouinard, 2004; Wardle, 1990).

Tricyclic antidepressants, most notably imipramine hydrochloride, have been studied in depth as antianxiety agents (Brown et al., 1991). Imipramine has been found to be more effective than benzodiazepines in the long run in treating panic, par-ticularly when it is accompanied by depression. Other tricyclic antidepressants such as trimipramine, amitriptyline, doxepin, nortriptyline, and maprotiline have also been documented as effective in the treatment of panic (Lydiard & Ballenger, 1987). In a study by Mavissakalian (2003) that compared imipramine with sertraline in panic dis-order, there was greater early improvement with imipramine but no enduring differ-ences beyond week eight of treatment. As an alternative to tricyclic antidepressants, the monamine oxidase inhibitors (MAOIs) have been successful with individuals who suffer from panic associated with atypical depressive features. MAOIs, while effective, carry a number of serious side effects and require strict dietary restrictions that exclude foods containing tyramine. MAOIs, like the tricyclic antidepressants, require an onset period before any therapeutic effects may be gained (Riederer, Lachenmayer, & Laux, 2004).

Additional compounds, such as beta-adrenergic blockers and serotonin reuptake inhibitors, have also been used to treat panic with only minimal or no success. SSRIs have emerged as the first-choice treatment as they have a beneficial side effect profile and are relatively safe. Such compounds as paroxetine, sertraline, citalopram, and fluoxetine have also been reported to have an improved indication for panic disorder in the United States and Europe (Cloos, 2005).

Integrated Treatments

An integrated treatment approach that combines pharmacotherapy with cognitive-behavioral therapy may be the optimal treatment regime, especially during treatment of panic during crisis situations. An analysis by Starcevic, Linden, and Uhlenhuth (2004) found that combined treatments worked better with more severe cases of panic. Patients with more prominent panic attacks and somatic symptoms were more likely to be treated with cognitive-behavioral therapy plus a benzodiazepine where as those who had significant depressive symptomatology and higher disability levels were more likely to receive cognitive-behavioral therapy, benzodiazepines, and an antidepressant.

The combination of cognitive-behavioral strategies and pharmacological agents have previously been reported as successful in treating panic disorder. A study in 1998 involved a randomized double-blind, placebo-controlled clinical trial with 326 subjects carefully assessed for a diagnosis of panic disorder (Barlow, Gorman, Shear, & Woods, 1998). Patients received imipramine (IMI), cognitive-behavioral therapy (CBT), or a combination. The results indicate that both treatments were significantly better than placebos, and individual CBT and IMI worked approximately equally well at the end of acute treatment and after 6 months of maintenance. Response to placebos was short-lived. Among those completing treatment, IMI produced a better response. Six months following treatment discontinuation, more patients responding to IMI, whether combined with CBT or not, had deteriorated compared with those responding to CBT alone or CBT combined with placebos where subjects tended to retain their gains.

These investigators concluded that there may be little advantage to combining drug and CBT, and each individual treatment works approximately equally well immediately following treatment and during maintenance, although, obviously, medication, especially benzodiazepines, has the quickest initial effect.

Follow-up data after termination indicates that CBT is more durable. When pharmacological agents are used in conjunction with nonpharmacological techniques, it is recommended that a multicomponent treatment be used, such as the one described by Craske and Barlow (1990). This treatment program consists of four major components: (1) education and corrective information concerning the nature, etiology, and maintenance of panic; (2) cognitive therapy techniques aimed at helping the patient identify, monitor, and alter faulty appraisals of threat that contribute to panic occurrence; (3) framing in methods of slow diaphragmatic breathing as a way of reducing or eliminating physical symptoms that often trigger panic attacks; and (4) interoceptive exposure exercises designed to reduce patients' fear of somatic sensations through repeated exposure to feared bodily sensations. It is suggested that it might also apply to emergency settings.

Bibliotherapy

One of the adjunct techniques that has been found to be helpful with anxiety-disordered individuals is the use of assigned readings on the topic of panic—bibliotherapy (Gould, Clum, & Shapiro, 1993; Lidrin et al., 1994). As a behavioral technique, bibliotherapy is a continuous reinforcement of many of the principles and concepts promoted in therapy regarding coping skills. Literature may also help individuals who are suffering from panic feel less isolation and become aware that others experience these symptoms and struggle with the same reactions.

There are a number of excellent self-help books available on the market for panic sufferers, among them are *Don't Panic* (Wilson, 1986) and *Coping with Panic* (Clum, 1990). Both of these books have been written by professionals skilled in cognitive-behavioral therapies. As a result, they are fine supplemental reading and supportive aids to many of the techniques described in this chapter. Individuals should be directed to read these books as they are receiving treatment and may even benefit from them following the termination of therapy. For a more comprehensive listing of self-help books along with annotation, the reader is referred to Dattilio and Salas-Auvert (2000).

Homework

Homework is a very important aspect of cognitive-behavioral treatment of panic (Leahy, 2005). Many of the coping skills that are taught require practice in order to become part of the individual's work repertoire of skills. Such homework assignments as practicing breathing exercises and cognitive coping skills are necessary to learn how to respond effectively when a spontaneous panic attack occurs.

Recording information on forms such as the "panic diary" developed by Dattilio and reprinted in Dattilio and Salas-Auvert (2000) is also vital in allowing both the client and the therapist to track the occurrence and progress with the clients' panic occurrences.

Finally, homework is also a prelude to the eventual coping skills that will be used in relapse prevention. Whereas homework assignments vary during the course of treatment, typical assignments may include practicing methods of progressive muscle relaxation training, breathing exercises, practicing challenging automatic thought statements during periods of automatic activity, self-exposure to stimuli that may cause automatic arousal, and/or recording catastrophic thought statements.

Exercise

In a recent study conducted by Broman-Fulks, Berman, Rabian, and Webster (2004), it was determined that both high- and low-intensity exercise reduced anxiety sensitivity, a known precursor to panic attacks. However, high-intensity exercise caused more rapid reductions and produced more treatment responders. It was only the high-intensity exercise that reduced the fear of anxiety-related bodily sensations. Exercise as a prescriptive measure should be used with caution and as an adjunct or an integrative mode of treatment.

Relapse Prevention

Panic relapse after treatment occurs in the majority of cases as a result of the discontinuation of skills practice and exposure as well as poor follow-up in therapy. In fact, clients often end treatment abruptly because their symptoms have subsided.

It is important that clients contract with the therapist to complete their treatment and include all the follow-up visits. The follow-up visits should focus on a skills check and anticipation of the use of techniques in the event of a spontaneous recurrence of panic symptoms. Other issues that should be addressed are psychosocial and internal stressors that may trigger panic. Finally, it is also recommended that clients be instructed not to delay in contacting the therapist for booster sessions when they have difficulty coping on their own. It is often an extreme delay that can unwittingly facilitate the return of the panic cycle in full force.

SUPPORT GROUPS

A distinction must be made between group psychotherapy and support groups. Support groups typically are groups of individuals who have been through treatment and need to rely on group meetings as booster sessions. These groups usually are conducted by a trained professional or a paraprofessional and are designed primarily to support patients in utilizing what they have learned in the course of treatment. Although topics such as backsliding and stumbling blocks are often discussed, emphasis is placed on a support system as opposed to any specific intervention or treatment (Dattilio & Salas-Auvert, 2000).

Recovered panic-disordered individuals may form their own patient support groups and conduct them primarily as leaderless groups. These may be beneficial to some degree, but a useful caveat is that nonprofessionals may face difficulties depending on the condition of other group members. These groups are not recommended unless there is professional supervision, and it may behoove clinicians to have their patients avoid groups that are not so monitored.

Typically, support sessions are conducted on a monthly basis. Members may attend to talk about achieving their goals or to celebrate their successes. Generally, they can attend group meetings as long as sessions are available. Group support systems are recommended for individuals who have had serious relapses, but only after they have reentered treatment. Some support groups may also involve the spouse or other relatives of a person with panic disorder, and these can be very helpful to family members in their struggle to understand panic. It is important to remember that support groups are not a substitute for effective treatment, but are designed to complement treatment.

FAMILY/SPOUSAL SUPPORT

Even though panic is a disorder of the individual, it undoubtedly has a ripple effect on families. However, little research exists on the role of relationships and their contribution to panic disorder. Marital and family difficulties were ranked high on lists of stressors by panic-disordered subjects who were surveyed by researchers Thorpe and Burns (1983). Clearly, families may play a major role in accelerating the treatment process as well. Much of the professional literature supports the concept of educating spouses and family members to the treatment of panic and contributing to their understanding of why and how the disorder develops (Barlow, 2002). It may also be important for treating clinicians to coach spouses and immediate family members on their roles in the treatment process. Such spouse involvement should be executed with care and only after it has been determined that the patient's spouse or other family member is not facilitating an unhealthy dependency that may be enabling the patient's disorder, particularly because research has indicated that marital relations play a key role in the development and maintenance of panic and agoraphobia (Goldstein & Chambless, 1978; Wolpe, 1970). Further studies have focused on the relationship characteristics of agoraphobics and their partners (Epstein & Dutton, 1997) and suggest that agoraphobics are in more maladjusted marriages than are other couples; however, agoraphobics differ from other groups in that their degree of marital maladjustment falls in the middle between that of highly distressed and of nondistressed couples (Arrindell & Emmelkamp, 1986; Lange & Van Dyck, 1992). Unfortunately, little in the literature addresses the benefits of including the spouse in treatment, and the results of doing so are mixed (Arnow, Taylor, & Agras, 1985; Barlow, O'Brien, & Last, 1984; Himadi, Boice, & Barlow, 1986). Spouses are often trained by the treating clinician on how to coach their partners through difficult periods, as well as how to support the recovery process in general. Clinicians can and should take the opportunity to address any relationship issues that may be contributing to the panic cycle (e.g., overprotectiveness and dependency) and assess the need for further conjoint therapy. Because no research studies are available on the use of marital or family therapy alone or with medication for the treatment of panic, no conclusions can be drawn about the efficacy of the approach.

CONCLUSION

The treatment of panic in crisis settings is ripe for the application of cognitive-behavioral interventions that build coping skills. The strategies described in this chapter are reasonable adjuncts and alternatives to the sole reliance on pharmacotherapy in treating panic in crisis settings. Cognitive-behavioral strategies may prove to be most efficacious when used in conjunction with pharmacotherapy (Barlow et al., 1998; Sharp, Power, & Simpson, 1996). It is recommended that the cognitive-behavioral strategies described herein be considered prior to the use of pharmacological agents whenever possible (Solkol, Beck, Greenberg, Wright, & Berchick, 1989). Medication may serve as an adjunct to CBT rather than the reverse. Continued research in this area is certainly warranted.

REFERENCES

Aguilera, D. C. (1990). *Crises intervention: Theory and methodology*, St. Louis, MO: Mosby.
Alford, B. A., Beck, A. T., Freeman, A., & Wright, F. (1990). Brief focused cognitive therapy of panic disorder. *Psychotherapy, 27*(2), 230–234.
American Psychiatric Association. (2000). *Diagnostic and statistical manual of mental disorders* (4th ed., text rev.). Washington, DC: Author.
Antony, M. M., Orsillo, S. M., & Roemer, L. (Eds.). (2001). *Practioners' guide to empirically based measures of anxiety*. New York: Kluwer Academic/Plenum Press.

Appleby, I. L., Klein, D. F., Sachar, E., & Levitt, M. (1981). Biochemical indices of lactate induced panic: A preliminary report. In D. F. Klein & J. G Rabkin (Eds.), *Anxiety: New research and changing concepts* (pp. 121–132). New York: Raven Press.

Argyle, N. (1988). The nature of cognitions in panic disorder. *Behaviour Research and Therapy*, 26, 261–264.

Arnow, B. A., Taylor, C. B., & Agras, W. S. (1985). Enhancing agoraphobia treatment outcomes by changing couple communication patterns. *Behavior Therapy*, 16, 452–467.

Aronson, T. A., & Logue, C. M. (1988). Phenomenology of panic attacks: A descriptive study of panic disorder patients' self-reports. *Journal of Clinical Psychiatry*, 49, 8–13.

Arrindell, W., & Emmelkamp, P. (1986). Marital quality and general life adjustment in relation to treatment outcome in agoraphobia. *Advances in Behaviour Research and Therapy*, 8, 139–185.

Ascher, M. (1984). Paradox in behavior therapy: Some data and some possibilities. *Journal of Behavior Therapy and Experimental Psychiatry*, 15(5), 187.

Ballenger, J. C., Burrows, G. D., & Dupont, R. L. (1988). Alprozolam in panic disorder and agoraphobia: Results from a multicenter trial: Efficacy in short-term treatment. *Archives of General Psychiatry*, 45, 413–422.

Bandura, A. (1977). Self-efficacy: Toward a unifying theory of behavioral change. *Psychological Review*, 84, 191–215.

Barlow, D. H. (2002). *Anxiety and its disorders* (2nd ed.). New York: Guilford Press.

Barlow, D. H., Gorman, J. M., Shear, M. K., & Woods, S. W. (1998, November). Study design and pretreatment attrition. In D. Barlow (Chair), *Results from the multicenter clinical trial on the treatment of panic disorder: Cognitive-behavior treatment versus imipramine versus their combination.* Symposium presented at the 32nd annual convention of the Association for Advancement of Behavior Therapy, Washington, DC.

Barlow, D. H., O'Brien, G. T., & Last, C. G. (1984). Couples treatment of agoraphobia in relation to marital adjustment. *Archives of General Psychiatry*, 36, 807–811.

Beck, A. T. (1987). *Anxiety inventory.* Philadelphia: Center for Cognitive Therapy.

Beck, A. T., & Emery, G., with Greenberg, R. L. (1985). *Anxiety disorders and phobias.* New York: Basic Books.

Beck, A. T., Freeman, A., & Associates. (1990). *Cognitive therapy of personality disorders.* New York: Guilford Press.

Beitman, B. D., DeRosear, L., Basha, I., Flaker, G., & Corcoran, C. (1987). Panic disorder with cardiology patients with atypical or non-anginal chest pain. *Journal of Anxiety Disorders*, 1(3), 277–282.

Borden, J. W., Clum, G. A., & Salmon, P. G. (1991). Mechanisms of change in the treatment of panic. *Cognitive Therapy and Research*, 15(4), 257–272.

Borkovec, T. D., & Grayson, J. B. (1980). Consequences of increasing the functional impact of emotional stimuli. In K. Blankstein, P. Pliner, & J. Polivy (Eds.), *Assessment and modification of emotional behavior* (pp. 328–343). New York: Plenum Press.

Boyd, J. H. (1986). Use of mental health services for the treatment of panic disorder. *American Journal of Psychiatry*, 143, 1569–1574.

Bradwejn, J., Koszycki, D., Payeur, R., Bourin, M., & Borthwick, H. (1992). Replication of action of cholecystokinin tetrapeptide in panic disorder: Clinical and behavioral findings. *American Journal of Psychiatry*, 149, 962–964.

Breir, A., Charney, D. S., & Heninger, G. B. (1984). Major depression in patients with agoraphobia and panic disorder. *Archives of General Psychiatry*, 41, 1129–1135.

Broman-Fulks, J. J., Berman, M. E., Rabian, B. A., & Webster, M. J. (2004). Effects of aerobic exercise on anxiety sensitivity. *Behavior Research and Therapy*, 42, 125–136.

Brown, C. S., Rakel, R. E., Well, B. G., Downs, J. M., & Akiskal, H. S. (1991). A practical update on anxiety disorders and their pharmacologic treatment. *Archives of Internal Medicine*, 151, 873–884.

Bruce, S. E., Vasile, R. G., Goisman, R. M., Salzman, C., Spencer, M., Macham, J. J., et al. (2003). Are benzodiazepines still the medication of choice for patients with panic disorder with or without agoraphobia? *American Journal of Psychiatry, 160*, 1432–1438.

Chambless, D. L., Caputo, G. C., Bright, P., & Gallagher, R. (1984). Assessment of fear in agoraphobia: The Body Sensations Questionnaire and the Agoraphobic Questionnaire. *Journal of Consulting and Clinical Psychology, 52*, 1090–1097.

Charney, D. S., Heninger, G. R., & Breier, A. (1984). Noradrenergic function of panic anxiety: Effects of yohimbine in healthy subjects and patients with agoraphobia and panic disorder. *Archives of General Psychiatry, 41*, 751–763.

Chouinard, G. (2004). Issues in clinical use of benzodiazepines: Potency, withdraw and rebound. *Journal of Clinical Psychiatry, 65*(Suppl. 5), 7–12.

Clark, D. M. (1986). A cognitive approach to panic. *Behaviour Research and Therapy, 24*, 461–470.

Clark, D. M., & Ehlers, A. (1993). An overview of the theory and treatment of panic. *Applied and Preventive and Preventive Psychology, 2*, 131–139.

Clark, D. M., Salkovskis, P. M., & Chalkley, A. J. (1985). Respiratory control as a treatment for panic attacks. *Journal of Behavior Therapy and Experimental Psychiatry, 16*, 23–30.

Cloos, J. M. (2005). The treatment of panic disorder. *Current Opinion in Psychiatry, 18*(1), 45–50.

Clum, G. A. (1990). *Coping with panic.* Pacific Grove, CA: Brooks/Cole.

Cohen, A. S., Barlow, D. H., & Blanchard, E. B. (1985). Psychophysiology of relaxation-associated panic attacks. *Journal of Abnormal Psychology, 94*, 96–101.

Craske, M. G., & Barlow, D. H. (1990). *Therapist guide for the mastery of anxiety and panic.* Albany: University of Albany, State University of New York, Center for Stress and Anxiety Disorders.

Crowe, R. R., Noyes, R., Pauls, D. L., & Slymen, D. J. (1983). A family study of panic disorder. *Archives of General Psychiatry, 40*, 1065–1069.

DaCosta, J. M. (1871). On irritable heart: A clinical study of a functional cardiac disorder and its consequences. *American Journal of Medical Science, 61*, 17–52.

Dager, S. R., Cowley, D. S., & Dunner, D. L. (1987). Biological markers in panic states: Lactate-induced panic and mitral valve prolapse. *Biological Psychiatry, 22*, 339–359.

Dattilio, F. M. (1986). Differences in cognitive responses to fear among individuals diagnosed as panic disorder, generalized anxiety disorder, agoraphobia with panic attacks and simple phobia. *Dissertation Abstracts International, 48*, O3A.

Dattilio, F. M. (1987). The use of paradoxical intention in the treatment of panic attacks. *Journal of Counseling and Development, 66*, 66–67.

Dattilio, F. M. (1990). Symptom induction and de-escalation in the treatment of panic attacks. *Journal of Mental Health Counseling, 12*(4), 515–519.

Dattilio, F. M. (1992a). Interoceptive sensations during sexual arousal and panic. *The Behavior Therapist, 15*(9), 231–233.

Dattilio, F. M. (1992b). "The SAEB system"—Crises intervention techniques with panic. In *Crisis intervention*, symposium presented at the 26th annual meeting of the Association for the Advancement of Behavior Therapy, Boston.

Dattilio, F. M. (1994a). SAEB: A method of conceptualization in the treatment of panic. *Cognitive and Behavioral Practice, 1*(1), 179–191.

Dattilio, F. M. (1994b). *The use of the SAEB system and symptom induction in the treatment of panic* [Videotape, 58 minutes]. Bristol, PA: Taylor & Francis.

Dattilio, F. M. (1994c). Paradoxical intention as a proposed alternative in the treatment of panic disorder. *Journal of Cognitive Psychotherapy, 8*(1), 33–40.

Dattilio, F. M. (2005, Spring). Anxiety tremors in a 13½-year-old female with idiopathic Parkinson's disease. *Journal of Neuropsychiatry and Clinical Neuroscience, 17*(2), 9–12.

Dattilio, F. M., & Berchick, R. M. (1992). Panic disorder with agoraphobia. In A. Freeman & F.

M. Dattilio (Eds.), *Comprehensive casebook of cognitive therapy* (pp. 89–98). New York: Plenum Press.

Dattilio, F. M., & Castaldo J. E. (2001). Differentiating symptoms of anxiety from relapse of Gullian-Barré Syndrome. *Harvard Review of Psychiatry, 9,* 260–265.

Dattilio, F. M., & Castaldo, J. E. (2006). Differentiating cognitive impairment from symptoms of anxiety in coronary artery bypass grafting encephalopathy. *Neuropsychiatric Disease and Treatment, 2*(1).

Dattilio, F. M., & Kendall, P. C. (1994). Panic disorder. In F. M. Dattilio & A. Freeman (Eds.), *Cognitive-behavioral strategies in crisis intervention* (pp. 46–66). New York: Guilford Press.

Dattilio, F. M., & Kendall, P. C. (2000). Panic disorder in F. M. Dattilio & A. Freeman (Eds.), *Cognitive-behavioral strategies in crisis intervention* (2nd ed., pp. 59–83). New York: Guilford Press.

Dattilio, F. M., & Salas-Auvert, J. A. (1999). Heart attack or panic attack? *ADAA Reporter, X*(3), 1–3.

Dattilio, F. M., & Salas-Auvert, J. A. (2000). *Panic disorder: Assessment and treatment through a wide-angle lens.* Phoenix, AZ: Zeig/Tucker.

Dell, P. F. (1981). Some irreverent thoughts on paradox. *Family Process, 20,* 37–42.

Diez, C., Gastó, C., & Vallejo, J. (1989). Desarrollo de conductas de evitación en un sujeto concrise de angustia anipicas [Development of behavioral avoidance in a subject with atypical anxiety crisis]. *Revista de Psiquíatría de la Facultad de Medicina de Barcelona, 16*(6), 329–332.

DiNardo, P. A., Barlow, D. H., Cerny, J., Vermilyea, B. B., Vermilyea, J. A., Himadi, W., et al. (1985). *Anxiety Disorders Interview Schedule—Revised (ADIS-R).* Albany: Phobia and Anxiety Disorders Clinic, State University of New York at Albany.

Dowd, E. T., & Trutt, S. D. (1988). Paradoxical interventions in behavior modification. In M. Hersen, C. Eisler, & D. Miller (Eds.), *Progress in behavior modification* (Vol. 12, pp. 96–130). New York: Pergamon Press.

Dunner, D. L. (1985). Anxiety and panic: Relationship to depression and cardiac disorders. *Psychosomatics, 26,* 18–21.

Edinger, J. D., & Jacobsen, R. (1982). Incidence and significance of relaxation treatment side effects. *The Behavior Therapist, 5,* 137–138.

Efran, J. S., & Caputo, C. (1984). Paradox in psychotherapy: A cybernetic perspective. *Journal of Behavior Therapy and Experimental Psychiatry, 15*(3), 235–240.

Ehlers, A., & Breuer, P. (1992). Increased cardiac awareness in panic disorder. *Journal of Abnormal Psychology, 101*(3), 371–382.

Epstein, N. B., & Dutton, S. S. (1997, November). *Relationship characteristics of agoraphobics and their partners.* Paper presented at the 31st annual meeting of the Association for Advancement of Behavior Therapy, Miami, FL.

Feske, U., & Goldstein, A. J. (1997). Eye movement desensitization and reprocessing treatment for panic disorder: A controlled outcome and partial dismantling study. *Journal of Consulting and Clinical Psychology, 65*(6), 1–10.

Frankl, V. E. (1975). Paradoxical intention and de-reflection. *Psychotherapy: Theory, Research and Practice, 12,* 226–237.

Frankl, V. E. (1984). Paradoxical intention. In G. R. Weeks (Ed.), *Promoting change through paradoxical therapy* (pp. 36–48). Homewood, IL: Dow Jones-Irwin.

Goldenberg, H. (1983). *Contemporary clinical psychology.* Pacific Grove, CA: Brooks/Cole.

Goldstein, A. J., & Feske, U. (1994). Eye movement desensitization and reprocessing for panic disorder: A case series. *Journal of Anxiety Disorders, 8,* 351–362.

Goldstein, R. B., Wickramaratne, P. J., Horwath, E., & Weissman, M. M. (1997). Familial aggregation and phenomenology of "early onset" (at or before age 20 years) panic disorder. *Archives of General Psychiatry, 54,* 271–278.

Gould, R. A., Otto, M. W., & Pollack, M. H. (1995). A meta-analysis of treatment outcome for panic disorder. *Clinical Psychology Review, 8,* 819–844.

Gould, R. A., Clum, G. A., & Shapiro, D. (1993). The use of bibliotherapy in the treatment of panic: A preliminary investigation. *Behavior Therapy, 24,* 241–252.

Gray, J. A. (1982). *The neuropsychology of anxiety.* Oxford, UK: Clarendon.

Greenberg, R. L. (1989). Panic disorder and agoraphobia. In J. Scott, J. M. G. Williams, & A. T. Beck (Eds.), *Cognitive therapy in clinical practice: An illustrative casebook* (pp. 25–49). London: Routledge & Kegan Paul.

Hamilton, S. P., Heiman, G. A., Haghighi, F. G., Mick, S., Klein, D. F., Hodge, S. E., et al. (1999). Lack of genetic linkage or association between functional serotonin transporter polymorphism and panic disorder. *Psychiatric Genetics, 9,* 1–6.

Heide, F. J., & Borkovec, T. D. (1983). Relaxation-induced anxiety: Paradoxical anxiety enhancement due to relaxation training. *Journal of Consulting and Clinical Psychology, 51,* 171–182.

Hibbert, G. A. (1984). Hyperventilation as a cause of panic attacks. *British Medical Journal, 288,* 263–264.

Himadi, W. G., Boice, R., & Barlow, D. H. (1986). Assessment of agoraphobia—II: Measurement of clinical change. *Behaviour Research and Therapy, 24*(3), 321–332.

Katon, W. (1992). *Panic disorder in the medical setting.* Rockville, MD: National Institute of Mental Health.

Katon, W., & Kleinman, A. M. (1980). Doctor-patient negotiation and other social science strategies in patient care. In L. Eisenberg & A. M. Kleinman (Eds.), *The relevance of social science for medicine* (pp. 253–259). Dordrecht, the Netherlands: D. Reidel.

Kendall, P. C., & Hammen, R. (1999). *Abnormal psychology.* Boston: Houghton-Mifflin.

Kendall, P. C., & Norton-Ford, J. D. (1982). *Clinical psychology: Scientific and professional dimensions.* New York: Wiley.

Kerr, W. J., Dalton, J. W., & Gliebe, P. A. (1937). Some physical phenomena associated with anxiety states and their relation to hyperventilation. *Annals of Internal Medicine, 11,* 961–992.

Kiselica, M. S., & Baker, S. B. (1992). Progressive muscle relaxation and cognitive restructuring: Potential problems and proposed solutions. *Journal of Mental Health Counseling, 14*(2), 149–165.

Knowles, J. A., Fyer, A. J., Vieland, V. J., Weissman, M. M., Hodge, S. E., Heiman, G. A., et al. (1998). Results of a genome-wide genetic screen for panic disorder. *American Journal of Genetics, 81,* 139–147.

Knowles, J. A., & Weissman, M. M. (1995). Panic disorder and agoraphobia. In J. M. Oldham & M. B. Riba (Eds.), *Review of psychiatry* (Vol. 14, pp. 383–404). Washington, DC: American Psychiatric Press.

Kocmur, M., & Zavasnik, A. (1991, April). Patients' experience of the therapeutic process in a crisis intervention unit. *Crises, 12*(1), 69–81.

Lange, A., & Van Dyck, R. (1992). The function of agoraphobia in marital relationship. *Acta Psychiatrica Scandinavica, 85,* 89–93.

Lazarus, A. A., & Mayne, T. J. (1990). Relaxation: Some limitations, side effects and proposed solutions. *Psychotherapy, 27*(2), 261–266.

Leahy, R. L. (2005). Panic, agoraphobia, and generalized anxiety. In N. Kazantzis, F. P. Deane, K. R. Ronan, & L. L'Abate (Eds.), *Using homework assignments in cognitive-behavior therapy* (pp. 193–218). New York: Routledge.

Ley, R. A. (1985). Blood, breath and fears: A hyperventilation theory of panic attacks and agoraphobia. *Clinical Psychology Review, 5,* 271–285.

Ley, R. A. (1986). Hyperventilation and lactate infusion in the production of panic attacks. *Clinical Psychology Review, 8,* 1–18.

Lidrin, D. M., Watkins, P., Gould, R. A., Clum, G. A., Asterino, M., & Tulloch, H. L. (1994). A comparison of bibliotherapy and group therapy in the treatment of panic disorder. *Journal of Consulting and Clinical Psychology, 62,* 865–869.

Liebowitz, M. R., Fryer, A. B., & Goman, J. M. (1986). Alprazolam in the treatment of panic disorder. *Journal of Clinical Psychopharmacology, 6,* 13–20.

Lum, L. (1981). Hyperventilation and anxiety state. *Journal of the Royal Society of Medicine, 74,* 1–4.

Lydiard, R. B., & Ballenger, T. C. (1987). Antidepressants in panic disorder and agoraphobia. *Journal of Affective Disorders, 13,* 153–168.

Margraf, J., & Ehlers, A. (1989). Etiology models of panic: Medical and biological aspects. In R. Baker (Ed.), *Panic disorder: Theory, research, and therapy.* Chichester, UK: Wiley.

Mavissakalian, M. R. (2003). Imipramine vs. sertraline in panic disorder: 24-week treatment completers. *Annals of Clinical Psychiatry, 15,* 171–180.

Meuret, A. E., Wilhem, F. H., & Roth, W. T. (2004). Respiratory feedback for treating panic disorder. *Journal of Clinical Psychology, 60,* 197–207.

Oppenheimer, B. S., & Rothschild, M. A. (1918). The psychoneurotic factor in irritable heart of soldiers. *Journal of the American Medical Association, 70,* 1919–1922.

Ottaviani, R., & Beck, A. T. (1987). Cognitive aspects of panic disorders. *Journal of Anxiety Disorders, 1,* 15–28.

Pitts, F. N., & McClure, J. N. (1967). Lactate metabolism in anxiety neurosis. *New England Journal of Medicine, 277,* 1329–1336.

Prince, M., & Putnam, J. J. (1912). A clinical study of a case of phobia: A symposium. *Journal of Abnormal Social Psychology, 7,* 259–292.

Raskin, M., Peeke, H. V., Dickman, W., & Pinsker, H. (1982). Panic and generalized anxiety disorders: Developmental antecedents and precipitants. *Archives of General Psychiatry, 39,* 687–689.

Regier, D. A., Boyd, J. H., Burke, J. D., Rae, D. S., Myers, J. K., Kramer, M., et al. (1988). One-month prevalence of mental disorders in the United States: Based on five epidemiologic catchment area sites. *Archives of General Psychiatry, 45,* 977–986.

Reiss, S., Peterson, R. A., Gursky, D. M., & McNally, R. J. (1986). Anxiety sensitivity, anxiety frequency and the prediction of fearfulness. *Behaviour Research and Therapy, 24,* 1–8.

Riedere, P., Lachenmayer, L., & Laux, G. (2004). Clinical applications of MAO-inhibitors. *Current Medical Chemistry, 11,* 2033–2043.

Roberts, A. R. (Eds.). (1990). *Crises intervention handbook: Assessment, treatment and research.* Belmont, CA: Wadsworth.

Rosenman, R. H. (1985). The impact of anxiety on the cardiovascular system. *Psychosomatics, 26,* 6–17.

Roy-Byrne, P., Craske, M. G., Stein, M. B., Sullivan, G., Bystritsky, A., Katon, W., et al. (2005). A randomized effectiveness trial of cognitive-behavioral therapy and medication for primary care panic disorder. *Archives of General Psychiatry, 62*(3), 290–298.

Sexton, T. L., Montgomery, D., Goff, K., & Nugent, W. (1993). Ethical, therapeutic and legal considerations in the use of paradoxical techniques: The emerging debate. *Journal of Mental Health Counseling, 15*(3), 260–277.

Shapiro, F. (1996). Eye movement desensitization and reprocessing: Evaluation of controlled PTSD research. *Journal of Behavior Therapy and Experimental Psychiatry, 27,* 209–218.

Shapiro, F. (1998). Eye movement desensitization and reprocessing (EMDR): Historical context, recent research, and future directions. In L. VandeCreek & T. Jackson (Eds.), *Innovations in clinical practice: A sourcebook* (Vol. 16, pp. 211–217). Sarasota, FL: Professional Resource Press.

Shapiro, F., & Forrest, M. S. (1997). *EMDR: The breakthrough therapy.* New York: Basic Books.

Sharp, D. M., Power, K. G., & Simpson, R. J. (1996). Fluvoxamine, placebo, and cognitive behaviour therapy used alone and in combination in the treatment of panic disorder and agoraphobia. *Journal of Anxiety Disorder, 10,* 219–242.

Sheehan, D. V. (1982). Panic attacks and phobias. *New England Journal of Medicine, 307,* 156–158.

Skerrit, P. W. (1983). Anxiety and the heart—A historical review. *Psychological Medicine, 13,* 17–25.

Skolnick, P., & Paul, S. M. (1983). New concepts in the neurobiology of anxiety. *Journal of Clinical Psychiatry, 44,* 12–19.

Solkol, L., Beck, A. T., Greenberg, R. L., Wright, F. D., & Berchick, R. J. (1989). Cognitive therapy of panic disorder: A nonpharmacological alternative. *Journal of Nervous and Mental Disease, 177,* 711–716.

Spitzer, R. L., & Williams, J. B. W. (1986). *Structured Clinical Interview for DSM-III-R, Upjohn Version (SCID-UP-R).* New York: New York State Psychiatric Institute, Biometrics Research.

Starcevic, V., Linden, M., & Uhlenhuth, E. H. (2004). Treatment of panic disorder with agoraphobia in an anxiety disorders clinic: Factors influencing psychiatrists' treatment choices. *Psychiatry Residency, 125,* 41–52.

Svensson, T. H. (1987). Peripheral, autonomic regulation of locus coeruleus noradrenergic neurons in the brain: Putative implications for psychiatry and psychopharmacology. *Psychopharmacology, 92,* 1–7.

Swinson, R. P., Soulios, C., Cox, B. J., & Kuch, K. (1992). Brief treatment of emergency room patients with panic attacks. *American Journal of Psychiatry, 149,* 944–946.

Telch, M. J., Lucas, J. A., Schmidt, N. B., Hanna, H. H., Jaimez, T. L., & Lucas, R. A. (1993). Group cognitive-behavioral treatment of panic disorder. *Behaviour Research and Therapy, 31*(3), 279–287.

Thorpe, G. L., & Burns, L. E. (1983). *The agorgaphobic syndrome.* New York: Wiley.

Von Korff, M., Shapiro, S., Burke, J. D., Teitelbaum, M., Skinner, E. A., German, P., et al. (1987). Anxiety and depression in a primary care clinic: Comparison of Diagnostic Interview Schedule, General Health Questionnaire, and practitioner assessments. *Archives of General Psychiatry, 44,* 152–156.

Wardle, J. (1990). Behavior therapy and benzodiazepines: Allies or antagonists? *British Journal of Psychiatry, 156,* 163–168.

Wayne, G. J. (1966). The psychiatric emergency: An overview. In G. J. Wayne & R. R. Koegler (Eds.), *Emergency psychiatric and brief therapy* (p. 321). Boston: Little, Brown.

Weiss, S. R. B., & Uhde, T. W. (1990). Annual models of anxiety. In J. C. Ballanger (Ed.), *Neurobiology of panic disorder* (pp. 3–27). New York: Wiley-Liss.

Weissman, M. M. (1993). Family genetic studies of panic disorder. *Journal of Psychiatric Research, 27*(Suppl. 1), 69–78.

Weissman, M. M., & Merikangas, K. R. (1986, June). The epidemiology of anxiety and panic disorders: An update. *Journal of Clinical Psychiatry, 47*(Suppl. 1), 1–7.

Westphal, C. (1871). Die Agoraphobie, eine Neuropathische Erscheinung [Agoraphobia, a neurological discovery]. *Archiv für Psychiatrie und Nervenkrankheiten, 3,* 138–161.

White, J., Keenan, M., & Brooks, N. (1992). Stress control: A controlled comparative investigation of large group therapy for generalized anxiety disorder. *Behavioral Psychotherapy, 20,* 97–114.

Wilson, R. (1986). *Don't panic: Taking control of anxiety attacks.* New York: Rawson.

Wolpe, J. (1958). *Psychotherapy by reciprocal inhibition.* Stanford, CA: Stanford University Press.

Zitrin, C. M., Klein, D. F., & Woerner, M. G. (1978). Behavior therapy, supportive psychotherapy, Imipramine and phobias. *Archives of General Psychiatry, 35,* 107–116.

Zung, W. W. K. (1975). A rating instrument for anxiety disorders. *Psychosomatics, 12,* 371–
    379.

SUGGESTED READINGS

Dattilio, F. M. (1994a). SAEB: A method of conceptualization in the treatment of panic. *Cognitive and Behavioral Practice, 1*(1), 179–191.
Dattilio, F. M., & Salas-Auvert, J. A. (2000). *Panic disorder: Assessment and intervention through a wide-angle lens.* Phoenix, AZ: Zeig/Tucker.
Wilson, R. (1986). *Don't panic: Taking control of anxiety attacks.* New York: Rawson.

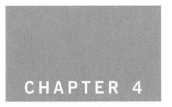

CHAPTER 4

Crisis Intervention Strategies for Treating Law Enforcement and Mental Health Professionals

Laurence Miller

So you *still* think helping people is easy, rewarding, and/or professionally satisfying? Well, it's still one hell of a way to make a living. Just ask a cop. Just ask yourself. Those of us in the public safety and mental health fields know that our clientele often do not welcome our interventions, do not follow our directions, and then blame us when things go wrong. Alternatively, they become desperate for our help and sometimes seem so needy that it feels like nothing we can do will make dent in their travail.

In training both police officers and mental health crisis professionals, I am struck by the similarities in what these two groups of professionals do on a daily basis (Miller, 2006b). For one thing, we both spend most of our time dealing with the outer reaches of human nature. That is why I usually begin my police academy classes by telling the officers:

"We both do the same kind of work, only I have the easy job. That is, we both deal with extremes of human emotion and behavior, but I get to do it in the relatively secure confines of an office or clinic, while you have to do it on the street. My customers are frequently challenging, sometimes annoying, occasionally threatening, but rarely overtly dangerous; your customers may kill you. I often have to make tricky diagnostic determinations and decide on an appropriate course of action, and so do you. But I typically have the luxury of hours or days to pore over records and interview my patient in a quiet room; you have to make a snap decision under noisy, confusing, or hazardous conditions. If I'm wrong, I can usually go back and try something else; if you're wrong, people may be injured or killed."

Is it any wonder that many of our colleagues in both the law enforcement and emergency mental health fields stress out, burn out, or are driven out of the crisis-response field altogether? Before this happens, though, we ought to offer—and take—a dose of our own medicine and apply the skills and techniques we use for others to our own wounded ranks. We do what we do, after all, because crisis intervention and trauma work involve the use of sharply honed action-oriented skills combined with concern for the human community. Stressful work is going to produce stress effects. Effectively helping the helpers is perhaps the greatest form of collegial and interdisciplinary respect (Miller, 1995, 1998a, 1998c).

Accordingly, this chapter describes the particular stresses and intervention strategies for two special groups of helpers that are most often on the front lines of crisis intervention: law enforcement and mental health professionals (Miller, 1994, 1998a, 1998c, 1999a, 1999c, 1999d, 2000a, 2003b).

STRESS AND COPING IN CRISIS INTERVENTION AND PUBLIC SAFETY PROFESSIONALS

Law Enforcement

Police officers regularly deal with the most violent, impulsive, and predatory members of society, putting their lives on the line and handling traumatic crises that most of us view from the sanitized distance of our newspapers and TV screens. In addition to the daily grind, officers are frequently the targets of criticism and complaints by citizens, the media, the judicial system, opportunistic politicians, hostile attorneys, "do-gooder" clinicians and social service workers, and their own administrators and law enforcement agencies (Blau, 1994; Miller, 1995, 2005a, 2006b).

While police officers generally carry out their sworn duties and responsibilities with competence and dedication, the stress load may sometimes be too much to handle, and every officer has his/her breaking point. For some, it may come in the form of a particular dramatic event, such as a gruesome accident or homicide, a vicious crime against a child, a close personal brush with death, the killing or wounding of a partner, the mistaken shooting of an innocent civilian, or an especially grisly accident or crime scene.

For other officers, there may be no single major trauma, but the identified mental breakdown occurs under the cumulative weight of a number of more moderate stresses over the course of the officer's career. In either case, an officer may feel that the department does not support him/her and that there is nowhere else to vent his/her frustration and distress. So the officer bottles up his/her feelings, becomes surly with coworkers and civilians, and grows hypersensitive to small annoyances on and off the job. As his/her isolation and feelings of alienation grow, health and home life begin to deteriorate, work becomes a burden, and the officer may ultimately feel that he is los-ing his mind, or going "squirrelly" (McCafferty, McCafferty, & McCafferty, 1992; Russell & Beigel, 1990).

Most police officers deal with both routine and exceptional stresses by using a variety of situationally adaptive coping and defense mechanisms, such as repression, displacement, isolation of feelings, humor, or just clamming up and toughing it out. Officers develop a closed society, and insular "cop culture" centering around "the job." Part of this closed-society credo is based on the shared belief that no civilian or outsider could possibly understand what police officers go through on a day-to-day basis (Anderson, Swenson, & Clay, 1995; Blau, 1994; Miller, 2006b; Woody, 2005).

According to one estimate (Sewell, Ellison, & Hurrell, 1988), after a traumatically stressful incident, such as a shooting, approximately one-third of officers have minimal or no problems, another third have moderate problems, and the final third have severe problems affecting the officer, his/her family, and the department. More recently, it has been debated whether police trauma produces an inordinate number of stress dis-abilities compared to other professions (Curran, 2003), but most authorities agree that stress reactions of some type are common. Surprisingly, however, despite the popular notion of rampantly disturbed police marriages, the empirical evidence does not sup-port a higher-than-average divorce rate for police officers than for a demographically matched population (Borum & Philpot, 1993; Miller, 1995, 2006b, 2007).

Up to two-thirds of police officers involved in shootings experience significant emotional reactions, which include a heightened sense of danger, flashbacks, intrusive imagery and thoughts, anger, guilt, sleep disturbances, withdrawal, depression, and other stress symptoms. But police often overlook the cumulative effect of more ordi-nary stressors, such as long overtime hours during disasters, dealing with child victims, attempting resuscitation on a victim who dies, or working a fatal accident scene where the officer knows the victim. Failure to resolve these issues often leads to a variety of maladaptive response patterns. Some officers begin to overreact to perceived or imag-ined threats, while others ignore clear danger signals. Some cops quit the force prema-turely, while others become discipline problems or show increased absenteeism, impaired work performance, stress disorders, substance abuse, or a host of other per-sonal problems that can interfere with functioning at home and on the job (Solomon, 1995; Solomon & Horn, 1986).

In some cases, the untreated aftereffects of a traumatic incident may persist for months or years in the form of anger, hostility, irritability, conflicts with authority, fatigue, impaired concentration, loss of self-confidence, or increased indulgence in food or substances. Many of these long-term effects interfere with work performance and threaten the stability of personal relationships. Ultimately, they may be responsi-ble for early retirement, burnout, or, in rare cases, suicide (Bohl, 1995; Cummings, 1996; Miller, 2005b, 2006a; Regehr & Bober, 2004).

In other cases, the delayed or prolonged stress reaction manifests itself in the form of "psychosomatic" symptoms such as headaches, chronic musculoskeletal pain syn-dromes, stomachaches, heart palpitations, or breathing disturbances. Typically, physi-cal symptoms are easier to justify as a cause of stress-related disability than "mental problems" for police officers, rescue workers, and others who are invested in their sense of toughness and resilience (Benedikt & Kolb, 1986; Hall, 1986; McFarlane, Atchison, Rafalowicz, & Papay, 1994; Miller, 1995, 1999b; Regehr & Bober, 2004; Toch, 2002; Woody, 2005).

Special pressures are experienced by higher-ranking officers, such as homicide detectives, especially those who are involved in the investigation of particularly brutal crimes, such as multiple murders or serial killings (Sewell, 1993). The normally expected societal protective role of the police officer becomes heightened at the same time as their responsibilities as public servants who protect individual rights become compounded by the pressures to solve the crime.

A multiple murder investigation forces an officer to confront stressors directly related to his/her projected role and image of showing unflagging strength in the face of adversity and frustration, responding competently and dispassionately to crises, and placing the needs and demands of the public above personal feelings. Moreover, the sheer magnitude and shock effect of many mass-murder scenes and the violence, muti-lation, and sadism associated with many serial killings, sometimes involving children, often exceed the defense mechanisms and coping capacities of even the most seasoned and hard-boiled investigator. Revulsion may be tinged with rage, all the more so when fellow officers have been killed or injured, or when the killer is known but the existing evidence is insufficient to support an arrest or conviction. The cumulative effect of fatigue compounds the problem, leading to case errors, deteriorating work quality, and the wearing down of the investigator's normal defenses, rendering him or her even more vulnerable to stress and burnout (Sewell, 1993).

Mental Health Clinicians

Doing crisis intervention and trauma therapy is not for the faint of heart; it is tough, demanding work that can take an exhausting toll on practitioners. If that were not enough, crisis therapy can be a dangerous profession, especially when caseloads include severely disturbed, potentially violent patients, usually seen in institutional psychiatric and forensic settings, but increasingly turning up in routine clinical practice as the demographics of 21st-century mental health practice continue to shift. Thera-pists and mental health care professionals are often threatened, sometimes stalked, and occasionally assaulted. Some are seriously injured, and a few of our colleagues have been killed (Miller, 1998a, 1998c).

Clinicians who work on a regular basis with traumatized patients and people in crisis may be subject to special stresses. Trauma workers are surrounded by the extreme intensity of trauma-inducing events and their aftermaths. Figley (1995) identi-fies several reasons why trauma therapists are especially vulnerable to what he terms *compassion fatigue*. First, empathy is a major personal resource for trauma workers to help the traumatized. While the process of empathizing with the trauma victim and family members helps to understand their experience, therapists themselves may be traumatized in the process. Second, many trauma therapists have experienced some traumatic event in their lives, and this unresolved trauma may be activated by reports of similar traumas in patients. There is thus a danger of the crisis worker's overgeneralizing from his/her own experiences and methods of coping, and overpromoting those methods with patients. Finally, special stresses are involved in working with traumatized children, where the identification factor is always high (James, 1989; Johnson, 1989; Miller, 1998b, 1999a, 1999c, 2000b; Miller & Schlesinger, 2000). In fact, the most stressful critical incident calls for police and emergency services personnel almost always involve injured children (Miller, 1995, 1998c, 2003b).

As the therapist begins to lose his/her objectivity and overidentify with patients, depression may develop. The therapist may start to "not give a damn" about patients—or anyone else. Therapists may be relieved when "difficult" patients cancel sessions (Moon, 1999). Crisis clinicians may walk around in fear and dread of their beepers and cell phones going off, announcing the next emergency they must respond to. The stress effects may spill over into the therapist's family life as he/she becomes more withdrawn and emotionally unavailable (Cerney, 1995). Alternatively, other therapists may become "trauma junkies," increasingly reinforced by the lurid thrill of working with such dramatic cases, but in the process sacrificing their clinical objectivity and effectiveness (Yassen, 1995).

McCann and Pearlman (1990) coined the term *vicarious traumatization* to describe the transformation that occurs within the therapist as a consequence of empathic engagement with patients' trauma experiences and their sequelae. These effects usually do not arise solely from one therapy relationship but are cumulative across time and number of helping relationships. The *burnout* literature (Ackerly, Burnell, Holder, & Kurdek, 1988; Deutsch, 1984; Gilliland & James, 1993; Pearlman & MacIan, 1995; Robinette, 1987; Rodolfa, Kraft, & Reiley, 1988) suggests that being younger or newer to trauma work is associated with the highest levels of burnout. As in any field, a certain selection process seems to operate in terms of personality structure, temperament, and cognitive style, so that a delicate balance emerges, in terms of clinical effectiveness, between being too fresh and callow versus being too encrusted and emotionally shriveled (Miller, 1993, 2003a).

Talbot, Dutton, and Dunn (1995) describe some of the distinctive features that make trauma and crisis work stressful for psychotherapists. First, there is the urgency and immediacy of the response. The crisis response is usually of an outreach or in-the-field nature, which means that the therapist has little or no control over many aspects of the situation: when it happens, where it happens, who will be there, and what services will be required. Typically, there is no advance notice, little time to prepare, limited time for individual interventions, lack of space, and unfamiliar, even dangerous surroundings.

In a crisis, therapists need to be able to work speedily and effectively to stabilize the situation. The cumulative volume of the work, both in terms of the number of people requiring attention in any one crisis and numerous successive crises, can exert a debilitating effect. In addition, emotional intensity is high and victims are often in a regressed and decompensated state. Victims themselves may perceive therapeutic interventions as intrusive and become resistant or hostile. Clinicians accustomed to structured therapeutic interactions may find themselves feeling overwhelmed when confronted by trauma victims whose needs are largely for basic empathy and containment. Often there is nothing to do but listen, and even this may be an extremely difficult task under chaotic circumstances. Also, there is typically little or no history regarding the precrisis or premorbid functioning of the victims. The crisis often occurs within an organizational context (e.g., the criminal justice system), that makes particular demands on first responders, which may be at odds with the needs and wishes of the victim or the clinician (Talbot et al., 1995).

The stresses of crisis intervention can affect mental health clinicians in a number of ways. In the aftermath of their interventions with victims of armed bank holdups, for example, clinicians often find themselves feeling isolated, angry, tense, confused, powerless, hopeless, anxious, emotionally exhausted, and overwhelmed with responsibility (Talbot et al., 1995). Patients' problems seem alternately insignificant or insurmountable, and the clinicians may begin to lose perspective and to overidentify with their patients. Clinicians may intellectualize, becoming overly rigid and inflexible in their thinking. Using denial as a protective strategy, clinicians are often unaware of the way in which the work has affected them, and the recollection among different emergencies becomes blurred.

These clinicians often feel exhausted, increase their alcohol use, suffer somatic symptoms such as headaches, gastrointestinal complaints, and sleep disturbances with nightmares, experience increased sensitivity to violence in general, and become emotionally demanding of family and friends. They become increasingly tense and distractible, expecting the phone to ring at any moment announcing yet another crisis or emergency (Talbot et al., 1995). As noted previously, we ought to be able to put our clinical money where our mouths are and see if we can effectively reach out to our colleagues in distress.

INTERVENTIONS WITH CRISIS INTERVENTION PERSONNEL: GENERAL CONSIDERATIONS

To avoid overly clinical-sounding connotations, mental health intervention services with emergency service and crisis personnel have often been conceptualized in such neutral terminology as *debriefing* or *stress management* (Anderson et al., 1995; Belles & Norvell, 1990; Miller, 1999e; Mitchell & Bray, 1990). In general, incident-specific, one-time interventions will be most appropriate for handling the effects of overwhelming trauma on otherwise normal, well-functioning personnel. Where posttraumatic sequelae persist, or where the psychological problems relate to a longer-term pattern of maladaptive functioning under relatively routine stresses, more extensive individual psychotherapeutic approaches are called for (Miller, 1995, 1998c, 2003b, 2006b).

CRITICAL INCIDENT STRESS DEBRIEFING

Although the "stress debriefing" approach has grown out of the general field of crisis intervention, and is an important element of all therapeutic work with traumatized patients, *critical incident stress debriefing* (CISD) has been organizationally formalized for law enforcement and emergency services primarily by Jeff Mitchell and his colleagues (Mitchell, 1983, 1988; Mitchell & Bray, 1990; Mitchell & Everly, 1996). CISD is now implemented in public safety departments throughout the United States, Britain, Europe, Australia, and other parts of the world (Dyregrov, 1989). CISD is often subsumed under the broader umbrella category of *critical incident stress management* (CISM), which includes a range of preventive and crisis intervention strategies, such as one-on-one defusings, large-scale demobilizations, and other approaches (Everly & Mitchell, 1997; Everly, Flannery, & Mitchell, 2000; Mitchell & Everly, 1996).

In many respects, CISD epitomizes the cognitive-behavioral approach to crisis intervention. It is a structured technique designed to promote the emotional processing of traumatic events through the ventilation and normalization of reactions, as well as preparation for possible future experiences (Everly & Mitchell, 1997; Mitchell & Everly, 1996). Flexible adaptations of CISD have included applications to individual, family, child, and group therapy (Everly et al., 2000; Johnson, 1989; Miller, 1998c, 1999e).

Structure of the Debriefings

A CISD typically is a peer-led, clinician-guided process, although the individual roles of clinicians and peers may vary from setting to setting. The staffing of a debriefing usually consists of one or more mental health professionals and one or more *peer debriefers*, that is, fellow police officers, firefighters, paramedics, or crisis clinicians who have been trained in the CISD process and who may have been through critical incidents and debriefings in their own careers.

A typical debriefing takes place within 24 to 72 hours after the critical incident and consists of a single group meeting that lasts 2 to 3 hours, although shorter or longer meetings may be dictated by circumstances. Group size may range from a handful to a roomful, the deciding factor usually being how many people will have time to fully express themselves in the number of hours allotted for the debriefing. Where large numbers of crisis workers are involved, such as in mass disaster rescues, several debriefings may be held successively over the course of days to accommodate all the personnel involved (Mitchell & Bray, 1990; Mitchell & Everly, 1996).

The formal CISD process consists of seven key phases:

1. *Introduction.* The introduction phase of a debriefing is the time in which the team leader—either a mental health professional or peer debriefer, depending on the composition of the group—gradually introduces the CISD process, encourages participation by the group, and sets the ground rules by which the debriefing will operate. Generally, these involve confidentiality, attendance for the full session, nonforced participation in discussions, and the establishment of a noncritical atmosphere.

2. *Fact phase.* During this phase, the group members are asked to briefly describe their job or role during the incident and, from their own perspective, provide some facts regarding what happened. The basic question is: "What did you do?"

3. *Thought phase.* The CISD leader asks the group members to discuss their first and subsequent thoughts during the critical incident: "What went through your mind?"

4. *Reaction phase.* This phase is designed to move the group participants from a predominantly cognitive and intellectual level of processing to a more emotionally expressive and cathartic mode: "What was the worst part of the incident for you?" It is usually at this point that the meeting gets intense, as members take their cue from one another ad begin to vent their distress. Clinicians and peer debriefers keep a keen eye out for any adverse reactions among the personnel.

5. *Symptom phase.* This begins the movement back from the predominantly emotional processing level to the cognitive mode. Participants are asked to describe cognitive, physical, emotional, and behavioral signs and symptoms of distress that appeared at the scene or within 24 hours of the incident; a few days after the incident; and continually, persisting even at the time of the debriefing. This allows for sharing and universalizing of potentially disorienting stress symptoms and reactions in a constructively intellectualized, problem-solving discussion. The question here is: "What have you been experiencing since the incident?"

6. *Education phase.* Continuing the move back toward cognitive processing, information is exchanged about the nature of the stress response and the expected physiological and psychological reactions to critical incidents. The clearest role for the mental health professional in this phase is as teacher and expert in traumatic stress effects. This serves to normalize the stress and coping responses and provides a basis for questions and answers.

7. *Reentry phase.* This is a wrap-up, during which any additional questions or statements are addressed, referral for individual follow-ups are made, and general group bonding is reinforced: "What have you learned?" "Is there anything positive that can come out of this experience that can help you grow personally or professionally?" "How can you help one another in the future?"

This is not to suggest that these phases always follow one another in unvarying, mechanical sequence. On the contrary, in practice I have found that once group participants feel comfortable with the debriefing process and start talking, the fact, thought, and reaction phases often blend together. Indeed, as Mitchell and Everly (1996) recognize, it would seem artificial and forced to abruptly interrupt someone expressing emotion just because it is not the "right phase." Initially, debriefings should adhere to the stepwise sequence, but as long as the basic rationale and structure of the debriefing are maintained, the therapeutic effect will usually result. In most cases, clinician-team leaders have to assertively step in only when emotional reactions become particularly intense, or where one or more group members begin to blame or criticize others.

Special Applications of CISD

For the past quarter century, the standard "Mitchell model" of CISD has been used with wide success all over the world, with diverse groups of emergency service, military, and civilian personnel (Everly & Mitchell, 1997; Everly et al., 2000; Miller, 1995, 1998c, 1999e, 2000a, 2005a, 2006b; Mitchell & Bray, 1990; Mitchell & Everly, 1996). In an effort to expand and refine its clinical applicability, in the past decade some new innovative adaptations of the basic CISD technique have begun to be applied in different settings and for diverse groups of crisis responders. This section describes some recent applications of the CISD approach to law enforcement and mental health professionals.

Law Enforcement

Police officers can be an insular group, often reluctant to talk to outsiders, especially "shrinks." They may be more resistant to showing weakness in front of their peers than are other emergency personnel. Officers typically work alone or with a partner, as opposed to firefighters and paramedics, who are trained to have more of a team mentality (Anderson et al., 1995; Blau, 1994; Kirschman, 1997; Peak, 2003; Reese, 1987; Solomon, 1995; Toch, 2002; Woody, 2005). This has led to some special adaptations of the CISD approach for law enforcement.

To keep the focus on the event itself and to minimize the singling out of individuals, many mental health and law enforcement professionals recommend that, following a critical incident, there be a policy of mandatory referral of all involved personnel to a debriefing or other appropriate mental health intervention (Horn, 1991; McMains, 1991; Mitchell, 1991; Reese, 1991; Solomon, 1988, 1990, 1995). The administrative policy should state that debriefings and other postincident interventions are confidential, the only exceptions being the usual duty-to-report considerations of danger to self or others, or disclosure of a serious crime. If such matters come up before, during, or after a debriefing, CISD team members should call the department psychologist or mental health services coordinator; this may be especially appropriate where the issue involves sensitive legal or political issues. Temporary administrative leave or light duty may be appropriate following high-profile situations, such as officer-involved shootings (Honig & Roland, 1998; Solomon, 1988, 1990, 1995).

When only one officer is involved in the critical incident (as in a shooting), or as a more focused, individualized follow-up to the general group debriefing, Solomon (1995) recommends that individual debriefings be conducted by a mental health professional. In an individual debriefing, the emotional impact of the incident is assessed and explored as thoughts, feelings, and reactions are discussed. A recommended format for individual debriefing sessions is to go over the incident "frame by frame" with the officer, while he/she verbalizes the moment-to-moment thoughts, perceptions, sensory details, feelings, and actions that occurred during the incident. This helps the officer become aware of, sort out, and understand what happened; get in touch with the perceptions and state of mind experienced during the incident; and understand why certain actions were taken or specific decisions were made. The frame-by-frame approach defuses inappropriate self-blame by helping the officer to differentiate what was under his/her control from what was not, and what was known at the time from what was impossible to know then but may appear painfully clear in hindsight (Solomon, 1990, 1995).

As a more general follow-up to standard debriefing for incidents that have had intense or wide-ranging psychological effects, Solomon (1995) recommends what he terms a *critical incident peer support seminar*, in which the involved officers come together for 2 or 3 days in a retreat-like setting to revisit their experience several months following the critical incident. The seminar is facilitated by mental health professionals and peer support officers.

Sewell (1993, 1994) has elaborated a CISD-type adaptation of the CISM model to the particular needs of homicide detectives who investigate multiple murders and other violent crimes. The major objectives of this process are (1) ventilation of intense emotions; (2) exploration of symbolic meanings; (3) group support under catastrophic conditions; (4) initiation of the grief process within a supportive environment; (5) reduction of the "fallacy of uniqueness"; (6) reassurance that intense emotions under catastrophic conditions are normal; (7) preparation for the continuation of the grief and stress process over the ensuing weeks and months; (8) preparing for the possible development of emotional, cognitive, and physical symptoms in the aftermath of a serious crisis; (9) education regarding normal and abnormal stress response syndromes; and (10) encouragement of continued group support and/or professional assistance.

Sewell (1994) regards such interventions as appropriate for two specific groups, at two specific times. First, the stress of the first responders who dealt with the trauma of the original scene must be confronted quickly and decisively. Second, the stress of involved investigators must be handled as needed throughout the course of the crime's investigation and prosecution. In the regular debriefing sessions, whether for the first responders or case investigators, attendance should be mandatory and must be supported by the brass. Where an officer needs additional debriefing or other mental health assistance, this should be administratively encouraged and nonstigmatized.

Perhaps the most comprehensive adaptation to date of the CISD process for law enforcement is the one by Bohl (1995), who explicitly compares and contrasts the phases in her program with the phases of the Mitchell model. In Bohl's program, the debriefing takes place as soon after the critical incident as possible. A debriefing may involve a single officer within the first 24 hours, later followed by a second, with a group debriefing taking place within 1 week to encourage bonding. This is to address the lower team orientation of most police officers who may not express feelings easily, even—or especially—in a group of their fellow officers.

The Bohl model makes no real distinction between the cognitive and emotional phases of a debriefing. If an officer begins to express emotion during the fact or cognitive phase, there is little point in telling him/her to stifle it until later. To be fair, as noted earlier, the Mitchell model certainly allows for flexibility and common sense in structuring debriefings, and both formats recognize the importance of responding empathically to the specific needs expressed by the individuals who attend the debriefing, rather than following an arbitrary set of rules.

In the emotion phase itself, what is important in the Bohl model is not the mere act of venting but, rather, the opportunity to validate feelings. Bohl does not ask what the "worst thing" was, because she finds the typical response of cops to be that "everything about it was the worst thing." However, it often comes as revelation to these law enforcement tough guys that their peers have had similar feelings. Still, some emotions may be difficult to validate. For example, guilt or remorse over actions or inactions may actually be appropriate, as when an officer's momentary hesitation or impulsive action resulted in someone getting hurt or killed. The question then becomes: "Okay, you think you screwed up, you feel guilty; now, what are you going to do with that guilt?" That is, "What can be learned from the experience to prevent something like this from happening again?"

The Bohl model inserts an additional debriefing phase, termed the *unfinished business phase*, which has no counterpart in the Mitchell model. Participants are asked, "What in the present situation reminds you of a past experience? Do you want to talk about that (those) other situation(s)?" This phase grew out of Bohl's observation that the incident that prompted the current debriefing often acts as a catalyst for recalling past events. Participants are reminded of prior critical incidents, probably none of which were followed by a formal debriefing. The questions give participants a chance to talk about incidents that may arouse strong and unresolved feelings. Bohl finds that such multilevel debriefings result in a greater sense of relief and closure than would occur by sticking solely to the present incident.

The education or teaching phase in the Bohl model resembles its Mitchell model counterpart in that participants are schooled about normal and abnormal stress reactions, how to deal with coworkers and family members, and what to anticipate in the near future. For example, an officer's child may have heard that his parent shot and killed a suspect and the child may be questioned or teased at school. How to deal with children's responses may therefore be an important part of this education phase (Anderson et al., 1995; Kirschman, 1997; Miller, 2007).

Unlike the Mitchell model, the Bohl model does not ask whether anything positive, hopeful, or growth-promoting has arisen from the incident. Officers who have seen their partners shot or killed, or who have had to deal with horrendous child abuse or other senseless brutality may find it difficult to see anything hopeful or positive in the experience, no matter how well they have handled this situation. Add to this the potential cumulative demoralization of past encounters with human nature's dark side, and it is understandable that expecting officers to extract some kind of "growth experience" from this kind of tragedy may seem like a sick joke. In my own experience, however, it seems to be the individual personality of the officer that contributes to postincident hope versus cynicism (Miller, 2003a).

A final non-Mitchell phase of the debriefing added by the Bohl model is the *round robin*. Each officer is invited to say anything he/she wants. The statement can be addressed to anyone, but others cannot respond directly; this is intended to give participants a feeling of safety. My own concern is that this may provide an opportunity for last-minute gratuitous sniping, which can chip away at the carefully crafted supportive atmosphere built up during the debriefing. In addition, in practice, there does not seem to be anything particularly unique about this round-robin phase to distinguish it from the standard reentry phase of the Mitchell model. Finally, adding more and more "phases" to the debriefing process may serve to decrease the forthrightness and spontaneity of its implementation. Again, clinical judgment and common sense should guide the process, but Bohl's (1995) model, as well as those of Sewell (1993, 1994) and Solomon (1988, 1990, 1995), represent important contributions toward tailoring the CISD approach to the specific needs of law enforcement. We need more research and more reports from the field.

Traumatized Psychotherapists

Concepts such as *vicarious traumatization* (McCann & Pearlman, 1990) and *compassion fatigue* (Figley, 1995) remind us of the cumulatively stressful effect on trauma therapists of working with successive cases of wounded and shattered patients. The very empathy we rely on to connect with our traumatized patients and establish a healing relationship also carries the risk of emotional contagion that may lead to therapeutic burnout or depression (Moon, 1999). Could applying a CISD approach to therapist critical incident stress provide a salubrious taste of our own medicine (Miller, 1998a)?

Talbot et al. (1995) argue that psychotherapists, more so than other crisis workers, require specifically "psychological" understanding and integration to be able to function and intervene effectively. These authors' own program (Manton & Talbot, 1990; Talbot et al., 1995) has evolved largely through their work with bank employee victims of armed holdups and the mental health clinicians who debrief them. In this model, the aim of *psychological debriefing* for mental health clinicians is to help them deal with the stresses of trauma work via ventilation, catharsis, and sharing of experiences, in order to achieve psychological mastery of the situation and prevent the development of more serious delayed stress syndromes. Particularly important for psychotherapists is the careful exploration of their identification with the victim's experience, which enables them to properly assimilate the burden of empathy. Finally, the therapists are helped to integrate the traumatic experience and make a transition back to everyday life.

In this model, the debriefing of the debriefers is attended by two or more psychologists who were not part of the original civilian debriefing; for clarity, I have referred to them as *secondary debriefers* (Miller, 1998a, 1998c). The therapist debriefing is held away from the crisis scene as soon as is practicable for all involved therapists to attend.

In Talbot et al.'s (1995) psychological debriefing model, the procedure incorporates the crisis event, the responses to that event by the psychologists, and the processes occurring in the debriefing itself. Its aim is to tie in and make sense of the crisis and the subsequent counseling so that a clear, total picture is formed. The secondary debriefer is consequently dealing with a number of different levels of the crisis: the event itself, the victims' responses to the event, the psychotherapists' responses to the event, the psychotherapists' responses to the victims, and each psychotherapist's personal and professional response to the events. In essence, the secondary debriefer assumes the role of clinical supervisor to help each therapist reach an understanding of the interventions that were made, assess those that were useful, explore possible alternatives, and decide on future actions.

The secondary debriefer needs to normalize the experiences of fearfulness and sadness that follow the traumatic event. Part of his/her responses may also involve what Talbot et al. call a *parallel process*, in which the psychotherapist is experiencing what the victims have experienced. Past unresolved issues may also come up, particularly if there have been violence or abuse experiences in the therapists' histories. Fully dealing with countertransference issues is usually beyond the scope of a single debriefing, but these should be followed up by further treatment if necessary (Maier & Van Ryboeck, 1995; Miller, 1998c).

In Talbot et al.'s (1995) system, to help make sense of the therapists' experiences in the original crisis and in the present debriefing, the secondary debriefer brings together his/her knowledge of the original crisis victims as individuals and as a group, and his/her understanding of the operative psychological processes. Because more psychological knowledge is often associated with more intellectualized and sophisticated defenses, the secondary debriefer, consistent with the supervisor-type role, may need to be somewhat more confrontive with the debriefed therapists than clinicians typically are with civilian victims or, for that matter, than debriefers might be with other crisis responders, such as police officers, firefighters, or paramedics. The ultimate goal is to tie in themes and personal issues, draw parallels, and put the incident into perspective.

Finally, as in a therapeutic session, the secondary debriefer needs to summarize, to contain, and to make sense of what occurred. Talbot et al. (1995) assert that it can be useful for the individual therapists to verbalize what they have gained and learned from working in the crisis and from the victim debriefings. To continue personally and professionally, psychotherapists need to have a sense of mastery of the experience, as well as the assurance of feeling valued, worthwhile, and positive about themselves and their work. Cognitive understanding and adaptive self-insight give psychotherapists mastery of the situation, objectivity, and a theoretical base from which to make interventions. This is essential for them to continue to function as effective trauma psychotherapists. The same recommendations apply to therapists in all specialties (Miller, 1992, 1993, 1998c).

Process Debriefing

As psychotherapists become more involved in the critical incident stress field, it is inevitable that we will see more psychologically sophisticated analyses of the cognitive-behavioral and psychodynamic processes involved in debriefing methods, along with more complex and nuanced intervention approaches. Ideally, this will not sacrifice the basic on-the-street adaptability and clinical user-friendliness of the stress debriefing model; indeed, it would be ironic if greater depth of understanding led to a more narrow range of practical applicability.

Dyregrov (1997) describes a CISD-type model of intervention that he terms *process debriefing*, incorporating the same basic structure as the Mitchell model but placing more emphasis on analyzing and addressing the group dynamics that actually take place in a debriefing. Characteristics of process debriefing include (1) strong mobilization of group support; (2) primary use of other group members to normalize reactions to stress; (3) active use of the group as a resource; (4) limiting the number of participants to 15 members per group; and (5) emphasis on the role of the group leader and coleader in providing a model of communication by the way they interact with one another.

In this sense, process debriefing seems to represent a species of cognitive-behavioral group therapy more than being a strict CISD approach. Indeed, while pointing out that formal mental credentials are no guarantee of therapeutic effectiveness, Dyregrov (1997) emphasizes the need for group leaders to have the necessary knowledge, training, and experience to positively influence the group experience. Accordingly, he cites several criteria for effective therapists, including sincerity in the helping relationship, provision of a safe and trusting atmosphere of nonpossessive warmth, and accurate, empathic, moment-by-moment understanding of the patient. Much of this will be familiar to practitioners of group therapy approaches (Courchaine & Dowd, 1994), and of course, much of the same criteria for clinical effectiveness apply to therapists in all areas of practice (Miller, 1993).

While a more intensive concern for group dynamics characterizes the content of process debriefing, the structure of the session itself stays fairly close to the Mitchell model, with some modifications. Dyregrov (1997) conceptualizes the nature and purpose of the introduction and fact phases of the debriefing in terms of an inclusive *relationship phase*, in which the trust, authority, and structure of the group are established. Other modifications include (1) the importance of pre-debriefing preparation by the leader and coleader, in terms of learning about the nature of the critical incident and the composition of the group; (2) an emphasis on the relationship between the leader and coleader during the debriefing in providing a model of healthy interaction; (3) the importance of *microcommunication*, such as voice inflection, eye contact, and nonverbal signals; (4) the importance of sensitively varying the intervention style for different groups (e.g., police officers, paramedics, nurses, or psychotherapists); and (5) the role of the physical environment or setting of the debriefing in influencing the group process.

As highly trained clinical practitioners, we can well empathize with therapists who feel that their rich and varied clinical skills are often underutilized in the structured setting of an emergency service debriefing. However, we must remember that the CISD model was developed precisely for its utility as a first-line, first-aid approach to mental health crisis intervention and trauma care. The melding of more sophisticated psychodynamic group therapy approaches with the CISD model is certainly to be welcomed, and it may in fact be an indispensable component for certain groups, such as traumatized psychotherapists (Miller, 1998a; Talbot et al., 1995).

But, *as* therapists, we need to take responsibility for knowing our patients, and for tailoring our interventions accordingly. With certain groups, cognitively and psychodynamically rich and sophisticated clinical interventions may be piercingly effective in drawing out inhibited feelings and leading to shared expression and resolution of shock and trauma. For other groups, however, the therapist's knowledge and skills must remain more under the surface, the debriefing appearing to occur smoothly and naturally, while the unseen influence of the clinician's knowledge, talent, and training produces no brilliant therapeutic fireworks but is effective precisely because it makes the whole process "look easy."

PSYCHOTHERAPY WITH CRISIS INTERVENTION PERSONNEL

Sometimes the psychic cuts go deeper, and the psychological field dressing of the CISD approach must be supplemented by more intensive and extensive individual psychotherapeutic modalities. And as with CISD approaches, the particular intervention strategy must be tailored the to clinical species of crisis intervention specialist we treat.

Police Officers and Emergency Services Personnel

Crisis personnel, police officers especially, have a well-deserved reputation for shunning mental health services, often repudiating its practitioners as softies and bleeding hearts who help get guilty criminals off with overelaborate psychobabble excuses. Other crisis personnel fear being "shrunk," having a view of psychotherapy as akin to brainwashing, a humiliating experience in which they are supposed to lie on a couch and sob about their toilet training. More commonly, the idea of needing "mental help" implies weakness, cowardice, and lack of ability to do the job. In the environment of many departments, some workers realistically fear censure, stigmatization, ridicule, impaired career advancement, and alienation from coworkers if they are perceived as the type who "folds under pressure." Moreover, others in the department who have something to hide may fear a colleague "spilling his guts" to the shrink and blowing the malfeasor's cover. In reality, attempts by personnel to seek mental health intervention of any type should be forthrightly supported by the departmental administration (Anderson et al., 1995; Blau, 1994; Miller, 1995, 2006b; Mitchell & Everly, 1996).

Trust and the Therapeutic Relationship

Trust is a crucial element in doing effective psychotherapy with police officers (Silva, 1991), a lesson that can be applied to clinical work with all emergency services personnel (Miller, 1995, 1998c, 2006b). Difficulty with trust seems to be an occupational hazard for workers in law enforcement and public safety, who generally have a strong sense of self-sufficiency and insistence on solving their own problems. Therapists who work with crisis personnel may at first need to put up with a lot of testing on the part of their patients: "Why are you doing this?" "What's in it for you?" "Who's going to get this information?" Patients may expose the therapist to mocking cynicism and criticism about the job, baiting the therapist to agree, and thereby hoping to expose the therapist's prejudices about the patient's profession (Silva, 1991).

The development of trust during the establishment of the therapeutic alliance depends on the therapist's skill in interpreting the patient's statements, thoughts, feelings, reactions, and nonverbal behavior. In the best case, the patient begins to feel at ease with the therapist and finds comfort and sense of predictability from the psychotherapy session. Silva (1991) outlines the following guidelines for the establishment of therapeutic trust:

- *Accurate empathy.* The therapist conveys his/her understanding of the patient's background and experience (but beware of premature false familiarity and phony "bonding").
- *Genuineness.* The therapist is spontaneous yet tactful, flexible yet creatively structured and adaptive, and tries to communicate as nondefensively as possible.
- *Availability.* The therapist is available, within reason, whenever needed, and avoids making promises and commitments he/she cannot keep.
- *Respect.* The therapist is both tough-minded and gracious and seeks to preserve the patient's sense of autonomy, control, and self-respect within the therapeutic relationship. Respect is shown by the therapist's overall attitude, language, and behavior, such as indicating regard for rank or job role by initially using formal departmental forms of address, such as "officer," "detective," "lieutenant," and so on, until trust and mutual respect allow the patient to ease formality. Here it is important to avoid two important traps: (1) overfamiliarity, patronizing, and talking down to the officer; or (2) trying to "play cop" or force bogus camaraderie by assuming the role of a colleague or field commander.
- *Concreteness.* Whether performing a rescue or conducting an investigation, officers and crisis responders value action and results. Here, the cognitive-behavioral model has the advantage of emphasizing active, goal-oriented, and problem-solving approaches.

Therapeutic Strategies and Techniques

Most law enforcement and emergency services personnel come under psychotherapeutic care in the context of some form of posttraumatic stress reaction or other incident that abruptly challenges the officer's coping resources. In general, the effectiveness of any intervention will be determined by the timeliness, tone, style, and intent of the intervention. Effective therapy with this class of patients generally follows the cognitive-behavioral guidelines of brevity, focus on specific symptomatology or conflict issues, and inclusion of direct operational efforts to resolve the conflict or to reach a satisfactory conclusion (Blau, 1994; Fullerton, McCarroll, Ursano, & Wright, 1992; Wester & Lyubelsky, 2005).

Blau (1994) recommends that the first meeting between the therapist and a police officer establish a safe and comfortable working atmosphere by the therapist's articulating (1) a positive regard for the officer's decision to seek help; (2) a clear description of the therapist's responsibilities and limitations with regard to confidentiality and privilege; and (3) an invitation to the officer to state his or her concerns.

A straightforward, goal-directed, problem-solving approach for this patient group includes (1) creating a sanctuary; (2) focusing on critical areas of concern; (3) identifying desired outcomes; (4) reviewing assets; (5) developing a general plan; (6) identifying practical initial implementations; (7) reviewing self-efficacy; and (8) setting appointments for review, reassurance, and further implementation (Blau, 1994).

Blau (1994) delineates a number of effective individual intervention strategies for police officers:

- *Attentive listening.* This includes good eye contact, an occasional nod, and genuine interest, without inappropriate comments or interruptions.
- *Being there with empathy.* This therapeutic attitude conveys availability, concern, and awareness of the turbulent emotions being experienced by the traumatized worker. It is also helpful to let the patient know, in a nonalarming manner, what he or she is likely to experience in the days and weeks ahead.
- *Reassurance.* This is valuable as long as it is reality oriented. It should take the form of reassuring the patient that routine matters will be handled, premises and property will be secured, deferred responsibilities will be handled by others, and organizational and command support will be provided.
- *Supportive counseling.* This includes effective listening, restatement of content, clarification of feelings, and reassurance, as well as community referral and networking with liaison agencies, as necessary.
- *Interpretive Counseling.* This type of intervention should be used when the patient's emotional reaction is significantly greater than the circumstances of the critical incident seems to warrant. In appropriate cases, this therapeutic strategy can stimulate the patient to search for underlying emotional stresses that intensify a traumatic event. In some cases, this may lead to ongoing psychotherapy.

Not to be neglected is the use of *humor.* While humor has a place in many forms of psychotherapy (Fry & Salameh, 1987), it may be especially useful in working with law enforcement and emergency services personnel (Fullerton et al., 1992; Silva, 1991). In general, if the therapist and patient can laugh together, it may lead to the sharing of more intimate feelings. Humor serves to bring a sense of balance and proportion to a traumatically warped and twisted world. Even sarcastic, gross humor may allow the venting of anger, frustration, resentment, and righteous indignation and thereby lead to constructive therapeutic work. As long as such humor does not degenerate into mean-spirited mockery of victims or colleagues, a mature attitude toward a traumatic event can actually frame the important existential lessons in terms of creative irony. "Show me a man who knows what's funny," Mark Twain said, "and I'll show you a man who knows what's not."

One caveat about humor, however: Many traumatized patients may be quite concrete and suspicious at the outset of therapy, and so the constructive therapeutic use of humor may have to await the formation of a therapeutic relationship that allows a certain degree of cognitive and emotional latitude. As in all effective cognitive-behavioral therapies, clinicians should respect the individual differences in cognitive style and coping resources of their patients and implement their interventions accordingly.

Case Study

"Don't get me wrong, I've seen plenty of dead bodies, fresh ones and ripe ones. But this was different. There was no reason for this, just no damn excuse. This was a little kid—this could have been *my* kid."

This statement came from a veteran police officer, Sgt. Williams, who was first on the scene following the shooting death of a young child by the boy's mentally handicapped older brother, who had been left unsupervised by the children's parents in the same house as an unsecured handgun. After police had responded to the emergency call, entered the home, and secured the scene, paramedics worked on the boy, but there was not much they could do; the child had apparently died instantly from a large-caliber bullet wound to the head. Operationally, this was not the worst death the emergency responders had ever seen; it was not the grisliest, nor even the most touch-and-go in terms of lifesaving attempts, as the child was pretty much gone before they arrived. The main traumatizing effect of this call was sheer existential indigestibility of the death circumstances: an innocent victim, even an incompetently innocent perpetrator set up for tragedy by stupidly careless adults who should have known better—there was "just no reason."

Our CISD team conducted two debriefings, the first involving a mix of police officers, paramedics, and radio dispatchers; the second with emergency room nurses and one medical resident who had handled the child at the emergency room. Most of the debriefed personnel seemed to benefit from the meeting, the main topic revolving around how crisis personnel can function coolheadedly during emergencies by discounting the horror around them, yet still retain their humanity. Aside from a follow-up phone call from one of the nurses, everybody seemed to get back to work and go on with their lives.

Except Sgt. Williams. The CISD team psychologist got a call about a week later that Williams needed to come in and "touch base" with him about a few things. After a period of clinical rapport building, Williams expressed that he had been having stomach cramps and insomnia since the incident, and had been "blaming myself" for the child's death, even though he knew logically that there was nothing he could have done. He also had experienced a few nightmares in which the bloody child was still alive and walking toward him, saying, "Why did you let me live like this?"

Williams revealed that when he was about 15, he was placed in charge of his 8-year-old brother at a lakeside family summer resort, while the parents went into the local town for the afternoon. Preoccupied with horsing around with his buddies, the youthful Williams lost track of his brother, who suffered a near-drowning incident with brain anoxia, leaving him moderately handicapped. Even though both witnesses and the local emergency room doctor said that the accident had happened almost instantly—the boy had slipped off a pier—Williams's family blamed him for a long time for "not being responsible," and Williams had internalized this guilt and shame.

Even years later, when the family and the brother himself had long since let Williams off the hook emotionally, he continued to ruminate about his lack of vigilance that "left my brother like that." Most recently, this feeling had been reinforced by the child shooting.

In psychotherapy, it was actually Sgt. Williams himself who easily made the connection. The following is a condensation of the therapeutic dialogue that took place over several sessions.

WILLIAMS: I'm dreaming about my little brother, aren't I?

THERAPIST: Why do you say that?

WILLIAMS: Because in the dream, the kid is yelling about me letting him "live like that." The kid on the call died, but my brother's still alive.

THERAPIST: What's the relationship with your brother like now?

WILLIAMS: He still lives with our folks. I see him from time to time.

THERAPIST: What I mean is . . .

WILLIAMS: Yeah, I know, does he blame me like they did.

THERAPIST: And?

WILLIAMS: To tell you the truth, we never actually talked about it.

THERAPIST: How come?

WILLIAMS: I dunno, can of worms, that whole thing.

THERAPIST: How old's your brother now?

WILLIAMS: 24.

THERAPIST: What's my next question?

WILLIAMS: Yeah, talk to him about it, but what do I do, just blurt it out?

THERAPIST: No, just spend some more time with your brother. If and when the conversation swings around to the past, gently raise the issue of how he's dealt with this thing his whole life.

WILLIAMS: What if I don't like the answer?

THERAPIST: This isn't a mandatory requirement. You don't have to do any of this. I'm just making this suggestion because you said you've been walking around with this on your head, and this may be a way to put it to rest, one way or the other.

WILLIAMS: OK, I'll think about it.

There were no therapeutic miracles in this case, and Sgt. Williams hesitated for several weeks before arranging a get-together with his brother. Meanwhile, a few sessions of individual psychotherapy, while probably not "resolving" the issue in a classically psychodynamic sense, did allow for a cognitive-behavioral normalization of the response and reframing of the issue in terms of old emotional baggage that could be compartmentalized and tolerated, as long as lessons learned from the past incident and the present could be applied to Sgt. Williams's current personal and professional life. Sgt. Williams went back to effective police work and shortly thereafter passed the qualifying exam to be promoted to lieutenant. At the conclusion of treatment, he had still not met with his brother, but he seemed a little more at ease at the prospect of doing so.

Crisis Intervention with Clinicians and Trauma Therapists

Ironic but true: Many therapists do not like therapy—for themselves, that is. To reach this group of helpers, special adaptations to the therapeutic model and process are necessary.

General Decompression and Self-Help Measures

It sounds deceptively obvious that all therapists should establish and maintain a balance between their professional and personal lives, but for trauma therapists this is especially important (Cerney, 1995). Some authorities recommend that a sense of civic responsibility expressed in social activism can be an outlet for frustration and serve to productively bind anxiety and focus energies (Comas-Diaz & Padilla, 1990; Yassen, 1995)—as long as such activism does not become an obsessive, self-destructive "crusade." Letting the public know one's views, beliefs, and ideals can be a potent antidote to the secretive and silencing nature of the trauma. What may seem like small acts of activism can also combat powerlessness, the feeling that "with all I do, I don't make a dent." Self-help also occurs in the shape of formal or informal support groups or incorporating stress-reduction activities and exercises into the therapist's daily life (Saakvitne & Pearlman, 1996).

Therapeutic Support for Traumatized Therapists

In cases in which therapists have been directly traumatized, as when assaulted in mental health or criminal detention facilities, institutional leaders can take the following steps to ensure that traumatized workers are not stigmatized and ostracized by their colleagues (Catherall, 1995). First, leaders must recognize that other employees may have an emotional reaction to the traumatized worker. Second, leaders must create regular opportunities for the group to meet and talk about their exposure to traumatic stress. It is most effective if someone in a position of authority takes responsibility for normalizing the experience. Finally, leaders must actively encourage the group to see the individual traumatized worker's reaction as a common group problem and deal with it on that basis.

In dealing with countertransferential reactions to aggressive and violent patients, Maier and Van Ryboek (1995) describe the following institutional policy and procedure. In this model, staff are expected to identify and share feelings with their peers and supervisors in forums provided by the clinical administration. Should these feelings interfere with the ability to provide effective and humane treatment to a patient, staff are expected to address the relevant issues. The formal personnel process may be utilized to shape the required change, including referral to the employee assistance program (EAP). If, over time, the staff member is unable to keep feelings of fear and anger from affecting his/her work performance, a change in work area or assignment may be in order.

Typically, nursing and mental health staff victims of workplace violence, such as assaults by patients, experience intense emotional reactions (Lanza, 1995, 1996; Miller, 1997). They want to talk about their reactions but feel it is "unprofessional" to do so. Victims typically do not expect to receive support from hospital administrators, despite their history of loyal service to the institution, and this may produce further anger and demoralization.

Blaming oneself is often a way to impute at least some kind of meaning and controllability to an otherwise incomprehensible catastrophic event. Self-blame can be functional if it involves attributions to one's specific behavior in a specific situation, rather than to enduring personality characteristics, the often-cited difference between *behavioral self-blame* and *characterological self-blame*. But even behavioral self-blame is not helpful if victims feel that they used appropriate precautions, followed all the safety rules, and bad things happened anyway; this may produce a sense of helplessness and failure. Both administrators and clinicians can help assaulted staff sort out the realities of safe conduct from runaway catastrophic fears and fantasies.

Building on a combination of the CISD model and individual cognitive-behavioral therapeutic approaches, Flannery and colleagues (Flannery, 1995; Flannery, Fulton, Tausch, & DeLotti, 1991; Flannery, Penk, Hanson, & Flannery, 1996; Flannery et al., 1998) have developed a comprehensive, voluntary, peer-help, systems approach, called the Assaulted Staff Action Program (ASAP), for health care staff who have been attacked by patients at work. ASAP provides a range of services including individual critical incident debriefings of assaulted staff, debriefings of entire wards, a staff victims' support group, employee–victim–family debriefing and counseling, and referrals for follow-up psychotherapy as indicated. The ASAP team structure is comprised of 15 direct-care staff volunteers. The ASAP team director is responsible for administering the entire program and for ensuring the quality of the services.

When combined with preincident training and stress management, this approach has proven helpful in the aftermath of patient assaults on employee victims and in significantly reducing the overall level of violence itself. In facilities where it has been applied, the ASAP program is reported to have reduced staff turnover, sick leave, industrial accident claims, and medical expenses as the overall assault rates have declined. The developers of the ASAP model point out that the costs associated with the entire program are less than that of one successful lawsuit.

Obviously, all these supportive measures depend on a certain degree of trust and cooperation within an organization. This may not always be forthcoming, however, or it may not go far enough. In more complex cases, or those involving more disabling traumatization, therapists may need more focused, individualized therapy.

Psychotherapy with Traumatized Therapists

Perhaps not surprisingly, the literature is sparse on therapeutic modalities for therapists themselves. Traumatized therapists who enter treatment require their own therapists to be accepting, nonjudgmental, and empathic, without becoming enmeshed or overawed—in other words, similar to the kind of therapist most effective in treating other traumatized patients. One of the most difficult issues traumatized therapists face is the assault on their perceptions of the world and its inhabitants (Cerney, 1995; Figley, 1995).

Cerney (1995) has treated a number of therapists suffering from secondary trauma, or vicarious traumatization, using a suggestive imagery technique (Grove & Panzer, 1991). Although there is no hypnotic induction per se, when patients are asked to form an image, they often spontaneously go into a suggestible trance state. When patients present a nightmare, flashback, or other type of intrusive thought or imagery, they are asked to "redream" the dream or go over the experience again. At the point at which the traumatic event is about to begin, the therapist suggests they freeze the scene so that they can program how the scenario is to proceed. They are then asked if they would like to enter the scene—be it dream, memory, or flashback—from the distance of a mature, safe perspective. Or they may bring anyone they wish into the scene with them and thereby restructure it in a less threatening and more empowering way.

Specific techniques aside, when working with traumatized clinicians, I have found the biggest challenge to be that of maintaining flexibility of the therapist's role. At one moment, clinicians will want the therapist to be a colleague with whom they can share "war stories"; the next moment, they may become helpless and dependent, expecting the therapist to offer them some brilliant insight into restoring their motivation and reviving their career. Complicating the process is the general sense of underlying stress and burnout we all feel in confronting the social and economic changes in mental health care.

In workshops and individual approaches, probably the most effective approach I have utilized is similar to that used with burnout cases from other professions: Find a new way to use your talents and abilities. As simplistic as this may sound, part of this approach comes from the field of rehabilitation, which emphasizes the concept of *transferable skills*. If therapists can forge new niches for themselves, such as teaching, writing, consulting, or social activism, and if they can learn not to put all their technical eggs in one professional basket, a creative diversification of practice may be an antidote to demoralization and burnout. Alternatively, passionate devotion to a single burning cause may be as effective, or more effective, in jump-starting the commitment process to renewed professional and personal growth. As we tell our patients, the proper solution depends on the nature of the problem and the nature of the person. This is true for ourselves as well.

Case Study

Therapist Smith was a 55-year-old married, male psychologist who began work at an inpatient psychiatric and substance abuse rehabilitation facility to supplement his private practice income, which was beginning to dwindle under the onslaught of health maintenance organization regulation. Therapist Jones was a 29-year-old, single female clinical social worker who had been a therapist and case manager at a shelter for abused women and children before beginning work as a clinician on the same unit as Smith at nearly the same time. Smith, after an almost 30-year career as an independent, outpatient clinical psychologist, resented the hospital job as an unwanted but necessary compromise to maintain his family's lifestyle. Jones, a 5-year veteran of domestic violence shelter work and suicide hotlines, saw the relatively "normal" psychiatric cases of the hospital as a professional respite from her prior steady clinical diet of acute crisis intervention work.

One afternoon, a cocaine- and alcohol-dependent bipolar patient, who had been discharged a week earlier when his insurance ran out, appeared abruptly at Smith and Jones's unit to visit a former roommate who was still hospitalized. Once on the unit, he produced a handgun and announced that he was there to "rescue" the former roommate. Smith emerged from his office cubicle and immediately had the gun shoved in his face. A few tense moments ensued, when Jones came around a corner and confronted the scene of Smith held at bay while the rest of the staff and patients stood around, unable to intervene for fear that Smith would be killed. Jones attempted to defuse the situation and talk down the disturbed intruder but apparently moved threateningly close and was stuck twice, on the head and cheek, by the barrel of the gun. Fortunately, the second blow resulted in the assailant losing his grip on the weapon, which fell to the floor, and he was immediately subdued by hospital staff using standard takedown procedures.

"I've had it with this crap," later exclaimed the uninjured but clearly traumatized Smith during a mandated EAP counseling session. Rather than deal with the potential violence of the hospital unit, he opted to go back to private practice, whatever the financial consequences might be, because "I sure as hell don't get paid enough to get shot." Still, for months, he experienced nightmares, anxiety, and depression, had trouble concentrating during his clinical sessions, became irritable and detached with friends and family, and eventually retired from practice about a year after the incident. Through it all, he refused any kind of therapeutic help himself because, "What good would it be to talk about it anyhow?"

EAP COUNSELOR: If one of your patients told you that, what would you say?

SMITH: Probably what you're going to say: "You have to try to process it, not let it fester, get it out of your system," or some crap like that.

EAP COUNSELOR: How about this crappy suggestion: Bury it as long as that lets you get on with your life and your work. If it doesn't bother you, treat it like mental shrapnel, that is, it's in there but it's not worth all the painful digging around to get it out. But if it continues to really distract you and screw up your daily life, then at some point, once other parts of your life have stabilized, consider a "second opinion."

SMITH: You're right, I've got to first make up my mind what I want to do, then I'll consider the "baggage." I just didn't think I'd be doing this at my age.

Jones spent a day at a local medical hospital being treated for a fractured cheek-bone. Less than a week later, she was back at work. She attended the mandated EAP counseling session but did not like the counselor so sought her own therapist through her company insurance plan. She attended this therapy for about 3 months, then felt she had worked through the traumatic event sufficiently to continue her career and life. She noticed a tendency to become overinvolved in her work, which she half-jokingly described to a coworker as "my intellectualized counterphobic defense," but was eager to move on in her career as a therapist and case manager.

THERAPIST: Overall, you seemed to have handled this event pretty well.

JONES: "Handle?" What do you mean, "handle"? Even now, every time I think about it, I almost pee in my pants—I could've been killed!

THERAPIST: But you're back at work.

JONES: Well, what am I supposed to do, just sit home and ruminate? Work gives me a chance to focus, to use my brain. But I still walk around edgy.

THERAPIST: That's PTSD 101. As far as classic symptoms and reactions, you're a case that follows the textbooks. And you'll probably follow the second half of the book that deals with recovery over the next few months. If work is your best therapy, then go for it. Just be careful not to get so intense that you burn yourself out.

JONES: No chance of that (*laughs*).

Individual psychodynamics aside, it is clear that Smith, already tired and demoralized from having to make a second-choice career move just to stay ahead financially, needed very little in the way of a traumatic event to propel him into full-scale burnout. Jones, on the other hand, although hardly happy about being pistol-whipped in the first few weeks of a new job, was able to assimilate this traumatic event by virtue of her prior experience with "hard-case" clientele, her ability to utilize adaptive defenses such as humor and sublimation, her willingness to seek help as necessary, and her goal-oriented ambition to advance in her career.

SUMMARY AND CONCLUSIONS

Law enforcement officers, rescue medics, trauma therapists, and other crisis personnel need to be mindful of their own needs as clinicians and as helping human beings who regularly deal with dark aspects of human nature and sometimes refractory types of psychotherapy patients. Continued education and training, interaction and cross-fertilization with peers, interdisciplinary collaboration, periodic diversion into pleasant activities, development of a sense of mission and purpose, and willingness to access help for ourselves when necessary can protect against premature burnout and contribute to our effectiveness as helpers and healers. The same recommendations apply equally to crisis responders in all fields (Miller, 1998c). We serve others best when we take care of ourselves.

REFERENCES

Ackerly, G. D., Burnell, J., Holder, D. C., & Kurdek, L. A. (1988). Burnout among licensed psychologists. *Professional Psychology: Research and Practice, 19,* 624–631.

Anderson, W., Swenson, D., & Clay, D. (1995). *Stress management for law enforcement officers.* Englewood Cliffs, NJ: Prentice Hall.

Becknell, J. M. (1995, March). Tough stuff: Learning to seize the opportunities. *Journal of the Emergency Medical Services,* pp. 52–59.

Belles, D., & Norvell, N. (1990). *Stress management for law enforcement officers.* Sarasota, FL: Professional Resource Exchange.

Benedikt, R. A., & Kolb, L. C. (1986). Preliminary findings on chronic pain and posttraumatic stress disorder. *American Journal of Psychiatry, 143,* 908–910.

Blau, T. H. (1994). *Psychological services for law enforcement.* New York: Wiley.

Bohl, N. (1995). Professionally administered critical incident debriefing for police officers. In M. I. Kunke & E. M. Scrivner (Eds.), *Police psychology into the 21st century* (pp. 169–188). Hillsdale, NJ: Erlbaum.

Borum, R., & Philpot, C. (1993). Therapy with law enforcement couples: Clinical management of the "high-risk lifestyle." *American Journal of Family Therapy, 21,* 122–135.

Catherall, D. R. (1995). Preventing institutional secondary traumatic stress disorder. In C. R. Figley (Ed.), *Compassion fatigue: Coping with secondary traumatic stress disorder in those who treat the traumatized* (pp. 232–247). New York: Brunner/Mazel.

Cerney, M. S. (1995). Treating the "heroic treaters." An overview. In C. R. Figley (Ed.), *Compassion fatigue: Coping with secondary traumatic stress disorder in those who treat the traumatized* (pp. 131–149). New York: Brunner/Mazel.

Comas-Diaz, L., & Padilla, A. (1990). Countertransference in working with victims of political repression. *American Journal of Orthopsychiatry, 60,* 125–134.

Courchaine, K. E., & Dowd, E. T. (1994). Groups. In F. M. Dattilio & A. Freeman (Eds.), *Cognitive-behavioral strategies in crisis intervention* (pp. 221–237). New York: Guilford Press.

Cummings, J. P. (1996, October). Police stress and the suicide link. *The Police Chief,* pp. 85–96.

Curran, S. (2003, January/February). Separating fact from fiction about police stress. *Behavioral Health Management,* pp. 3–4.

Deutsch, C. J. (1984). Self-reported sources of stress among psychotherapists. *Professional Psychology: Research and Practice, 15,* 833–845.

Dyregrov, A. (1989). Caring for helpers in disaster situations: Psychological debriefing. *Disaster Management, 2,* 25–30.

Dyregrov, A. (1997). The process in psychological debriefing. *Journal of Traumatic Stress, 10,* 589–605.

Everly, G. S., Flannery, R. B., & Mitchell, J. T. (2000). Critical incident stress management: A review of the literature. *Aggression and Violent Behavior, 5,* 23–40.

Everly, G. S., & Mitchell, J. T. (1997). *Critical incident stress management (CISM): A new era and standard of care in crisis intervention.* Ellicott City, MD: Chevron.

Figley, C. R. (1995). Compassion fatigue as secondary traumatic stress disorder: An overview. In C. R. Figley (Ed.), *Compassion fatigue: Coping with secondary traumatic stress disorder in those who treat the traumatized* (pp. 1–20). New York: Brunner/Mazel.

Flannery, R. B. (1995). *Violence in the workplace.* New York: Crossroad.

Flannery, R. B., Fulton, P., Tausch, J., & DeLoffi, A. (1991). A program to help staff cope with psychological sequelae of assaults by patients. *Hospital and Community Psychiatry, 42,* 935–942.

Flannery, R. B., Hanson, M. A., Penk, W. E., Goldfinger, S., Pastva, G. J., & Navon, M. A. (1998). Replicated declines in assault rates after implementation of the Assaulted Staff Action Program. *Psychiatric Services, 49,* 241–243.

Flannery, R. B., Penk, W. E., Hanson, M. A., & Flannery, G. J. (1996). The Assaulted Staff Action Program: Guidelines for fielding a team. In G. R. VandenBos & E. Q. Bulatao (Eds.), *Violence on the job: Identifying risks and developing solutions* (pp. 327–341). Washington, DC: American Psychological Association.

Freeman, A., & Dattilio, F. M. (1994). Introduction. In F. M. Dattilio & A. Freeman (Eds.), *Cognitive-behavioral strategies in crisis intervention* (pp. 1–22). New York: Guilford Press.

Fry, W. F., & Salameh, W. A. (Eds.). (1987). *Handbook of humor and psychotherapy*. Sarasota, FL: Professional Resource Exchange.

Fullerton, C. S., McCarroll, J. E., Ursano, R. J., & Wright, K. M. (1992). Psychological response of rescue workers: Firefighters and trauma. *American Journal of Orthopsychiatry, 62,* 371–378.

Gilliland, B. E., & James, R. K. (1993). *Crisis intervention strategies* (2nd ed.). Pacific Grove, CA: Brooks/Cole.

Grove, D. J., & Panzer, B. I. (1991). *Resolving traumatic memories: Metaphors and symbols in psychotherapy*. New York: Irvington.

Hall, W. (1986). The Agent Orange controversy after the Evatt Royal Commission. *Medical Journal of Australia, 145,* 219–255.

Honig, A. L., & Roland, J. E. (1998, October). Shots fired: Officer involved. *The Police Chief*, pp. 65–70.

Horn, J. M. (1991). Critical incidents for law enforcement officers. In J. T. Reese, J. M. Horn, & C. Dunning (Eds.), *Critical incidents in policing* (rev ed., pp. 143–148). Washington, DC: U.S. Government Printing Office.

James, B. (1989). *Treating traumatized children: New insights and creative interventions*. New York: Free Press.

Johnson, K. (1989). *Trauma in the lives of children: Crisis and stress management techniques for counselors and other professionals*. Alameda, CA: Hunter House.

Kirschman, E. (1997). *I love a cop: What police families need to know*. New York: Guilford Press.

Lanza, M. L. (1995). Nursing staff as victims of patient assault. In C. R. Figley (Ed.), *Compassion fatigue: Coping with secondary traumatic stress disorder in those who treat the traumatized* (pp. 131–149). New York: Brunner/Mazel.

Lanza, M. L. (1996). Violence against nurses in hospitals. In G. R. VandenBos & E. Q. Bulatao (Eds.), *Violence on the job: Identifying risks and developing solutions* (pp. 189–198). Washington, DC: American Psychological Association.

Maier, G. J., & Van Ryboek, G. J. (1995). Managing countertransference reactions to aggressive patients. In B. S. Eichelman & A. C. Hartwig (Eds.), *Patient violence and the clinician* (pp. 73–104). Washington, DC: American Psychiatric Press.

Manton, M., & Talbot, A. (1990). Crisis intervention after an armed hold-up: Guidelines for counselors. *Journal of Traumatic Stress, 3,* 507–522.

McCafferty, R. L., McCafferty, E., & McCafferty, M. A. (1992). Stress and suicide in police officers: Paradigm of occupational stress. *Southern Medical Journal, 85,* 233.

McCann, I. L., & Pearlman, L. A. (1990). *Psychological trauma and the adult survivor: Theory, therapy, and transformation*. New York: Brunner/Mazel.

McFarlane, A. C., Atchison, M., Rafalowicz, E., & Papay, P. (1994). Physical symptoms in posttraumatic stress disorder. *Journal of Psychosomatic Research, 38,* 715–726.

McMains, M. J. (1991). The management and treatment of postshooting trauma. In J. T. Reese, J. M. Horn, & C. Dunning (Eds.), *Critical incidents in policing* (rev ed., pp. 191–198). Washington, DC: U.S. Government Printing Office.

Miller, L. (1992). Cognitive rehabilitation, cognitive therapy, and cognitive style: Toward an integrative model of personality and psychotherapy. *Journal of Cognitive Rehabilitation, 10*(1), 18–29.

Miller, L. (1993). Who are the best psychotherapists? Qualities of the effective practitioner. *Psychotherapy in Private Practice*, 12(1), 1–18.

Miller, L. (1994). Civilian posttraumatic stress disorder: Clinical syndromes and psychotherapeutic strategies. *Psychotherapy*, 31, 665–664.

Miller, L. (1995). Tough guys: Psychotherapeutic strategies with law enforcement and emergency services personnel. *Psychotherapy*, 32, 592–600.

Miller, L. (1997). Workplace violence in the rehabilitation setting: How to prepare, respond, and survive. *Florida State Association of Rehabilitation Nurses Newsletter*, 7, 4–6.

Miller, L. (1998a). Our own medicine: Traumatized psychotherapists and the stresses of doing therapy. *Psychotherapy*, 35, 137–146.

Miller, L. (1998b). Psychotherapy of crime victims: Treating the aftermath of interpersonal violence. *Psychotherapy*, 35, 336–345.

Miller, L. (1998c). *Shocks to the system: Psychotherapy of traumatic disability syndromes*. New York: Norton.

Miller, L. (1999a). Treating posttraumatic stress disorder in children and families: Basic principle and clinical applications. *American Journal of Family Therapy*, 27, 21–34.

Miller, L. (1999b). "Mental stress claims" and personal injury: Clinical, neuropsychological, and forensic issues. *Neurolaw Letter*, 8, 39–45.

Miller, L. (1999c). Posttraumatic stress disorder in child victims of violent crime: Making the case for psychological injury. *Victim Advocate*, 1, 6–10.

Miller, L. (1999d). Workplace violence: Prevention, response, and recovery. *Psychotherapy*, 36, 160–169.

Miller, L. (1999e). Critical incident stress debriefing: Clinical applications and new directions. *International Journal of Emergency Mental Health*, 1, 253–265.

Miller, L. (2000a). Law enforcement traumatic stress: Clinical syndromes and intervention strategies. *Trauma Response*, 6(1), 15–20.

Miller, L. (2000b). Traumatized psychotherapists. In F. M. Dattilio & A. Freeman (Eds.), *Cognitive-behavioral strategies in crisis intervention* (2nd ed., pp. 429–445). New York: Guilford Press.

Miller, L. (2003a, May). Police personalities: Understanding and managing the problem officer. *The Police Chief*, pp. 53–60.

Miller, L. (2003b). Law enforcement responses to violence against youth: Psychological dynamics and intervention strategies. In R. S. Moser & C. E. Franz (Ed.), *Shocking violence II: Violent disaster, war, and terrorism affecting our youth* (pp. 165–195). New York: Thomas.

Miller, L. (2005a, April). Critical incident stress: Myths and realities. *Law and Order*, p. 31.

Miller, L. (2005b). Police officer suicide: Causes, prevention, and practical intervention strategies. *International Journal of Emergency Mental Health*, 7, 23–36.

Miller, L. (2006a, March). Practical strategies for preventing officer suicide. *Law and Order*, pp. 90–92.

Miller, L. (2006b). *Practical police psychology: Stress management and crisis intervention for law enforcement*. Springfield, IL: Thomas.

Miller, L. (2007). Police families: Stresses, syndromes, and solutions. *American Journal of Family Therapy*, 35, 21–40.

Miller, L., & Schlesinger, L. B. (2000). Survivors, families, and co-victims of serial offenders. In L. B. Schlesinger (Ed.), *Serial offenders: Current thought, recent findings, unusual syndromes* (pp. 309–334). Boca Raton, FL: CRC Press.

Mitchell, J. T. (1983). When disaster strikes . . . the critical incident stress process. *Journal of the Emergency Medical Services*, 8, 36–39.

Mitchell, J. T. (1988). The history, status, and future of critical incident stress debriefing. *Journal of the Emergency Medical Services*, 13, 47–52.

Mitchell, J. T. (1991). Law enforcement applications for critical incident stress teams. In J. T. Reese, J. M. Horn, & C. Dunning (Eds.), *Critical incidents in policing* (rev ed., pp. 201–212). Washington, DC: U.S. Government Printing Office.

Mitchell, J. T., & Bray, G. P. (1990). *Emergency services stress: Guidelines for preserving the health and careers of emergency services personnel.* Englewood Cliffs, NJ: Prentice-Hall.

Mitchell, J. T., & Everly, G. S. (1996). *Critical incident stress debriefing: An operations manual for the preservation of traumatic stress among emergency services and disaster workers* (2nd ed.). Ellicott City, MD: Chevron.

Moon, E. (1999, February). How to handle the high cost of caring. *Professional Counselor*, pp. 18–22.

Palmer, C. E. (1983). A note about paramedics's strategies for dealing with death and dying. *Journal of Occupational Psychology, 56*, 83–86.

Peak, K. J. (2003). *Policing in America: Methods, issues, challenges* (4th ed.). Upper Saddle River, NJ: Prentice Hall.

Pearlman, L. A., & MacIan, P. S. (1995). Vicarious traumatization: An empirical study of the effects of trauma work on trauma therapists. *Professional Psychology: Research and Practice, 26*, 558–565.

Reese, J. T. (1987). Coping with stress: It's your job. In J. T. Reese (Ed.), *Behavioral science in law enforcement* (pp. 75–79). Washington, DC: Federal Bureau of Investigation.

Reese, J. T. (1991). Justification for mandating critical incident aftercare. In J. T. Reese, J. M. Horn, & C. Dunning (Eds.), *Critical incidents in policing* (rev. ed., pp. 213–220). Washington, DC: U.S. Government Printing Office.

Regehr, C., & Bober, T. (2004). *In the line of fire: Trauma in the emergency services.* New York: Oxford University Press.

Robinette, H. M. (1987). *Burnout in blue: Managing the police marginal performer.* New York: Praeger.

Rodolfa, E. R., Kraft, W. A., & Reiley, R. R. (1988). Stressors of professionals and trainees at APA-approved counseling and VA medical center internship sites. *Professional Psychology: Research and Practice, 19*, 43–49.

Russell, H. E., & Beigel, A. (1990). *Understanding human behavior for effective police work* (3rd ed.). New York: Basic Books.

Saakvitne, K. W., & Pearlman, L. A. (1996). *Transforming the pain: A workbook on vicarious traumatization.* New York: Norton.

Sewell, J. D. (1993). Traumatic stress in multiple murder investigations. *Journal of Traumatic Stress, 6*, 103–118.

Sewell, J. D. (1994). The stress of homicide investigations. *Death Studies, 18*, 565–582.

Sewell, J. D., Ellison, K. W., & Hurrell, J. J. (1988, October). Stress management in law enforcement: Where do we go from here? *The Police Chief*, pp. 94–98.

Silva, M. N. (1991). The delivery of mental health services to law enforcement officers. In J. T. Reese, J. M. Horn, & C. Dunning (Eds.), *Critical incidents in policing* (pp. 335–341). Washington, DC: Federal Bureau of Investigation.

Solomon, R. M. (1988, October). Post-shooting trauma. *The Police Chief*, pp. 40–44.

Solomon, R. M. (1990, February). Administrative guidelines for dealing with officers involved in on-duty shooting situations. *The Police Chief*, p. 40.

Solomon, R. M. (1995). Critical incident stress management in law enforcement. In G. S. Everly (Ed.), *Innovations in disaster and trauma psychology: Applications in emergency services and disaster response* (pp. 123–157). Baltimore: Chevron.

Solomon, R. M., & Horn, J. M. (1986). Post-shooting traumatic reactions: A pilot study. In J. T. Reese & H. A. Goldstein (Eds.), *Critical incidents in policing* (rev. ed., pp. 383–394). Washington, DC: U.S. Government Printing Office.

Talbot, A., Dutton, M., & Dunn, P. (1995). Debriefing the debriefers: An intervention strategy to assist psychologists after a crisis. In G. S. Everly & J. M. Lating (Eds.), *Psycho-*

traumatology: Key papers and core concepts in posttraumatic stress (pp. 281–298). New York: Plenum Press.

Toch, H. (2002). *Stress in policing.* Washington, DC: American Psychological Association.

Wester, S. R., & Lyubelsky, J. (2005). Supporting the thin blue line: Gender-sensitive therapy with male police officers. *Professional Psychology: Research and Practice, 36,* 51–58.

Woody, R. H. (2005). The police culture: Research implications for psychological services. *Professional Psychology: Research and Practice, 36,* 525–529.

Woody, R. H. (2006). Family interventions with law enforcement officers. *American Journal of Family Therapy, 34,* 95–103.

Yassen, J. (1995). Preventing secondary traumatic stress disorder. In C. R. Figley (Ed.), *Compassion fatigue: Coping with secondary traumatic stress disorder in those who treat the traumatized* (pp. 178–208). New York: Brunner/Mazel.

SUGGESTED READINGS

Blau, T. H. (1994). *Psychological services for law enforcement.* New York: Wiley.

Figley, C. R. (Ed.). (1995). *Compassion fatigue: Coping with secondary traumatic stress disorder in those who treat the traumatized.* New York: Brunner/Mazel.

Gilliland, B. E., & James, R. K. (1993). *Crisis intervention strategies* (2nd ed.). Pacific Grove, CA: Brooks/Cole.

Miller, L. (1998). *Shocks to the system: Psychotherapy of traumatic disability syndromes.* New York: Norton.

Miller, L. (2006). *Practical police psychology: Stress management and crisis intervention for law enforcement officers.* Springfield, IL: Thomas.

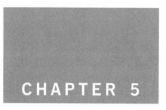
The Crisis-Prone Patient
THE HIGH-AROUSAL CLUSTER B
PERSONALITY DISORDERS

**Gina M. Fusco
Arthur Freeman**

*K*risti paced feverishly back and forth. Four quick paces to the center of the room, then back to the hallway again, each time her breathing increasing in intensity. Her chest was constricted so tight she had trouble catching her breath. Why won't her hands stop shaking? Her stomach was like a roller coaster, flipping up and down, and churning over and over again. Her mind raced. "Damn!" She was losing control. She was in fact as one of her favorite characters in a TV show once said, "officially spiraling." Her thoughts only propelled her further into the catastrophic emotional oblivion she was feeling. "Why did he do this to me *again*!" Rage and desperation surged throughout her system. She allowed revengeful thoughts to brew. "I'll show him!" and "He'll never be happy without me!" Kristi repeatedly checked her watch. Yes, she was sure. He said he would call at 8:00 tonight! Exasperated, it was just too much to bear. At 8:10 P.M., 28-year-old Kristi gazed with tears streaming down her cheeks at her forearms. She dramatically reminisced at her brief meeting of the young man 2 days ago whom she met, spent the night with, and with whom she shared her deepest fears. She knew it was more than the high they had from the alcohol and the cocaine. What a powerful emotional and physical connection! "Didn't he feel it too!?" Defeated, she scanned the length of her arms and momentarily registered the faded scars that at one time or another, encapsulated each of her life's ongoing disappointments. There was nothing better for her. Ever. This was what life had to offer. Resigned, she forfeited the splinters of hope she had left, and cut her arms repeatedly.

Kristi represents a group of patients who experience overwhelming emotional states that impact and impair adaptive and healthy coping and problem-solving strategies during stressful and potential "crisis" situations. Overwhelmed by powerful emotional and cognitive impressions of loss, attack, and invalidation, these individuals have few resources to manage stressors. Lacking an integrated internal compass to provide guidance and predictability, Kristi resorts to what she knows helps her to feel not better per se but *different*. Devoid of any futuristic thinking, Kristi sees no hope, no control, and no self-efficacy to manage what seems to be a lifelong road ahead of sheer and utter disappointment. Her intense emotions seem even to cause physical pain and discomfort. Reacting to the emotional tidal wave, Kristi impulsively engages in self-injury as a coping strategy. Her transitory shame and recognition of prior acts of self-injury are no match for her intense emotional pain. For Kristi, engaging in self-injury perpetuates an already established and well-reinforced behavioral cycle. Not only is her experience reinforced by the physiological and emotional changes she experiences after she self-injures, but the reinforcement of the maladaptive behavior confirms and solidifies what she already knows, she is worthless and unable to manage any other more adaptive way. Her overwhelming emotional states block any positive cognitive processing. Subsequently, she repeats what she has already established as her "way of handling things." Millon described personality pathology as a bad one-act play that repeats itself over and over without modification or more adaptive endings. This is exemplified by the inflexible adaptiveness demonstrated by Kristi's behavior (Millon & Davis, 2000).

Psychotherapists know this patient. Typically presenting as manifesting one of the four D's—discomfort, dysfunction, dyscontrol, and disorganization—these patients apparently have difficulty in resolving their stress and resultant difficulty through the use of more adaptive internal or external resources. Identified as the crisis-prone patient (Freeman & Fusco, 2000) who usually meets criteria for the Axis II, cluster B personality disorders (borderline, antisocial, narcissistic, and histrionic) (American Psychiatric Association, 2000), these patients problem-solve poorly, have limited or minimal coping strategies, and generally have problems managing in an adaptive, proactive healthy way normal, common life stressors and much less high-stress experiences. Rather, common stressors can in effect become life crises, either as a single episode or as a cascading series of crises or "brushfires." When unable to manage these crises, psychotherapy may be sought. In extreme cases, crisis intervention is needed. Patients with this pattern of mismanaging stressful situations require a different therapeutic approach than patients who throughout their lives have coped well, seem to recoup, learn, and return to at least their prior level of coping.

The crisis-prone patient typically has a premorbid history of high arousal, sensitivity, and emotional dyscontrol and dysregulation. The excitability and crisis-prone style of these individuals is emblematic of the cluster B patient (Millon, 1999). Crisis prone, although a tempting heuristic to be applied to cluster B personality disorders in general, should not be utilized in isolation as a specific diagnostic descriptor but, rather, as a description of those patients who lack coping and problem-solving ability, and exhibit high-arousal characteristics. In diagnosing personality disorders, the necessary and sufficient DSM-IV-TR (American Psychiatric Association, 2000) criteria should be met.

These patients often have a long history of maladaptive coping strategies leading to overt and unhealthy behaviors, which over time may have caused the patient to engage in self-harm, unhealthy relationships, difficulty in social and vocational arenas, and frequent overwhelming intrapersonal distress. Their baseline is compromised, and they are generally more susceptible to being overwhelmed or unable to cope. For these individuals, "being in crisis is a way of life" (Freeman & Fusco, 2000, p. 28). The high-arousal individual is either in a crisis, on the verge of a crisis, or has a crisis looming just over the horizon, and occurring in the not too distant future. Complicating matters, crises are exacerbated by the bidirectionality of the patient's being excitable, dramatic, and easily aroused and agitated. His/her experience of life as a series of the *crises du jour* creates the ongoing expectation that life is unfair, unpredictable, and often out of control. Whether there is an addictive quality to having crises (and thereby being in a state of high arousal) or the tendency for self-defeating and self-victimizing, these patients may demand much time, effort, energy, and attention from their therapists.

COUNTERTRANSFERENCE

Frequently the therapist may experience negative reactions and feelings within the therapeutic context. Freeman and Fusco (2005) describe countertransference stress as the fleeting session-to-session reactions of the therapist to the patient, and counter-transference structure, as a more stable reaction that goes beyond the single session but rather becomes the typical way in which the therapist experiences the patient. Typical to crisis-prone patients, therapists more readily adopt a countertransference structure that may include negative assumptions, feelings, and helplessness. This negative structure creates the backdrop for which episodic countertransference stress occurs. Because session-to-session stress is expected, a negative countertransference structure causes an often intense, exaggerated reaction from the therapist. If the stress had occurred in isolation, it would not likely cause powerful emotional reactions. Typical session stress may in fact become the proverbial "straw that breaks the therapist's back." Therapists must ensure that, when working with these patients, ongoing examination and evaluation of their internal experiences are explored, and, if necessary, processed through supervision or peer review.

We want to differentiate between two types of patients. The first is the patient who is in crisis due to some natural disaster or traumatic life circumstance. The other type is the crisis-prone patient for whom waking in the morning and having to cope with life's daily events is fraught with potential crises and the resulting angst. The focus of this chapter is on the latter type. These patients, in addition, have met the DSM-IV-TR criteria of a personality disorder within the cluster B spectrum.

The format of this chapter is to examine the cluster B personality disorders in the context of Millon's conceptualization of the multiaxial model (Millon & Davis, 2000) and then offer a cognitive-behavioral therapy (CBT) model to assist the clinician in understanding, applying, and preparing for both the crisis work and the ensuing treatment. In addition, we suggest specific crisis intervention models and techniques. At times, an individual may not fall definitively within a single diagnostic category. By recognizing the cluster B spectrum, wherein elements of all the disorders may be present, one can assign the individual to the cluster. In keeping with the dimensional perspective, patients who demonstrate personality disorder features or traits may also benefit from the overall conceptualization. For the purposes of this chapter, however, we approach each diagnosis separately because individuals will generally respond to the stress of crisis in a typical or predictable manner that is consistent with their disorder and respective schema.

PERSONALITY DISORDERS

Personality disorders are defined as "an enduring pattern of inner experience and behavior that deviates markedly from the expectations of the individual's culture, . . . is inflexible and pervasive, . . . leads to distress and impairment, . . . can be traced back at least to adolescence or early adulthood, is stable and of long duration, and leads to distress or impairment" (American Psychiatric Association, 2000, p. 689). In addition, this pattern is manifested in two or more of the following: cognition, affect, interpersonal functioning, and impulse control. Patients diagnosed with these disorders have typically experienced difficulties in their relationships, socialization, employment, and overall functioning.

Inasmuch as their style is egosyntonic (i.e., internally consistent with the individual's schema), they generally avoid psychotherapy. Referrals are frequently sought when they are experiencing a crisis and/or through family or external pressure. Confounding to the clinician and to those around them, they verbalize the pain and discomfort experienced in the crisis but ironically often appear reluctant or unable to change what they do, how they feel, or what they think. The nature of their crises may involve fundamental safety issues related to suicidal and homicidal threats, gestures, or attempts, which clearly complicates the treatment process. Typically other-blaming, they generally interpret crises that they encounter in life as a product of other people's negative behavior, neglect, or ill will, and therefore they negate or diminish their own ability to influence the given situation. Given the long-term nature of the patients' characterological problems, they are often experts at being in crisis.

Consistent with personality disorders, these individuals often demonstrate a sincere bewilderment as to how they end up in crisis situations despite their frenetic lifelong crisis-laden experiences. Although patients with personality disorders may be aware of the self-defeating nature of their personality problems (e.g., overdependence, lack of empathy, dramatics, excessive avoidance, and demands for attention), they are perplexed as to how to change these patterns. They may make statements indicating they have no or little control over their behaviors and reactions. Their descriptions of their behaviors may be contradictory in that they recognize they are doing the behavior, but the responsibility of the behavior seems to be a function of something separate or distinct from them. Acceptance and responsibility becomes a difficult hurdle, as the very ego-syntonic nature prevents further insightful and cognitive self-awareness. Still other patients may have the motivation to change but do not have the skills to do so.

In sum, patients with a cluster B personality disorder who are experiencing crisis may have little idea about how they got to be the way they are; how they contribute to their stress, crises, perceived life problems; and ultimately, how to change.

Individuals vary in their reactions to crisis. Some individuals are surprised and taken aback when an apparently common situation erupts into a crisis. Up to that point they may have had no inkling of what may have been clear, obvious, and readily observed by others. They may have missed the cues that others might have seen as warning signs of an escalating situation. Other crisis-prone individuals are aware of potential difficulty but see the trigger or threshold point as being far more distal than it actually is. Still others are aware of the nature and extent of the crisis but choose to manage crises by ignoring the problems and hoping that the crises will abate spontaneously. There are also those that see themselves as innocent victims of a malevolent world. Still others seem to take a masochistic delight in pushing life situations as far as they can to precipitate crises, thereby satisfying their self-fulfilling prophesies about the evils of the world. Finally, some individuals appear to be in no objective crisis but nevertheless live the life of "Chicken Little" and perceive the world as a source of crises.

MILLON'S MULTIAXIAL PERSPECTIVE: THE PSYCHOLOGICAL IMMUNE SYSTEM

The multifaceted composite of all the available information regarding patient's presentation is known as the case conceptualization (Millon & Davis, 2000). Without an overall understanding of the patient, opportunities to enter into an understanding of the patient's typical way of functioning may be missed. To gain a better understanding of how the personality functions within a holistic perspective, Millon and Davis state that the five axes within DSM are the means with which "the various symptoms and personality characteristics of a given patient can be brought together to paint a picture that reflects the functioning of the whole person" (p. 5). Defining the case conceptualization of a crisis-prone patient with an understanding of the basic premise behind the diagnostic classification system will be helpful in understanding the complex interaction between the clinical disorders listed on Axis I, the personality disorders listed on Axis II, and, particular to the crisis patient, the psychosocial stressors listed on Axis IV. Millon and Davis (2000) state that "the model increases clinical understanding by ensuring that all possible inputs to the psychopathology of the given subject receive attention" (p. 7).

Millon and Davis analogize the personality as one's psychological immune system. The personality, in effect, is made up of one's coping repertoire and ability to adapt and therefore creates immunity to invading stressors or, in keeping with the analogy, bacteria. Throughout development, one faces crises and challenges. As development occurs, the system learns to respond, shift, adapt, and cope. However, if the system is overwhelmed by stressors insurmountable to the existing coping system, the system cannot effectively manage. For example, a developing preschooler with the support of his parents learns to cope with a new babysitter. The child builds resiliency and coping ability to adapt and manage change and disappointment at losing the familiar baby sitter. However, if the child faces abuse or neglect, his coping ability may not be able to tolerate the extreme stress, and subsequently he will be overwhelmed, permanently changed, or constricted. For those with trauma in their histories, their coping strategies or "immune system" becomes belabored with prior failed attempts to cope, poorly learned adaptive skills, and ineffectual problem solving. The system in effect becomes disabled and therefore vulnerable to stressors which can easily overwhelm the already handicapped system. Each stressor, whether considered traumatic or a common everyday stress, burdens an already taxed system and subsequently creates symptomology related to what is in effect, system overload. In sum, if one's immune and coping systems or personality (Axis II) are compromised, then when faced with stressors or challenges (Axis IV), the result is distress, impairment, or dysfunction (Axis I). This is represented in the equation and is fundamental to multiaxial diagnosis and case conceptualization: Axis II + Axis IV = Axis I (Millon & Davis, 2000). Thus if the coping system is impaired, the patient is crisis prone, that is, unable to manage the usual stressors of life and ultimately vulnerable to additional stressors that can overwhelm an already compromised system.

Consistent with the cluster B personalities, many patients have trauma histories. In concert with a hyperactive reactive central nervous system, these patients have a lowered threshold and limited tolerance to stress (Stone, 1993). The hyperaroused patient may be unable to withstand even the mildest of stimuli. Freeman and Fusco (2005) write as an exaggeration, "such a patient may complain about the molecules of air constantly bombarding his exposed skin, thereby making him exquisitely sore" (p. 332).

As one means of conceptualizing the concept of extreme sensitivity, Freeman and Fusco (2005) conceptualize the crisis-prone patient as someone who is precariously balanced on one leg at the apex of a mountain peak. They are vulnerable to even the slightest breeze or wind change which can quickly cause a loss of balance. The patient's life is focused on maintaining his/her precarious balance so as to not fall to the rocks below and be destroyed. What this individual lacks is a "stable base" from which he/she can address life stressors.

Ball, Links, Strike, and Boydell (2005) demonstrated that for those individuals who demonstrate severe persistent mental illness, no clear precipitant may even be evident to identify as the onset or precursor of a crisis. Internal fluctuation, readily identified as mood lability or changes within cluster B personalities, may also cause a loss of balance. Therefore, one must fight to maintain his/her balance to avoid certain calamity, disaster, and what in his/her view amounts to be imminent demise.

Following the metaphor, the goal of crisis work and psychotherapy is to help establish a "stable base" or platform paralleling the more flexible and adaptive approach to managing the breezes of life. If the patient had a metaphorical "terrace" on which to stand, his/her balance would be better and he/she would not have to spend so much life energy on staying in place. By building a platform of consistent problem-solving and coping skills, the patient is no longer the overwhelmed subject of the slightest breeze, stress, or crisis that had previously shook his/her very core. Necessary to building this stable base is a strong therapeutic relationship that shares the building of such a base as a work in progress, both demanding of the therapist and of the patient.

SOURCES OF LIFE STRESS

Clearly, stress can come from any source inasmuch as stress is subjectively experienced. Most commonly, however, for the crisis-prone individual life operates by the equation "STRESS = DISTRESS." There appears to be no discrimination of stressful events; therefore, the patient tends to respond with the same reaction to any perceived pressures. The stressor event or circumstances typically include interpersonal relationship problems or discord, occupational difficulties, and family conflicts. The sequelae of the crisis can include substance abuse, eating disorders, depression, anxiety disorders, suicidal ideation and action, self-injurious behaviors, or behavior injurious to others. In some cases there can be a loss of reality significant enough to be labeled as psychosis.

Part of the difficulty for the crisis-prone individual comes from the normal and reasonable reaction that, when under stress, individuals perceive they have or will lose control of voluntary behavior. There is an automaticity to their responses that allows an escape from the stressful and/or crisis situations. This might be fight, flight, or freeze. Getting the patient in crisis to take back control of thoughts and actions is essential. This is complicated by the patient's vulnerability, compromised immune system, and maladaptive strategies to cope.

The role of child sexual abuse, complex abuse, and early developmental trauma has been shown to be associated with significant adult pathologies, including personality disorders (Johnson, Smailes, Cohen, Brown, & Bernstein, 2000). Ratican (1992) notes that child sexual abuse is an etiological factor in the more severe of psychopathologies including dissociative disorders, anxiety disorders, eating disorders, sexual disorders, mood disorders, substance abuse, and personality disorders. Given the high association between borderline personality disorder and child sexual abuse, some researchers have suggested that the disorder be reconceptualized as a specific posttraumatic disorder or as an early developmental trauma syndrome (Sansone, Sansone, & Levitt, 2004). Specifically van der Kolk (2005), in conjunction with the National Child Traumatic Stress Workgroup on Diagnosis, has proposed a new diagonosis, developmental trauma disorder, which captures the multiplicity of trauma exposures over critical developmental stages and the subsequent long-term pervasive effects of such repeated traumatic events. Studies have shown the high prevalence rates of child maltreatment and sexual abuse to range from 3 to 31% (Finkelhor et al., 1986). More recently, national rates of childhood maltreatment were measured to occur in 11.9% of children (U.S. Department of Health and Human Services, 2004), and that childhood maltreatment is often an etiological factor with cluster B personality disorders (Allen, 2004). It is therefore imperative that clinicians be knowledgeable about these different types of trauma when assessing for the internalizing and externalizing symptomatology consistent with childhood trauma and the associated developmental effects. Commonalities exist between both the internalizing and externalizing manifestations of trauma-related symptoms, suggesting there is a shared etiological basis or origin. Trauma affects the individual as a whole, including biological substrates and cognitive, emotional, affective, social, and interpersonal domains. Creating vulnerability and compromising the developing immune system or personality may in effect interact and or activate dormant genetic material predisposing one to developing symptoms or, in more severe cases, disorders (Leckman, 1998). The numerous manifesting symptoms that frequently represent the reason for a crisis referral may in fact be linked. A suggested metaphor that includes trauma as the "core" or "body" of the symptoms can be analogized to that of a spider. Existing as the central body, trauma creates the potential developmental pathways to numerous high-risk symptoms or disorders which are comparable to the "legs" of the spider. The body or central organizing factor is the personality (compromised by trauma) which provides the foundation to each of the legs. All are related to each other, as the central body guides all the legs through and within the environment. Thus, with those patients who have experienced trauma, comorbidity is typically present.

PSYCHIATRIC COMORBIDITY AND HIGH-RISK BEHAVIORS

Lambert (2003) stated, "Psychiatric comorbidity between personality disorders and commonly co-occurring conditions such as addiction and mood disorders increases the risk of completed suicide, as does a history of child sexual abuse and antisocial traits" (p. 74). In addition, Oquendo et al. (2003) demonstrated that those with comorbid lifetime posttraumatic stress disorder (PTSD) and depression more frequently attempted suicide than those without PTSD. Supporting the Oquendo et al. study, Soloff, Fabio, Kelly, Malone, and Mann (2005) identified that high-lethality suicide attempters with a borderline personality disorder diagnosis were more likely to have major depressive disorder, comorbid antisocial personality disorder, and family histories of substance abuse. Studies have also demonstrated the shared etiological factors between long-standing dysthymic disorders and cluster B personality disorders (Riso, Klein, Ferro, & Kasch, 1996). Sansone et al. (2004) connect an individual's trauma history, which may include observing or being exposed to the violation of body boundaries (either self or other inflicted), to the characteristic of dehumanizing and devaluing of oneself prevalent with self-injurious behaviors. Clinicians therefore need to be fully trained in the assessment of trauma, the internalizing and externalizing factors related to trauma, and the powerful empirical evidence that demonstrates the prevalence.

VULNERABILITY FACTORS

In addition to trauma, there are other factors that lower the threshold and thereby increase the individual's vulnerability and problem-solving difficulties, thus maintaining the crisis situation. These are all circumstances, situations, or deficits that have the effect of decreasing the patient's ability to cope effectively with life stressors. The patient may lose options or fail to see available options and as a result end up in crisis. Alone or in combination these factors may increase the patient's suicidal thinking or actions, lower threshold for anxiety stimuli, or increase the patient's vulnerability to depressogenic thoughts and situations (Freeman & Simon, 1989). These factors include:

1. *Acute illness.* This may range from a severe and debilitating illness to more transient illnesses such as headaches, virus infections, irritable bowel syndrome, and so on.
2. *Chronic illness.* When the health problem is chronic, there can be an acute exacerbation of suicidal thinking.
3. *Deterioration of health.* There may a loss of activity due to aging.
4. *Hunger.* During times of food deprivation, the individual is often more vulnerable to a variety of stimuli. Recent studies have shown strong evidence linking mood disorders to those with an eating disorder (Woodside & Staab, 2006). Studies have also indicated that in times of hunger, individuals should not attempt to shop for food because of the probability of over purchasing food.
5. *Anger.* When individuals are angry, they can lose problem-solving ability. They may also lose impulse control or overrespond to stimuli that they are usually able to ignore.
6. *Fatigue.* In a similar fashion, fatigue decreases both problem-solving strategies and impulse control and can therefore increase feelings of hopelessness.
7. *Loneliness.* When individuals see themselves as isolated, leaving this unhappy world may seem to be a reasonable option. They may have made the determination that they would not be missed if they were not in this world.
8. *Major life loss.* Following the loss of a significant other through death, divorce, or separation, individuals often see themselves as having reduced options, or they do not care about what happens to them. They may begin to question their purpose and future direction without the other.
9. *Poor problem-solving ability.* Certain individuals may have impaired problem-solving ability. This deficit may not be obvious until the individual is placed in situations of great stress. The ability to deal with minor problems may never test the individual's ability to manage more complicated issues or a crisis.
10. *Substance abuse.* The abuse of many substances can cause two types of problems: acute, in which the patient's judgment is compromised during periods of intoxication, and more chronic, in which judgment may be impaired more generally.
11. *Chronic pain.* Chronic pain may have the effect of causing the individual to see suicide as one method for achieving release from the pain. They may have viewed each treatment failure as cause or additional reason to commit suicide.
12. *Poor impulse control.* Certain patients have poor impulse control because of organic (hyperactivity) or functional problems. Patients with bipolar illness, borderline, antisocial, or histrionic personality disorders may all have impulse control deficits.

13. *New life circumstance.* Changing jobs, marital status, homes, or family status are all stressors create psychological vulnerability. Assessment of the vulnerability factors may help to explain crisis behaviors, intense reactions to crises, suicidal ideation, and actions that predict the possibility of bouts of suicidal ideation or other poor coping strategies.

14. *Trauma.* Trauma, either current or in the past, can compromise the coping system, making the individual even more disposed to additional trauma.

THE CBT APPROACH

In recent years, CBT has been utilized in the treatment of personality disorders, (e.g., Beck, Freeman, Davis, & Associates, 2004; Linehan, 1993) and crisis intervention (e.g., Dattilio & Freeman, 2000).

The CBT perspective, interventions, and techniques are designed to understand how a stimulus is perceived, interpreted, categorized, and responded to. For the cluster B, crisis-prone patient, quickly accessing schematic material is essential in formulating a workable and helpful series of interventions and an overall treatment plan (Freeman & Fusco, 2004).

The structure of agenda setting is essential in crisis work. The therapist must work with the patient to set an agenda for every session, to help focus the therapy work, and to help the patient to make better use of time, energy, and available skills. We emphasize that often the reason individuals are in crisis is that they have lost their ability to organize and problem-solve. By setting an agenda, the therapist models a problem-solving focus and an imposed structure creates a sense of safety and predictability for the patient. The collaboration with the patient in crisis is not likely to be 50:50, but may be 70:30 or even 90:10, with the therapist providing most of the energy and structure within the session. Having the patient use the session time for abreaction and endless review of the crisis situation without taking a problem-solving approach is not recommended.

UNDERSTANDING THE ROLE OF SCHEMATA

The personality disorder is probably one of the most striking representations of Beck's concept of schema (Beck, Rush, Shaw, & Emery, 1979; Beck, Freeman, & Associates, 1990; Beck et al., 2004; Freeman, 1993; Freeman, Pretzer, Fleming, & Simon, 1990; Layden, Newman, Freeman, & Byers-Morse, 1993). Highly idiosyncratic, the specific rules that govern and influence information processing and behavior can be classified into a variety of useful categories, such as personal, familial, cultural, religious, gender, or occupational schemata. Normally, schemata can be inferred from behavior or assessed through a complete and thorough intake, interview, and history-taking process. Thoughts are directly derived from the belief systems and often provide the inroad or identification of the schemata. As a result of maladaptive schemata, one's automatic thoughts are cognitively distorted.

For the patient in crisis, the clinician needs to adapt his/her interview style to include an in-depth evaluation eliciting activated schemata related to the current situation and its related and precipitating factors. Through Socratic questioning, the clinician can elicit the automatic thoughts or processes engendering the distress felt by the patient that may lead to a crisis. Active schemata govern the usual integration of information and result in everyday behavior. Inactive schemata become active when the individual experiences subjective distress or a crisis. At that threshold point, these dormant schemata become active and govern behavior. When the crisis situation (subjectively or objectively perceived) is no longer present, the inactive schemata will typically recede to their previous state of dormancy (Freeman & Fusco, 2000).

In addition, schemata may be classified as noncompelling or compelling. A noncompelling schema is one that the individual believes in but can relatively easily challenge and/or surrender. Compelling schemata are not easily challenged and are modified only with great difficulty, or not at all. When a crisis-prone patient presents in crisis, typically the activated schema is of a compelling nature, therefore more difficult to question or challenge. Moreover, due to the interpersonal difficulties embodied within the individual with a personality disorder, once activated, these compelling schemata create an intense and at times provocative atmosphere. Stress-related schemata may in fact impair any rational processing of the situation, including automatic thoughts and statements that may include, "I'll never make it," or "I can't cope!" (Freeman & Fusco, 2004). Complicated and competing schemata often coexist. Fusco and Apsche (2005) state that those with borderline personalities and often cluster B patients, "typically maintain numerous schema that may be in opposition to each other or incongruent" (p.77). Table 5.1 shows a sample of typical schemata of the cluster B disorders which may be activated within a crisis.

SCHEMATIC SHIFT POTENTIAL

For effective crisis intervention, it is imperative to assess the patient's ability to address, challenge, and dispute the schematic material that has initiated and supported the crisis response. This in turn allows the crisis intervention to be targeted toward the appropriate level in which the patient is functioning. The ability to shift or alter schemata can be viewed as a continuum that includes schematic paralysis, schematic rigidity, schematic stability, schematic flexibility, and schematic instability. They can each be defined in the following way:

• *Schematic paralysis.* In this state, the beliefs are ossified. The individual will maintain the beliefs regardless of the situation, context, or requirements of the circumstance.

• *Schematic rigidity.* The rules at this state are dogmatic. Individuals will not easily change what they do or how they respond. They can, in crisis situations, alter the beliefs, but when the crisis abates, they return to their dogmatic insistence that things be the way they expect things to be.

TABLE 5.1. Typical Schemata of the Cluster B Disorders

Antisocial personality disorder

I need to look out for myself.
Other people are patsies or wimps.
I need to be the aggressor or I will be the victim.
Rules are for others.
I am entitled to break the rules.
If I don't push others, I won't get what I want.
Take it, you deserve it.
Get the other guy before he gets you.

Borderline personality disorder

I am not sure who I am.
I will eventually be abandoned.
My pain (psychic) is so intense that I cannot bear it.
My anger controls me, I cannot modulate my behavior.
My feelings overwhelm me, I cannot modulate my feelings.
He/she is so very, very good that I am so lucky; or (alternately and quickly)
    he/she is so very, very awful that I cannot bear them.
When I am overwhelmed I must escape (by flight or suicide).
I am not able to control my life.
No one can help me or understand me.

Histrionic personality disorder

Appearances are important. Beauty is the most important in judging others.
I am basically unattractive.
I need and am entitled admiration from others in order to be happy.
People are judged on external appearances. I must be noticed.
If I can't captivate people, I am helpless.
I must never be frustrated in life.
I must get everything I think that I want.
Emotions should be expressed quickly and directly.

Narcissistic personality disorder

I am more special than others, so therefore, I deserve special things.
I'm superior and others should acknowledge this.
I'm above the rules.
If other's don't recognize my superiority, they should be punished.
If I'm not on top, I'm a flop.
Strive at all costs to demonstrate superiority.
I must have my way in every interaction.
I must not be, in any way, foiled in seeking pleasure or status.
I should only have to relate to special people like me.
No one should have more of anything than I have.
Few people can really understand me.

Note. Data from Beck, Freeman, and Associates (1990) and Beck, Freeman, Davis, and Associates (2004).

• *Schematic stability*. The individual whose rules are stable is far more steady and predictable. Predictability does not necessarily imply that his/her functioning is improved. Individuals with stable schemata will predictably respond to stress over many different times or situations. During a crisis, their schemata may be altered; however, they will largely respond in a predictable fashion.

• *Schematic flexibility*. Flexibility is required for creativity and problem solving. These individuals may look for new answers to old problems. When confronted by crisis, they look for new ways to cope.

• *Schematic instability*. These individuals are in a state of chronic chaos. They have poor problem-solving strategies. Life is filled with unexpected assaults to which they respond without attempting to develop a coping strategy. They may appear more erratic and unpredictable to others as their schemata continually fluctuate as a response to internal and external influences. These individuals may be thought of as having a more externalized locus of control.

THE ROLE OF EMOTIONS IN THE CRISIS-PRONE PATIENT

Cluster B personalities often appear "dramatic, emotional, or erratic" (American Psychiatric Association, 2000, p. 685). Emotional dysregulation is a central feature for these disorders and typically will drive or be implicated in the escalation or activation of a crisis. Significant contributions to the understanding of emotional dysregulation within the borderline personality structure is provided by Linehan's dialectical behavior therapy view (Linehan, 1993). Linehan states that emotional dysregulation is likely to be linked to temperament, and that this dysfunction causes an intense response to stressful events. In addition, returning to a nonactivated emotional homeostasis does not occur quickly. Emotion, for this group of patients, was invalidated by their environments and significant others, never allowing appropriate and healthy processing of emotional material. Thus, the interaction between the emotional volatility and invalidating environment creates intense dysregulation and inadequate emotional control (Linehan, 1993).

Beck et al. (2004) note emotions are related to basic cognitive structures and strategies, "the affects related to pleasure and pain play a key role in the mobilization and maintenance of the crucial strategies . . . survival and reproductive strategies appear to operate in part through their attachment to the pleasure–pain centers" (p. 29). Within a crisis, powerful emotions activate compelling schemata that, through a distorted perceptual filter, create maladaptive behaviors and coping strategies. Given that a deficit in cognitive problem solving and decision making is implicated in those with suicidal behaviors (Links, Bergmans, & Cook, 2003), impairment in these areas warrants further evaluation. Links, Bergmans, and Cook provide a comprehensive review of current studies that examine problem solving in the realm of suicidal patients. In addition to others, they cite Izard (2002), O'Leary, (2000), and Greenberg and Paivio (1997) as providing important contributions to the literature. Izard (2002) identified emotions as having a potent influence on cognitive processing, including perception, association, processing, retrieving, and action. Izard identifies emotions as the "primitives of awareness" (p. 797), which can therefore affect the mind in its problem solving, facilitation of prosocial behaviors, and the overall activation and motivation of thought and action. Emotions ultimately can preempt or thwart information processing, thereby preventing adaptive problem solving. O'Leary (2000) implicated retrieval problems in accessing prior learned material for those diagnosed with borderline personality disorder. Thus it is not so much the ability to learn but, rather, the ability to recall or retrieve the material. Greenberg and Pavio (1997) describe the functional participation of emotions in the guidance and enhancement of problem solving and decision making. The authors state that emotions in effect establish the priority of goals and the end or final goal (Greenberg & Paivio, 1997). Keeping in mind the Beck et al. (2004) premise, the emotional priority overriding the cognitive system is likely related to seeking pleasure or avoiding pain. Therefore interventions, especially crisis strategies, need to focus on the profound influence emotions serve in problem solving and cognitive processing.

CRISIS INTERVENTION

Imperative in crisis intervention is to ascertain the safety of the patient, both to him- or herself and to others. The treatment, depending on the nature of the situation, can either be a one-time intervention or a series of brief therapy sessions designed to assist the patient to return to a previous higher level of adaptive functioning.

Discerning and manifesting relative schemata assists the therapist in examining the advantages and disadvantages to maintaining schemata and introduces ways to dispute/alter strongly held schemata (through assimilation and accommodation). Overall, the immediate goals of CBT in crisis intervention are:

1. Evaluating and assessing the immediacy of the crisis situation.
2. Assessing the individual's coping repertoire to deal with the crisis.
3. Generating options of thought, perception, and behavior (includes problem-solving skills).

Roberts's Crisis Intervention Model

Roberts (1994, 2000) introduced a comprehensive seven-stage crisis intervention model that can be utilized as a general approach to crisis intervention. By utilizing the model (keeping in mind the cluster B high-arousal personality), Roberts's model synthesizes effective treatment intervention and ongoing psychotherapy.

Stage 1: Plan and Conduct a Crisis Assessment

First, the patient's safety is paramount. Chioqueta and Stiles (2004) note that "personality disorders are associated with suicide risk" (p. 128). Is the patient in immediate danger? The assessment of a high-arousal, crisis-prone patient needs to incorporate major evaluation strategies. Freeman and Fusco (2000) provide the following guidelines for those patients who may require emergent or urgent intervention.

SUICIDE THINKING CONTINUUM AND THE ROLE OF HOPELESSNESS

The assessment of risk to self and others is a complicated, necessary, and often difficult process. The therapist directly elicits information from the patient to assist in defining the overall level of intervention that will ensure the safety and physical integrity of the patient and others. Suicidal and homicidal behavior, threats, or undiminished ideation will require a change in treatment plan to include the potential for hospitalization, family sessions, psychiatric consultation, emergency services intervention, and commitment (Freeman & Fusco, 2004). Lambert (2003) strongly cautions against underestimating what may seem to be "manipulative" or "contigency-based" suicidal gestures as a means of secondary gain, as many of these patients at one time do have suicidal intent.

- *Thoughts.* Refers to individuals experiencing fleeting thoughts of suicide or homicide. These are relatively harmless and do not include any intent.
- *Ideation.* Refers to actual *ideas* about harming oneself or others. They are more formed ideas rather than fleeting thoughts. How frequent are the thoughts? How intense? What is the frequency? What is the duration?
- *Cognitive urge.* Indicates that the patient is experiencing thoughts to continue the process of planning or moving forward to harm themselves or others. Thoughts such as "How should I go about figuring out how to do this?" may occur.
- *Plan.* Have patients established a plan as to how they may harm themselves or someone else? What are the specifics involved with the plan? Does it involve others? Does the patient have access to the plan? If the patient has identified a plan, it is essential to determine and assess its actual lethality (Roberts, 1994). Brent (1987) demonstrated a strong relationship between the medical lethality of the plan chosen and suicide intent. Roberts (1994) writes that, in general, those plans considered to be more lethal include concrete, specific, and dangerous methods. In addition, the author states, "Suicidal plans generally reveal the relative risk in that the degree of intent is typically related to the lethality of the potential method (e.g., using a gun or hanging infers higher intent, whereas overdosing or cutting infers lower intent)" (Roberts, 2000, p. 140). This, however, is not a blanket statement, as all suicidal plans have the potential to be lethal and should be considered as such.
- *Behavioral urge.* Behavioral urges occur when the patient actually moves from the cognitive realm into the behavioral realm. The person may begin procuring items to complete his/her plan. A behavioral urge may include the patient holding and considering his/her means to complete the plan (e.g., picking up a bottle of pills and considering its effects).
- *Intent.* Refers to whether the individual has the actual intention to die or harm others. Has the patient identified that he/she actually intends to die or kill someone

else? Is the patient experiencing thoughts of hopelessness, a key predictor of suicide? (Beck, 1986).

• *Attempt/gesture.* Has the patient made an attempt to kill him/herself or someone else? What was the result of the attempt? What are the patient's thoughts that he/she survived the attempt? Gestures can be construed as either an episode of self-injury or a "practice" run to plan a larger attempt. Empirical studies have suggested that, "an early history of repeated 'gestures' progresses to death" (Soloff et al., 2005, p. 388).

• *Second attempt.* Patients who have made a prior attempt are more likely to make a second attempt (Reinecke, 2000).

• *Impulsivity.* At any point along the continuum, if the patient has a history of impulsivity, which may or may not include substance abuse, the patient may immediately progress from a fleeting suicidal thought to actually making an attempt. By its nature, impulsivity increases the risk one may commit an act of harm. Research has clearly implicated impulsivity in self-harm in substance abuse disorders and in cluster B personality disorders (Casillas & Clark, 2002). Careful assessment of impulsivity and substance abuse is essential.

• *Hopelessness.* Individuals who are self-injurious and suicidal exhibit hopelessness. The literature has been clear that there is a powerful association with hopelessness and completed suicide (e.g., Beck, Brown, Berchick, Stewart, & Steer, 1990; Soloff, Lynch, Kelly, Malone, & Mann, 2000). The strength of the research necessitates clinicians to incorporate questions regarding whether hopelessness is present and applying the individual's responses to the overall conceptualization. Similar to impulsivity, hopelessness can propel an individual to make an attempt or gesture, providing little to no time for intervention. In combination with the trait of impulsivity, a lethal outcome could result. A powerful study by MacLeod et al. (2004) clearly identified the role of the lack of future or positive thinking for those with personality disorders. The study identified that negative future thinking seemed to "set the stage" as a background vulnerability for providing no buffer to manage triggering events such as interpersonal conflict so often apparent in cluster B disorders. Those with cluster B personalities demonstrated lower positive future thinking and lacked a basic inability to enact a compensating plan. The authors suggest teaching planning skills as a means of "arming" the patient for ongoing stressors and situations (MacLeod et al., 2004).

• *Comorbid psychopathology.* Compounding symptoms associated with high-risk behaviors present with disorders such as mood, psychiatric, and personality disorders that add to the overall risk of suicide (Reinecke, 2000). These symptoms require the clinician to be sure a complete and adequate evaluation, history, and mental status exam are completed.

IMPULSE CONTROL

Impulsivity can propel a passing inclination to actualizing behavior. Those with the cluster B personalities may have neuropsychological and psychophysiological mechanisms that inhibit or lower impulse control (Besteiro-Gonzalez, Lemos-Giraldez, & Muniz, 2004). The impulse control is a hierarchical sequence that requires the therapist to help the patient manage each step within the sequence. The ultimate goal is to build the platform or base of the psychoeducational skill to assist in ameliorating the present crisis, and the future crisis can become an arena in which to practice crisis resolution.

The first step in the sequence is to ascertain the individual's motivation to control his/her life crises. If the motivation is poor or limited, that is, if the patient believes that the crises are not his/her fault but due to the malice of others or to the confluence of the planets, little more can be done with the patient. Until the therapist helps to generate the motivation for change, a key question must be, "What is the value to you of being in crisis?" The therapist should stay with that question and not be sidetracked into discussions of all the "thems" that create the crises. The patient must be motivated to do something about the "its" rather than the "thems."

Once there is some motivation to change, the next step is to determine the patient's ability to solve problems. Keep in mind the powerful influence emotions have on cognitive processing. Any of several problem-solving protocols can be used, including the work of Nezu and Nezu (1989) and Nezu and D'Zurilla (1981). For many patients, the basic work of Spivak, Platt, and Shure (1976) can be used. The problem-solving training is a major part of the therapy work and will continue throughout the other stages. The individual's level of frustration (threshold) must be established. The question here is, "At what point do you stop trying?" or "At what point do you revert to the same old techniques for coping with crises that haven't worked in the past?" In addition, posing to the patient, "What has worked for you before?" encourages the patient to be receptive to the fact that he/she has been able to manage prior events. Once the threshold and vulnerability factors have been addressed, the therapist can work with the patient to identify a crisis on which to practice.

The choice of a specific crisis situation is essential. Here again, the patient or therapist may want to deal with broad crisis situations or even classes of crises. This must be resisted. Using a specific situation allows for clear delineation of goals, problems, and interventions. Once this is done, the process continues.

The simple problem-solving technique of looking at the pros and cons of crisis management is introduced. This is done for two reasons. The first is to identify the relative weighting of how the individual sees the goals and purposes of crisis management. The second is to model how one can look at choices and options. The weighting may be against taking a crisis management approach, for instance, "I shouldn't have to be the one to change." The therapist can look at the advantages and disadvantages with the patient.

The patient's resistance or impediments to change must be evaluated. Too often, the best therapeutic work is sabotaged because scant attention was paid to the possible impediments. These include impediments from four sources: the patient (skills, psychopathology, abstract thinking), the therapist (skills, ability), the pathology (level of psychopathology and ability to relate interpersonally), and the environment (brief or time-limited sessions that do not allow for comprehensive treatment, unsafe situations).

The next step is to identify and select a more appropriate, prosocial, assertive coping response or behavior. The premise is that having a patient give up one behavior without having an appropriate replacement will ultimately lead to relapse. It is said that nature abhors a vacuum. This is especially true when you ask a patient to stop one behavior without having a substitute to fill the void.

The therapist and patient must plan a careful implementation of the new behavior and then experiment with it in a careful and controlled manner. After a reasonable trial (to be determined by the patient and therapist), the new behavior can be evaluated in terms of how well the new coping behavior meets the needs of the individual and the circumstances.

If the new behavior is successful, the therapist and patient can then choose another crisis issue to be resolved. The patient may not be able to generalize his/her success, and each crisis situation may have to be dealt with separately.

If the new behavior is unsuccessful, there are three key areas to review:

1. Did the patient have the ability to control the crisis?
2. Were the impediments and resistances dealt with?
3. Was the alternative crisis-management strategy appropriate?

Stage 2: Establish Rapport and Rapidly Establish Relationship

Roberts (2000) suggests that the second stage is integrated throughout stage 1. Indeed, without rapport, patients in crisis may or may not be willing to share what may be their most frightening and tightly held schemata related to the crisis. They may be embarrassed, ashamed, or even fearful of their own responses. Roberts states that the main task of the interviewer is to convey genuine respect, acceptance, and reassurance. In addition, safety is a predominant issue, particularly if the individual has been a victim of a crime or, for some, has a history of trauma.

Cluster B personalities typically seek treatment due to ongoing and intense relationship problems, and when stressed they manifest the "hallmarks of psychiatric impairment . . . in establishing social networks that provide adequate support in stressful times" (Bender, Farber, & Geller, 2001, p. 552). The authors conclude that attachment difficulties and less secure attachment are associated with higher-level cluster B personality traits of histrionic, borderline, antisocial, and narcissism. When examining the specific cluster B disorders, Gacano, Meloy, and Berg (1992) noted that for those within the cluster B spectrum, borderline and narcissistic subgroups had a greater capacity for attachment and were more anxious than the antisocial group. Bender et al. (2001) note that those individuals who are insecurely attached are more likely to remain focused on the negative aspects of therapy, have difficulty accessing mental images within therapy to be utilized during a crisis, and have difficulty coping with heightened emotions outside the therapeutic session. Kolden et al. (2005) integrate results from their prior study and conclude that those patients high in cluster B traits felt more open and involved in the session when they were not interpersonally distressed. When distressed interpersonally, therapists reported that they used more explicit direction and structure. It is therefore imperative that the clinician is knowledgeable regarding the differential diagnosis of the cluster B disorders, in addition to the general difficulty with attachment that clearly presents within a crisis situation.

Stage 3: Examine Dimensions of the Problem in Order to Define It

Roberts (2000) suggests that the clinician attempt to identify (1) the precipitating event which began the crisis; (2) previous coping methods; and (3) danger and lethality. He suggests that these areas are should be explored through open-ended questions and focus on the *now* of the situation, rather than the *how* of the situation (Roberts, 2000).

Freeman and Fusco (2000) suggest providing a structured and reframed synopsis of the patient's dilemma(s). Confusion and disorganization often render patients unable to define their problem. The therapist works to assist the patient to focus on the specific areas creating problems rather than deal with the vagaries of their actual symptoms. This provides a directive approach to setting the stage for treatment plans that outline and generate options. If the therapist focuses more on the identification of problems, the patient will most likely gain some relief at having his/her issues clearly identified. However, the clinician must be sure not to focus on an overly specific problem too early as he/she may miss bigger, more complicated, or dangerous problems. A specific problem list is helpful (Freeman & Fusco, 2000).

Stage 4: Encourage an Exploration of Feelings and Emotions

Roberts (2000) suggests that this step is closely associated with step 3, in that by defining the dimensions of the problem, related high-arousal emotions are typically identified. Exploration of emotions is encouraged in a supportive, accepting, and nonjudgmental stance. Active and reflective listening is key to creating a safe, empathic atmosphere for the patient to express and experience his/her feelings (Roberts, 2000).

Many crisis-prone patients are highly sensitive and are driven to react or change their state of discomfort (seeking pleasure and avoiding pain) by altering the felt experience. Linehan (1993) notes that the emotional dysregulation that exists for the borderline population is a result of a pervasively invalidating environment. She, as well as Roberts (2000), supports validating and accepting within management of a patient in crisis. Dialectical treatment incorporates the basic tenets of acceptance and change (Robins & Chapman, 2004).

Stage 5: Generate and Encourage Alternatives; Explore and Assess Past Coping Attempts

Roberts (2000) suggests that the clinician and the patient examine prior coping strategies together. Similar to the psychological "immune system" metaphor, Roberts suggests that those individuals who demonstrate resiliency will likely manage and cope well. However, those who are not resilient tend to have low self-esteem and efficacy, poor social supports, and lack necessary problem-solving skills. It is imperative that the patient explore alternatives and related consequences and revisit previous partial solutions, the "paths not chosen," in prior crisis situations. Roberts also states that the clinician may need to be more proactive and direct in helping the crisis patient to conceptualize alternatives, particularly if he/she as overwhelmed with emotional states.

Freeman and Fusco (2000) suggest the following:

1. Identify support networks, friends, family, church, employee assistance programs (EAPs), employees, support groups, 12-Step groups, sponsors, and hotlines.

2. If possible and if the patient agrees (if emergency, no waiver is needed), bring support network into initial evaluation to activate or challenge held beliefs regarding worth and other issues. When seeing a patient in crisis for the first time, most likely a family member or friend has come along to the session.

3. Help identify the patient's own internal resources and strengths which may be overlooked (schema activation). The patient may readily identify held beliefs ("I can't do anything right"; "I'm a loser, no one loves me"; "There's no hope," "I'd be better off dead than trying something new"; etc). These beliefs offer data and information about areas to challenge, dispute, or modify.

4. Call on previous challenges that the patient was able to overcome (maintaining employment despite debilitating illness, completing a course, taking care of children, getting self up and dressed, caring for home, etc.).

5. Imagine a role model managing the problem and ask "How is X able to do this?" Be specific. For instance, "How would your best friend handle this?"

Stage 6: Develop and Formulate an Action Plan

Within this stage, Roberts (2000) states, "The basic premise underlying a cognitive approach to crisis resolution is that the ways in which external events and a person's cognitions of the events turn into personal crisis are based on cognitive factors" (p. 20). Roberts describes cognitive mastery as including the client understanding how and why the crisis occurred, the event's idiosyncratic meaning and the cognitive errors or distortions that are activated within the crisis, and, finally, the cognitive restructuring or challenging of dysfunctional thinking.

Freeman and Fusco (2000) suggest in developing a positive plan of action:

1. Elicit commitment from the patient to the plan of action.
2. Bring supports in to provide backup and motivation to complete the plan.
3. Advocate for the patient—for instance, in accessing social services or treatment options or providing alternative options of support (shelters, etc.).
4. Use imagery (imagine completion of goals, seeing self attempting and completing stepwise tasks).
5. Be concrete and specific in identifying future plans and related goals. The more specific the goals, the more the patient can affirm that he/she is actually accomplishing something.

Stage 7: Follow-Up

The key to successful crisis intervention is follow-up (Roberts, 2000). Patients often require booster sessions or, in some cases, referral to ongoing psychotherapy to assist in continuing treatment progress. Roberts suggests that the clinician remain aware of therapeutic factors related to crisis and trauma, such as the avoidance found within those with PTSD. Orbach (1999) states that although time-limited cognitive-behavioral therapies are efficacious while engaged in the process, over the long term, it did not show continued effectiveness for those with suicidality and depression. This clearly indicates the need for booster sessions and for the patient to be assured that additional sessions may be necessary and in some instances encouraged.

TREATMENT INTERVENTIONS AND TECHNIQUES

Several cognitive and behavioral techniques can be used by the therapist to help question both the distortions and the schemata that underlie them. These techniques can be taught to the patients to help them respond in more functional ways. A rule of thumb in treating severely depressed or overwhelmed patients would be that the more severe the dysfunction, the greater the proportion of behavioral to cognitive interventions the therapist will use (see Figure 5.1). The precise mix of cognitive and behavioral techniques will depend on the patient's level of functioning.

Self-Monitoring

Self-monitoring is a method in which patients can learn more about themselves and is an intrinsic aspect to cognitive-behavioral treatment and crisis intervention. Self-monitoring can be described to patients as watching and viewing themselves to see what and how they respond, think, feel, and react physically to certain events or situations. The goal of self-monitoring is to learn to predict a situation in which the patient may become distressed, and to know typically how he/she may react. This is particularly important for crisis-prone patients who many times are unaware of the impending crisis.

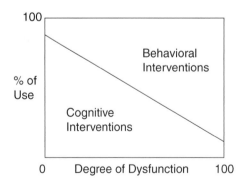

FIGURE 5.1. Use of cognitive and behavioral interventions.

Homework

Therapy, of necessity, must take place beyond the confines of the consulting room. It is important for the patient to understand that the extension of the therapy work to the nontherapy hours allows for a greater therapeutic focus. The homework can be cognitive and/or behavioral. It might involve having the patient complete an activity schedule (an excellent homework for the first session), complete several dysfunctional thought records, or try new behaviors. The homework needs to flow from the session material rather than being tacked onto the end of the session simply because cognitive therapy "should" include homework. The more meaningful and collaborative the homework, the greater the likelihood the patient will comply with the therapeutic regimen. The homework should be reviewed at the next session. If the homework is not part of the session agenda, the patient will quickly stop doing the homework. The more the patient is helped to do homework, the better. When therapy ends, everything will be homework for the patient.

As the crisis-prone patient will likely have ongoing therapeutic contact, homework specific to the crisis can be implemented within the overall treatment plan. Initially, self-monitoring should be incorporated as a basic and ongoing intervention. Homework assignments can include the Incident Chart (Fusco & Freeman, 2004) or the more traditional Dysfunctional Thought Record (Beck, 1995). In addition, working with an integrated self-directed goal sheet can encourage and help with patient assertion. Integrating Meichenbaum and Turk's (1987) work, Freeman and Fusco (2005) suggest the following:

1. Homework needs to be collaboratively developed.
2. Tasks should be simple.
3. Provide the client with a choice.
4. Specify what will be done, when, and how.
5. Engage significant others in the task.
6. Directly, in a stepwise fashion, teach self-monitoring skills.
7. Specify contingencies that follow adherence or nonadherence.
8. Offer mild countersuggestions about the completion of the task.
9. Anticipate disappointments, difficulties, and obstacles.
10. Provide feedback on adherence and the accuracy of performance.
11. Record positive behaviors rather than negative behaviors.
12. Assign "do" tasks rather than "don't" tasks.

MAINTENANCE OF PROGRESS

For most individuals, coping with potential crises is a lifelong endeavor. This does not necessarily mean that they must come for therapy on a weekly basis. For some patients a session once a month as a "check-in" session to review and manage the problems and solutions of the past month will suffice. For other patients, a check-in phone call on some scheduled basis may be required. For some patients the therapy sessions might be "as needed." For others, therapy is an essential part of their lives.

SUMMARY

The patient in crisis experiences discomfort, dysfunction, dyscontrol, and disorganization—one in great measure or several in combination. For patients who are experiencing a crisis and have adequate intrapersonal and interpersonal resources, a crisis period need not be a time for only negative results or consequences. These patients may take advantage of their experiences to formulate positive change, growth, and adaptation to life's circumstances. However, for those patients diagnosed with a cluster B personality disorder or who are crisis-prone, additional stressors—whether internal or external—can create a "crossover" through threshold or trigger points. With their psychological immune systems compromised, thresholds for these patients are invariably lower than for those who are not crisis-prone. This is particularly so for the cluster B patient. Sensitive, erratic, and at times subject to extreme periods of lability, these patients often respond to stressors from an emotional standpoint, thus interfering with adaptive and positive problem solving. Unarmed with adequate coping or modulating strategies to manage these emotional states, an already vulnerable system can be thrown into crisis by minimal amounts of stress. High-arousal patients such as these usually have additional vulnerability factors that compound and complicate an already chaotic system. These include those factors from the patients themselves, their environment, supports or inadequate supports, and—characteristic to these disorders—unstable relationships.

By understanding and eliciting the patient's primary or underlying schematic material related to their personality style derived from a comprehensive case conceptualization, the therapist can approach each crisis situation armed with an understanding of the cognitive processes in which the patient is reacting. For the cluster B patient, all these disorders will react in an egosyntonic, emotionally charged manner. It will be difficult for these patients to comprehend their role in the crisis and, likewise, their ability to effect change within the crisis.

By applying the revised stages of change proposed by Freeman and Dolan (2001), the therapist can understand and conceptualize the readiness or ability for the patient to engage in schematic shifts. Often these patients are operating within schematic paralysis and are therefore not open to shifting, adapting, or assimilating change to schemata. Being challenged with therapeutic interventions aimed at cognitive distortions, patients can begin to create options for themselves rather than making negative assumptions that no other choices are available to them. This is particularly true for the suicidal patient who has designated death as the only option to manage unbearable pain. By creating a continuum of options other than suicide, the patient can begin to see the alternatives, rather than the sheer hopelessness that creates, feeds, and worsens suicidal ideation.

For the cluster B patient, the application of the defined schematic patterns will often assist the therapist in defining, creating, and refining therapeutic interventions. By framing basic schematic representations in a nonpejorative style to the patient, the patient can therefore feel understood. For example, to the narcissistic patient, the therapist might say, "You have special needs right now that you feel aren't getting met. Maybe there are some other options or means to explore having those needs met."

This statement reframes the narcissist's basic schematic pattern of being different or special; however, it also creates an inroad to intervention by suggesting options. In other words, we encourage therapists to use the personality pathology as a guide or aid in creating therapeutic interventions. Thorough evaluation, assessment, and triage of the patient are imperative to crisis intervention. This includes a comprehensive suicide and homicide inquiry. As many cluster B patients often react in a dramatic or emotional style, threats of harm to themselves or others can be easily made. We strongly advise that all threats be taken seriously and that the clinician should apply the patient's history and current mental status to the conceptualization and determination of the lethality of the patient. Roberts (2000) provides an excellent crisis intervention model from which to form relevant and practical treatment interventions.

All assessments should also include whether the patient can demonstrate good impulse control. By utilizing the cognitive-behavioral therapy approach encouraging self–other monitoring, patients can learn to target their own impulses by being aware or cognizant of their escalation. They will then create for themselves a choice of behaviors to utilize as a response to the impulse and also to avert a crisis. For those patients largely more depressed or dysfunctional and unable to access their cognitive resources as readily, more behavioral treatment approaches are encouraged.

Throughout treatment, challenging dysfunctional beliefs through myriad techniques creates options and alternatives and ultimately fosters hope for the patient, The method of these challenges is an opportunity for the therapist to utilize creativity and apply the patient's strengths to the task set forth. For the cluster B crisis-prone patient, the therapist can utilize and reframe schematic personality patterns to guide and cognitively intervene, thwart, and divert a crisis situation into an opportunity to collaboratively generate options and alternatives and attempt new coping strategies, ultimately improving the patient's quality of life.

REFERENCES

Allen, J. (2004). *Traumatic relationships and serious mental disorders*. Chichester, UK: Wiley.

American Psychiatric Association. (2000) . *Diagnostic and statistical manual of mental disorders* (4th ed., text rev.). Washington, DC: Author.

Ball, J., Links, P., Strike, C., & Boydell, K. (2005). "It's overwhelming . . . everything seems to be too much": A theory of crisis for individuals with severe persistent mental illness. *Psychiatric Rehabilitation Journal*, 29(1), 10–17.

Beck, A. (1986). Hopelessness as a predictor of eventual suicide. *Annals of the New York Academy of Science*, 487, 90–96.

Beck, A., Brown, G., Berchick, R., Stewart, B., & Steer, R. (1990). Relationship between hopelessness and ultimate suicide: A replication with psychiatric outpatients. *American Journal of Psychiatry*, 147, 190–195.

Beck, A. T., Freeman, A., & Associates. (1990). *Cognitive therapy of personality disorders*. New York: Guilford Press.

Beck, A. T., Freeman A., Davis, D., & Associates. (2004). *Cognitive therapy of personality disorders* (2nd ed.). New York: Guilford Press.

Beck, A. T., Rush, A. J., Shaw, B. E., & Emery, G. (1979). *Cognitive therapy of depression*. New York: Guilford Press.

Beck, J. (1995). *Cognitive therapy: Basics and beyond*. New York: Guilford Press.

Bender, D., Farber, B., & Geller, J. (2001). Cluster B personality traits and attachment. *Journal of the American Academy of Psychoanalysis and Dynamic Psychiatry, 29*(4), 551–563.

Besteiro-Gonzalez, J. L., Lemos-Giraldez, S., & Muniz, J. (2004). Neurological, psycho-physiological, and personality assessment of DSM-IV clusters of personality disorders. *European Journal of Psychological Assessment, 20*(2), 99–105.

Brent, D. (1987). Correlates of the medical lethality of suicide attempts in children and adolescents. *Journal of the American Academy of Child and Adolescent Psychiatry, 26*, 87–91.

Casillas, A., & Clark, L. (2002). Dependency, impulsivity, and self-harm: Traits hypothesized to underlie the association between Cluster B personality and substance use disorders. *Journal of Personality Disorders, 16*(5), 424–437.

Chioqueta, A., & Stiles, T. (2004) Assessing suicide risk in cluster C personality disorders. *Crisis, 25*(3), 128–133.

Dattilio, F. M., & Freeman, A. (Eds.). (2000). *Cognitive-behavioral strategies in crisis intervention* (2nd ed.). New York: Guilford Press.

Finkelhor, D., Araji, S., Baron, L., Browne, A., Peters, S. D., & Wyatt, G. E. (1986). *Sourcebook on child sexual abuse*: Newbury Park, CA: Sage.

Freeman, A., & Dattilio, F. (Eds.). (2000). *Cognitive-behavioral strategies in crisis intervention, 2nd ed*. New York: Guilford Press.

Freeman, A., & Dolan, M. (2001). Revisiting Prochaska and DiClemente's stages of change theory: An expansion and specification to aid in treatment planning and outcome evaluation. *Cognitive and Behavioral Practice, 8*(3), 224–234..

Freeman, A., & Fusco, G. M. (2000). Treating high-arousal patients: Differentiating between patients in crisis and crisis-prone patients. In F. Dattilio & A. Freeman (Eds.), *Cognitive-behavioral strategies in crisis intervention* (pp. 27–58). New York: Guilford Press.

Freeman, A., & Fusco, G. M. (2004). *Borderline personality disorder: A therapist's guide to taking control*. New York: Norton.

Freeman, A., & Fusco, G. M. (2005). Borderline traits. In N. Kazantis, F. Deane, K. Ronan, & L. L'Abate (Eds.), *Using homework assignments in cognitive behavior therapy* (pp. 329–353). New York: Routledge.

Freeman, A., Pretzer, J., Fleming, B., & Simon, K. M. (1990). *Clinical applications of cognitive therapy*. New York: Plenum Press.

Freeman, A., Pretzer, J., Fleming, B., & Simon, K. M. (2004). *Clinical applications of cognitive therapy* (2nd ed.). New York: Springer.

Freeman, A., & Simon, K. M. (1989). Cognitive therapy of anxiety. In A. Freeman, K. M. Simon, L. Beutler, & H. Arkowitz (Eds.), *Comprehensive handbook of cognitive therapy* (pp. 347–366). New York: Plenum Press.

Fusco, G. M., & Apsche, J. (2005). Cognitive behavioral therapy. In A. Freeman, M. Stone, & D. Martin (Eds.), *Comparative treatments for borderline personality disorder* (pp. 75–104). New York: Springer.

Fusco, G. M., & Freeman, A. (2004). *Borderline personality disorder: A patient's guide to taking control*. New York: Norton.

Gacano, C., Meloy, J., & Berg, J. (1992). Object relations, defensive operations, and affective states in narcissistic, borderline, and antisocial personality disorder. *Journal of Personality Assessment, 59*(1), 32–49.

Greenberg, L. S., & Paivio, S. C. (1997). *Working with emotions in psychotherapy*. New York: Guilford Press.

Izard, C. E. (2002). Translating emotion theory and research into preventative interventions. *Psychological Bulletin, 128*, 796–824.

Jakubowski, P., & Lange, A. J. (1978). *Responsible assertive behavior*. Champaign, IL: Research Press.

Johnson, J., Smailes, E., Cohen, P., Brown, J., & Bernstein, D. (2000). Associations between four types of childhood neglect and personality disorder symptoms during adolescence and early adulthood: Findings of a community-based longitudinal study. *Journal of Personality Disorders*, *14*(2), 171–187.

Kolden, G., Klein, M., Strauman, T., Chisholm-Stockard, S., Heerey, E., Schneider, K., et al. (2005). Early psychotherapy process and cluster B and C personality pathology: Similarities and differences in interactions with symptomatic and interpersonal distress. *Psychotherapy Research*, *15*(3), 165–177.

Lambert, M. (2003). Suicide risk assessment and management: Focus on personality disorders. *Personality Disorders*, *16*(1), 71–76.

Layden, M. A., Newman, C. F., Freeman, A., & Byers-Morse, S. (1993). *Cognitive therapy of borderline personality disorder*. Boston: Allyn & Bacon.

Leckman, J. (1998). Understanding developmental psychopathology: How useful are evolutionary accounts? *American Academy of Child and Adolescent Psychiatry*, *37*(10), 1011–1021.

Linehan, M. (1993). *Cognitive behavioral treatment of borderline personality disorder*. New York: Guilford Press.

Links, P., Bergmans, Y., & Cook, M. (2003). Psychotherapeutic interventions to prevent repeated suicidal behavior. *Brief Treatment and Crisis Intervention*, *3*(4), 445–464.

MacLeod, A., Tata, P., Tyrer, P., Schmidt, U., Davidson, K., & Thompson, S. (2004). Personality disorder and future-directed thinking in parasuicide. *Journal of Personality Disorders*, *18*(5), 459–468.

Meichenbaum, D., & Turk, D. (1987). *Facilitating treatment adherence: A practitioner's handbook*. New York: Plenum Press.

Millon, T., & Davis, R. (2000). *Personality disorders in modern life*. New York: Wiley.

Nezu, A. M., & D'Zurilla, T. J. (1981). Effects of problem definition and formulation on the generation of alternatives in the social problem-solving process. *Cognitive Therapy and Research*, *5*, 265–271.

Nezu, A. M., & Nezu, C. M. (1989). *Clinical decision making in behavior therapy: A problem-solving perspective*. Champaign, IL: Research Press.

O'Leary, K. (2000). Borderline personality disorder. Neuropsychological testing results. *Psychiatric Clinics of North America*, *23*, 41–60.

Oquendo, M., Friend, J., Halberstam, B., Brodsky, B., Burke, A., Grunebaum, M., Malone, K., & Mann, J. (2003). Association of co-morbid posttraumatic stress disorder and major depression with greater risk for suicidal behavior. *American Journal of Psychiatry*, *160*(3), 580–582.

Orbach, I. (1999). Brief cognitive therapy for depressed and suicidal adolescents: A critical comment. *Clinical Child Psychology and Psychiatry*, *4*, 593–596.

Prochaska, J. O., & DiClemente, C. C. (1982). Transtheoretical therapy: Toward a more integrative model of change. *Psychotherapy: Theory Research and Practice*, *20*, 161–173.

Prochaska, J. O., & DiClemente, C. C. (1983). Stages and processes of self-change of smoking: Toward an integrative model of change. *Journal of Consulting and Clinical Psychology*, *5*, 390–395.

Prochaska J. O., & DiClemente, C. C. (1992). Stages of change in the modification of problem behaviors. In M. Hersen, R. M. Eisler, & P. M. Miller (Eds.), *Progress in behavior modification* (pp. 184–214). Sycamore, IL: Sycamore Press.

Ratican, K. (1992). Sexual abuse survivors: Identifying symptoms and special treatment considerations. *Journal of Counseling and Development*, *71*(1), 33–39.

Reinecke, M. (2000). Suicide and depression. In F. Dattilio & A. Freeman (Eds.), *Cognitive behavioral strategies in crisis intervention, 2nd ed.* (pp. 84–125). New York: Guilford Press.

Riso, L., Klein, D., Ferro, T., & Kasch, K. (1996). Understanding the comorbidity between early onset dysthymia and cluster B personality disorders: A family study. *American Journal of Psychiatry, 153*(7), 900–907.

Roberts, A. (1994). *Crisis intervention handbook.* New York: Oxford University Press.

Roberts, A. (2000). *Crisis intervention handbook* (2nd ed.). New York: Oxford University Press.

Roberts, A., & Everly, G. (2006). A meta-analysis of 36 crisis intervention studies. *Brief Treatment and Crisis Intervention, 6*(1), 10–21.

Robins, C., & Chapman, A. (2004). Dialectical behavior therapy: Current status, recent developments, and future directions. *Journal of Personality Disorders, 18*(1), 73–89.

Sansone, R., Sansone, L., & Levitt, J. (2004). Borderline personality disorder: Self-harm and eating disorders. In J. Levitt, R. Sansone, & L. Cohn (Eds.), *Self-harm behavior and eating disorders: Dynamics, assessment, and treatment* (pp. 61–73). New York: Brunner-Routledge.

Shneidman, E. S. (1993). Suicide as a psychache. *Journal of Nervous and Mental Disease, 181,* 145–147.

Slaiku, K. (1990). *Crisis intervention* (2nd ed.). Boston: Allyn & Bacon.

Soloff, P. H., Fabio, A., Kelly, T., Malone, K., & Mann, J. (2005). High-lethality status in patients with borderline personality disorder. *Journal of Personality Disorders, 19*(4), 386–399.

Soloff, P. H., Lynch, K. G., Kelly, T. M., Malone, K. M., & Mann, J. J. (2000). Characteristics of suicide attempts of patients with major depressive episode and borderline personality disorder: A comparative study. *American Journal of Psychiatry, 157,* 601–608.

Spivak, G., Platt, J. J., & Shure, M. B. (1976). *The problem solving approach to adjustment.* San Francisco: Jossey-Bass.

Stone, M. (1993). *Abnormalities of personality.* New York: Norton.

U.S. Department of Health and Human Services, Administration for Children, Youth, and Families. (2004). *Child maltreatment 2002: Reports from the states to the National Child Abuse and Neglect Data System.* Washington, DC: U.S. Government Printing Office.

van der Kolk, B. (2005). Developmental trauma disorder. *Psychiatric Annals, 35*(5), 401–408.

Woodside, B., & Staab, R. (2006). Management of psychiatric comorbidity in anorexia nervosa and bulimia nervosa. *CNS Drugs, 20*(8), 655–663.

SUGGESTED READINGS

Freeman, A., & Fusco, G. M. (2004). *Borderline personality disorder: A therapist's guide to taking control.* New York: Norton.

Fusco, G. M., & Freeman, A. (2004). *Borderline personality disorder: A patient's guide to taking control.* New York: Norton.

Kreisman, J. J., & Straus, H. (1989). *I hate you, don't leave me: Understanding the borderline personality disorder.* New York: Avon Books.

Linehan, M. M. (1993). *Cognitive-behavioral treatment of borderline personality disorder.* New York: Guilford Press.

Mason, P. T., & Krieger, R. (1998). *Stop walking on eggshells: Taking your life back when someone you care about has borderline personality disorder.* Oakland, CA: New Harbinger.

Millon, T. & Davis, R. (2000). *Personality disorders in modern life.* New York: Wiley.

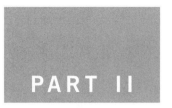

PART II

Medically Related Crises

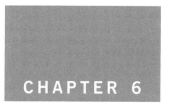

CHAPTER 6

Traumatic Brain Injury

Mary R. Hibbard
Wayne A. Gordon
Lynne M. Kothera

*I*ndividuals often present to mental health professionals in psychological crisis following a significant traumatic event. While the origins of these traumatic events can vary—for example, a motor vehicle accident (MVA), a pedestrian accident, a sports-related accident, a whiplash injury, a serious fall or an act of violence (abuse, assault, etc.)—many individuals report a combination of anxiety and stress-related symptoms. The events surrounding the trauma will, by definition, place the individual at increased risk of having experienced a simultaneous, and potentially undiagnosed, traumatic brain injury (TBI) (Moore, Terryberry-Spohr, & Hope, 2006) with rates of anxiety as high as 29% in individuals who had experienced a TBI at the time of the precipitating event (Epstein & Ursano, 1994). The physical, cognitive, and affective changes following TBI will complicate the clinical presentation of anxiety symptoms, and necessitate shifts in traditional cognitive-behavioral approaches to assessment and treatment. An understanding of TBI is essential for clinicians to be able to effectively diagnose and treat individuals with dual diagnoses of anxiety and TBI. This chapter provides (1) an overview of the prevalence, etiology, and functional changes following TBI; (2) approaches to screening for a TBI; (3) the psychiatric disorders observed following TBI; and (4) suggested modifications of cognitive-behavioral approaches to assessment and treatment of individuals with dual diagnoses of an anxiety disorder and a TBI. Case studies highlight suggested modifications in assessment and treatment approaches.

TRAUMATIC BRAIN INJURY: THE SILENT EPIDEMIC

TBI, especially less severe (also known as mild) brain injury, has been called the silent epidemic (Marino, 1999; Tellier et al., 1999). TBI is the leading cause of death and disability in the United States, with an estimated 1.5–2 million such injuries occurring annually. Each year, brain injuries result in approximately 1 million emergency room visits, 230,000 hospitalizations, and 151,000 deaths (Woo & Thoidis, 2000). In addition, 80,000 TBI survivors will experience the onset of long-term disability each year with as many as 6.5 million Americans currently living in the United States with TBI-related challenges (Centers for Disease Control and Prevention, 2004; Martin & Johnstone, 2006). To gain perspective on the impact of TBI in the United States, one needs only to compare the prevalence of TBI with other medical conditions: AIDS—350,000 people currently living in the United States; breast cancer—182,000 women and 1,000 men will be diagnosed each year; and 7,800 Americans will sustain spinal cord injuries every year (Marino, 1999). TBI is more frequently diagnosed in men, with peak ages of occurrence noted in adolescence and young adulthood and in persons over the age of 75. The leading causes of TBI are MVAs, violence, and falls (Centers for Disease Control and Prevention, 2004; National Institutes of Health, 1999; Woo & Thoidis, 2000).

UNDERSTANDING TBI

TBI occurs when there is a significant blow to the head that results in either a loss of consciousness or a period during which mental status is altered and/or the person feels "dazed and confused." Many individuals subsequently experience changes in physical functioning, thinking, mood, and behavior. TBI exists along a continuum of severity typically estimated either by the duration of loss of consciousness (LOC) or by the duration of time that the person experiences an altered mental status following the blow to the head. Severity of brain injury can also be inferred from the depth and/or length of coma that ensues following a blow to the head.

Approximately 15% of individuals who are diagnosed with TBI will have experienced a *moderate to severe injury* (Centers for Disease Control and Prevention, 2004). The vast majority of these individuals are hospitalized, with many of these individuals experiencing coma of varying duration following TBI. Typically, such individuals receive intensive medical and rehabilitation services to address their residual cognitive, physical, and emotional symptoms and, thus, are "known" to the medical system. The remaining 85% of individuals who experience a TBI will have a *mild injury*. A mild injury is defined as

> the occurrence of an injury to the head arising from blunt trauma or acceleration or deceleration forces with one or more of the following conditions attributable to the head injury: any period of observed or self-reported transient confusion disorientation or impaired consciousness, dysfunction of memory around the time of injury or loss of consciousness

lasting less than 30 minutes; and observed signs or other neurobiological or neuropsychological dysfunction such as seizures, irritability, lethargy or vomiting following the head injury, headaches, dizziness, irritability, fatigue or poor concentration. (Centers for Disease Control and Prevention, 2004, p. 4)

Many individuals with a mild TBI present to local emergency rooms or local physicians' offices for evaluation, are diagnosed with a "concussion," and are told that they will be "fine" in several days. An even larger number of individuals with mild TBI fail to seek medical attention and therefore remain undiagnosed (Bernstein, 1999; Gerberding & Binder, 2003; Gordon et al., 1998). Although the negative consequences of a mild brain injury tend to dissipate over time, approximately 15% of such individuals will continue to experience residual cognitive, physical, and emotional changes (Uzzell, 1999). Lack of proper identification of the underlying brain injury pathology in these individuals often results in persons developing secondary affective reactions (i.e., depression and/or anxiety) due to their lack of understanding of new cognitive functioning difficulties in everyday activities. It is of little surprise, then, that individuals with potentially undiagnosed TBI often present to the mental health professional with predominant anxiety or depressive symptoms posttrauma (Holtzer, Burright, Lynn, & Donovick, 2000; Koren, Arnon, & Klein, 1999).

Of specific focus to this chapter, the most common anxiety disorder reported after an MVA is posttraumatic stress disorder (PTSD) (Blanchard et al., 1995; Koren et al., 1999; Mayou, Bryan, & Duthie, 1993). Unfortunately, screening for a potential coexisting TBI was not included in these studies, leaving the issue of undiagnosed TBI unanswered. Given that anxiety disorders in general and PTSD in particular are common diagnoses following a known TBI (Ashman et al., 2004; Bryant & Harvey, 1999; Hibbard, Uysal, Kepler, Bogdany, & Silver, 1998; Ohry, Rattock, & Solomon, 1996; Rattock, 1996; Silver, Rattock, & Anderson, 1997), the potential for an undiagnosed TBI in at least a proportion of individuals presenting to mental health settings following an MVA appears likely.

THE ETIOLOGY OF TBI

When an individual experiences a TBI, there is a traumatic blow to the head or rapid movement of the head resulting in damage or destruction of brain tissue. Two types of injuries to the head resulting in brain injuries are commonly seen: an open-head injury and a closed-head injury (Bernstein, 1999). In *open-head injury*, the individual experiences a blow to the head in which the skull is penetrated. Damage following an open-head injury tends to be more localized, with subsequent impairment limited to the areas of the brain damaged by the path of the object entering the head and the specific location within the brain at point of impact. The most common etiologies of an open-head injury are gunshot wounds and the person being hit by a falling object (Centers for Disease Control and Prevention, 2004; National Institutes of Health, 1999).

In *closed-head injury*, damage to the brain occurs due to inertial forces created within the brain (Bernstein, 1999). A closed-head injury can result from any event in which the brain is set in rapid motion within the skull and then comes to an abrupt stop (e.g., during a car crash or on unexpected impact during a sports event). In these types of injuries, inertia throws the head forward, creating equal momentum in the opposite direction resulting in rotational movement of the brain against the spinal cord and within the skull itself. These rapid movements cause the brain to move in two or more different directions at once, causing stretching and tearing of nerve cells throughout the brain and bruising of near and distant brain (Bagley, Grossman, & Lenkinski, 1998; Cecil et al., 1998). The head does not have to actually hit a surface to incur a closed-brain injury. For example, in a whiplash injury, the head is "whipped" forward and back and from side to side causing the brain to collide at high velocity with the rough inner surfaces of the skull. The extent of damage is usually related to the initial severity or force of the blow and the part of the head that has been hit. For example, the unbelted passenger's head that is slammed into a car windshield during a high-speed impact will probably result in a more severe brain injury than a seat-belted passenger's head who is involved in a similar MVA during a lower-speed impact. The most common etiologies of closed-head injury are MVA, pedestrian accidents, sports accidents, falls, and violence (shaken baby syndrome, abuse, assault, etc.) (Centers for Disease Control and Prevention, 2004; National Institutes of Health, 1999).

TYPICAL SEQUELAE OF TBI

The impact of brain injury on an individual's functioning will depend on many factors: the severity of the initial injury, the areas of the brain that have been damaged, the rate and completeness of physiological recovery, the nature and extent of deficits post-injury, the individual's awareness of these changes, and the unique meaning these changes have to an individual. Typically, functional changes are grouped into three major domains: physical, cognitive, and affective or behavioral changes. Most individuals experience symptoms across the three domains; however, the relative severity of symptoms and the degree of interference in completing everyday activities will vary from person to person.

The most common *physical changes* reported by an individual after brain injury include extensive fatigue, clumsiness, decreased or altered sensory functioning (i.e., changes in hearing, vision, smell and touch), difficulties with sleep, body temperature changes, seizures, and change in appetite and weight. The *cognitive changes* will significantly interfere with everyday functioning and successful resumption of many former life roles. These symptoms include impaired attention and concentration, reduced processing speed, word-finding difficulties, altered academic abilities (i.e., errors in simple math computation, spelling, reading, and comprehension), decreased memory and learning abilities, and impaired executive functioning (i.e., reduced ability to plan, sequence, prioritize, think flexibly or abstractly, or problem-solve). *Affective changes* following TBI include changes in mood, and alterations in behavioral control and interpersonal relationship. Mood changes typically reflect symptoms of depression, mood lability, and anxiety. Behavioral changes include an inability to manage the unexpected and a reduced ability to control anger. Impaired interpersonal communication (e.g., an inability to follow conversations, being rude, interrupting people, and talking too fast or too slowly), while more subtle, may have a serious impact on the person's ability to develop and maintain meaningful relationships (Arlingthuas, Shoaib, & Price, 2005; Martin & Johnstone, 2006).

SCREENING FOR A PRIOR TBI

When an individual presents to the mental health professional with an anxiety disorder secondary to a traumatic event, screening for a prior TBI should be a routine part of the intake interview. The purpose of this screening is to rule out a possible but heretofore unidentified TBI. Traumatic events during which a possible TBI might have occurred include MVA, pedestrian accidents, sports-related accidents, whiplash injuries, serious falls, and a prior history of abuse or assault (Gordon et al., 1998; Gordon, Haddad, Brown, Hibbard, & Sliwinski, 2000).

If, upon questioning, an individual reports that the traumatic event involved a blow to the head accompanied by either a period of loss of consciousness or an altered mental state, the clinician is encouraged to probe for potential physical, cognitive, and affective symptoms (outlined in the previous section of this chapter) that the individual may be experiencing since the traumatic event. When changes are reported, the probability of a previously undiagnosed TBI at the time of the trauma is significantly increased.

Joint discussion of this probable secondary diagnosis is an important therapeutic intervention. In our clinical experiences, an individual whose TBI remains undiagnosed is often quite aware of his/her affective distress (and hence is seeking psychological help); however, the individual remains perplexed and frightened by the seemingly random and unexplained changes in his/her physical, cognitive, and affective functioning since the traumatic event. The process of relating these functional changes to a possible undiagnosed TBI is often comforting to the individual who, until then, felt he/she was truly "going crazy." A referral for neuropsychological evaluation should be discussed with the individual at this juncture. A neuropsychological evaluation serves to confirm the diagnosis of TBI and will provide a specific profile of the individual's cognitive strengths and weaknesses, which can then be integrated in effective treatment planning (Pelham & Lovell, 2005).

PSYCHIATRIC DISORDERS FOLLOWING TBI

In addition to known physical, cognitive, and behavioral changes that occur following TBI, the majority of individuals with TBI are frequently diagnosed with one or more newly acquired DSM Axis I (American Psychiatric Association, 1994) disorders. Co-occurring depression and anxiety are the most prevalent Axis I disorders (Ashman et al., 2004; Deb, Lyons, Koutzouis, Ali, & McCarthy, 1999; Hibbard et al., 1998; Jorge, Robinson, Strarkstein, & Arndt, 1994; Jorge et al., 2004; Mooney & Speed, 2001; Wallace & Bogner, 2000). The presence of a psychiatric disorder poses additional challenges for an individual with TBI as he/she attempts to reintegrate back into the community and resume former life roles (Hibbard et al., 2004).

During the 1980s, psychiatric challenges following TBI were clinically described by family members and care providers, with depressive symptoms reported in 6–77% of TBI survivors (Brooks, Campsie, Symington, Beattie, & McKinley, 1986; Kinsella, Moran, Ford, & Ponsford, 1998; Rutherford, Merritt, & McDonald, 1979; Van Zomeren, & Vandenberg, 1985) and anxiety symptoms reported in 18–60% of TBI survivors (Brooks et al., 1986; Dikman, McLean, & Temkin, 1989; Tyerman & Humphrey, 1984). In the past two decades, research efforts have shifted to the use of psychiatric diagnoses using DSM-IV criteria (American Psychiatric Association, 1994) to diagnose post-TBI emotional disturbances. The most prevalent Axis I disorder following TBI is major depression, with the frequency of this disorder unrelated to time postonset or severity of injury. Major depression was noted in 26% of individuals at 1 year (Jorge et al., 1994), 50–77% at 3 to 5 years (Fann, Katon, Uomto, & Essleman, 1995; Van Reekum, Bolango, Finlayson, Garner, & Links, 1996; Varney, Martz, & Roberts, 1987), and 61% at 8 years (Hibbard et al., 1998). While robust rates of resolution have been reported (Fann et al., 1995; Hibbard et al., 1998; Van Reekum et al., 1996), elevated rates of major depression are noted decades after the injury (Koponen et al., 2002).

While the prevalence of anxiety disorders following TBI have been less well evaluated, they are also frequent reactions following TBI and often coexist with depression post-TBI (Hibbard et al., 2004). At 1 year post-TBI, generalized anxiety disorder (GAD) was found in 11% of individuals (Jorge et al., 1994). More than 20% of individuals at 3 and 5 years post-TBI (Fann et al., 1995; Van Reekum et al., 1996) and 9% of individuals at 8 years post-TBI (Hibbard et al., 1998) were diagnosed with new onset of a GAD, with a range of GAD reported to fall between 3 and 28% across studies (Koponen et al., 2002; Hiott & Labbate, 2002). Panic disorders post-TBI seem to increase over time post injury (i.e., 4–6% at 3 and 5 years post-TBI (Fann et al., 1995; Van Reekum et al., 1996) and 14% at 8 years post-TBI (Hibbard et al., 1998). Across studies, the prevalence of panic disorders is reported to range from 4 to 17% across studies (Koponen et al., 2002; Hiott & Labbate, 2002). Obsessive–compulsive disorder (OCD) and phobia are less frequently documented post TBI with ranges of 2–15% for OCD and 1–10% for phobias reported across studies (Hibbard et al., 1998; Hiott & Labbate, 2002; Koponen et al., 2002).

Of current interest to this chapter, PTSD following TBI has received considerable research attention. The specific issue debated in earlier literature was whether an individual with no recall of a traumatic event (due to a loss of consciousness at the time of TBI onset) could meet full criteria for PTSD (Bontke, 1996; Sbordone & Liter, 1993). At present, there is general agreement that individuals with TBI often experience PTSD; however, some individuals having attenuated PTSD symptoms reported frequency rates of PTSD post TBI range from 3 to 30% post TBI (Hibbard et al., 1998; Hiott & Labbate, 2002; Koponen et al., 2002; McMillan, 2001; Ohry et al., 1996; Silver et al., 1997). When these anxiety disorders develop post-TBI, they are more likely to coexist with other Axis I disorders (Hibbard et al., 1998; Silver et al., 1997) and appear to be more chronic in nature.

MODIFICATIONS OF COGNITIVE-BEHAVIORAL ASSESSMENT FOR INDIVIDUALS WITH TBI AND ANXIETY DISORDERS

Individuals with potentially undiagnosed TBI are likely to present to mental health settings with anxiety symptoms. Additional diagnostic considerations are necessary when assessing such individuals. A multimethod approach is suggested which includes obtaining pertinent information from a variety of sources about the TBI, the events surrounding the trauma, and functional changes since the TBI (Hibbard, Grober, Stein, & Gordon, 1992; Hibbard, Gordon, Stein, Grober, & Sliwinski, 1993). Suggested areas of investigation include the following:

• *A detailed history of events surrounding the traumatic episode.* Due to a potential loss of consciousness or alteration in memory surrounding the trauma, information from multiple sources may be necessary to round out a detailed history of the actual event. Direct questioning of the individual and his/her family and a review of available medical documentation should be utilized to maximize the clinical picture. Specific issues to explore include the individual's last memories before the traumatic event, the earliest memories following the event, a description of events that occurred after the trauma, and feeling/reactions of the individual during the traumatic event itself (Gordon et al., 2000). This information is important for later planning of cognitive and behavioral interventions.

• *An evaluation of TBI related changes.* It is important to identify the nature and relative severity of physical, cognitive, and behavioral challenges experienced by the individual secondary to the TBI. These self-reports should be corroborated by other family members' impressions as well as a neuropsychological evaluation whenever possible. Test results should be incorporated into treatment planning (Gordon et al., 2000).

• *Pretrauma psychosocial factors.* Essential areas to be explored include prior personality traits, previous stressful events and subsequent coping abilities, prior sexual or physical abuse, and prior substances/drug usage.

• *A structured clinical interview to determine DSM-IV diagnoses.* The cornerstone of the assessment remains the structured clinical interview to determine whether the individual meets criteria for a DSM-IV Axis I diagnosis (American Psychiatric Association, 1994). Individuals with TBI are more likely to exhibit comorbid Axis I disorders (i.e., major depression and an anxiety disorder) (Hibbard et al., 1998; Hibbard et al., 2004; Ashman et al., 2004). As a result, the clinician should screen for these coexisting psychiatric difficulties as well.

The clinician should also be aware of the potential overlap of symptoms that can occur in individuals who present with TBI and comorbid Axis I psychopathology. More specifically, anxiety disorders, major depression, and TBI can *all* result in symptoms of fatigue, sleep difficulties, problems with concentration, sensitivity to noise, and irritability. However, clear differences do exist in symptoms among the various diagnoses. For example, TBI may result in a loss of actual recall of the traumatic event itself yet results in a reexperiencing phenomenon (i.e., flashbacks and nightmares) reflective of the event, numbing of general responsiveness, or hyperarousal seen in individuals with PTSD (Silver et al., 1997). In a similar fashion TBI may result in avoidance of select behaviors and situations relevant to the trauma itself without the person's being cognizant of why he/she is avoiding these behaviors/situations. Conversely, anxiety disorders and major depression do not typically result in severe impairments to memory, attention, information-processing speed, executive functioning, and/ or affective control; these symptoms are commonly observed following TBI. Hence, the clinician needs to assess the full range of affective, cognitive, and behavioral symptoms when attempting to diagnose coexisting TBI and other comorbid Axis I psychopathology.

COGNITIVE-BEHAVIORAL TREATMENT OF ANXIETY DISORDERS IN INDIVIDUALS WITH TBI

Cognitive-behavioral therapy has been suggested as an effective approach to treatment of major depression and anxiety in the general population (Kocsis, 2000; McGinn, 2000), in those individuals coping with health challenges (Boyce, Gilchrist, Tulley, & Rose, 2000; Cuijpers, 1998; Markowitz, Speilman, Scarvalone, & Perry, 2000), and in those individuals coping with acquired brain injury (Hibbard et al., 1992; Meed & Tate, 2000; Blanchard et al., 2003). Based on earlier work by the present authors in treating individuals with depression following stroke (Hibbard et al., 1992), specific modifications of cognitive-behavioral therapy approaches are suggested when working with individuals with TBI. These modifications include embedding cognitive remediation strategies within therapy sessions to enhance treatment effectiveness, addressing an individual's mourning of real losses secondary to brain injury, and the importance of involving family members as therapeutic helpers within treatment. (For a specific listing of these modifications, the patient is referred to Hibbard et al., 1992.) Because many individuals with TBI and anxiety disorders also present with comorbid major depression (Hibbard et al., 1998), these principles are especially relevant.

Traditional approaches to treatment of anxiety disorders include the use of behavioral exposure techniques, anxiety management techniques, and antianxiety medications (Rothbaum & Foa, 1992). When addressing anxiety disorders in individuals with TBI, additional treatment considerations must include the extent with which compensatory strategies need to be used within treatment (Hibbard et al., 1992; Hibbard et al., 1993). In general, the more severe the cognitive impairments, the greater the emphasis on the use of compensatory strategies within treatment. The severity of coexisting cognitive deficits will also have an impact on the selection of behavioral techniques and anxiety management tools utilized.

Two well-known behavioral approaches traditionally used in the treatment of anxiety disorders are useful intervention strategies for individuals with acquired brain injury: exposure and anxiety management techniques (Rothbaum & Foa, 1992). Both approaches are highlighted below.

Exposure

Exposure techniques are used when an anxiety disorder involves excessive avoidance; treatment is intended to activate and modify the fear structure (Rothbaum & Foa, 1992). Exposure-based procedures share a common approach in that all strategies utilize confrontation of the feared situations. These techniques can be classified along three dimensions: the medium of exposure (imagined or *in vivo*), the length of exposure (short vs. long), and the level of arousal during exposure (low vs. high). At one end of the continuum is systematic desensitization (Wolpe, 1973), during which an exposure is imagined, brief, and minimally arousing. At the other end of the continuum is *in vivo* flooding (Marks, 1987), during which an exposure is prolonged and designed to elicit high levels of anxiety. In individuals with TBI, exposure techniques must be considered within the context of the individual's recall of the precipitant event and the cognitive limitations of the individual secondary to TBI. For example, in an individual with severe cognitive impairments and no recall of the events surrounding the trauma, systematic desensitization techniques would not be utilized. The individual's avoidant behaviors would be better addressed using *in vivo* flooding combined with both antianxiety medications and anxiety management techniques.

Anxiety Management

Anxiety management techniques focus on anxiety reduction by provision of skills to control fears in an individual (Rothbaum & Foa, 1992) and may include all or some of the following techniques: relaxation training (Bernstein & Borkovec, 1973; Jacobsen, 1938), stress inoculation training (Meichenbaum, 1974), cognitive restructuring (Beck, 1972), guided self-dialogue (Meichenbaum, 1974), breathing retraining (Clark, Salkovskis, & Chaukley, 1985; Wolpe, 1985), and distraction (Wolpe, 1973). Perhaps the most widely used technique is deep muscle relaxation training (Wolpe, 1985). Cognitive restructuring, guided self-dialogue, and breathing relaxation techniques appear to be the most effective tools for symptom control post-TBI because these approaches will minimize the person's potential limited attention span and memory difficulties. Relaxation training and stress inoculation approaches may offer the least effective approaches to anxiety reduction given these cognitive challenges for many individuals following TBI. Each of latter techniques is described below:

• *Cognitive restructuring* (Beck, Rush, Shaw, & Emery, 1979) is used when the goal of treatment is to challenge and restructure an individual's automatic thoughts into more rational self-statements. In this paradigm, a therapist provides an A–B–C (where A = antecedent, B = belief, C = consequence) model to address automatic thoughts, has the individual focus on these automatic subjective thoughts, helps the individual assess the rationality of the beliefs, and consequently assists the individual to challenge and replace these beliefs with more rational self-statements. Once learned in a neutral setting, these techniques are then applied to avoidant experiences.

• *Guided self-dialogue* (Meichenbaum, 1974) is utilized when the goal of treatment is to focus on internal self-statements (i.e., what an individual is saying to oneself) and creation of dialogue substitution. In this approach, the therapist teaches the individual to focus on internal dialogues in order to identify irrational, faulty, or negative statements. More rational and facilitative self-statements are then substituted. Unique statements to use in confrontation and management of anxiety, for coping with feelings of being overwhelmed, and for reinforcement are generated and then applied to the specific avoidant problem. Self-statements generated during the session are written on cue cards and practiced within and outside the session. Use of individualized cued cards is particularly helpful for individuals who present with cognitive difficulties following TBI.

• *Breathing relaxation techniques* (Clark et al., 1985) are utilized as a behavioral countercondition to anxiety. In this approach, the individual is taught to practice taking a normal breath, exhaling slowly while saying the word *calm*, pausing briefly between breaths, and performing a distraction counting task (i.e., counting to 4 slowly), before taking the next breath. The entire sequence is practiced during the session, and the individual is asked to practice the exercise between sessions. Breathing techniques can then be applied later in treatment when imaginary or *in vivo* exposure techniques are implemented. These techniques are extremely useful for individuals with TBI but these individuals typically require written cue cards to help remember and/or sequence this multi-step task.

CASE STUDIES

Two vignettes are presented here to illustrate the challenges presented when assessing and treating anxiety disorders in individuals with coexisting TBI. Modifications in traditional cognitive-behavioral approaches based on the nature and severity of an individual's cognitive functioning secondary to a TBI are highlighted. In vignette 1 (Ms. D.), an individual's TBI was undiagnosed at the time of the initial referral for treatment for severe anxiety symptoms. Identifying the TBI required shifts in both assessment and cognitive-behavioral treatment approaches. In vignette 2 Mr. S. was subsequently diagnosed with anxiety disorder during the course of treatment for his major depression. In this vignette, the individual's severe memory impairments required significant modification of traditional cognitive-behavioral approaches to address his anxiety disorder.

Vignette 1

Client's name:	Ms. D.
Reason for referral:	Severe anxiety secondary to MVA
Time posttrauma:	4 months

Description of Traumatic Event

During a winter ski vacation, Ms. D. was involved in an MVA. She was a front-seat passenger in a van that skidded on a mountain road, turned over, and fell into a ditch overhanging the mountain edge. She was brought by ambulance to a local hospital where she was diagnosed with a concussion and soft tissue injuries of her neck secondary to whiplash. Neuroradiological evaluations (CT scans, MRI) were negative. On subsequent follow-up by her local physicians, a variety of postaccident physical complaints were identified: impairments in her walking, severe photophobia (i.e., sensitivity to light), frontal headaches, occipital head pain, numbness and tingling in her left hand and foot, a retinal hemorrhage, and a temporal mandibular joint (TMJ) disorder.

Prior Psychosocial History

Ms. D. was a 49-year-old married female who was involved in a long-standing and stable marriage. She had four grown children with two still living at home. Ms. D. was a college graduate who worked as the general office manager for her husband in his large real estate office. In that capacity, she oversaw a staff of five persons. She has been unable to return to work since her MVA. Her medical history was negative for drug or alcohol abuse and/or prior emotional difficulties.

Recall of Events Surrounding the Trauma

Since Ms. D. was involved in an MVA in which she was diagnosed with a concussion, the possibility that Ms. D. was experiencing residual functional changes of a TBI as well as anxiety symptoms was explored in further detail. On detailed questioning about events related to her MVA, Ms. D. related the following story: "I remembered getting into a van at the top of a mountain, and falling asleep as the van slowly went down a rather sharp and winding mountain road. The next thing I remember is being jolted awake by the jerky movements of the van as it careened down a twisty part of the road. The van flipped over and then headed over the side of the mountain. I don't know what happened next, but the next thing I remember is that the van had come to a standstill and was now hovering off the top of a cliff with the front half of the van dangling freely above a deep ravine. I remember feeling totally overwhelmed with the fear that if I moved, the van would topple off the cliff and kill us all." In reviewing Ms. D.'s report, she was certain that she had hit her head during the MVA but was unsure if she experienced a loss of consciousness. She did remember that she felt "dazed and confused" and had terrible headaches and severe neck pains for several days following the MVA.

Brain Injury Symptoms

Given her positive history of a blow to the head, combined with an altered mental state postevent, questions about potential TBI-related changes were explored (Gordon et al., 2000). The patient reported a variety of physical complaints: headaches, dizziness and vertigo, balance and coordination problems, a weight gain of 25 pounds since the MVA, neck and TMJ pain, sensitivity to light, numbness and tingling in her left extremities, and fatigue and sleep disturbances. Her cognitive complaints included significant problems with concentration, memory, thinking, and decision making. She spontaneously reported that she often would go through the day "unable to accomplish anything because she was totally unable to structure herself." Her affective changes were her largest complaints with frequent symptoms of anxiety and depression reported.

The patient was referred for a neuropsychological evaluation in order to determine her relative cognitive strengths and weaknesses. Test findings suggested that Ms. D. was functioning in the high average range of intelligence. Testing also validated her self-reports of significant deficits in the domains of visual and verbal memory, motor planning, attention, and organization secondary to a mild TBI.

DSM-IV Diagnosis

Using a structured clinical interview for DSM-IV diagnoses (American Psychiatric Association, 1994) the patient met criteria for major depression. She endorsed severe depressive symptoms on the Beck Depression Inventory (Beck, 1987) (BDI = 36). The patient was also diagnosed with PTSD. Her PTSD symptoms included intrusive symptoms (a recurrent nightmare about falling off a bridge while she was driving a car). Her nightmares were accompanied by panic (palpitations) and autonomic (profuse sweating) responses. The frequency of her nightmares had gradually increased with a growing dread of going to bed at night for fear of having the nightmare. Her avoidance symptoms included efforts to avoid any activity that involved being in a car; that is, she would take subways or walk whenever possible and avoid car trips where travel over a bridge was required to reach a destination. In addition, she began to notice her conscious avoidance of any physical structure that had height (a small walk bridge in a park, an escalator in a store, a ramp, etc.). Her hyperarousal symptoms included severe sleep difficulties, problems with concentration, marked irritability, and an exaggerated startle response. Her symptoms worsened rather than improved over the prior 2 months, resulting in her self-referral for medication and psychological treatment. The patient had seen her local physician who had prescribed an antidepressant for her mood and a sleep medication to address her sleep disturbance 2 weeks prior to her initial intake interview with the current therapist.

Initial Diagnoses

Axis I: Major depression, PTSD
Axis III: Mild TBI
GAF: 60

Formulation of Cognitive-Behavioral Treatment Plan

Ms. D. presented with PTSD symptoms of avoidant behaviors, nightmares, and hypervigilance related to her MVA. Ms. D. also presented with major depression and mild to moderate cognitive impairments in memory, attention, and executive functioning secondary to her TBI. Given Ms. D.'s combined affective and cognitive profile, a multimodal approach to treatment was formulated (Hibbard et al., 1992; Hibbard et al., 1993), which included an initial combination of pharmacological treatment, anxiety management techniques, and compensatory strategies for her cognitive challenges with the later use of exposure techniques to address her avoidant behaviors.

Initial Phase of Treatment

Ms. D.'s ongoing level of depression and her response to prescribed medications for mood and sleep were monitored during weekly cognitive-behavioral psychotherapy sessions. Treatment of her PTSD focused on detailed education about PTSD and the relationship of her PTSD to her traumatic MVA. The initial anxiety management technique introduced in session was breathing relaxation exercises. Ms D. had minimal trouble learning this technique; however, cue cards were written and used in both her subsequent sessions and when she was practicing this technique as a homework assignment. Cognitive restructuring and guided self-dialogue were next introduced. Sessions focused on helping Ms. D. understand the A–B–C paradigm and learn basic techniques to reality test and reformulate her self-statements within neutral or less affective-laden situations in her everyday life. For example, Ms. D. presented to treatment with the preconceived and automatic thought that she was unable to do "anything" around the house. While many of her ongoing difficulties in everyday functioning were due to cognitive failures, her reactions to these failures were extreme and only served to further limit her abilities to organize herself following her TBI. Early sessions were spent in helping Ms. D. cognitively organize her day-to-day activities. A daily planner was introduced into session as a compensatory tool for her executive functioning difficulties. Sessions were spent in preplanning activities she wanted to accomplish daily and having her write them in her planner. She was then taught how to use her planner as an ongoing organizer of her daily activities. Once the patient was able to use her planner more effectively at home, sessions shifted to identifying her automatic thoughts related to her reduced level of current functioning. These critical self-statements were reanalyzed, less critical counterstatements were created, and alternative approaches to minimize her cognitive confusion during such situations were developed. All facilitative statements were written on cue cards and organized by areas of potential problems encountered in her home (problems in cooking, problems when shopping, difficulties on the phone, etc.). To enhance her recall and use of these facilitative cue cards, she was asked to review the cards each morning and prior to any activity that had previously challenged her. As a source of potential reinforcement, she was also asked to record *any and all* tasks she accomplished each day, regardless of the relative merit of the accomplishment.

Middle Phase of Treatment

This phase of intervention focused on Ms. D.'s automatic thoughts as related to avoidant situations and the creation of self-statements to deal with her fears. Personal statements were created in session for use during attempts to engage in previously avoided activity and when she experienced increased anxiety while engaging in the activity. All self-statements were written on cue cards and placed in her daily planner. A hierarchy of avoidant activities was generated, with the least anxiety-producing events becoming the primary target for between session assignments. For Ms. D., these activities included walking over slightly elevated ramps and walk bridges in her local community park. Relaxation and use of previously generated self-statements were combined with systematic desensitization techniques to address Ms. D.'s imagined reactions to avoidant situations within session.

Final Phase of Treatment

Engaging in previously avoided activities in the community via *in vivo* assignments was the focus of the final phase of treatment. Using the hierarchy of avoidant activities, Ms. D.'s *in vivo* assignment was to have her initially walk up and over an elevated ramp followed by a slightly higher walk bridge in her local community park on a daily basis. Ms. D. was asked to review the anxiety management techniques practiced in session before leaving her house and then utilize her cue cards as reinforcement during her actual attempts at an activity. These repeated assignments exposed Ms. D. to previously avoided activities in order to flood her, thereby decreasing her overall fear of the activity. Ms. D.'s successes in engaging in these activities between sessions were reviewed during each subsequent session with the effectiveness of her anxiety management tools examined. Once a "comfort" zone for engaging in a select activity was achieved, the next avoidant activity in her hierarchy was addressed. Over several months, Ms. D. was able to engage in most activities she had been avoiding since her MVA. Her most positive outcomes were her ability to bike over a bridge at the end of a large reservoir (a favorite weekend route for Ms. D. and her husband) and sit in her husband's car as he drove out of the city over a large connecting bridge. She continued to apply anxiety management techniques when engaging in formerly avoided events; however, she is now able to rely on her own self-generated statements rather than reading her cue cards to successfully engage in these activities.

Vignette 2

Client's name: Mr. S.
Reason for referral: Severe depressive symptoms secondary to MVA
Time post trauma: 6 months

Description of Traumatic Event

Mr. S. was involved in an occupational accident in which he fell 30 feet from the bucket of a tree-cutting truck when it accidentally overturned. During the accident, Mr. S. was ejected from the bucket and fell onto a cement sidewalk. Because Mr. S. was unable to provide an adequate history, his family and available medical records were reviewed. On family interview, it was determined that Mr. S. was rendered unconscious at the time of the accident. He remained in a coma for approximately 3 hours after the accident. Mr. S. was taken to a local hospital by ambulance and admitted to the intensive care unit for 1 month. This was followed with an additional month of rehabilitation. According to Mr. S.'s medical records, he experienced a closed-head injury, a basilar skull fracture, four fractured spinal vertebrae, a fractured scapula, and nerve damage to his left hand secondary to his fall. Neuroradiological evaluations (CT scan findings) documented bilateral frontal-lobe contusions, a left subarachnoid hemorrhage, and the basilar skull fracture. Mr. S. evolved from coma in a state of extreme agitation, which required medication. At 6 months post-TBI, the patient presented with numerous complaints including decreased sensation and movement of his left hand, severe frontal and occipital headaches, visual disturbances, depression, irritability, and severe memory loss.

Prior Psychosocial History

Mr. S. was a 35-year-old male who was living with a significant other for the past 6 years. He had three small children by this relationship. Mr. S. completed 11th grade and immigrated to the United States from the Caribbean after being recruited by a major league team to play professional baseball. He left baseball after 3 years due to shoulder injuries sustained during play. He had worked as a tree cutter for the past 7 years, rising to the rank of foreman at the time of his injury. He has been unable to return to work since his TBI. His medical history was negative except for moderate social use of alcohol on weekends before his accident.

Recall of Events Surrounding the Accident

Because Mr. S. had a clearly documented severe TBI, attempts to delineate his recall of events were pursued. Mr. S. had no recall of events occurring 3 weeks prior to his work-related accident. Upon interview, the first thing Mr. S. remembered was being in his apartment after discharge from the rehabilitation facility 1 month earlier. Hence, a period of probable amnesia (lack of continuous memory) for approximately 3 months was noted, a pattern not atypical of individuals who sustain more severe brain injuries. As a result of his severe memory deficits, Mr. S. would ask repeatedly for information about his accident and an explanation for his current functional difficulties.

Brain Injury Symptoms

Because Mr. S. had a documented severe TBI, he and his mate were interviewed in order to determine Mr. S.'s current functional difficulties. On self-report (Gordon et al., 2000), the patient admitted to numerous and severe physical complaints: headaches, dizziness, difficulty lifting heavy objects, a loss of smell, balance and coordination problems, moving slowly, poor sleep, and blurred vision. His cognitive complaints focused primarily on his decreased memory. In contrast, his mate reported significantly more cognitive problems in attention, memory and learning, thinking, decision making, and executive functioning. Mr. S. endorsed many affective changes since his TBI with symptoms reflective of severe anxiety and depression. His mate agreed with the patient's self-report but also reported that Mr. S. had poor control of his behavior and emotions (e.g., throwing things, cursing at others, and difficulty coping with change). A neuropsychological evaluation had been completed 1 month prior to his initial intake interview. Testing suggested that Mr. S. was functioning in the low average range of intellectual functioning. Testing further validated the patient's self reports by documenting significant deficits across all cognitive domains assessed: attention, memory, information processing speed, executive functioning, and language abilities.

DSM-IV Diagnosis

Using a structured clinical interview for DSM-IV diagnoses (American Psychiatric Association, 1994), the patient initially met criteria for a major depression. He endorsed severe depressive symptoms on the Beck Depression Inventory (Beck, 1987) (BDI = 45).

Initial Diagnoses

Axis I: Major depression
Axis III: Severe TBI
GAF: 40

Mr. S. was referred to a psychiatrist for medication evaluation and placed on an antidepressant for his depression, a mood stabilizer for his affective dyscontrol, and a sleep medication. In addition, the patient was seen for weekly cognitive-behavioral psychotherapy and two sessions per week of cognitive remediation. This combined approach (Hibbard et al., 1992; Hibbard et al., 1993) resulted in a modest reduction in the severity of his depression and increased learning of compensatory tools for his severe memory and executive functioning deficits. During the course of treatment, a second Axis I diagnosis was made based on behavioral information that emerged within the context of treatment. Mr. S. was subsequently diagnosed with a phobia when it was observed that the patient was exhibiting particular avoidant behaviors. For example, Mr. S. would frequently cancel appointments because the "elevator in his apartment building was broken." As he was able to climb stairs without difficulty, his reasons for canceling were challenged. Mr. S. replied that he could not take the stairs to exit his apartment because he was "too nervous." In addition, when Mr. S. came to sessions, he would sit as far from the office window as possible. Due to the severity of his memory deficits, Mr. S. never voiced concerns about his avoidant behaviors or the underlying anxiety related to these activities. Quite by accident, the therapist requested Mr. S. to look out of the window of her office at activities that were occurring on the street below. This request was met with an immediate and excessive anxiety reaction and a strong resistance to look downward. Mr. S. could not explain why this was occurring, and lacked the insight to relate his behaviors to the etiology of his TBI (i.e., a fall from a height of 30 feet).

Mr. S.'s mate was interviewed about these behaviors and validated his avoidance of looking out of any window, his refusal to ride down on an escalator, and his adamant refusal to use the stairs to exit his fifth-floor apartment. (This latter behavior was particularly troublesome because the elevator was often broken, and it thus raised an issue about safety for the family in case of fire.) A further concern (i.e., Mr. S.'s willingness to fly given his difficulty with heights) was particularly relevant to treatment planning as relocation to his native country (via plane) was anticipated following his rehabilitation. Prior to his TBI, the patient had had no difficulty with the stairs or flying.

Mr. S.'s phobic symptoms had remained "hidden" during the early months of treatment due to the severity of his depression and memory deficits. Furthermore, his self-limited involvement with activities in his community offered the patient minimal opportunities to become aware of the functional limitations of his avoidant behaviors. He had simply restricted his activities to minimize situations in which anxiety reactions would occur. In the brain injury literature, two competing theories are proposed for the later development of avoidant reactions despite the fact that the person may be totally amnestic to the traumatic event. One theory posits that behaviors may be "pseudomemories" derived from the patient learning details about the accident subsequent to the event (Bryant, 1996). The alternative hypothesis is that symptoms are reflective of "nonverbal" or "nondeclarative memory" traces for the events surrounding the trauma, which in turn become the basis for postevent avoidant behaviors (Bryant, 1996; Layton & Wardi-Zonna, 1995). In Mr. S.'s situation, his lack of memory of events surrounding his fall would suggest that his avoidant symptoms were more reflective of the later hypothesis.

Revised Diagnoses

Axis I: Major depression, phobia
Axis III: Severe TBI
GAF: 45

Formulation of Cognitive-Behavioral Treatment Plan

Due to the severity of his memory and other cognitive deficits, a multimodal approach was utilized to treat Mr. S.'s severe depression and significant cognitive impairments. This approach combined traditional cognitive-behavioral interventions, a heavy emphasis on the use of psychopharmacological interventions, and aggressive cognitive remediation. Treatment of Mr. S.'s avoidant behaviors and anxiety symptoms related to his phobia for heights were introduced later in treatment. Pharmacological interventions, limited exposure treatment, breathing relaxation training, and behavioral management training for his family were utilized to address his phobic responses.

Initial Phase of Treatment

The initial emphases of cognitive remediation was to reorient Mr. S. to the reasons for his current functional limitations and teach Mr. S. to use a daily planner to record pertinent information about his TBI, his cognitive and mood difficulties, his daily activities, and his taking of prescribed medications for his mood. Mr. S.'s ongoing level of depression and his continued compliance with taking his medications for mood, behavioral control, and sleep were monitored during weekly cognitive-behavioral psychotherapy sessions. Mr. S. was taught to use a daily planner to record all his daily activities and keep track of whether he was taking his medication. Cognitive-behavioral psychotherapy focused on behavioral strategies to increase his social activities and enhance his self-esteem. Cognitive restructuring was utilized to help Mr. S. limit his critical self-statements about "being totally useless," with all counter-responses written in his daily planner for later recall and practice within session. His daily planner entries were reviewed in sessions to evaluate the extent of his social involvement, medication compliance, and created self-facilitating statements.

Middle Phase of Treatment

This phase of intervention focused on treatment of Mr. S.'s phobia. Initial sessions focused on providing the family with education about a phobia and its relationship to Mr. S.'s accident. Introduction to anxiety management techniques was limited to training of breathing relaxation exercises. Due to the severity of Mr. S.'s memory deficits, each step in the relaxation exercises were written out, placed in Mr. S.'s daily planner, and then reviewed with Mr. S. following each written step during subsequent sessions. Once he was able to independently locate the written instructions in his daily planner and follow the steps required in the breathing relaxation exercise by himself, he was assigned daily practice sessions at home. Compliance with home practice was monitored through review of Mr. S.'s daily planner entries. Due to the severity of the patient's memory impairments, guided self-dialogue was not attempted.

The next phase of treatment focused on creating a hierarchy of avoidant activities with information obtained from both Mr. S. and his mate. For Mr. S., the hierarchy of anxiety-producing activities included walking down stairs, riding down escalators, and looking down from places of increasing height (e.g., looking out of windows on higher floors of a building or from balconies). Because his memory impairments precluded Mr. S. from remembering events surrounding his initial accident, systematic desensitization was not attempted. However, *in vivo* exercises were utilized in combination with antianxiety medications and breathing exercises to help Mr. S. engage in previously avoided activities. On consultation with Mr. S.'s psychiatrist, "as needed" antianxiety medication was prescribed with Mr. S. instructed to take the medication before attempting *in vivo* exposure techniques in session.

Sessions were preplanned in which Mr. S. would practice *in vivo* exposure with his therapist. On such days, Mr. S. wrote in his daily planner to take the antianxiety medication 1 half hour before coming to session. For each session, relaxation breathing was practiced in the safety of the therapist's office. Mr. S. was then escorted to the targeted avoidant activity. Using the hierarchy of avoidant activities, the initial target for *in vivo* practice was escorting Mr. S. down a short flight of stairs within the same building. Initially, Mr. S. clung to the stairwell wall, walked sideward down the steps in a hesitant fashion, and began to hyperventilate. Distraction techniques (e.g., focusing on a distant point, rather than looking down to the bottom of the stairs), breathing exercises, and direct supervision by the therapist enabled Mr. S. to resume a more normalized stair-descending approach. The therapist gradually faded her direct supervision but remained at the top of the stairs for more distant supervision and support. Over time, the flights of stairs within the building were increased.

Once Mr. S. became comfortable with descending stairs, assignments were extended to his own apartment house where he was asked to take the antianxiety medication 30 minutes before practicing descending flights of stairs with his mate. Once comfortable with this routine, he was encouraged to do the activity independently. His weekly progress was monitored by reviewing entries in his daily planner about the number of flights of stairs he had descended each week. Flooding (i.e., repeat exposure to stair decent activities), combined with antianxiety medications and anxiety management strategies, decreased his overall fear of this activity. Once a "comfort" zone for this activity was achieved, the next avoidant behavior in his hierarchy was focused on (i.e., looking down from heights). *In vivo* practice within the session was again utilized for this task. Initially, Mr. S. was escorted to a second-story window and asked to look at distant objects at eye level across the street. He was then asked to slowly drop his line of vision while practicing relaxation/breathing exercises. This approach was repeated at gradually greater heights (higher stories of the building) and then transferred to practice overlooking edges of balconies. Premedication, relaxation techniques, and direct supervision were combined for all *in vivo* exposure events. Over a relatively short period of time, Mr. S. was able to descend stairs and tolerate a considerable downward gaze from various heights. He continued to show significant anxiety, however, when asked to redirect his gaze directly downward from a considerable height.

Final Phase of Treatment

Because discharge from rehabilitation was imminent and plane tickets had already been purchased for his planned relocation to his country of origin, several additional treatment strategies were implemented to maximize Mr. S.'s ability to engage in a plane trip without an extreme phobic reaction. His psychiatrist was consulted to increase his dose of "as-needed" antianxiety medications in anticipation of his upcoming plane flight. Mr. S and his mate were seen in joint session to discuss behavioral strategies to help Mr. S. control his anxiety during the flight. Breathing exercises were reviewed with his mate taught to coach Mr. S. proactively during the flight. Additional distracter strategies were suggested to minimize Mr. S.'s awareness of being in the plane itself (and therefore flying at a considerable height). These strategies included reserving a plane seat without a window, seating Mr. S. in the middle of a row, bringing other family members along on the trip, use of headsets with Mr. S.'s favorite music and alerting the plane personnel to the specific needs of Mr. S. Additional behavioral management strategies included increased use of medication and the most optimal timing of such medication relative to the plane flight itself. In summary, a combination of behavioral management techniques, breathing exercises, and medication allowed Mr. S. to successfully return to his homeland without an exacerbation of his phobic symptoms.

CONCLUSION

This chapter provides a clinical understanding of TBI, including its prevalence, etiology, and functional changes. The importance of screening for TBI in individuals presenting with anxiety disorders is stressed. Frequent and coexisting psychopathologies following TBI are highlighted. Suggestions to broaden traditional cognitive-behavioral assessment and shift cognitive-behavioral treatment when treating individuals with combined cognitive and psychiatric challenges are discussed and illustrated via vignettes of individuals with varying severities of TBI. It is hoped that this chapter has served to heightened clinical sensitivity to the potential of a comorbid TBI in individuals who present with anxiety disorders post trauma. A broader approach, which incorporates cognitive strategies, is essential if treatment of anxiety disorders in individuals with TBI is to be effective.

ACKNOWLEDGMENTS

Preparation of this chapter was supported by the Rehabilitation Research and Training Center on TBI Interventions (Grant No. H 133B040033) and the New York Traumatic Brain Injury Model System (Grant No. H 133A020501) from the National Institute on Disability and Rehabilitation Research, U.S. Department of Education, to the Department of Rehabilitation Medicine, Mount Sinai School of Medicine, New York, New York.

REFERENCES

American Psychiatric Association. (1994). *Diagnostic and statistical manual of mental disorders* (4th ed.). Washington, DC: Author.

Arlinghaus, K. A., Shoaib, A. M., & Price, T. R. P. (2005). Neuropsychiatric assessment. In J. M. Silver, T. W. McAllister, & S. C. Yudofsky (Eds.), *Textbook of traumatic brain injury* (pp. 59–78). Arlington VA: American Psychiatric Press.

Ashman, T. A., Speilman, L. A., Hibbard, M. R., Silver, J. M., Chandra, T., & Gordon, W. (2004). Psychiatric challenges in the first 6 years after traumatic brain injury. *Archives of Physical Medicine and Rehabilitation, 85*(4, Suppl. 2), S36–S42.

Bagley, L. J., Grossman, R. I., & Lenkinski, R. E. (1998). Proton magnetic resonance spectroscopy for diction of axonal injured patients. *Journal of Neurosurgery, 88,* 795–801.

Beck, A. (1987). *Beck Depression Inventory: Manual.* San Antonio, TX: Psychological Corporation.

Beck, A. T. (1972). *Depression: Cause and treatment.* Philadelphia: University of Pennsylvania Press.

Beck, A. T., Rush, A. J., Shaw, B. F., & Emery, G. (1979). *Cognitive therapy for depression.* New York: Guilford Press.

Bernstein, D. A., & Borkovec, T. D. (1973). *Progressive relaxation training.* Springfield, IL: Research Press.

Bernstein, D. M. (1999). Recovery from mild head injury. *Brain Injury, 13*(3), 151–172.

Blanchard, E. B., Hickling, E. J., Devineni, T., Veazey, C. H., Galovski, T. E., Mundy, E., et al. (2003). A controlled evaluation of cognitive behavioral therapy for posttraumatic stress in motor vehicle accident survivors. *Behaviour Research and Therapy, 41,* 79–96.

Blanchard, E. B., Hickling, E. J., Taylor, A. E., Loos, W. R., Forneris, C. A., & Jaccard, J. (1995). Who develops PTSD from motor vehicle accidents. *Behaviour Research and Therapy, 34*(1), 1–10.

Bontke, C. F. (1996). Controversies: Do patients with mild brain injuries have posttraumatic stress disorders too? *Journal of Head Trauma Rehabilitation, 11*(1), 95–102.

Boyce, P., Gilchrist, J., Tulley, N. J., & Rose, D. (2000). Cognitive behavior therapy as a treatment for irritable bowel syndrome: A pilot study. *Australian and New Zealand Journal of Psychiatry, 34,* 300–309.

Brooks, N., Campsie, L., Symington, C., Beattie, A., & McKinley, W. (1986). The five year outcome of severe blunt head injury. *Journal of Neurology, Neurosurgery and Psychiatry, 46,* 336–344.

Bryant, R. A. (1996). Posttraumatic stress disorder, flashbacks, and pseudomemories in closed head injury. *Journal of Traumatic Stress, 9,* 621–629.

Bryant, R. A., & Harvey, A. (1999). The influence of traumatic brain injury on acute stress disorders and post traumatic stress disorder following motor vehicle accident. *Brain Injury, 13,* 15–22.

Cecil, K. M., Hills, E. C., Sandel, E., Smith, D. H., McIntosh, T. K., Mannon, L. J., et al. (1998). Proton magnetic resonance spectroscopy for detection of axonal injured patients. *Journal of Neurosurgery, 88,* 795–801.

Centers for Disease Control and Prevention. (2004). Heads up: Facts for physicians about mild traumatic brain injury (MTBI). Available at *www.ede.gov/migrated_Content/Brochure_and_Catagues/Tbi_mtbi_facts_for_physicians.pdf*

Clark, D. M., Salkovskis, P. M., & Chaukley, A. J. (1985). Respiratory control as a treatment for panic attacks. *Journal of Behavioral Therapy and Experimental Psychiatry, 9,* 109–114.

Cuijpers, P. (1998). Prevention of depression in chronic medical disorders: A pilot study. *Psychological Reports, 82,* 735–738.

Deb, S., Lyons, I., Koutzoukis, C., Ali, I., & McCarthy, G. (1999). Rates of psychiatric illness 1 year after traumatic brain injury. *American Journal of Psychiatry, 156*, 374–378.

Dikmam, S., McLean, A., & Temkin, N. (1989). Neuropsychological and psychosocial consequences of minor head injury. *Journal of Neurology, Neurosurgery and Psychiatry, 49*, 1227–1233.

Epstein, R. S., & Ursano, R. J. (1994). Anxiety disorders. In J. M. Silver, S. C. Yudofsky, & R. E. Hales (Eds.), *Neuropsychiatry of traumatic brain injury* (pp. 3–46). Washington, DC: American Psychiatric Press.

Fann, J. R., Katon, W. J., Uomoto, J. M., & Essleman, P. C. (1995). Psychiatric disorders and functional disability in outpatients with traumatic brain injuries. *American Journal of Psychiatry, 152*(1), 1493–1499.

Gerberding, T. L., & Binder, S. (2003). *Report to Congress on mild traumatic brain injury in the United States: Steps to prevent a serious public health problem.* Atlanta, GA: Center for Disease Control and Prevention, National Center for Injury Prevention and Control.

Gordon, W. A., Brown, M., Sliwinski, M., Hibbard, M. R., Patti, N., Weiss, M., et al. (1998). The enigma of hidden TBI. *Journal of Head Trauma Rehabilitation, 13*(6), 1–18.

Gordon, W. A., Haddad, L., Brown, M., Hibbard, M. R., & Sliwinski, M. (2000). The sensitivity and specificity of self report symptoms in individuals with traumatic brain injury. *Brain Injury, 14*, 21–33.

Hibbard, M. R., Ashman, T. A., Speilman, L. A., Chun, D., Chavatz, H., & Melvin, S. (2004). Relationship between depression and psychosocial functioning and health following traumatic brain injury. *Archives of Physical Medicine and Rehabilitation, 85*(4, Suppl. 2), S43–S53.

Hibbard, M. R., Gordon, W. G., Stein, P. S., Grober, S., & Sliwinski, M. (1993). A multimodal approach to the diagnosis of post-stroke depression. In W. A. Gordon (Ed.), *Advances in stroke rehabilitation* (pp. 185–214). Stoneham, ME: Andova.

Hibbard, M. R., Grober, S. E., Stein, P. N., & Gordon, W. G. (1992). Poststroke depression. In A. Freeman & F. M. Dattilio (Eds.), *Comprehensive casebook of cognitive therapy* (pp. 303–310). New York: Plenum Press.

Hibbard, M. R., Uysal, S., Kepler, K., Bogdany, J., & Silver, J. (1998). Axis I psychopathology in individuals with traumatic brain injury. *Journal of Head Trauma Rehabilitation, 13*(4), 24–39.

Hiott, D. V., & Labbate, L. (2002). Anxiety disorders associated with traumatic brain injuries. *Neurorehabilitation, 17*, 345–355.

Holtzer, R., Burright, R. G., Lynn, S. J., & Donovick, P. J. (2000). Behavioral differences between psychiatric patients with confirmed versus unconfirmed brain injuries. *Brain Injury, 14*(11), 959–973.

Jacobsen, E. (1938). *Progressive relaxation.* Chicago: University of Chicago Press.

Jorge, R. E., Robinson, R. B., Moser, D., Tateno, A., Crispo-Facorro, B., & Arndt, S. (2004). Major depression following traumatic brain injury. *Archives of General Psychiatry, 61*, 42–50.

Jorge, R. E., Robinson, R. G., Starkstein, S. E., & Arndt, S. W. (1994). Influences of major depression on one-year outcome. *Journal of Neurosurgery, 81*, 726–733.

Kinsella, G., Moran, C., Ford, B., & Ponsford, J. (1988). Emotional disorders and its assessment within severely head injured populations. *Psychological Medicine, 18*, 57–63.

Kocsis, J. H. (2000). New strategies for treating chronic depression. *Journal of Clinical Psychiatry, 61*(11), 42–45.

Koponen, S., Taiminen, T., Portin, R., Himanen, L., Isoniemi, H., Heinonen, H., et al. (2002). Axis I and II psychiatric disorders after traumatic brain injury: A 30-year follow up. *American Journal of Psychiatry, 159*, 1315–1321.

Koren, D., Arnon, I., & Klein, E. (1999). Acute stress response and post traumatic stress disorder in traffic accident victims: A one-year prospective follow-up study. *American Journal of Psychiatry, 156*(3), 367–373.

Layton, B. S., & Wardi-Zonna, K. (1995). Posttraumatic stress disorder with neurogenic amnesia for the traumatic event. *Clinical Neuropsychologist, 9,* 2–10.

Marino, M. (1999). CDC report shows prevalence of brain injury. *Brain Injury Association's TBI Challenge, 3*(3), 1.

Markowize, J. C., Spielman, L. A., Scarvalone, R. A., & Perry, S. W. (2000). Psychotherapy adherence of therapists treating HIV positive patient's depressive symptoms. *Journal of Psychotherapy Practice and Research, 9,* 75–80.

Marks, I. M. (1987). Flooding and allied treatments. In W. Agras (Ed.), *Behavior modification: Principles and clinical applications* (pp. 151–213). Boston: Little, Brown.

Martin, T. A., & Johnstone, B. (2006). Traumatic brain injury and the older adult. In S. Bush & T. A. Martin (Eds.), *Geriatric neuropsychiatry: Practice essentials* (pp. 301–323). New York: Taylor & Francis.

Mayou, R., Bryan, B., & Duthie, R. (1993). Psychiatric consequences of road traffic accidents. *British Medical Journal, 307,* 646–651.

McGinn, L. K. (2000). Cognitive behavioral therapy of depression: Theory, treatment and empirical status. *American Journal of Psychotherapy, 15,* 865–877.

McMillan, T. C. (2001). Error in diagnosing post-traumatic stress disorder after traumatic brain injury. *Brain Injury, 15,* 39–46.

Meed, J., & Tate, R. (2000). Evaluation of an anger management therapy programme following acquired brain injury: Preliminary study. *Neuropsychological Rehabilitation, 10,* 185–201.

Meichenbaum, D. (1974). *Cognitive behavior modification.* Morristown, NJ: General Learning Press.

Mooney, G., & Speed, J. (2001). The association between mild traumatic brain injury and psychiatric conditions. *Brain Injury, 15,* 865–877.

Moore, E. L., Terryberry-Spohr, L., & Hope, D. A. (2006). Mild traumatic brain injury and anxiety sequelae: A review of the literature. *Brain Injury, 204*(2), 117–132.

National Institute of Health. (1999). Rehabilitation of persons with traumatic brain injury. *Journal of the American Medical Association, 282*(10), 974–983.

Ohry, A., Rattock, J., & Solomon, Z. (1996). Posttraumatic stress disorder in brain injury patients. *Brain Injury, 10*(9), 687–695.

Pelham, M. F., & Lovell, M. R. (2005). Issues in neuropsychological assessment. In J. M. Silver, T. W. McAllister, & S. C. Yudofsky (Eds.), *Textbook of traumatic brain injury* (pp. 159–174). Arlington, VA: American Psychiatric Press.

Rattock, J. (1996). Do patients with mild brain injuries have posttraumatic stress disorder too? *Journal of Head Trauma Rehabilitation, 11*(1) 95–96.

Rothbaum, B. O., & Foa, E. B. (1992). Cognitive-behavioral treatment of posttraumatic stress disorder. In P. A. Saigh (Ed.), *Posttraumatic stress disorder: A behavioral approach to assessment and treatment* (pp. 85–11). New York: Pergamon.

Rutherford, W. H., Merritt, J. D., & McDonald, J. R. (1979). Symptoms at one year following concussion from minor head injury: A relative's view. *Brain Injury, 10,* 225–230.

Sbordone, R. L., & Liter, J. C. (1993). Mild traumatic brain injury does not produce post traumatic stress disorder. *Brain Injury, 9,* 405–412.

Silver, J. M., Rattok, J., & Anderson, K. (1997). Posttraumatic stress disorder and traumatic brain injury. *Neurocase, 3,* 1–7.

Tellier, A., Della Marva, L. C., Winn, A. C., Grahovac, S., Morris, W., & Brennan-Barnes, M. (1999). Mild head injury: A misnomer. *Brain Injury, 13,* 463–475.

Tyerman, A., & Humphrey, M. (1984). Changes in self-concept following severe head injury. *International Journal of Rehabilitation Research, 7,* 11–23.

Uzzell, B. P. (1999). Mild traumatic brain injury. Much ado about something. In N. R. Varney &

S. R. J. Roberts (Eds.), *The evaluation and treatment of mild traumatic brain injury* (pp. 1–14). Mahwah, NJ: Erlbaum.

Van Reekum, R. M., Bolango, I., Finlayson, M. A., Garner, S., & Links, P. S. (1996). Psychiatric disorders after traumatic brain injury. *Brain Injury, 10*(5), 319–327.

Van Zomeren, A., & Vandenberg, W. (1985). Residual complaints of patients two years after severe head injury. *Journal of Neurology, Neurosurgery and Psychiatry, 48,* 21–28.

Varney, N. R., Martz, J. S., & Roberts, R. J. (1987). Major depression in patients with closed head injuries. *Neuropsychology, 1,* 7–8.

Wallace, C. A., & Bogner, J. (2000). Awareness of deficits: Emotional implications for person with brain injury and their significant others. *Brain Injury, 14,* 549–62.

Wolpe, J. (1973). *The practice of behavior therapy.* New York: Pergamon Press.

Wolpe, J. (1985). Deep muscle relaxation. In A. S. Bellack & M. Hersen (Eds.), *Dictionary of behavior therapy techniques.* New York: Pergamon Press.

Woo, B. H., & Thoidis, G. (2000). Epidemiology of traumatic brain injury. In B. Woo & S. Nesathurai (Eds.), *The rehabilitation of people with traumatic brain injury* (pp. 13–17). Malden, MA: Blackwell Science.

SUGGESTED READINGS

Ashman, T. A., Speilman, L. A., Hibbard, M. R., Silver, J. M., Chandra, T., & Gordon, W. (2004). Psychiatric challenges in the first 6 years after traumatic brain injury. *Archives of Physical Medicine and Rehabilitation, 85*(4, Suppl. 2), S36–S42.

Gordon, W. A., Haddad, L., Brown, M., Hibbard, M. R., & Sliwinski, M. (2000). The sensitivity and specificity of self report symptoms in individuals with traumatic brain injury. *Brain Injury, 14,* 21–33.

Hibbard, M. R., Ashman, T. A., Speilman, L. A., Chun, D., Chavatz, H., & Melvin, S. (2004). Relationship between depression and psychosocial functioning and health following traumatic brain injury. *Archives of Physical Medicine and Rehabilitation, 85*(4, Suppl. 2) S43–S53.

Hibbard, M. R., Gordon, W. G., Stein, P. S., Grober, S., & Sliwinski, M. (1993). A multimodal approach to the diagnosis of post-stroke depression. In W. A. Gordon (Ed.), *Advances in stroke rehabilitation* (pp. 185–214). Stonington, ME: Andova.

Hibbard, M. R., Uysal, S., Kepler, K., Bogdany, J., & Silver, J. (1998). Axis I psychopathology in individuals with traumatic brain injury. *Journal of Head Trauma Rehabilitation, 13*(4), 24–39.

Silver, J. M., Rattok, J., & Anderson, K. (1997). Posttraumatic stress disorder and traumatic brain injury. *Neurocase, 3,* 1–7.

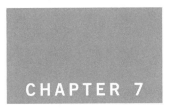

CHAPTER 7

Substance Misuse and Dependency
CRISIS AS PROCESS OR OUTCOME

Sharon Morgillo Freeman
Misti Storie

The Drug Abuse Warning Network (DAWN) is a public health surveillance system that monitors drug-related emergency department (ED) visits for selected metropolitan areas and provides estimates of use for the United States. It is a product of the Substance Abuse and Mental Health Services Administration (SAMHSA), U.S. Department of Health and Human Services. In 2003 it is estimated that there were 627,923 drug-related ED visits nationwide, according to 260 of the 518 hospitals that submitted usable data (Substance Abuse and Mental Health Services Administration, 2003a). Further, upon arriving in the ED, individuals are abusing an average of 1.7 drugs per visit, ranging from illicit drugs, alcohol, prescription and over-the-counter (OTC) pharmaceuticals, nonpharmaceutical inhalants, and dietary supplements (Substance Abuse and Mental Health Services Administration, 2003). The data indicate that not only are EDs in the United States being overwhelmed by drug-related visits, but also the individuals presenting themselves for such visits are abusing more than one substance at a time. This alarming data begs the question: Can these individuals be identified and helped? To help individuals with substance abuse problems, a therapist must understand what leads to substance misuse disorders, what crises are likely to complicate these disorders, and what crises increase the likelihood that misuse and dependence will continue.

Mood-altering substances are generally chosen by an individual based on three criteria: ease of access, rapid onset of action, and activation of the brain reward system (Freeman, 2004; Koob & Bloom, 1988; Koob & Le Moal, 1997; O'Brien, 2001). Most substances increase cell firing in the ventral tegmentum and stimulate dopamine (DA) release in the nucleus accumbens by decreasing presynaptic gamma-aminobutyric acid (GABA) release on the dopaminergic cells (Portenoy & Payne, 1992). A person experiences this DA release in the nucleus accumbens as a "rush" of a sense of well-being. The "rush" is highly rewarding and reinforcing. Therefore, the person is likely to repeat the experience in order to achieve the pleasurable effect again (Portenoy & Payne, 1992). It is important to remember that the process of chasing the "rush" of a substance does not in and of itself warrant the diagnosis of a substance-related disorder. In addition, many people have the impression that substance use + problems = substance dependence. However, these two factors are only half of the diagnosis. To meet the criteria for dependence in the fourth edition, text revision of *Diagnostic and Statistical Manual of Mental Disorders* (DSM-IV-TR), the person must experience tolerance, withdrawal, significant negative consequences related to substance use, and, most important, loss of control over his/her use (American Psychiatric Association, 2000).

Interestingly, the factors that lead to substance dependence are often similar to the factors that lead to a patient's relapse. We know, for example, that stress is one of the most powerful triggers of relapse, even after prolonged periods of abstinence from drugs or alcohol (Volkow, 2005). At the slightest provocation, stress-related neurotransmitters are released in the brain, producing unpleasant emotions that make the person want to resort to drugs again. Because life is filled with stressors, persons experiencing withdrawal from drug(s) are constantly having their stress system activated (Kreek & Koob, 1998). For example, respondents to a survey in New York City reported post-9/11 attack rates of depression and posttraumatic stress disorder (PTSD) were approximately twice the baseline levels previously documented in a 1999 benchmark national study. Rates of depression jumped from 4.9% of the population in 1999 to 9.7% after 9/11. Similarly, rates for PTSD jumped to 7.5%, when only 3.6% of the population qualified for a diagnosis of PTSD in 1999 (Vlahov et al., 2004). When looking at rates of new substance use, the researchers found that 3.3% of respondents who did not use substances during the week before 9/11 started smoking cigarettes after 9/11. Further, 19.3% of this cohort started drinking alcohol and 2.5% began using marijuana after 9/11. Overall, the percentages of respondents who smoked, consumed alcohol, and used marijuana increased 9.7%, 24.6%, and 3.2%, respectively, after the attacks. Furthermore, persons with problematic dependence on drugs or alcohol reported relapse or an increase of substance use after 9/11 (Vlahov et al., 2004). This behavior is predictable because people usually return to coping mechanisms that are familiar to them during times of stress.

Early life experience can also have a dramatic effect on the development of problematic alcohol consumption. Neurobiological markers have been found indicating that highly stressed monkeys later consumed more alcohol as young adults than their less stressed peers (Fahlke et al., 2000). It is not clear whether this hypersensitivity (1) exists before the person starts taking drugs and contributes to his/her initial drug use;

(2) results from the effects of chronic drug misuse on the brain; or (3) is a combination of both (Kreek, 1984). Other research indicates that the nervous system of persons addicted to psychoactive substances may be hypersensitive to chemically induced stress, suggesting that the nervous system may also be hypersensitive to emotional stress (Stocker, 1999). Stress hormones, such as corticotropin-releasing factor (CRF), are released in the body in small amounts throughout the day, but when the person is under stress, the level of these hormones increases dramatically. In the brain, CRF is released into the blood, which carries the CRF to the pituitary gland, located at the base of the brain. There, CRF stimulates the release of another hormone, adrenocorticotropin hormone (ACTH), which, in turn, triggers the release of other hormones—principally cortisol—from the adrenal glands (Stocker, 1999). CRF and ACTH may be among the chemicals that serve dual purposes as hormones and neurotransmitters. Researchers posit that if, indeed, these chemicals also act as neurotransmitters they may be involved in producing the emotional responses to stress (Kreek & Koob, 1998). If the stressor is mild, the pituitary gland inhibits the further release of CRF and ACTH, and they return to their normal levels. If the stressor is intense, the pituitary gland signals the brain to release more CRF, which outweighs the inhibitory signal from cortisol.

Another stress chemical in the brain is beta-endorphin. Beta-endorphin is released in response to stressors in efforts to increase the body's alertness, energy, and pain control in response to extreme stressors. Both alcohol and stress are known to increase the release of beta-endorphin in the pituitary gland and the brain. Research indicates that dysfunction in the activity of the pituitary beta-endorphin system *predates* the development of alcoholism in high-risk individuals and develops *after the onset* of substance dependence for low-risk individuals (Dai & Thavundayil, 2005; Addiction Technology Transfer Center, 2004). In a study conducted by Freeman (2005) at the University of Pennsylvania, it was discovered that 47% of individuals admitted to the inpatient substance dependency treatment program had a history of previously undiagnosed brain trauma and/or PTSD. Either or both of these disorders may affect a person's ability to respond to treatment as usual due to the symptoms inherent in each disorder, such as distractibility, irritability, difficulty attending to topics leading to difficulty learning, mistrust issues, and motivational problems.

TYPES OF CRISIS IN SUBSTANCE-MISUSING PERSONS

Legal

Indirect legal crises occur as a result of substance misuse, as well as direct consequences to substance use. Examples of indirect crises include loss of child custody and loss of living quarters (eviction), whereas public intoxication, presence of paraphernalia, assault, reckless endangerment, and parole violations are examples of direct consequences. In fact, the Bureau of Justice Statistics (2005) reports that among inmates with substance abuse or dependence in 2002, 68% of their criminal charges were for driving under the influence (DUI) convictions, paraphernalia charges, and drug dealing in the months immediately prior to their incarceration.

Alcohol is a known factor in 60–70% of homicides, 40% of suicides, 40–50% of fatal motor vehicle accidents, 60% of fatal burns, 60% of drownings, and 40% of fatal falls (Miller, Lestina, & Smith, 2001). Based on annual averages from SAMHSA's National Surveys on Drug Use and Health in 2002, 2003, and 2004, an estimated 1.2 million adults age 18 or older were arrested for serious violent or property offense in the past year (Office of Applied Studies, 2003, 2004, 2005b). Adults who had been arrested for serious violent or property offenses in the past year were more likely than their counterparts to have abused marijuana, cocaine, crack cocaine, hallucinogens, methamphetamines, heroin, and prescription drugs (Office of Applied Studies, 2005a).

Accident-Related Injuries

Alcohol and drug abusers are three to four times as likely to be hospitalized for an injury (Miller et al., 2001). Alcohol use is a predictor of injury severity in vehicle crash injuries increasing the person's scores on the Injury Severity Scale by 30% (Waller, Hill, Maio, & Blow, 2003). Alcoholics are more injury prone in general than nondrinkers and average 20–24% more emergency room visits than nonalcoholics. Heavy alcohol and drug users are also more likely to have impulsive behaviors, which increase risk taking, and depression, which increases self-injurious behaviors resulting in overdose and suicide attempt/completion (Rees, Horton, Hingson, Saitz, & Samet, 2002).

Relationships

Long-term substance misuse can negatively effect cognitive, emotional, and behavioral changes in functioning. These changes may be due to physiological alterations in brain functioning, adaptation to their environment in order to maintain their pattern of use, or a combination of both of these factors. Couples with one substance-misusing partner experience increased stress and decreased levels of enjoyment both with one another and with life in general. The partner who does not use substances may feel abandoned or unappreciated as the substance use escalates because more time is being dedicated to the substance abuse than to the couple. The probability of violence increases proportionally with the choice of substances (legal/illegal), the length of time using the substance, and an individual's comorbid personality structure. The lack of time, energy, and nurturance to the relationship often results in emotional distance and resentments that are difficult to deescalate without external assistance.

Intimate Partner Violence

Intimate partner violence (IPV) refers to verbal, psychological, and/or physical violence between two members of an intimately involved couple. Couples in relationships that involve substances have a much higher rate of verbal and physical violence within the relationship (O'Farrell, Fals-Stewart, Murphy, & Murphy, 2003). Psychoactive substances are both a risk factor and coping mechanism for stress and violence, as well

TABLE 7.1. Danger Signals in Couples with Substance Use Problems

1. Many arguments about the substance or things related to the substance, such as money problems, staying out late, not taking care of responsibilities in the home.

2. "Covering" for a partner who has been drinking or using drugs too much by making excuses for him/her (such as reporting to a boss or coworker that the substance user is "sick" and won't be at work).

3. A partner reporting that he/she uses substances to reduce tension or stress related to arguments and fights in the home about the substance itself.

4. Substance use is the only or one of the few things the partners like to do together.

5. Episodes of domestic violence or "angry touching" by either partner when a partner has been using substances.

6. Finding that one or both partners need to be intoxicated or high to show signs of affection or to talk about problems in their relationship.

7. The relationship or family as a whole becomes isolated from friends and relatives to hide the substance problem.

Note. Reprinted with permission from William Fals-Stewart.

as a precipitant. Psychoactive substance use exacerbates problems that already exist and is often an additional source of conflict (Quigley & Leonard, 2000). The increase in stress related to the escalation in violence has the ripple effect of increasing substance use as a coping mechanism to deal with the stress. In later stages, the substance use eventually becomes the primary issue for arguments and fighting. The resultant vicious cycle (substance use causes conflict → the conflict leads to more substance use as a way of reducing stress → conflict about the substance use escalates → more substance use occurs) becomes the couple's only mechanism of communication (Freeman, in press). Therefore, any therapist who suspects substance misuse as a component of marital or couple discord must conduct additional screening for misuse and/or violence in the situation. This reciprocal relationship between alcohol consumption and violence may be further exacerbated by the presence of underlying personality disorders and/or Axis I disorders, such as bipolar disorder or schizophrenia. Some of the common danger signals (identified by Fals-Stewart, 2003) that substance misuse may be causing harm in a couple's relationship are listed in Table 7.1.

Once a couple has been identified as suffering from IPV, they should be evaluated for substance misuse problems. If substance misuse is identified, the individual with the disorder should be referred to specialized therapy for substance disorders in addition to therapy for violence/aggression. This combination therapy approach has been shown to decreases male-perpetrated IPV as much as 50% (Caetano, Schafer, Fals-Stewart, Farrell, & Miller 2003).

Non-Relationship-Related Violence

The propensity for violence does not end with IPV. People who use mood-altering substances are impairing the function of the frontal lobe of the brain as soon as they ingest the substance. The frontal lobe of the brain is responsible for executive function and therefore governing socially acceptable behavioral choices as well as mediating impulsivity. Thus a person who has impairment of the frontal lobe is at high risk for making impulsive, inappropriate, and potentially dangerous decisions based on emotion. Prolonged use of substances increases the likelihood that a person will become irritable, paranoid, and self-absorbed. These characteristics combined with decreased impulse control are a formula for disaster. Once the person becomes involved with the use of illegal substances, the additional criminal factor adds another dimension placing the individual at even higher risk for violence. The individual is therefore at risk for violence aimed at him/herself as well as others.

Medical

Every psychoactive substance has the potential to create myriad short-term and long-term medical complications. Table 7.2 outlines the consequences for the primary substances of abuse (Storie, 2005).

Financial

A financial crisis usually begins with the use of family finances to cover the costs of substance procurement. This causes a crisis when the rent or mortgage is chronically late or even lapses to the point of foreclosure or eviction. Further, because cash reserves have been exhausted to pay for a costly drug habit, the user will begin to use credit cards excessively to pay for daily expenses. This dangerous pattern often leads to bankruptcy, repossession of purchases, and/or resorting to theft.

Co-Occurring Disorders

Persons who misuse substances to the point of developing dependence may exhibit symptoms and behaviors similar to those exhibited by persons with an Axis II (personality) disorder, such as antisocial personality disorder (ASP). In a study by Rounsaville et al. (1998), the majority of individuals with substance use disorder (57%) met criteria for at least one comorbid Axis II disorder. Cluster B disorders made up 45.7% of the individuals, with 27% of those being ASP diagnoses and 18.4% being borderline personality disorder (BPD) diagnoses. In addition, when the researchers included substance-related symptoms, there was a substantial increase in diagnosed cases, especially for ASP and BPD, which increased to 19.2% and 11.4%, respectively (Rounsaville et al., 1998). Differentiation between symptoms caused by substance abuse and resulting from an Axis II disorder requires a careful evaluation of the person's history of substance use and history of behavioral manifestation of disordered behavior patterns.

DSM-IV-TR recommends excluding Axis II symptoms that are accounted for by an Axis I disorder; this includes substance use disorders. Table 7.3 (Freeman, 2005) outlines those parallel presentations that often confuse the diagnostic picture with substance-misusing persons and persons with personality disorders.

TABLE 7.2. Short- and Long-Term Medical Complications of Psychoactive Substances

Substance	Short-term consequences	Long-term consequences
Alcohol	High blood pressure, irregular heartbeat, delusions, hostility, paranoia, staggering, slurred speech, memory loss, irritability, impaired judgment, disorientation, alterations in perception	Permanent memory loss, thiamine deficiency, esophageal reflux, stomach lining deterioration, hemorrhaging, ulcers, kidney inflammation, impotence, calcium depletion, reduction in white blood cells, cirrhosis of the liver, jaundice, diabetes
Amphetamine/ methamphetamine	Disconnected thought and speech patterns, anxiety, irritability, hallucinations, paranoia, aggression, insomnia, loss of appetite	Hypertension, stroke, brain hemorrhage, seizures, aneurysm, cardiac arrest, chronic psychotic illness, permanent damage to dopamine and serotonin neurons, death
Cocaine	Increased heart rate and blood pressure, insomnia, loss of appetite, elevated temperature, seizures, sudden cardiac arrest, anxiety, hallucinations, paranoia, nosebleeds, chronic cough, shortness of breath, nausea	Brain hemorrhaging, stroke, convulsions, severe headaches, depression, dental erosion, inflammation of heart muscles, irregular heartbeat, ulcers, liver failure, nasal septum damage, asthma, lung disease, erectile dysfunction, gastrointestinal complications, coma, death
Heroin	Bobbing head, suppression of cough, reduction in respiratory functions, decrease in blood pressure, slurred speech, constipation, nausea, vomiting, itching, inability to urinate, impaired judgment	Increased risk of infection, abnormal ovarian function, erectile dysfunction, asthma, liver or kidney disease, collapsed veins, abnormal levels of cortisol, chronic constipation, cardiovascular malfunction, severe skeletal-muscle breakdown, contraction of an infectious disease, death
Phencyclidine (PCP)	Slurred speech, numbness to extremities, muscular rigidity, increased heart rate and blood pressure, dramatic increase in blood pressure, nausea, vomiting, homicidal/suicidal behaviors	Coma, death, neuronal degeneration, permanent memory loss, speech and cognitive dysfunction, psychosis, chronic anxiety and agitation, respiratory failure, convulsions, seizures
MDMA	Nausea, vomiting, increased heart rate and blood pressure, elevated body temperature, dehydration, loss of appetite, seizures, convulsions, paranoia, panic attacks	Destroying of axons and terminals for serotonin, dopamine, and norepinephrine, decrease in blood flow, memory loss, short attention span, verbal reasoning difficulties, chronic muscle pain, chronic psychotic episodes

(continued)

TABLE 7.2. *(continued)*

Substance	Short-term consequences	Long-term consequences
Marijuana	Increased blood pressure and heart rate, headaches, numbness, increased appetite, tremors, sedation, decrease in REM sleep, impaired critical thinking skills, short-term memory impairment, paranoia, anxiety, hallucinations	Deficits in long-term memory and cognitive functioning, psychosis hallucinations, lungs more vulnerable to disease, disruption of menstrual cycles, increased absorption of carbon monoxide, irregular heartbeat, lowering of body temperature, respiratory illness, cellular abnormalities in lungs
Anabolic steroids	Increase in blood pressure, disruption of menstruation, deepening of voice for females, increase of blood cholesterol, water retention, sleep disturbances, increase in aggression, hallucinations, frightening dreams	Mania, psychosis, major depression, clogged arteries, heart attack, stroke, jaundice, liver tumors, cysts of blood in the liver, liver cancer, rupture and hemorrhage of the liver, stunted growth for adolescents, infertility, enlarged prostate

Individuals with substance misuse problems may have brain damage due to the primary effect of the substance(s) or due to consequences related to their use (e.g., motor vehicle accidents and other injuries to the head). These individuals can be poor historians as well: minimizing the impact of their use and behaviors or no longer enjoying the cognitive capability to provide an accurate history. It is in the patient's, and therapist's, best interest to obtain corroborating information about the patient's substance use patterns. Therefore, some basic guidelines to follow when gathering information about this population include the following:

1. Avoid relying on patient self-report for information. This information is likely skewed, protected, and limited despite a presentation of cooperation.

2. Obtain collateral information from as many sources as possible connected with the patient. For example, information should be gathered from family, friends,

TABLE 7.3. Parallel Diagnostic Presentation: Personality Disorder and Substance Dependence Disorder

1. There is often support system exhaustion (family, employment, financial, social).
2. Among the primary reactions and defenses are "other blaming."
3. The changes in behavior can usually be traced to early to mid teens.
4. Both disorders tend to progress over time as behaviors and drug use escalate.
5. There is often exacerbation and remissions with frequent crises.
6. There are often many apparently manipulative interactions.
7. Both disorders are at risk for affective disorders and exhausted support systems.
8. There is inadequate/limited/poor problem-solving skills.
9. There are multiple failure experiences in all aspects of life and with substance use.

medical practitioners, and previous therapists, as well as the patient's pharmacy. There is much information to be learned from a pharmacy-generated history of prescriptions (e.g., multiple prescribers, early refills, choices of prescription category, and treatment of medical consequences of misuse).

3. Construct a timeline of the patient's substance misuse patterns, consequences, and behaviors (Sobell & Sobell, 1992, 2005). This technique allows the patient to identify his/her own use progression, as well as behavioral escalation, in a non-threatening, collaborative manner.

4. Obtain a thorough medical history and physical evaluation that includes a liver panel and evaluation of gamma glutamyltransferase (GGT) enzymes in alcohol-misusing persons.

5. Evaluate the patient for possible neurological problems. Many substance-misusing persons have suffered head trauma, may have mild mental retardation, or may have a history of learning disabilities that have never been diagnosed. These problems may offer a neurological explanation for the maladaptive presentation (Freeman, 2005).

Substance misuse causes an alteration in the user's brain chemistry, which affects change in his/her perceptual experiences. To create this change in perception, the substance must act on neurotransmitters in the person's brain and either increase or decrease his/her normal mechanism of function. For example, the effects of some mood-altering chemicals on aggressive behavior may be mediated or diminished by glutamate and GABA (Freeman & Rathbun, 2006). Severe Axis I psychiatric disturbances are associated with abnormalities in serotonin and/or dopamine levels. Misuse of stimulants, most notably cocaine and methamphetamine, can produce aggressive effects by increasing the bioavailability of both dopamine and norepinephrine in the brain at the level of the synapse. Interestingly, nicotine has been found to have some antiaggressive effects, possibly because of its mediating effect on serotonin (Seth, Cheeta, Tucci, & File, 2002). The therapist should keep in mind that people with cluster B personality disorders are prone to substance misuse and drug-seeking or manipulative behaviors. All "controlled" or potentially addictive medications as treatment options for aggression or anxiety would therefore be relatively contraindicated (Freeman & Rathbun, 2006). The person who either has developed similar behavioral presentations or has an underlying personality disorder should be carefully evaluated before prescribing a pharmacological intervention.

METHODS OF COUNSELING CRISES IN SUBSTANCE-MISUSING PERSONS

Motivational Interviewing

Therapists used to believe that to motivate a person to change he/she was required to "hit bottom." This was often accomplished through aggressive confrontation of the substance-abusing person in order to "break him/her down" and increase his/her level of discomfort with current behaviors. If the person did not respond to the confrontation, which usually included an ultimatum, he/she was deemed "unready" to seek help, and family members were encouraged to abandon the person to the disease until he/she was ready to seek treatment. Researchers discovered that the vast number of people who were deemed "not ready" were in fact ready to change and would have responded positively to less aggressive tactics for change motivation if exercised (Prochaska & DiClemente, 1984). The "intervention" technique as described previously is still used, but it has been modified to better assist the person with identifying his/her own motivators for change. Prochaska and DiClemente developed a simple and useful model for understanding the stages of change that a person experiences in the therapeutic process. The stages-of-change (SOC) model includes precontemplation, contemplation, preparation, action, and maintenance stages (Prochaska & DiClemente, 1984).

The SOC model is currently the most recognizable and most used model in substance treatment. However, Freeman and Dolan (2001) improved on the original by addressing five additional stages. With the expansion from a 5-stage model to a 10-stage model, the therapist can pinpoint the situation and behavioral manifestations of change more clearly (Freeman & Dolan, 2001). Freeman and Dolan's 10-stage model (Table 7.4) includes the components of noncontemplation, anticontemplation, precontemplation, contemplation, action planning, action, lapse activation and redirection, relapse and redirection, termination, and maintenance. The additional stages reflect the experiences of clients and therapists both in and out of the therapeutic process. The modified-component SOC model may be applied to a variety of crisis situations, such as substance misuse, parasuicidal behaviors, and pathological gambling.

TABLE 7.4. Revised Stages Of Change Compared to Stages of Change

Prochaska & DiClemente	Freeman & Dolan
Precontemplation	Noncontemplation: "I didn't realize. . . "
Precontemplation	Anticontemplation (willful or nonwillful): "Leave me alone!"
Precontemplation	Precontemplation: "I am willing to think . . . "
Contemplation	Contemplation: "I need to do something about . . . "
Preparation	Action planning: "What can I do?"
Action	Action: "I need a plan"
Not included	Prelapse (redirection—cognitive and metacognitive): "I keep thinking about using . . . "
Not included	Lapse (redirection—behavioral): "slip"
Not included	Relapse (redirection—cognitive and behavioral): "I slipped again . . . "
Maintenance	Maintenance: "I have been sober for ___ months now."

Impediments to Change

Most people have good intentions when making a major change decision about their behavior. Good intentions are important, but ability and utility are essential. In most cases in which there is substance misuse involved, the patient is blamed and considered "bad," "in denial," or "noncompliant" if he/she fails to achieve success the first or second time that he/she seeks treatment. Interestingly, we do not apply these same terms to someone who has difficulty managing his/her diabetic diet or cardiac diet but tend to use it more with people who have difficulty managing their substance use behaviors. There are many different reasons why one person is successful and another is unsuccessful. Rather than blaming the patient for exhibiting the hallmarks of human nature, it is more beneficial to reevaluate the potential for change in the willing patient.

The Freeman Impediments to Change Scale—Substance Misuse version (Figure 7.1) was developed by Freeman, Freeman, and Roya and identifies the most commonly found problems with treating a person with a substance misuse disorder (Freeman, 2005). The scale is divided into four main factors with 10–11 subfactors related to each item listed. The four main areas of impediments are (1) patient factors, (2) practitioner/therapist factors, (3) environmental factors, and (4) pathology factors. For example, inability to access care due to financial factors is listed as an environmental factor. The Freeman Impediments to Change Scale—Substance Misuse version allows for the therapist's evaluation of impediments in an objective, nonjudgmental, and targeted fashion. Once the impediment(s) have been objectively identified, it is then a matter of developing a treatment plan incorporating or targeting these obstacles in the treatment. If an limited support network is a mitigating factor, this factor will continue to exert negative pressure on the progress of this patient until the therapist and patient evaluate this problem, develop goals, and reduce the impact.

Strategies for Change

The addition of a mood-altering substance to a system that is already unstable can create a potentially volatile situation rapidly. Therefore, it is critical that ground rules are established regarding safety at the beginning of the therapy relationship. Safety issues that are commonly encountered include (1) suicidal crises (often in the middle of the night), (2) legal crises involving arrests for driving under the influence or potential loss of custody of minor children, and (3) verbal abuse or physical violence toward one's partner, the therapist, or others. Therapists should be aware of their own prejudices regarding these issues, as well as their own boundaries before agreeing to treat these individuals. The patient must clearly agree to the safety rules as established in the initial session before treatment can begin. In addition it is critical with these individuals that the therapist does not bend, break, or alter the rules once established. Should the therapist break the rules, his/her credibility, as well as the therapy, itself is called into question. It also sends a signal to the individual that agreed-on rules are arbitrary and meaningless as long as the excuse has some modicum of face validity.

Instructions: For each of the following impediments, identify the contribution of that issue to the problems being encountered in therapy. It will be essential for the therapist to review all the areas with the patient.

0 = no importance; 1 = some importance; 2 = moderate importance; 3 = great importance; 4 = major importance

Patient Factors					
1	Skill deficit regarding techniques to control substance use and/ or comply with therapeutic regimen/expectations	0	1	2	3	4
2	Negative cognitions regarding previous treatment experience or abstinence failure(s)	0	1	2	3	4
3	Negative cognitions regarding the consequences to others about altering substance use	0	1	2	3	4
4	The patient experiences secondary gain from disease symptoms	0	1	2	3	4
5	The patient experiences significant primary gain from substance use	0	1	2	3	4
6	Fear of changing one's actions, thoughts, feelings	0	1	2	3	4
7	Motivation to discontinue substance use has not reached contemplative stage	0	1	2	3	4
8	General negative set regarding ability to control use or stop use	0	1	2	3	4
9	Limited or restricted self-monitoring/monitoring of others	0	1	2	3	4
10	Patient frustrated with lack of treatment progress over time/or perceived stigma of being in therapy	0	1	2	3	4
11	Insufficient personal resources (physical, cognitive, or intellectual) to control substance use	0	1	2	3	4
Practitioner/Therapist Factors					
1	Insufficient therapist skill/experience with substance use	0	1	2	3	4
2	Patient and practitioner distortions are congruent	0	1	2	3	4
3	Limited or insufficient socialization of patient to treatment generally and to specific treatment model	0	1	2	3	4
4	Incomplete or absent collaboration and working alliance	0	1	2	3	4
5	Insufficient or inadequate data regarding individuals history	0	1	2	3	4
6	Therapeutic narcissism	0	1	2	3	4
7	Timing of intervention was not aligned with patient and/or did not match motivation level	0	1	2	3	4

(continued)

FIGURE 7.1. Freeman Impediments to Change Scale—Substance Misuse. Copyright by Arthur Freeman and Sharon Morgillo Freeman. Reprinted by permission.

8	Therapy goals are unstated, unrealistic, or vague: There is misalignment of patient goals with therapy goals	0	1	2	3	4
9	Evaluation of developmental process does not take temporal factor of substance abuse into account or is overestimated	0	1	2	3	4
10	Generalized negative beliefs (discriminatory) about substance use or unrealistic expectations of patient	0	1	2	3	4
11	Insufficient flexibility and creativity in treatment planning	0	1	2	3	4
Environmental Factors						
1	Environmental stressors preclude changing	0	1	2	3	4
2	Significant others actively or passively sabotage therapy	0	1	2	3	4
3	Agency reinforcement of pathology and illness via compensation or benefits	0	1	2	3	4
4	Cultural or family issues regarding help seeking	0	1	2	3	4
5	Significant family pathology and/or active substance use in the home	0	1	2	3	4
6	Demands made by family members or significant others directly conflict with the therapeutic plans or activities	0	1	2	3	4
7	Unrealistic or conflicting demands on patient by institutions or other external source	0	1	2	3	4
8	Financial factors limit change (inability to access care)	0	1	2	3	4
9	System homeostasis	0	1	2	3	4
10	Inadequate or limited support network	0	1	2	3	4
Pathology Factors						
1	Patient flexibility severely restricted resulting in movement constraints in treatment compliance	0	1	2	3	4
2	Significant medical/physiological problems	0	1	2	3	4
3	Difficulty in establishing trust	0	1	2	3	4
4	Autonomy press	0	1	2	3	4
5	Severe impulsive response pattern independent of substance use	0	1	2	3	4
6	Confusion, dementia, or limited cognitive ability	0	1	2	3	4
7	Symptom profusion	0	1	2	3	4
8	Dependence on external controls	0	1	2	3	4
9	Severe self-devaluation	0	1	2	3	4
10	Severely compromised energy	0	1	2	3	4

FIGURE 7.1. *(continued)*

Excuse making is a common problem for individuals with substance misuse crises. Their partner or parent may have developed a habit of "covering" for them. This behavior is protective in nature—protective of the person's dignity, as well as protective of family assets (as in calling the employer to excuse the partner's absence from work) (Freeman, in press). The protective partner has usually been "trained" by the substance-misusing person through conversations and discussions that include rescuer/victim roles, misuse–forgiveness behaviors, begging–lying–forgiveness conversations, and brief periods of sobriety that "prove" that the behavior was "just a slip." These circular conversations establish an atmosphere of reward conditioning (interval reward). For the family member, the occasional "win" is the positive reinforcement that conditions the family member to "just hang in there for a little while longer."

The therapist will most likely witness many of these circular conversations in therapy sessions. Maintaining neutrality and avoiding blame is critical to the ongoing motivational process of changing behavior (O'Farrell et al., 2003). In other words, if the therapist is seen as judgmental, the substance-misusing individual, and most likely his/her partner or parent, will begin to protect each other and return to older, more familiar methods of coping, despite previous periods of misuse and anger. Change will occur slowly and retention in therapy is needed to effect this change. The old adage "You can't treat them if you don't see them" definitely fits for these individuals. Given that partners of substance-misusing individuals are often hungry for answers to "fix" the problem, the therapist can use this information as a means to educate those significant others involve in treatment.

Abstinence from substance use is always an integral part of session goals and focus, with the therapist reinforcing abstinence behavior in each session. Abstinence coaching and counseling can be viewed as an overriding format with behavioral, emotional, and cognitive issues as the specific foci for each session. Figure 7.2 shows this process in action:

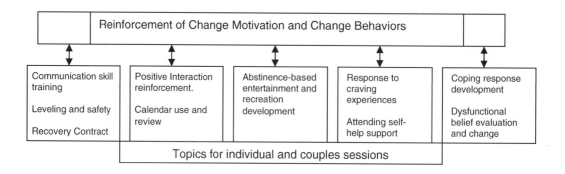
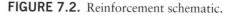

FIGURE 7.2. Reinforcement schematic.

Cognitive Techniques

Clarifying Idiosyncratic Meaning

The substance-misusing population often has a sublanguage that is unique to a geographic location, substance type, or substance subculture. The therapist should not assume to know what the person's words or statements mean. Asking for clarification ensures that the therapist understands exactly what is being communicated. This technique also models the need for active listening skills and a way to verify assumptions.

Questioning the Evidence

Many people function and behave without thinking about the meaning or evidence behind their "routine" behaviors and responses to events or feelings. It is important to examine the source of data and question the evidence that has been collected in support of dysfunctional views. For example, a wife believed that expressing her concern about her husband's alcohol use would upset him and be viewed as nagging. The husband, on the other hand, felt that his wife's silence indicated a lack of concern and/or disapproval of him in general.

Examining Options and Alternatives

The therapist helps to examine all possible alternatives to a response or situation. Using the simple statement "And what else might that mean . . . ?" or "What other things have you done to . . . ?" helps the person develop a list of alternate behaviors for specific situations.

Decatastrophizing

Individuals with substance misuse problems have often experienced catastrophic events and consequences. They may feel overwhelmed when a problem recurs because it awakens the memory of past experiences. Helping the person develop strategies to evaluate responses to potential problems with a series of data-collection exercises and reality testing is basic to therapy.

Assessing Advantages and Disadvantages

This strategy helps the individual gain balance and perspective regarding his/her view of an issue. The individual can evaluate, for example, the advantages and disadvantages of dressing in a certain way that may be acceptable in his/her subculture and unacceptable in his/her long-term recovery view. This technique can also be used to reinforce the cognitive-behavioral therapy (CBT) process altogether by evaluating the advantages and disadvantages of thinking in a certain way ("I will be ridiculed for saying 'no' to the offer of a drink") or feeling a certain way ("She *makes* me mad—I can't help it!").

Scaling

This is an excellent technique for individuals who have dichotomous responses and thinking patterns. The therapist helps the couple view things along a continuum in order to help them gain perspective and distance from the automatic all-or-nothing responses.

Self-Instruction

This is another very simple technique that reinforces the CBT experience and parallels components of many self-help groups, such as Alcoholics Anonymous (AA). Basically self-instruction is talking to oneself. Using the AA adages, such as "this too shall pass" and "keep it simple," are examples of such self-instruction techniques that provide the person with a guide to responding to cues and triggers.

Behavioral Techniques

Activity Scheduling

Individuals with substance use problems often feel overwhelmed in daily life and catastrophize over simple situations. They usually have minimal opportunities to experience positive outcomes and rewards to behavioral changes they have tried. Using a calendar provides a visual cue that is very helpful outside the therapy office by offering an opportunity to plan between sessions and to maintain a record of events that are recovery based. The visual properties provides the person with a mechanism of reinforcement that is both subtle and simple.

Social Skills Training

A lack of basic social, conversational, and interaction skills is not uncommon in this population. Many times the individual has cut off relationships with non-substance-misusing persons and, therefore, feels awkward about integrating into new social groups. Training may include job interview skills, such as handshaking, dressing, and expected courtesy during the interview. Changing language patterns, such as reduction in profanity or slang, may be needed with some people.

Assertiveness Training

Development of assertive techniques for the patient, and often his/her partner, is essential to the recovery plan. Individuals who have aggressive tendencies are often paired with partners who have developed significant passive tendencies. The therapist would need to help each individual to moderate these styles in order to improve communication between themselves and others.

Behavioral Rehearsal/Role Playing

Substance misuse often results in a decrease in the individual's ability to think abstractly. This is due to both acute and chronic changes in brain function. Behaviors and cognitions regress to a level of immaturity and, therefore, concrete operations. Due to this regression in cognitive structure, the use of role play becomes an important intervention technique. It allows the person to experience an alternative behavior/ thinking pattern and to practice the new behavior before being put to the test in an actual situation. Through behavioral rehearsal, the person actually practices the new behavior *in vivo* and identifies problems to be worked on ahead of time.

Table 7.5 lists an overview of CBT techniques for substance-misusing persons.

Adjunctive Interventions

Therapists working with substance-misusing individuals should be familiar with the community and medical support systems that are integral for successful recovery. For example, the support of AA has been the cornerstone of recovery since the early 1930s and remains one of the most well-known lay recovery networks in the world. Recently, other recovery groups have developed that offer community support to these individuals, including SMART Recovery. Often participation in a recovery network is a man-

---

TABLE 7.5. CBT Techniques for Substance-Misusing Persons

1. Maintain a high degree of structure in therapy generally and each session specifically.
2. Limit demands for patient problem solving *unless and until* the problem solving skills are in place.
3. Use a concrete rather than abstract approach (aphorisms useful).
4. Substance of choice will often point to schematic structure.
5. Focus on purpose and meaning of substance misuse.
6. Identify schemata that fuel substance misuse.
7. Identify the patient enablers (personal, institutional, or group).
8. Work to disempower enablers.
9. Identify patient supporters.
10. Patient must agree to change.
11. Therapeutic goals must be realistic and proximal.
12. Therapy must be directive.
13. Therapy must include psychoeducation without being boring or "preachy."
14. The patient must learn to identify automatic thoughts (ATs) related to craving.
15. The patient must learn to identify ATs related to seeking (drive) behavior.
16. The patient must learn to identify ATs related to using substances.
17. Extensive use of self-instructional techniques.
18. Need to develop and maintain motivation.
19. Identify and develop prescriptions for vulnerability factors.
20. Identify threshold for substance use.
21. Focus on the therapeutic relationship.
22. Be aware of both negative and positive countertransference.

datory part of a recovery contract, especially for those who have legal requirements for treatment. Support networks provide the individual with a ready-made social group that is abstinence focused, and therefore, likely to reinforce the change motivation and behavior process.

In noncounseling settings, brief interventions can be as effective as lengthier interventions when it is impractical to provide a 1-hour intervention. These short, targeted 5- to 15-minute interventions conducted by a medical professional during a routine health exam have been proven to increase a person's awareness of a substance misuse problem enough to initiate a contemplation or action stage of change. Other brief interventions, for example have included "motivational feedback" provided to college students through e-mail, which draws their attention to their risk status in a nonthreatening manner (Saunders, Kypri, Walters, Laforge, & Larimer, 2004).

Another intervention that is becoming more common in treating these individuals is the addition of medication management for control of cravings for substances. These medications include acamprosate (Campral), vivitrex (Vivitrol), bupronex (Suboxone), and the soon to be released modafanil (Provigil) and topiramate (Topamax), to name a few. Therapists should be familiar with each of these medications regarding their indication, expected action, and potential side effect profiles in order to help individuals make informed decisions about taking the medication or maintaining their use. For many individuals, the advent of the availability of medications that interrupt the craving processes are akin to the invention of antibiotics for infection treatment. Others may not be good candidates for these medications due to the side effect profiles or other problems with their use.

CASE STUDY

Brenda is a 36-year-old married attorney who arrives for an evaluation of her alcohol use at the demand of her husband. Brenda is very quiet in the session, initially expressing embarrassment that she has been identified as having an alcohol abuse problem. The therapist observes that Brenda is very thin (67 inches, 118 pounds) with pale skin, dark circles under her eyes, and mild tremor in her hands. Brenda reports that she is at risk for losing her job at her firm due to having missed several court appearances and not turning in important paperwork. She becomes tearful as she discusses each new consequence and crisis related to her alcohol problems. The goal of this session is to move Brenda from the stage of precontemplation to contemplation or action stage of change.

THERAPIST: You said on your intake sheet that you are coming in for an evaluation of your drinking problems. Why do you think that you might have a drinking problem?

BRENDA: My husband said I had to come in here or else . . .

THERAPIST: Or else?

BRENDA: Or else he will leave me (*begins to cry*). I know I have a problem, but I am sure I can handle it.

THERAPIST: When did you first think you might have a drinking problem?

BRENDA: About three years ago, that was when I was put on probation at work the first time.

THERAPIST: The first time?

BRENDA: Yes, this is the second time I have been in trouble. I somehow managed to pull things together for a couple of years and then . . . well, it all fell apart!

THERAPIST: What do you mean by "pull things together"? [Clarifying idiosyncratic meaning]

BRENDA: I stopped drinking.

THERAPIST: How long did you stay away from alcohol during the time you "pulled things together?"

BRENDA: About a month, month and a half maybe. I really thought I could control it. I made bets with myself that I could drink just one or two. Before long I was right back where I started.

THERAPIST: And where was that? [Making the abstract more concrete]

BRENDA: A bottle of wine every night and a few martinis during lunch. I go through a fifth of vodka in a day or two.

THERAPIST: What else are you using? [Directive question aimed to evaluate reasons for her slim build and other physical symptoms such as high blood pressure and red eyes/nose]

BRENDA: What do you mean?

THERAPIST: Are you using anything else in addition to the alcohol? Any other substances?

BRENDA: Yes (*embarrassed*). I use cocaine.

THERAPIST: How much cocaine are you using?

BRENDA: I have to smoke every day to keep going.

THERAPIST: When you say smoke, are you freebasing crack cocaine? [Clarifying]

BRENDA: yes.

THERAPIST: Each time you freebase, how much are you using? [Clarification of amount used]

BRENDA: I buy a dime each time.

THERAPIST: And how much cocaine will a dime get you these days? [Clarification of amount used. Most early users use a "nickel" bag—$5 worth. A "dime" is $10 worth and the actual amount is usually a quarter of a gram.]

BRENDA: About a quarter gram . . .

THERAPIST: How long does a quarter of a gram last you?

BRENDA: About an hour if I go slow.

THERAPIST: I noticed that you are pretty thin and your nose is red. Have you had other medical problems related to the cocaine? For example, heart problems? [Evaluating for possible impending medical crisis]

BRENDA: A couple of times my heart started racing and I was afraid it would burst in my chest. I went to my doctor and he said I have high blood pressure and gave me medication for the palpitations and the blood pressure.

THERAPIST: Do you take your medications? [Evaluating patient's compliance to medical treatment as well as possible medical complications]

BRENDA: No, I forget pretty often.

THERAPIST: Let me summarize what we know so far. You have told me that you are drinking a bottle of wine every night, a few martinis during lunch, and a fifth of vodka every day or two. You are using a quarter of a gram of cocaine a day. You are at risk of losing your job and have significant medical problems related to your use. What would you like to do at this point? [Determining level of motivation]

BRENDA: I would like to quit using everything! [Contemplation stage]

THERAPIST: What happens when you have tried to quit everything? [Evaluating impediments to change]

BRENDA: I can't do it! I have tried and tried! No one believes me! [Impediments are fear of failing again]

THERAPIST: Have you tried checking in to a hospital to be detoxified from chemicals?

BRENDA: No way! I'm not that bad! I can't miss work and who would take care of things! [Impediment to change: fear of additional consequences if she seeks treatment]

THERAPIST: Are you taking care of things now? [Decatastrophizing]

BRENDA: No.

THERAPIST: Would you like me to help you quit everything? [Motivation to change—moving to action stage]

BRENDA: That's why I'm here!

THERAPIST: I am worried about your medical condition. I think you need to be monitored in a hospital when you quit everything. Would you like me to help you find a place to go?

BRENDA: (bursting into tears again) I can't believe this is happening to me! I can't believe this! [Catastrophic thinking]

THERAPIST: Would you like me to help you find a place to go?

BRENDA: (sighing) Yes. I know it is the best thing. [Action stage]

THERAPIST: Here are some options. (Lists options.)

BRENDA: OK. What do we do now? [Action stage]

THERAPIST: Will your husband help you get to the hospital? [Evaluation of support system and patient's perception of support]

BRENDA: I think so. He says he'll help me do whatever it takes.

At this point the therapist reviews admission procedures and contacts the facility to arrange for admission. In the aforementioned situation, Brenda's case becomes complicated when the therapist pushes for additional data. The husband and Brenda both identified alcohol problems; however, Brenda had some symptoms that were observable that indicated there might be other substances involved. Identifying the full extent of her substance use allowed for a better evaluation of her medical status, which was significantly compromised. It is not unusual for individuals who misuse substances to be diagnosed and treated for medical complications related to their use. Brenda had cardiac complications as well as hypertension. She also had tremors of her hands. These symptoms indicate a dysregulation of her autonomic nervous system. Given these symptoms she was at risk for seizures if she discontinued the alcohol use abruptly. The therapist knew that it was not likely that she would be able to locate and admit herself to a treatment facility once she left the office and therefore arranged for an appropriate location that would monitor her during her detoxification phase. Obtaining Brenda's agreement required careful questioning that was nonjudgmental based on the data she was providing. Brenda felt respected and listened to and therefore was more amenable to the therapist's recommendations. This helped to move Brenda from a contemplative stance to action. Involving her husband set the stage for couples therapy in the future as well as evaluating her support system.

SUMMARY

Substance use and misuse disorders affect hundreds of thousands of individuals in the United States alone each year. As a result, these individuals often require immediate, empirically based assistance from ED professionals, behavioral health specialists, and general practitioners due to medical crises, relationship crisis, and financial crisis. In addition, many individuals end up in U.S. prisons and jails for serious legal violations directly or indirectly related to their substance misuse.

Individuals, families, and couples that present for therapy in an outpatient setting in crisis require multiple skill level assistance. Therapists treating these individuals also require multiple skill level training and understanding. CBT models, including motivational interviewing and SOC theory, along with specific CBT techniques, can be matched to the individual's motivation and ability to change. The therapist must be adept at identifying strengths that may help a person to change as well as the many potential impediments to change that may stall or thwart the therapeutic efforts. Establishing and keeping clear therapeutic rules and boundaries, utilizing various behavioral and cognitive techniques during sessions, and enacting adjunctive interventions all increase the potential for a positive outcome and crisis resolution.

REFERENCES

Addiction Technology Transfer Center. (2004). *Alcoholism: The science made easy* [Electronic version]. Kansas City, MI: Author.

American Psychiatric Association. (2000). *Diagnostic and statistical manual of mental disorders* (4th ed., text rev.). Washington, DC: Author.

Bureau of Justice Statistics. (2005, July). *Substance dependence, abuse, and treatment of jail inmates, 2002* (NCJ 209588).

Caetano, R., Schafer, J., Fals-Stewart, W., Farrell, T., & Miller, B. (2003). Intimate partner violence and drinking: New research on methodological issues, stability and change and treatment. *Alcoholism: Clinical and Experimental Research, 27*(2), 292–300.

Dai, X., & Thavundayil, J. (2005). Differences in the peripheral levels of ß-endorphin in response to alcohol and stress as a function of alcohol dependence and family history of alcoholism. *Alcoholism: Clinical and Experimental Research, 29*(11), 1965–1975.

Fahlke, C., Lorenz, J. G., Long, J., Champoux, M., Soumi, S. J., & Higley, J. D. (2000). Rearing experiences and stress-induced plasma cortisol as early risk factors for excessive alcohol consumption in nonhuman primates. *Alcoholism: Clinical and Experimental Research, 24*(5), 644–650.

Fals-Stewart, W. (2003). The occurrence of interpartner physical aggression on days of alcohol consumption: A longitudinal diary study. *Journal of Consulting and Clinical Psychology, 71*(1), 41–52.

Freeman, A., & Dolan, M. (2001). Revisiting Prochaska and DiClemente's stages of change: An expansion and specification to aid in treatment planning and outcome evaluation. *Cognitive and Behavioral Practice, 8*(3), 224–234.

Freeman, S. M. (2004). The relationship of opioid treatment in chronic pain conditions: Implications on brain reward response. *Journal of Addiction Nursing, 15*, 3–10.

Freeman, S. M. (2005). Substance misuse disorders. In A. Freeman & S. M. Freeman (Eds.), *Cognitive behavior therapy in nursing practice* (pp. 113–144). New York: Springer.

Freeman, S. M. (in press). Cognitive behavioral treatment of couples and relationship problems: Substance misuse as a complication. In A. Freeman (Ed), *Cognitive behavior therapy with couples*. New York: Rowman & Littlefield.

Freeman, S. M., & Rathbun, J. M. (2006). Psychopharmacologic options for antisocial personality disorder. In F. Rotgers & M. Manniaci (Eds.), *Comparative treatment of antisocial personality disorders* (pp. 179–190). New York: Springer.

Koob, G. F., & Bloom, F. E. (1988). Cellular and molecular mechanisms of drug dependence. *Science, 242*(4879), 715–723.

Koob, G. F., & Le Moal, M. (1997). Drug abuse: Hedonic homeostatic dysregulation. *Science, 278*(5335), 52–58.

Kreek, M. J. (1984). ACTH, cortisol, and b-endorphin response to metyrapone testing during chronic methadone maintenance treatment in humans. *Neuropeptides, 5*, 277–278.

Kreek, M. J., & Koob, G. F. (1998). Drug dependence: Stress and dysregulation of brain reward pathways. *Drug and Alcohol Dependence, 51*, 23–47.

Miller, T. R., Lestina, D. C., & Smith, G. S. (2001). Injury risk among medically identified alcohol and drug abusers. *Alcoholism: Clinical and Experimental Research, 25*(1), 54–59.

O'Brien, C. (2001). Drug addiction and drug abuse. In J. G. Hardman, L. E. Limbird, & A. G. Gilman (Eds.), *Goodman & Gilman's the pharmacological basis of therapeutics* (pp. 621–643). New York: McGraw-Hill.

O'Farrell, T. J., Fals-Stewart, W., Murphy, M., & Murphy, C. M. (2003). Partner violence before and after individually based alcoholism treatment for male alcoholic individuals. *Journal of Consulting and Clinical Psychology, 71*(1), 92–102.

Office of Applied Studies. (2003). *Results from the 2002 National Survey on Drug Use and*

Health: National findings (DHHS Publication No. SMA 03-3836, NSDUH Series H-22). Rockville, MD: Substance Abuse and Mental Health Services Administration.

Office of Applied Studies. (2004). *Results from the 2003 National Survey on Drug Use and Health: National findings* (DHHS Publication No. SMA 04-3964, NSDUH Series H-25). Rockville, MD: Substance Abuse and Mental Health Services Administration.

Office of Applied Studies. (2005a). *The NSDUH Report: Illicit drug use among persons arrested for serious crimes* [Online]. Retrieved December, 15, 2005, from *oas.samhsa.gov/2k5/arrests/arrests.htm*

Office of Applied Studies. (2005b). *Results from the 2004 National Survey on Drug Use and Health: National findings* (DHHS Publication No. SMA 05-4062, NSDUH Series H-28). Rockville, MD: Substance Abuse and Mental Health Services Administration.

Portenoy, R. K., & Payne, R. (1992). Acute and chronic pain. In J. H. Lowinson, P. Ruiz, R. B. Millman, & J. G. Langrod (Eds.), *Substance abuse: A comprehensive textbook* (2nd ed., pp. 691–721). Philadelphia: Lippincott Williams & Wilkins.

Prochaska, J. O., & DiClemente, C. C. (1984). *The transtheoretical approach: Crossing the traditional boundaries of therapy.* Homewood, IL: Irwin.

Quigley, B. M., & Leonard, K. E. (2000). Alcohol and the continuation of early marital aggression. *Alcoholism: Clinical and Experimental Research, 24*(7), 1003–1010.

Rees, V. W., Horton, N. J., Hingson, R. W., Saitz, R., & Samet, J. H. (2002). Injury among detoxification individuals: Alcohol users greater risk. *Alcoholism: Clinical and Experimental Research, 26*(2), 212–217.

Rounsaville, B. J., Kranzler, H. R., Ball, S., Tennen, H., Poling, J., & Triffleman, E. (1998). Personality disorders in substance abusers: Relation to substance use. *Journal of Nervous and Mental Disease, 186*(2), 87–95.

Saunders, J. B., Kypri, K., Walters, S. T., Laforge, R. G., & Larimer, M. E. (2004). Approaches to brief interventions for hazardous drinking in young people. *Alcoholism: Clinical and Experimental Research, 28*(2), 322–329.

Seth, P., Cheeta, S., Tucci, S., & File, S. E. (2002). Nicotinic—Serotonergic interactions in brain and behaviour. *Pharmacology and Biochemistry of Behaviour, 71*(4), 795–805.

Sobell, L. C., & Sobell, M. B. (1992). Timeline followback: A technique for assessing self-reported alcohol consumption. In R. Z. Litten & J. Allen (Eds.), *Measuring alcohol consumption: Psychosocial and biological methods* (pp. 41–72). New Jersey: Humana Press.

Sobell, M. B., & Sobell, L. C. (2005). Guided self-change model of treatment for substance use disorders. *Journal of Cognitive Psychotherapy: An International Quarterly, 19*(3), 199–210.

Stocker, S. (1999). Studies link stress and drug addiction. *NIDA Notes, 14*(1). Retrieved December, 10, 2005, from *www.drugabuse.gov/NIDA_Notes/NNVol14N1/Stress.html*

Storie, M. (Ed.). (2005). *The basics of addiction counseling: Desk reference and study guide.* Alexandria, VA: NAADAC, the Association for Addiction Professionals.

Substance Abuse and Mental Health Services Administration. (2003). *Drug Abuse Warning Network, 2003: Area profiles of drug related mortality* (DAWN Series D-27; DHHS Publication No. (SMA) 05-4023). Rockville, MD: Author.

Vlahov, D., Galea, S., Ahern, J., Resnick, H., Boscarino, J. A., Gold, J., et al. (2004). Consumption of cigarettes, alcohol, and marijuana among New York City residents six months after the September 11 terrorist attacks. *American Journal of Drug and Alcohol Misuse, 30*(2), 385–407.

Volkow, N. (2005). *Message from the Director: The effects of stress on drug abuse.* Retrieved December, 15, 2005, from *www.drug abuse.gov/about/welcome/MessageStress905.html*

Waller, P. F., Hill, E. M., Maio, R. F., & Blow, F. C. (2003). Alcohol effects on motor vehicle crash injury. *Alcoholism: Clinical and Experimental Research, 27*(4), 695–704.

SUGGESTED READINGS

Barry, K. L. (1999). *Brief interventions and brief therapies for substance abuse. A treatment improvement protocol (TIP) Series #34.*

Rockville, MD: U.S. Department of Health and Human Services, Substance Abuse and Mental Health Services Administration Center for Substance Abuse Treatment.

Beck, A., Wright, F., Newman, C. & Leise, B. (1993). *Cognitive therapy of substance abuse.* New York: Guilford Press.

Carroll, K. (1998, April). *A cognitive behavioral approach: Treating cocaine addiction, Manual 1 of therapies for treating drug addiction* (NIH Publication No. 98-4308). Washington, DC: National Institute on Drug Abuse.

Miller, W., & Rollnick, S. (2002). *Motivational Interviewing* (2nd ed.): Preparing people for change. New York: Guilford Press.

O'Farrell, T., & Fals-Stewart, W. (2006). *Behavioral couples therapy for alcoholism and drug abuse.* New York: Guilford Press.

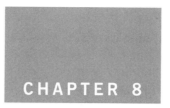

CHAPTER 8

Crisis with Medical Patients

Frank M. Dattilio
Elizabeth A. Davis
Robert M. Goisman

*I*n the previous editions of the book, the chapters on medical crisis addressed medical patients who experienced crisis with psychiatric illnesses (DiTomasso & Kovnat, 1994; DiTomasso, Martin, & Kovnat, 2000). Although this is a common problem, which reportedly exists in primary care settings (Marsland, Wood, & Mayo, 1976; Robinson, 1998), many medical conditions cause a crisis legitimately without the presence of a psychiatric component. Medical illnesses actually contribute to stress-related mental health disorders that occur subsequent to the original medical illness. Therefore, crises that surround medical illness can exist with or without a psychiatric component.

This chapter focuses on the use of cognitive-behavioral strategies with patients who maintain a diagnosable physical illness that in turn contributes to subsequent mental stress reaction or illness. In addition, the issue of those with primary psychiatric diagnoses also carrying a physical diagnosis is addressed.

Even though a medical illness in and of itself does not necessarily constitute a crisis in general, it may contribute to the exacerbation of symptoms, or the environmental surroundings that contribute to a crisis situation, depending on the course and severity of the illness. The manner in which an individual who is afflicted with a medical illness responds to it usually makes the difference in a crisis state. Sometimes, depending on the circumstances, surrounding issues regarding a particular medical illness may exacerbate the normal amount of stress that accompanies the illness in and of itself.

A perfect example is the case of Bob, who developed cancer. This condition by itself would be a stressor, but the mere fact that Bob's cancer was one that is so unusual for a male caused additional stress for Bob, particularly when he proceeded to explain his illness to others. Bob discovered a painful lump in his breast and underwent a mammogram and a subsequent biopsy. He was subsequently diagnosed with stage 2 breast cancer. The American Cancer Society estimates that nearly 270,000 cases of breast cancer are diagnosed each year, but fewer than 1%, or only 1,690 of them, involve males. Such a low incidence makes male breast cancer one of the rarest cancers in the country. It also explains the generally low level of public awareness about the illness. Bob stated that the most awkward thing for him was when he explained to people that he had breast cancer. More than half of the males would say, "Yeah, right!" or "I didn't know men could get that. Does that mean you'll have a mastectomy?" Most people were in shock, particularly the women with whom Bob shared this news. Bob also struggled with feeling "odd," due to the unusual affliction. He often struggled with the atypical reaction that most individuals had to his statements, which somewhat detracted from the normal course of condolence or support that others typically offer. This situation put Bob in somewhat of a crisis, particularly because he had to deal with the social aspect of the rarity of his cancer, as well as the fact that he faced dealing with a malignancy that could very well threaten his life.

Most medical crises typically involve the psychological and emotional aspects that surround the medical affliction. For example, individuals who struggle with a sense of insecurity and loss of control prior to their illness may find that this matter is exacerbated once they learn of their physical fate. The issue of one's sense of security and control is probably one of the most primary areas of concern found among those who are experiencing a medical crisis (Eppersen-Sebour, 1990; Parad & Parad, 1990). Further, Feinstein and Carey (1999) discuss the issues of "reality stressors," which center around patients with health problems and the effect it can have on their job, marital status, family, and even financial situation. Coping mechanisms and coping skills for life-threatening illnesses are usually not tested until the individual is afflicted. It would be fair to say that the majority of individuals who experience medical crisis never prepared themselves for the impact of such a condition, particularly when that condition affects their ability to function and/or immobilization. Such conditions serve as personal threats to one's sense of stability and control and wreak havoc with their family and their daily functioning by creating psychological turmoil and physical restriction. Much of the professional literature in the past has focused on the crippling effect of a medical condition on an individual's ability to cope and how being overwhelmed can greatly contribute to the individual's physical and mental deterioration (Dohrenwend & Dohrenwend, 1982; Taylor, 1986).

The addition of psychological counseling in the treatment of patients with a medical illness has been addressed heavily in the professional literature (Feldman & Christensen, 2003; Roberts, Kiselica, & Fredrickson, 2002; Williams, Pollin, & Koocher, 1999). For the cognitive-behavioral therapist, techniques and interventions that address cognition, emotion, and behavior are paramount to aiding the individual suffering from the medical crisis and in dealing with the situation in the most appropriate manner possible. The role of dysfunctional beliefs and attitudes that are often based on misinterpretation of the severity of the situation may clearly contribute to a crisis state. There is a denial, or naivete, that individuals sometimes maintain that "such an illness will never happen to me." This renders them particularly vulnerable because they never prepare for the coping mechanisms involved and what they would need to do at the point that they might be assigned such a diagnosis. The fact of the matter is that physical illnesses are very much a part of life and no one is immune to serious illness. A fine example of this is outlined by DiTomasso and Mills (1990), who address the failure that individuals engage in to seek follow-up after diagnosis of a disease and noncompliance with treatment recommendations. The authors go on to discuss how these factors contribute greatly to crisis in medical patients. Denial is often a common defense mechanism for most people receiving a diagnosis of a serious medical illness. Denial can often serve to exacerbate a crisis situation further down the line. Medical conditions that are ignored often develop into serious pathology and precipitate crises that might have been averted in many instances (DiTomasso et al., 2000). Kahana, Kahana, Harel, and Rosner (1988) emphasized that all the self-defining constructs and coping skills that an individual has developed over a lifetime will often be seriously challenged upon being diagnosed and possibly cause them to be overwhelmed in the face of a medical crisis.

Furthermore, researchers indicate that a strong relationship between cognitions, affect, and behavior, and how well people weather illness and health problems contributes greatly to how they deal with a crisis at hand. This issue has been given increasing attention in the medical and psychological literature (Baum & Posluszny, 1999). These researchers suggest that the perception of a medical illness may precipitate a crisis that, in turn, may exacerbate the original medical condition. As a consequence of the medical condition at hand, a crisis may complicate and undermine a recovery by creating a vicious cycle for the patient, even long after the patient recovered from his/her illness. This is particularly so when a person is recovering from a serious medical illness in which many of the symptoms overlap with symptoms of anxiety and stress (Dattilio & Castaldo, 2001; Dattilio, 2001). A prime example of this is Bert, the individual presented below, who experienced a heart attack but subsequently developed anxiety and panic over the affliction and continuously experienced false alarms that frequently landed him in the emergency room. Because Bert was unable to attend adequately to the anxiety and the stress produced by his fear of having another heart attack, he eventually ended up experiencing a subsequent infarction.

Bert, a 55-year-old actuary, was driving home from work when he experienced a sudden increase in heart rate, along with difficulty breathing. Thinking that perhaps he needed some fresh air, he began to roll down the window and, as he did, his symptoms spontaneously worsened. He then experienced a hot flash that emanated through his body like an electrical shock. As this occurred, he began to sweat profusely and experienced a tingling sensation in his hands and his forearms. These symptoms caused him to immediately recall a previous experience that he had had when he suffered a heart attack approximately 1½ years earlier while playing tennis with his wife.

Bert's immediate thought was, "Oh, God, I'm having another heart attack. This one's going to kill me." As the symptoms escalated, Bert became increasingly distressed and was unable to concentrate due to being overwhelmed by his condition. He decided to drive directly to the local hospital and went directly to the emergency room, where he received immediate attention after alerting the attendants about what he was experiencing.

The emergency room physicians performed an arterial blood gas determination, along with an electrocardiogram. Both tests yielded results that were negative for a myocardial infarction. After careful observation and a consultation with a hospital cardiologist, it was determined that Bert had experienced a panic attack. Even though he was still quite shaken, he was initially relieved, although this event recurred six or seven times throughout the subsequent year. Much of what Bert struggled with was being able to differentiate between panic attacks and heart attacks because they were so similar in nature. Unfortunately, Bert never consulted a psychologist or psychiatrist for his condition and kept "slugging it out," as he put it. This, unfortunately, led to a subsequent heart attack in which he was later convinced that he had heart disease and was hospitalized. It was only at this point that a psychiatric consult was ordered and Bert was informed that he had likely driven himself to a second heart attack by overreacting to his anxiety and panic symptoms. Bert then decided to seek mental health treatment for himself and learned to manage his stress more effectively.

As in the brief aforementioned example, intense levels of stress often may further exacerbate an existing illness, which may further compromise an individual's ability to cope. The issue of psychological components has been studied more recently, particularly focusing on the use of interventions (Rose, 1991). Therefore, early intervention with patients in crisis, as in the case cited here, usually equals the best results. However, this situation is difficult because many medical patients are usually in a tailspin and, on learning of their diagnosis, are not always receptive to mental health treatment during the initial phase of their illness (Gilliland & James, 1997). The afflicted patient may be more physically and psychologically healthy earlier in the phase and, therefore, may be able to collaborate in implementing a coping style for dealing with his/her illness. Early treatment intervention may also help to preclude the formation of negative cognitions regarding the treatment outcome (DiTomasso et al., 2000). These authors mention a "cognitive set," which is formed by repeated failures on the part of the patient afflicted in attempting to cope with his/her illness. Sometimes, patients who experience such failures may undermine their own beliefs about the realistic likelihood of a positive outcome, forcing them into a downward spiral. Therefore, the notion of an early intervention may optimally offer assessment, or serve as a prophylaxis, and offset the potential difficulty of psychological exacerbation. The use of cognitive-behavioral strategies or techniques such as cognitive restructuring and behavioral control have been found to be effective in short-term intervention approaches to helping individuals deal with crisis (Parad & Parad, 1990; Dattilio, 2001).

To do this, however, one must first understand the causes of crises and how they typically ensue in a medical crisis situation. There is likely a sequence of events that occur with medical crises that contribute to the full blossoming of the psychological crisis. Feinstein and Carey (1999) discuss the special meaning that a crisis holds for individual patients, and how that crisis is crucial in driving the patient's reaction to a full-blown trauma. Therefore, the areas that must be addressed and considered are precipitating events, cognitions, emotions, behaviors, and the impact of the physical symptoms on the patient.

PRECIPITATING EVENTS

Precipitating events may be both emotional and physical. Therefore, one has to examine the surrounding emotional events and psychological factors that coexist with any physical symptoms contributing to the crisis. Certainly, the combined effects of any of these are also important factors. What is particularly important, and is addressed later, is how individuals interpret those events and the schemata that surround the particular event. Therefore, if an individual has been under a certain amount of stress with regard to family problems, or work-related issues, and subsequently experiences symptoms that are either cardiovascular or neurological, they may easily connect the two and develop the schema that one caused the other. They could also develop the schema that the two are unrelated but are simply co-occurring.

COGNITIONS

Cognitions are probably one of the most important factors affecting the escalation of crisis in medical patients. Many of the cognitions include negative attitudes, assumptions, maladaptive beliefs, cognitive distortions, distorted use of information, and misinterpretation.

Maladaptive Assumptions

These are distorted assumptions or beliefs that may activate underlying schemata previously learned by an individual. This may have a powerful effect on the escalation of catastrophic thoughts, unleashing a cascade of emotion and behavior. An example would be, "Any pain or medical illness will absolutely lead to a serious condition." This could easily influence an individual's reaction to the news of medical problems and/or the progression of the medical problem, and affect the manner in which the individual adjusts to it. This typically goes hand in hand with insufficient information. This concept supports the old adage: "A little information can be a dangerous thing." Not having all the facts can be very harmful and patients are often encouraged to wait until they have all the information before deciding how to react.

Cognitive Distortions

These are distorted beliefs about one's health that can easily affect the perception of an event or worsen the implications of the perceived event, depending on the circumstances. Patients who catastrophize about the meaning of a diagnosed medical problem might be expected to react in a more extreme manner, contributing to further cognitive distortions. An example of this might be assuming that the early development of symptoms of diabetes necessarily means that an individual will immediately suffer from permanent blindness or the loss of a limb.

Insufficient Information

Often, a patient's lack of information about a particular medical condition greatly contributes to his/her distress, particularly because the patient may have a tendency to "fill in the gaps" and make matters worse when it is not necessary. Even some negative fantasies and distortions may run wild, which can contribute to reducing the individual's ability to cope. The lack of information is a vital issue, particularly as it relates to early cognitive theory and the discussion of thoughts based on erroneous information. Nowhere does this ring more true than with physical illness.

BEHAVIORS

Certainly, the behavior of a patient greatly contributes to the course of a crisis and how this may exacerbate a medical condition. There are several factors that are contained in the behavioral component that should be considered.

Poor Coping Strategies

This is often indicated by impulsive behaviors, jumping to conclusions, and overreacting. Individuals need to attempt to remain calm until they have all the information and final test results of their illness. Learning to cope by taking it one step at a time is vitally important to dealing with any subsequent disposition.

Insufficient Social and Family Support

Support networks are essential, particularly when first receiving news of the medical condition. Individuals who do not have such support tend to feel isolated and are left to deal with the situation by themselves. This loneliness, in fact, may also contribute to depression and escalation of cognitions and catastrophization, particularly because they do not have the support network to help "anchor" them, or ground them in reality, and remind them to keep things intact and not blow them out of proportion. Individuals who are stricken with a medical illness are more likely to recover and to weather any crisis surrounding their illness as opposed to those individuals without family support.

TREATMENT STRATEGIES

There are a number of cognitive therapy strategies that are designed specifically to aid patients in testing the reality of their cognitions. These strategies can be classified as either cognitive or behavioral in approach, but some overlap may occur.

Cognitive Techniques

Downward Arrow

This term, first coined by Beck et al. (1979), is phrased because of its actual use of downward-pointing arrows to aid clients in understanding the logic and sequencing of their reasoning. The therapist follows a client's statement by asking, "If so, then what?" This elicits a sequence of thoughts and beliefs, which aids in uncovering the client's underlying assumptions.

Idiosyncratic Meaning

This is the process of clarifying a statement made by the client so that the therapist may have a high level of understanding of the client's perceived grasp of reality.

Labeling of Distortions

By labeling distortions, clients are able to identify automatically any dysfunctional thoughts and monitor their cognitive patterns. Through this type of monitoring a more accurate route toward change occurs. For a more detailed description, see Burns (1980, 1989).

Questioning the Evidence

Once the patient learns to question the actual evidence, the process of substantiation is initiated and becomes an automatic procedure following any irrational thought statement. This process allows clients to decide whether their statements are based on erroneous information.

Examining Options and Alternatives

This entails going back over all the possible options and alternatives that exist in attempts to avoid the trap of seeing "no way out" of a circumstance or situation. The specific task is to work until the individual is generating new options.

Reattribution

Placing all the blame on oneself is a common occurrence observed with patients, particularly in the guilt-ridden or depressed cases. Reattribution merely involves the individual appropriately distributing responsibility to the rightful parties and dispelling the notion that any single individual is responsible for everything.

Decatastrophizing

Patients who engage in catastrophic thinking tend to focus on the most extreme negative outcome of any given situation. Decatastrophizing involves aiding these individuals in balancing out their focus on the worst anticipated state by reestimating the situation and asking, "So what's the worst thing that might occur? And if so, would this be so horrible?"

Advantages and Disadvantages

In attempts to have patients sway from dichotomous thought patterns, instructing them to list advantages and disadvantages of a situation allows them to change their perspective and balance out the alternatives.

Paradox or Exaggeration

This technique may be viewed as the inverse of decatastrophizing. It involves the therapist taking an issue or idea to the extreme for the patient, allowing the latter to view the absurdity of an overinflated viewpoint. This often aids the patient in developing a more balanced perspective on the issue.

Turning Adversity to Advantage

Taking an unfortunate situation and using it as an advantage can be very helpful. For example, being rejected by the school of one's choice may be an indirect route toward a more promising alternative.

Replacement Imagery

Freeman (1986) describes a more detailed account of how this is used. In essence, the fact that many individuals experience negative dreams and images does indicate that the power of imagery is strong. Patients can therefore be helped to change the direction of those dreams and images to positive, more successful coping scenes.

Behavioral Techniques

While the mechanics involved with cognitive-behavioral therapy involve the primary use of cognitive techniques such as those stated earlier, behavioral techniques are also used as supportive measures and as means for collecting information in facilitating change. The following behavioral techniques are the ones most frequently used in a cognitive-behavioral approach.

Assertiveness Training

A large component of assertiveness training involves both cognitive processes and behavioral practice. The latter, in essence, consists of the therapist teaching or modeling for the patient desired behaviors in social situations. This is used particularly often for anxiety disorders such as social phobia or agoraphobia. The term *in vivo* is used to indicate that the behaviors are acted out in real life.

Behavioral Rehearsal

This is the behavioral counterpart to cognitive rehearsal. The difference lies with the behaviors themselves being the subjects rehearsed (e.g., asserting oneself in public or getting up and going to work). Feedback from the therapist to the patient is then given as a means of guidance and development of effective responses and styles. This also involves the reinforcement of existing skills.

Graded Task Assignments

This is the process of establishing a hierarchy of events that involve the target behaviors, whether approaching a parent or overcoming a fear of meeting new people. The specific tasks are arranged in steps from least anxiety producing or threatening to most anxiety producing. This allows for a gradual approach to facing the threatening object/event.

Bibliotherapy

The prescription of reading assignments has always been a strong characteristic of cognitive therapy. Readings frequently assigned to patients are books designed for the general public, such as *Feeling Good* or the *Feeling Good Handbook* (Burns, 1980, 1989), *Cognitive Therapy and the Emotional Disorders* (Beck, 1976), *Own Your Own Life* (Emery, 1984), *Talk Sense to Yourself* (McMullin & Casey, 1975), *Woulda, Coulda, Shoulda* (Freeman & DeWolf, 1990), and *The Worry Cure* (Leahy, 2006). These readings are assigned as an adjunct to therapy to serve as supportive and educational tools to augment the therapeutic process.

Relaxation and Meditation

The use of programs including progressive muscle relaxation, meditation, and focused breathing has proven to be helpful to anxiety patients in learning to distract themselves and gain control over their anxiety.

Overbreathing and the encouragement of hyperventilation are effective techniques for helping patients learn that they can master breathing control and regulate anxiety symptoms.

Social Skills Training

This involves reviewing and instructing the patient in behaviors that are necessary for social interaction (e.g., maintaining conversations with others, posture, eye contact, and assertiveness skills; in addition, developing techniques for self-expression and conveying individual thoughts and opinions).

Homework

One of the most important features of cognitive-behavioral therapy is the use of homework assignments (Kazantzis, MacEwan, & Dattilio, 2005). Because the actual therapy sessions are limited to only 1 or 2 hours per week in the office, it is imperative that activities in support of the treatment continue outside the sessions. The emphasis is placed on self-help assignments that serve as a continuation of what was addressed in the preceding session. This is also an integral part of the collaborative process between the patient and the therapist. Assignments typically include those techniques listed above. The assignments are tailored to the specific problem and are a result of the collaborative process that occurs during the process of treatment.

Cognitive-Behavioral Strategies for Intervening with Medical Crisis

The cognitive-behavioral approach to treatment is ideal for addressing situations in crises, particularly those with medical crises (Kaupp, Rapoport-Hubschman, & Spiegel, 2005). The fact that CBT is a collaborative and empirical approach also rests its premise on evidence-based efforts to address the problem at hand. In many respects, this is exactly "what the doctor ordered" in that it helps provide individuals with some sense of structure and an organized paradigm to follow in dealing with crisis situations, particularly with regard to medical situations. The aspect of the psychoeducational component is ideal for understanding the complete essence of the medical condition, as well as how the individual is responding to the medical crisis. CBT has a variety of techniques for addressing crisis and helping individuals work through their particular issue (Edelman & Kidman, 1999). Some of the techniques were mentioned earlier in this chapter.

In general, of course, the better the patient's adaptation before an emergency, the better the patient will fare in an acute crisis. Many of the interventions discussed herein are most useful if practiced long before a crisis occurs (i.e., as part of daily management of chronic illness or as part of ongoing CBT). These interventions, if learned in a more relaxed setting when the patient is not in crisis, will be much more easily applied than those which the patient is attempting to use for the first time when an adverse medical event has already occurred.

Regarding these adaptation strategies, one general class of interventions is the area of stress management. There is ample literature addressing the use of relaxation methods as a general approach to living with chronic illness, pain, or even insomnia (Benson, 1975; National Institutes of Health, 1995). These methods include not only the traditional progressive muscle relaxation but also meditation, self-hypnosis, some martial arts techniques, and other allied interventions (Christensen & Boone, 2003). In addition to being of specific benefit for those disorders in which anxiety plays a significant role, patients who practice these methods daily often report an increased sense of well-being. Similarly, assessment of one's lifestyle regarding nicotine, alcohol, caffeine, exercise, and so on may lead to an increased sense of wellness.

Another general class of interventions includes cognitive restructuring methods. Typical cognitions in chronic illness can include "I can't cope," "I am a failure," "I should be doing more," and so on (Moorey 1996, p. 458). While it must be recognized by providers as well as by patients that some illnesses do confer realistic limitations, it is also the case that cognitive restructuring may be useful to correct exaggerated or overly defeatist responses. Standard cognitive techniques such as evidence gathering and hypothesis testing, automatic thought recording, and analysis of patterns of distortions may lead to significant relief. These methods are also useful in chronic pain, even during an acute exacerbation (Smith & Beers, 2003).

A third class of interventions regards decreasing medication noncompliance. Approximately 40% of patients do not follow treatments recommended during medical visits (DiMatteo, 2003), so it is reasonable to estimate that a significant percentage of acute medical crises are caused or exacerbated by patients not adhering properly to treatment regimens. Here also, cognitive restructuring may be useful, in this case by tracking one's thoughts about taking medications. Such cognitions may include "People who take medications are weak," "I'll get dependent on the drug," and so on (Wright, Basco, & Thase, 2006, pp. 217–218); these cognitions can be addressed by the same methods described above. Behavioral methods such as associating medication-taking with other more routine, high-frequency behaviors (e.g., brushing one's teeth) may also be useful (DiMatteo, 2003). Finally, addressing the pros and cons of medication compliance versus noncompliance may also help.

A fourth series of interventions centers on assessment and management of substance abuse. There is extensive literature on the assessment of readiness for change (Prochaska & DiClemente, 1992; Miller & Rollnick, 1991), and clinicians are advised to use these or other methods before attempting to take too definitive a stance on this issue with their patients, lest the patient–clinician relationship be jeopardized or terminated altogether. Yet, there is little doubt of the ubiquity of substance abuse in the average ambulatory care practice (Clark, 2003), so that practitioners cannot indefinitely avoid bringing this issue to their patients' attention on the grounds that "the time is not right yet." The onset of a medical crisis may trigger an acute episode of substance use, or conversely acute or chronic substance abuse or withdrawal may lead to a medical emergency (Clark, 2003). Interventions can include lifestyle changes, psychoeducation, motivational interviewing as a treatment, 12-step programs, cognitive restructuring (Beck, Wright, Newman, & Liese, 1993), and contingency contracting.

As described above, all these methods are best taught and applied *in advance* of a crisis. Learning new behaviors and coping skills is not best done under conditions of maximum arousal and anxiety, so that the patient who is skillful at using relaxation methods and cognitive disputation under everyday circumstances will have a tremendous advantage if in a crisis over the patient trying to use progressive muscle relaxation for the first time while experiencing crushing chest pain radiating down the left arm. Similarly, ongoing attention to substance use issues will decrease the need for the practitioner to consider detoxification as well as acute medical intervention for the patient in medical crisis.

If, however, there has been no opportunity (or patient motivation) to utilize any of these strategies first, the clinician still may be able to help the patient decrease the acute burden of illness posed by a medical crisis. For example, breathing retraining (Dattilio, 2001) is useful in acute panic, and the clinician may be able to "talk a patient down" if the patient is hyperventilating due to anxiety while acutely medically ill. Similarly, the use of guided imagery or visualization (Christensen, 2003. Orme-Johnson, Walton, & Lonsdorf, 1995) with the patient may counteract terrifying images which the patient may be having. Psychoeducation in the broad sense (i.e., careful, step-by-step explanation of what is transpiring) may also decrease the likelihood that the patient will misunderstand and exaggerate the dangerousness of diagnostic or treatment procedures. Finally, careful assessment of acute substance intake may decrease the likelihood of prolongation of a medical inpatient stay due to complications of substance abuse.

Following is a full-length case that illustrates the use of cognitive-behavioral techniques with a complicated example of medical/psychiatric crisis.

CASE STUDY

Katerina is a 55-year-old German-born woman with a history of multiple hospitalizations for psychotic depression. Katerina has been followed for the past 5 years on a weekly basis for psychotherapy and medication management. She is treated at a public teaching clinic where resident psychiatrists rotate during their training. Katerina's mother was reportedly a member of Hitler's Youth Group. Her Ukrainian father served in the Polish Army during the Occupation. Katerina was placed in foster care at age 3 after her parents divorced and remained there until age 8, at which point her father retrieved her and relocated to the United States. Unfortunately, Katerina would never see her mother again despite multiple efforts to do so.

Katerina's sexual abuse by her father began immediately upon her arrival in the United States. Although "fondling" would continue throughout her adult life, this abuse, which included oral and digital genital stimulation not leading to intercourse, was more systematic in her prepubertal years. Showing appropriate assertiveness and feeling as though she "had nothing to lose," she began threatening her father with "alerting the authorities" even at the risk of "being shoved and struck with a belt." Based on her experience of separation from family, life in an impoverished, war-torn German town with abusive foster parents, the commonplace presence of weapons in the household, and her father's unpredictable advances, she began carrying a knife in response to a core belief of helplessness in a world that contained unpredictable threats. Her father's stated desire that he wished she was a boy led also to a core belief of basic defectiveness.

Katerina completed high school in a parochial institution in good standing. She was unable to complete college-level classes due to her core belief of worthlessness, which led her to put her father's needs and wishes before her own. Feeling she could not measure up to his expectations for her as both a student and a financial contributor to the household, she adopted dichotomous thinking, whereby she was overcome by a sense of failure that she had not met certain exceptional goals, thus she could not gain independence. Consequently, Katerina became employed as an IBM punchcard clerk for a large insurance company for the next 17 years and ceased further striving for advancement.

In her early 20s she began to suffer depression and anxiety as she grappled with the frustrations of failed attempts to reunite with her mother and complex identity problems. She wore masculine clothing, some of which were borrowed from her father, and she used an alias when socializing with gay women. Subsequently, seeking out relief and clarification, she joined "Recovery, Inc.," an early form of CBT emphasizing "will training" for "nervous minds" started by Low (1950) in the early 20th century.

Meanwhile, despite her efforts, Katerina would experience increasing sadness, irritability, sleep problems, and decreasing productivity at work. After multiple relationships with women and men throughout her 20s, she felt disappointed in both. Also, realizing she had no professional future, she believed she was a great financial burden to her father. She became angry with the church as she realized she would be expected to deny her sexual orientation and would have to lie during confession about her quest to seek comfort and sexual companionship with women as well as men. These feeling of alienation only confirmed her core belief of basic defectiveness.

These identity problems and the continuing sexual abuse set the stage for Katerina's first hospitalization for psychosis and suicidal ideation at age 37. Additional precipitants of her psychosis included being informed by the German government of her mother's death, her father's failing health, and an unexpected visit by her sister whom she had not seen for more than 40 years. Over the next 18 years there were three additional hospitalizations for relapsing psychosis. Each episode was characterized by paranoia involving a meddling government agency—that the U.S. government was monitoring her telephone calls, or the Internal Revenue Service (IRS) was somehow after her. During one episode, she left home abruptly without a coat or shoes despite cold weather after an altercation with her father. She walked for miles feeling confused and afraid before asking a bystander to call 911 on her behalf.

In 2005 Katerina's father began to suffer complications of diabetes, including multiple strokes, seizures, and renal failure. Katerina, now 54 years old, avoided calling an ambulance, even when her father would fall or lose consciousness, fearing she may dishonor his lifelong wish to avoid medical involvement (which he saw as a personal encroachment) and incur medical costs. She finally was compelled to recruit her tenant to help pick his 200-pound 5'4" frame off the floor and seek medical intervention. The risk of making her father angry and disappointed overwhelmed her common sense for making a necessary intervention, thus perpetuating her core belief of helplessness and ineffectiveness.

After hospitalization and brief rehabilitation, her father was sent home with little services—the little he did get would soon be discontinued after he refused basic care and frightened visiting nurses with abusive comments. He would spend a few more months thereafter at home unbathed, incontinent, and unclothed from the waist down. Although he had given many indications that he had become demented and was completely unable to care for himself, Katerina would continue to see her father as threatening, willfully stubborn, and powerful. His belligerence, likely a symptom of delirium, would instead be viewed by his daughter as the characteristic protests of a fiercely individualistic and resourceful man.

Katerina's fortune telling and other distortions were addressed in therapy. The therapist explored the cognitive distortion that Katerina expected her father to get angry with her and ultimately blame her for "incurring large ambulance bills," such that this presumed outcome was far more intolerable than the risk of losing him altogether to catastrophic illness. A severity assessment was made with the patient, whereby the possible outcomes of her actions and beliefs were elucidated. First, she believed her father would physically attack her in his effort to maintain his independence. She imagined that he would feel that she had dishonored him by ignoring his wishes to avoid medical interventions. She also wondered if she appeared somehow duplicitous by trying to get rid of him in order to satisfy some selfish need. As if caught in between a rock and a hard place, she imagined he thought she was unable to care adequately for him or the household as any other adult would, and thus could never care for herself once he died.

Despite some risk that she might feel criticized or flee treatment, a probability assessment was performed looking at how likely a terrible outcome would be. The likelihood of his hurting her physically given his profound weakness was addressed in an effort to reassure her that she was safer than she was as a child. Given his seemingly obvious confused state, the therapist challenged Katerina's certainty regarding his ability to have such complex thoughts about her at the time he collapsed. These efforts to reframe her automatic thoughts set the stage for her gradual acceptance that she was not entirely helpless and that she would have some control over ascertaining her own limits in caring for her father.

As her father became increasingly ill, Katerina reported in one of her routine visits that she had experienced postmenopausal vaginal bleeding, prompting her primary care physician to refer her for an urgent pelvic ultrasound. According to Katerina, the ultrasound revealed fibrosis in the lower quadrant that obscured her ovary, raising concern for cancer. Katerina, however, became preoccupied with incidental gallstones. She began to "prepare" herself for the presumably necessary gallbladder surgery by reading a book on surgery; she also considered visiting an alternative medicine specialist for "hair analysis" and a holistic nutritionist to receive "specific recommendations."

This was an escape behavior, but as it did not interfere with necessary medical care, the therapist elected not to confront the patient on this matter. At this point multiple conflicting demands required prioritization. Katerina gave many indications of her underlying distress. A common cold with sore throat gave rise to catastrophic thinking as evidence for the "cancer spreading." Defiantly she stated that she would never relinquish her ovary or uterus because these were critical to her "being" a woman—a view that seemed consistent both with her father's libertarian, do-not-violate-me views and her own attempts to preserve her sense of self. She also bemoaned the unfairness of contracting cancer of the uterus, as she "was not promiscuous, never married, and bore no children."

Katerina became focused on the various tests and procedures that she was expected to endure in order to make a diagnosis. She made an appointment to visit a gynecological oncologist for further evaluation. This inevitable pelvic exam, she admitted, would be difficult, especially because the gynecologist was unfamiliar to her. She and the therapist reviewed her automatic thoughts around these expectations—she complained that she was inexperienced with such exams, as if this was another task she might fail, and she anticipated the actual speculum would be painful in the way she often found intercourse to be. She assumed no one would care about her feelings or physical comfort during the exam. An attempt was made to refocus her beliefs using a probability assessment, first asking her to comment on her past experience as an indicator of what would happen now. What became evident was that she more often than not had succeeded in the exam with her trustworthy primary care physician (PCP). She kept her appointment and later reported having undergone a painful endometrial biopsy successfully, the results of which were unremarkable, and found the unexpected presence of a reassuring resident helpful. She stated that her workup had at this point been completed.

Meanwhile, Katerina continued to wonder about the fate of her gallstones. When asked, "What do the gallstones mean to you? . . . What might be the consequence of having them?", she replied concretely, "They are the reason for the occasional nausea and reflux I have had over the years." These questions were intended by the therapist to elicit automatic thoughts associated with this seemingly lesser somatic preoccupation. However, the patient's response suggested that the gallstones served as a distraction from her worry that she was going to be either killed or stripped of her identity, thus confirming her core belief of defectiveness and worthlessness.

Katerina's PCP was contacted to clarify the patient's reports of her alarming symptoms, the apparent incompleteness of her workup, and the seemingly minimal management of the "obscured ovary." The PCP revealed that it was not clear when the vaginal bleeding actually occurred, despite Katerina's claims of immediacy. In fact, according to the PCP, Katerina had "waited months" to address the bleeding. The ovary was indeed visualized on the ultrasound, but it demonstrated some ambiguous, "irregular" contours that were most likely benign. Even though Katerina's physicians were not worried, this condition raised concern in her mind. She continued to await the "silent killer," as if to overregister the possibility that she had cancer. As with the gallstones, she demonstrated selective attention and her tendency toward maximization and minimization persisted as part of her overall catastrophic outlook. She acknowledged the therapist's inquiry into why she was not reassured by the negative test results with a response more characteristic of her father's mistrust in the medical establishment. She also reflected on her own core belief that something was amiss and that this health scare may have been a beacon for her sense of inadequacy and helplessness.

Following this crisis, Katerina's father collapsed at a bank. He required cardiac resuscitation and emergent dialysis. He had explicitly declined dialysis in the preceding months. Because his affairs were not in order, Katerina was forced to make decisions on behalf of her father that left her second-guessing her intentions to keep him alive. After he was transferred from the intensive care unit (ICU) to a nursing facility, Katerina was faced with a likely permanent separation for the first time since her childhood. Guilty, she began to feel responsible for her father's new-onset facial droop and complete aphasia and attributed these to having signed consent for the placement of a central line in his neck and the endotracheal tube; these automatic thoughts of "I must take responsibility" coexisted with her ongoing belief in herself as defective and incompetent. As a likely cerebrovascular event was not described in his discharge summary (although it was acknowledged at the nursing home), Katerina supposed that these procedures must have caused mechanical damage to his vocal cords. At this point the therapist intervened by educating the patient on medical practices and cause and effect in attempt to help her reassess the reality of her associations. Furthermore, she found it difficult to reconcile the inconsistencies of the medical record, an understandable position. This explanation seemed to reassure the patient, as she began to recognize the depth of her father's poor condition and that he had accrued so many years of ill health due to his own personal neglect independent of her decisions.

With her father gone, Katerina became increasingly concerned about her own health. She embarked on a health kick of sorts, monitoring her blood sugar with her father's glucose meter multiple times a day, hoping to avoid the inevitability of developing the disease that would ultimately kill her father. She discussed her dietary changes in detail, as well as the quality of her bowel movements during her therapy. Nonetheless, Katerina faced a sudden setback 2 months after her father's hospitalization.

She called just after Christmas to cancel a therapy appointment, revealing that she had been struck by a car 48 hours prior to calling. Without calling an ambulance or visiting an emergency room, she found that she had to drag herself home after the driver and a witness abandoned her. Despite her intense pain and some nausea, Katerina called her PCP's office, not to schedule an emergency visit but to cancel a routine appointment that had been scheduled because she "had had a bad fall." She declined any offers to be seen by a nurse practitioner in an urgent care visit. This delay in reporting of emergent matters began to surface as a theme in the treatment. She believed that by delaying medical attention, she could avoid showing the world she truly was inadequate in caring for herself, in the event that she had suffered only superficial injuries. Katerina agreed, with prompting from her concerned therapist, to visit an emergency room for orthopedic and neurological evaluation. Again, however, she declined the offer of a taxi and opted to wait another few hours for her tenant to return from work. She was evaluated and diagnosed with a broken arm and a broken foot.

Over the course of phone discussions, Katerina revealed the events of the Christmas night she was struck. She was walking home late at night from her father's nursing home, angry that her father was "hoarding" items in his drawer that "belonged to the nursing home"—his method, according to her, of seeking equality for the money he must now pay the nursing home. She also revealed her ambivalence about visiting at all. She had wanted to go to a local clubhouse instead where she could socialize and eat a prepared meal. However, believing that this was "likely his last Christmas," she chose to visit him.

She claimed she was trying "to beat the light" and noticed a car speeding toward her while she was crossing the intersection. She was knocked down but denied having hit her head. Her first thoughts were "I am going to die" and "my sister is going to inherit our father's money." These automatic thoughts reflected her core belief of basic defectiveness. As if to telepathically broadcast the patient's belief that she was incompetent and stupid, the driver reportedly got out of the car, first to inquire about her status; he then angrily stated, "this was stupid" and drove away, leaving her to get home on her own.

Deeply ashamed of the incident and of her conflicting thoughts, Katerina believed she somehow deserved such an outcome. Thus she decided not to tell anyone about the accident for fear that she would be chastised. Identifying with the driver's statements and then imagining her father's disappointment, the patient did not seek medical care despite acute pain; she assumed the emergency room doctors would also spend time criticizing her rather than evaluating her physically. She feared that if she filled out a police report, she would only be humiliated further by its futility, as she could not (responsibly) remember the details of the accident. Indeed, her PCP would later anger her with pressing inquiries about any intentional self-harm.

Katerina later acknowledged the pluses and minuses about the prospect of her father's return home, despite her worries that the "inheritance" was dwindling and her longing to have him close to her. For convenience, she convalesced on the couch near the dining area where her father once slept, stating concretely, "He will have to wait to come home because I need the couch." She avoided bathing for fear of hurting herself further. She began to document multiple episodes of hypoglycemia and reported her sugars routinely during her phone therapy. She also found herself wanting to return to some sort of formal Christian religion in order to forgive others and to have her father "saved." She began to watch Christian TV shows and sent away for literature. Meanwhile, she began to call "on-call" members of Recovery, Inc., to help her manage her "nervousness" and negative thoughts.

What emerged from her intense loneliness and fear was evidence for an ongoing manic episode, characterized by markedly decreased sleep, irritability, pressured speech, racing thoughts, paranoia, a sense of entitlement, and impulsiveness. Katerina kept a detailed log of each pill she took and blood sugar readings. She attempted correspondence with 50 old acquaintances, writing letters to former friends, family, and fellow patients, spent long hours on the phone, often giving and taking advice and finding herself easily angered and argumentative, thus alienating those whom she wished to draw closer. She became preoccupied with social injustices and perceived slights. She expressed her belief that her phone conversations were being monitored and that she was being cheated out of her pension, her life insurance, and her Medicare benefits, all in support of her having "worked for nothing" while others get free handouts. She became reluctant to exercise her broken limbs. She relied on home health aides to be bathed. She craved contact and requested that her psychiatrist call her daily to help "monitor" her symptoms and "listen."

The focus of treatment was aimed at supporting Katerina emotionally as she faced losing her father and coping with her own health problems, both real and perceived. Her complex of symptoms has also required both pharmacological and behavioral treatment. Her acute mania called for medication changes, namely, increasing the dose of quetiapine, the initiation of valproic acid, and the removal of an antidepressant, in an attempt to target her sleep disturbance, her acute paranoia, her impulsivity, and her racing thoughts. Throughout her treatment, the approach to Katerina's ongoing sleep problems (in addition to trials with sedating medications) was the employment of sleep hygiene techniques, including omitting caffeine and decreasing environmental stimulants before bedtime.

Katerina's paranoia and anxiety about her physical health, as well as her resistance to using new medications, were quite amenable to cognitive techniques. Expressing automatic thoughts, especially fortune telling and catastrophizing, Katerina has been convinced that certain adversities would eventuate. For example, regarding medication changes, she assumed that certain side effects belonging to one medication would occur with another, regardless of whether or not she had ever experienced such adverse effects. These misappropriations were attenuated using psychoeducation, as well as hypothesis testing and realistic appraisal.

A similar approach was taken when helping Katerina cope with confrontations she was having during her manic episode. Initially she was encouraged to use time delay and distraction—methods consistent with the self-soothing slogans employed by Recovery, Inc. Eventually, through use of the Socratic method and hypothesis testing, Katerina's expectations were addressed and she could determine alternative methods to having her needs met by others. First, her therapist would ask her what she was hoping for by interacting with a particular person, usually her sister who lived across the country or her ex-boyfriend who was also a fellow patient and had been helping her with chores. These expectations would then be reframed based on the history of the given relationship and the other party's limitations in terms of understanding Katerina's situation. As she began to see the discrepancies, Katerina was better able to distance herself from the interactions and either use time delay or rely on professional help for accomplishing certain tasks. Eventually, as her medications took effect and she gained mobility, she found herself feeling less driven by urgency and impulsivity.

In addition to utilizing such Recovery, Inc., statements as, "a nervous person may want approval but does not *need* it" or "the favorite pastime for a nervous person is self-torture," Katerina would also readily call another Recovery, Inc., member for a prescribed 5-minute period to perform an analysis of a situation that had been causing anxiety and distress. These cognitive-behavioral techniques, both self-prescribed and introduced in therapy, have helped Katerina manage her difficult transition as she must face the prospect of living without her father.

Interestingly, Katerina learned a valuable lesson from her father's departure. As a challenge to her cognitive distortions, his improved health and good mood have underscored for her the irreconcilable difference between the care he is requiring in the nursing home and what she would have been able to provide for him at home. As she recovered from the injuries of her car accident and her mania resolved, Katerina had a chance to receive closer monitoring. Together with the therapist, she examined the pros and cons of having her father return home or remain in the nursing home. Therapy helped to clarify her automatic thoughts and core beliefs. For example, feeling less trapped and helpless, she realized the cost to her own health of caring for her ill father.

CONCLUSION

The aforementioned case is an excellent example of how CBT is used with a psychiatric patient struggling with a medical crisis. Cases such as Katrina's are often quite arduous to monitor and may be accompanied by many complications. As stated earlier in this chapter, medical crisis can arise as the result of a preexisting mental illness, or a mental health diagnosis can spawn as a result of a medical illness. Either way, the two make for complications when treating cases such as Katrina. Sufficient medical diagnosis is necessary when treating such cases because of the potential for misdiagnosis and further complication. Therefore, in such situations, the treating mental health professional, if not a physician or medical personnel him/herself, should have access to a physician or medical specialist. As long as this is established through the use of CBT techniques, patients may learn to better manage their crisis so that their overall condition does not exacerbate.

REFERENCES

Baum, A., & Posluszny, D. M. (1999). Health psychology: Mapping biobehavioral contributions to health and illness. *Annual Review of Psychology, 50,* 137–163.

Beck, A. T. (1976). *Cognitive therapy and the emotional disorders.* New York: International Universities Press.

Beck, A. T., Rush, A. J., Shaw, B. F., & Emery, G. (1979). *Cognitive therapy of depression.* New York: Guilford Press.

Beck, A. T., Wright, F. D., Newman, C. F., & Liese, B. F. (1993). *Cognitive therapy of substance abuse.* New York: Guilford Press.

Benson, H. (1975). *The relaxation response.* New York: Avon.

Burns, D. (1980). *Feeling good: The new mood therapy.* New York: Signet.

Burns, D. (1989). *The feeling good handbook.* New York: Morrow.

Christensen, J. F. (2003). Suggestion and hypnosis. In M. D. Feldman & J. F. Christensen (Eds.), *Behavioral medicine in primary care: A practical guide* (2nd ed., pp. 45–53). New York: Lange Medical Books/McGraw-Hill.

Christensen, J. F., & Boone, J. L. (2003). Stress and disease. In M. D. Feldman & J. F. Christensen (Eds.), *Behavioral medicine in primary care: A practical guide* (2nd ed., pp. 299–311). New York: Lange Medical Books/McGraw-Hill.

Clark, W. D. (2003). Alcohol and substance use. In M. D. Feldman & J. F. Christensen (Eds.), *Behavioral medicine in primary care: A practical guide* (2nd ed., pp. 173–185). New York: Lange Medical Books/McGraw-Hill.

Dattilio, F. M. (2001). Cognitive-behavioral treatment of panic complicated by medical illness. *Psychotherapy, 38*(2), 212–265.

Dattilio, F. M., & Castaldo, J. E. (2001). Differentiating symptoms of panic from relapse of Guillain-Barré Syndrome. *Harvard Review of Psychiatry, 9,* 260–265.

DiMatteo, M. R. (2003). Patient adherence. In M. D. Feldman & J. F. Christensen (Eds.), *Behavioral medicine in primary care: A practical guide* (2nd ed., pp. 150–154). New York: Lange Medical Books/McGraw-Hill.

DiTomasso, R. A., & Kovnat, K. D. (1994). Medical patients. In F. M. Dattilio & A. Freeman (Eds.), *Cognitive-behavioral strategies in crisis intervention* (pp. 325–344). New York: Guilford Press.

DiTomasso, R. A., Martin, D. M., & Kovnat, K. D. (2000). Medical patients in crisis. In F. M. Dattilio & A. Freeman (Eds.), *Cognitive-behavioral strategies in crisis intervention* (2nd ed., pp. 409–428). New York: Springer.

DiTomasso, R. A., & Mills, O. (1990). The behavioral treatment of essential hypertension: Implications for medical psychotherapy. *Medical Psychotherapy, 3,* 125–134.

Dohrenwend, B. D., & Dohrenwend, B. P. (1982). Some issues in research on stressful life events. In T. Millon, C. Green, & R. Meagher (Eds.), *Handbook of clinical health psychology* (pp. 91–101). New York: Plenum Press.

Edelman, S., & Kidman, A. D. (1999, July–August). Description of a group cognitive-behaviour therapy programme with cancer patients. *Psycho-Oncology, 8*(4), 306–314.

Emery, G. (1984). *Own your own life.* New York: Signet.

Epperson-SeBour, M. (1990). Psychosocial crisis services in the Maryland emergency services system. In H. J. Parad & L. G. Parad (Eds.), *Crisis intervention book 2: The practitioner's sourcebook for brief therapy* (pp. 209–226). Milwaukee: Family Service America.

Feinstein, R. E., & Carey, L. (1999). Crisis intervention in office practice. In R. E. Feinstein & A. A. Brewer (Eds.), *Primary care psychiatry and behavioral medicine: Brief office treatment and management pathways* (pp. 430–447). New York: Springer.

Feldman, M. D., & Christensen, J. F. (Eds.). (2003). *Behavioral medicine in primary care: A practical guide* (2nd ed.). New York: Lange Medical Books/McGraw-Hill.

Freeman, A. (1986). Understanding personal cultural and family schemata in psychotherapy. *Journal of Psychotherapy and the Family, 2*(3/4), 79–99.

Freeman, A., & DeWolf, R. (1990). *Woulda, coulda, shoulda.* New York: Morrow.

Gilliland, B. E., & James, R. K. (1997). *Crisis intervention strategies* (3rd ed.). Pacific Grove, CA: Brooks/Cole.

Kahana, E., Kahana, B., Harel, Z., & Rosner, T. (1988). Coping with extreme trauma. In J. P. Wilson, Z. Harel, & B. Kahana (Eds.), *Human adaptation to extreme stress: From the Holocaust to Vietnam* (pp. 55– 80). New York: Plenum Press.

Kaupp, J. W., Rapoport-Hubschman, N., & Spiegel, D. (2005). Psychosocial treatments. In J. L. Levenson (Ed.), *American psychiatric publishing textbook of psychomatic medicine* (pp. 450–469). Washington, DC: American Psychiatric Publishing.

Kazantzis, N., MacEwan, J., & Dattilio, F. M. (2005). A guiding model for practice. In N. Kazantzis, F. P. Deane, K. R. Ronan, & L. L. L'Abate (Eds.), *Using homework assignments in cognitive-behavior therapy* (pp. 357–404). New York: Brunner-Routledge.

Leahy, R. (2006). *The worry cure.* New York: Random House.

Low, A. A. (1950). *Mental health through will training. A system of self-help in psychotherapy as practiced by Recovery, Incorporated.* Glencoe, IL: Willett.

Marsland, D. W., Wood, M., & Mayo, F. (1976). A data bank for patient care, curriculum, and research in family practice: 526,196 patient problems. *Journal of Family Practice, 3,* 25.

McMullin, R. E., & Casey, B. (1975). *Talk sense to yourself: A guide to cognitive restructuring therapy.* New York: Counseling Research Press.

Miller, W. R., & Rollnick, S. (1991). *Motivational interviewing: Preparing people to change addictive behavior.* New York: Guilford Press.

Moorey, S. (1996). When bad things happen to rational people: cognitive therapy in adverse life circumstances. In P. M. Salkovskis (Ed.), *Frontiers of cognitive therapy* (pp. 450–469). New York: Guilford Press.

National Institutes of Health. (1995). *NIH Technology Assessment Conference on Integration of Behavioral and Relaxation Approaches into the Treatment of Chronic Pain and Insomnia.* Bethesda, MD: National Institutes of Health.

Orme-Johnson, D., Walton, K., & Lonsdorf, N. (1995). Meditation in the treatment of chronic pain and insomnia. In National Institutes of Health, *NIH Technology Assessment Conference on Integration of Behavioral and Relaxation Approaches into the Treatment of Chronic Pain and Insomnia* (pp. 27–31). Bethesda, MD: National Institutes of Health.

Parad, H. J., & Parad, L. G. (1990). Crisis intervention: An introductory overview. In H. S. Parad & L. G. Parad (Eds.), *Crisis intervention book 2: The practitioner's sourcebook for brief therapy* (pp. 3–66). Milwaukee: Family Service America.

Prochaska, J. O., & DiClemente, C. C. (1992). The transtheoretical approach. In J. C. Norcross & M. R. Goldfried (Eds.), *Handbook of psychotherapy integration* (pp. 301–334). New York: Basic Books.

Roberts, S. A., Kiselica, M. D., & Fredrickson, S. A. (2002). Quality of life of persons with medical illnesses: Counseling's holistic contribution. *Journal of Counseling and Development*, *80*(4), 422–432.

Robinson, P. (1988). Behavioral health services in primary care: A new perspective for treating depression. *Clinical Psychology: Science and Practice*, *5*(1), 77–93.

Rose, D. S. (1991). A model for psychodrama psychotherapy with the rape victim. *Psychotherapy*, *28*(1), 85–95.

Smith, G. T., & Beers, D. (2003). Pain. In M. D. Feldman & J. F. Christensen (Eds.), *Behavioral medicine in primary care: A practical guide* (2nd ed., pp. 312–320). New York: Lange Medical Books/McGraw-Hill.

Taylor, S. E. (1986). *Health psychology.* New York: Random House.

Williams, J., Pollin, L., & Koocher, G. P. (1999). Medical crisis counseling on pediatric intensive care unit: Case examples and clinical utility. *Journal of Clinical Psychology in Medical Settings*, *6*(3), 249–258.

Wright, J. H., Basco, M. R., & Thase, M. E. (2006). *Learning cognitive-behavior therapy: An illustrated guide.* Washington, DC: American Psychiatric Association Press.

SUGGESTED READINGS

Christensen, J. F., & Boone, J. L. (2003). Stress and disease. In M. D. Feldman & J. F. Christensen (Eds.), *Behavioral medicine in primary care: A practical guide* (2nd ed., pp. 299–311). New York: Lange Medical Books/McGraw-Hill.

Dattilio, F. M. (2001). Cognitive-behavioral treatment of panic complicated by medical illness. *Psychotherapy*, *38*(2), 212–265.

Feinstein, R. E., & Carey, L. (1999). Crisis intervention in office practice. In R. E. Feinstein & A. A. Brewer (Eds.), *Primary care psychiatry and behavioral medicine: Brief office treatment and management pathways* (pp. 430–447). New York: Springer.

Feldman, M. D., & Christensen, J. F. (Eds.). (2003). *Behavioral medicine in primary care: A practical guide* (2nd ed.). New York: Lange Medical Books/McGraw-Hill.

Robinson, P. (1988). Behavioral health services in primary care: A new perspective for treating depression. *Clinical Psychology: Science and Practice*, *5*(1), 77–93.

CHAPTER 9

Acute and Chronic Pain

Sharon Morgillo Freeman

Pain is real when you get other people to believe in it. If no one believes in it but you, your pain is madness or hysteria.

—WOLF (1990, p. 254)

*L*ong-term, unremitting pain drains a person's resources and support systems both emotionally and physically. Many patients who experience chronic pain are often heard to say, "I can't live like this anymore!" An estimated 9% of U.S. adult population suffers from moderate to severe pain (American Pain Society, 1999). More than two-thirds of pain sufferers have been living with their pain for more than five years. One in three describe their pain as "the worst it can be." For one-third of sufferers, pain was so severe, they felt they "couldn't function as normal people" and sometimes felt so bad "they wanted to die" (American Pain Society, 1999). Two-thirds said their over-the-counter (OTC) medications were not effective, and 52% of those taking prescription medications said they were not effective (American Pain Society, 1999).

Patients are reluctant to seek help from a behavioral health specialist because they interpret referral to mean that others think they are "crazy," or faking their pain, or that their pain is somehow their fault (Fishman, 2004). Pain experience has both a physical and an emotional component. Pain activates emotions such as anger, anxiety, fear, and depression. In turn, these emotions activate pain perception. This is due to the neurophysiological and neuroanatomic structures in humans and points to the importance of managing both components of a person's pain experience. In addition, the experience of pain is often accompanied by a traumatic event, such as the pain from injuries sustained in a motor vehicle accident. Therefore, the pain management specialist must be prepared to treat and/or understand both of these critical components of pain. To do otherwise would most likely result in frustration for the patient and treatment provider due to continued suffering and possibly increased pain.

PAIN DEFINITIONS

Acute pain is directly related to tissue damage and has an obvious source; it can last for a moment (hitting your thumb with a hammer) or for months, as in the case of a severe injury (crash, shark bite, burns). Acute pain is limited in duration and usually responds to pharmacological treatment. Pain becomes chronic when it has persisted for 6 months or longer. Common examples of chronic pain include such processes as sickle cell disease, arthritis, cancer, fibromyalgia, headache, or back pain, or following traumatic injuries and burns.

Chronic pain often does not have an identifiable physical cause and is not amenable to physical interventions. In some cases the pain has exacerbations and remissions, or it may be present all the time. It is not unusual for chronic pain sufferers to fall into a cycle of pain, inactivity, sleeplessness, anger, hopelessness, and depression. Thomas (2005) reported that patients who are anxious and depressed experience more pain, have a greater frequency of hospital admissions, and use more negative coping strategies. They also have a greater tendency to be underconfident in their ability to cope with pain and believe that control of their pain is left to chance.

The gate control model, originally proposed by Melzack and Wall (1965), is currently the most utilized pain generation theory. These authors hypothesize that a spinal gating mechanism regulates the degree of pain transmission to the brain. Information from the periphery passes down descending fibers from the cortex, thalamus, and other parts of the brain to "prime" the nervous system to receive the stimulus interpreted as pain. Psychological factors such as emotion, cognitions, beliefs about self, and pain as well as expectations about pain relief all play a role in the perception and experience of a painful stimulus. Thus emotional and cognitive processes can affect the amount and quality of pain experience by altering the influence of the spinal gating mechanism and directly modulate pain experience (Thomas, 2005).

VOLUNTARY CONTROL OVER BRAIN ACTIVATION

Individuals control, albeit unwittingly, activation of specific brain mechanisms all the time. Voluntary activities activate certain brain regions resulting in the expression of the behavior "requested" by the individual. The use of voluntary control of heart rate, skin conductance, and muscle tone is used in biofeedback training for individuals with anxiety, for example. Biofeedback and relaxation training through guided imagery has been used to help individuals reduce pain perception and suffering. It has only recently been discovered that individuals can learn to directly control activation of certain regions of the brain that lead to pain perception to the point of changing the quality of severe, chronic clinical pain (deCharms et al., 2005). Subjects were monitored using guided training while undergoing functional magnetic resonance imagery (fMRI) while noxious stimuli were applied. The individuals were noted to be able to learn to control areas of the rostral anterior cingulate cortex (rACC), a region that is associated with pain perception and regulation. When the subjects induced increases or decreases in rACC functional magnetic resonance imaging (fMRI) activation there was a corresponding change in pain perception caused by the pain stimuli (deCharms, et al., 2005). In addition, the researchers discovered that patients suffering from chronic pain syndromes who were trained in the same techniques reported ongoing decreases in their levels of chronic pain.

COMMON FORMS OF PAIN DISORDERS SEEN IN CLINICAL PRACTICE

Common pain disorders seen in clinical practice include the following:

- *Headache:* tension headache, vascular headache, migraine.
- *Low back pain:* sciatica (leg pain due to an irritated nerve in the spine).
- *Arthritis pain:* osteoarthritis, rheumatoid arthritis.
- *Neurogenic pain:* trigeminal neuralgia, shingles, amputated "phantom" pain.
- *Fibromyalgia syndrome (FMS):* a chronic medical condition, characterized by widespread body and muscle pain and uncontrollable fatigue. Fibromyalgia may be accompanied by many other problems such as irritable bowel, headaches, sleep disorder, and cognitive impairments. Conditions that may fall into the same category of syndromes as FMS are chronic fatigue syndrome (CFS) and myofascial pain syndrome (MPS).
- *Irritable bowel syndrome* (IBS; also called spastic colon): People with IBS have digestive tracts that react abnormally to certain substances or to stress, leading to symptoms such as cramps, gas, bloating, pain, constipation, and diarrhea.
- *Gastrointestinal tract disorders* (Crohn's disease, diverticulitis, regional enteritis, granulomatous ileitis, ileocolitis): *Crohn's disease* is a chronic inflammation of the intestinal wall that may affect any part of the digestive tract. Common symptoms include chronic diarrhea (which sometimes is bloody), cramping abdominal pain, fever, loss of appetite, and weight loss. *Diverticulitis* is an inflammation of one or more diverticula, which are small mucosal pockets in the wall of the colon that may fill with stagnant fecal material or undigested food particles. Obstruction of the neck of the diverticulum may result in the distention secondary to mucus secretion and overgrowth of normal colonic bacteria. The thin-walled diverticulum, consisting solely of mucosa, is susceptible to vascular compromise and, therefore, is at risk for perforation. Walled-off infection can progress to abscess formation and possibly rupture resulting in generalized peritonitis and even death.

- *Ethyromyalgia:* a rare syndrome of paroxysmal vasodilation with burning pain, increased skin temperature, and redness of the feet and, less often, the hands.
- *Rheumatoid arthritis:* a chronic systemic disease primarily of the joints, marked by inflammatory changes in the synovial membranes and articular structures and by muscle atrophy and rarefaction of the bones.

PAIN-RELATED CRISES

Patients who suffer from chronic pain syndromes suffer secondary problems that can become overwhelming and even catastrophic. Pain causes time off work, financial burdens, disruption or discontinuation of function and roles, and family separations. This enormous toll taken on the person as a direct result of disabling pain increases his/her sense of helplessness, depression, and fear of the future. The growing sense of helplessness generates anger and frustration and may be complicated by the development of avoidance behaviors for social activity, intimacy, self-care such as exercise, and involvement in pleasurable activities.

Chronic pain conditions are associated with high rates of suicide (Fishbain, 1996; Fishbain, Cutler, Rosomoff, & Rosomoff, 2000). Chronic pain also increases the risk for aggressive behaviors, including violent ideation (Bruns & Disorbio, 2000). Antagonistic relationships with the individual and his/her peers at work, at home, and with the prescriber can escalate the patient's sense of frustration, leading to an increase in angry feelings and outbursts of temper. Patients have described the enormous amounts of paperwork and office visits as "attempts to avoid getting me help." People who have premorbid difficulties with temper and impulsivity are at even higher risk than those without these conditions. This would include those patients who have experienced angry outbursts or violence in the past as well as those persons who have cluster B Axis II (personality) disorders or who drink or use substances to cope with stress.

PAIN ASSESSMENT MEASURES

Formal checklists and rating scales help clinicians and patients describe the quality and intensity of pain experiences. They also allow for data comparison during therapy to evaluate changes subsequent to cognitive and behavioral interventions. The following list of instruments and checklists is intended to give the reader a basic overview of instruments available and is not by any means all inclusive.

- *Full or Short Form McGill Pain Questionnaires (MPQ; Melzack & Wall, 1965).* The MPQ is the best known and most widely used instrument and is available in several languages. This multidimensional measure assesses the severity of pain experienced and provides separate assessment of affective and sensory pain ratings. The MPQ contains 20 sets of verbal pain descriptors containing 78 adjectives. The adjectives are divided into four groups: *discriminative* (e.g., "throbbing, pinching, burning"), *affective–motivational* (e.g., "exhausting and blinding"), *cognitive–evaluative* (e.g., "miserable and annoying") and *miscellaneous* (e.g., "nagging and spreading"). The words are rank-ordered in each row of three to six choices. The number of words chosen and the mean rank of the words chosen evaluate the intensity and dimension of pain levels.

• *General Health Questionnaire (GHQ; Goldberg & Williams, 1988)*. The GHQ assesses anxiety and depression. It is a measure of current mental health and since the 1970s has been extensively used in a variety of settings and cultures. The GHQ was originally developed as a 60-item instrument but a range of shortened instruments includes the GHQ-30, the GHQ-28, the GHQ-20, and the GHQ-12. The scale asks whether the individual has experienced a particular symptom or behavior recently. Each item is rated on a 4-point scale and (e.g., when using the GHQ-12) it gives a total score of 36 or 12 based on the selected scoring methods. The most common scoring methods are bimodal (0–0–1–1) and Likert scoring styles (0–1–2–3). The GHQ-12 is brief, simple, and easy to complete, and its application in research settings as a screening tool is well documented.

• *Coping Strategies Questionnaire (CSQR; Gil, Abrams, Phillips, & Keefe, 1989; Rosenthiel & Keefe, 1983)*. The CSQR assesses a range of positive and negative pain coping strategies. The questionnaire contains seven scales of coping strategies. For example, the Catastrophizing scale contains six items that indicate maladaptive negative cognitions (e.g., "It's terrible and I feel it's never going to get any better" or "I worry all the time about whether it will end"). The items are scored on a 7-point Likert scale (0 = "never think or feel that," 6 = "always think or feel that"), and the scores are summed to range from 0 to 36.

• *Pain Self-Efficacy Questionnaire (PSEQ; Nicholas, 1989)*. The PSEQ is a 10-item self-report instrument that uses a 7-point scale to measure and assess how confident patients feel about functioning in daily life despite their pain. This instrument was developed specifically for patients with chronic pain problems.

• *Pain Anxiety Symptoms Scale (PASS; McCracken, Zayfert, & Gross, 1992)*. The PASS is a 40-item self-report measure that consists of four subscales measuring aspects of pain-related anxiety and avoidance: cognitive anxiety, fearful appraisal, escape avoidance, and physiological anxiety. Strahl, Kleinknecht, and Dinnel (2000) obtained data showing that pain anxiety, along with contributions of self-efficacy and coping strategies, strongly determines the physical, social, emotional, and role functioning in chronic rheumatoid arthritis patients. PASS scores correlated negatively with the amount of weight lifted and carried during a physical capacity evaluation, and they accounted for additional variance when measures of trait anxiety, depression, and pain severity were controlled. They suggested that patients with high PASS scores might have a fear of injury that causes them to avoid potentially painful physical exertion (Bruns & Disorbio, 2000).

• *Multidimensional Pain Inventory (MPI; Kerns, Turk, & Rudy, 1985)*. The MPI is a 61-item, self-report questionnaire that assesses functional pain impairment along 13 dimensions. The dimensional scales under the first section cover pain severity, activity interference, perceived life control, affective distress, and perceived level of social support. Section II assesses perceived responses of significant others and Section III assesses engagement in various activities of daily living. The response pattern is then coded into one of file profiles (e.g., "dysfunctional coper" or "adaptive coper").

• *Sickness Impact Profile (SIP; Bergner, Bobbitt, Carter, & Gilson, 1981)*. The SIP is a 136-item self-report questionnaire that measures impairment and disability along 12 functional dimensions: ambulation, mobility, body care and movement, social interaction, communication, alertness, emotional behavior, sleep and rest, eating, work, home management, and recreation. The test has been shown to correlate well with patient's reports of pain and physical examination measures.

• *Pain Beliefs and Perceptions Inventory (PBPI; Williams & Thorn, 1989)*. The PBPI is a 16-item patient self-report questionnaire that measures various beliefs and perceptions about pain. The responses are scored, summed, and then averaged to reflect ratings in one of four factors or scales. The scales are termed *Pain Mysterious; Pain Perception; Pain Consistency; and Self-Blame*. Normative means and standard deviations are provided at the bottom of the instrument and are based on a mixed sample of 213 patients with chronic pain conditions.

CHRONIC PAIN, COGNITIVE ERROR GENERATION, AND MOOD DISORDERS

Chronic pain tends to drain a person's energy and resources. The person may begin to feel helpless to the pain experience and stop believing that his/her life will ever improve. Feelings of helplessness, worthlessness, and self-denigration lead to social and behavioral withdrawal, and low energy, guilt, and anxiety begin to predominate his/her daily life. It is therefore not surprising that people who have long-term unremitting pain develop depression at higher rates than those without chronic pain. The estimated prevalence of major depressive episodes in persons with chronic pain are approximately 30% (De Vellis, 1993). Patients with long-term unremitting pain can provoke feelings of frustration, anger, and hopelessness in even the most seasoned clinician. Particularly difficult issues include anxiety disorders such as posttraumatic stress disorder, suicidality, opiate medication misuse, and chronic noncompliance (Wasan, Wootton, & Jamison, 2005). The presence of physical symptoms exacerbates mood disturbances two- to threefold. This may in part be related to the shared mechanisms involved in the serotonin and norephinephrine neurotransmitter systems. Both selective serontonergic and serotonin/norepinephrine reuptake inhibitors have been shown to relieve comorbid physical symptoms associated with posttraumatic stress disorders, depression, and pain (Bailey, 2003; Gallagher & Verma, 1999; Hamner & Robert, 2005; Strahl et al., 2000; Wasan et al., 2005).

Another component that affects pain perception, management, and expectation is anxiety. People with chronic pain may develop fear/anxiety when movement or their usual activities increase the pain (Craig & Bushnell, 1994). As a person decreases movement, he/she limits activities, which increases worry about losing control over his/her life, ability to work, and ability to socialize. People who are anxious focus more on painful symptoms, and this reinforces the sense of having no control, which can result in panic and possibly depression. Panic and anxiety may lead to beliefs that the situation is hopeless and/or that the individual is useless (Thomas, 2005). The anxiety/panic/belief generation/anxiety vicious cycle is quickly established. Depression and anxiety influence the way people think, which in turn influences pain behavior. According to Rosenthiel and Keefe (1983) catastrophizing is particularly prevalent in patients with chronic pain and may account for chronic pain's generation persistence (Vlaeyen, Geurts, Koler-Snijders, Boeren, & van Eck, 1995) and relapse after rehabilitation (Coughlan, Ridout, Williams, & Richardson, 1995).

People with anxiety are less likely to be able to generate rational cognitions and planning regarding their pain experience and behavior. For example, Eccelston (1994) found that intense pain experience interfered with the person's ability to attend to situations, access memory, and maintain conversations (Eccelston, 1994). Other cognitive errors include overgeneralization across experience, personalization (assuming personal responsibility with a tendency toward self-denigration), and selective abstraction of the negative aspects of the situation. According to Linton (1994), patients with chronic pain who do not catastrophize, self-blame, or self-denigrate function substantially better than those who engage in the use of these cognitive errors. There are five specific areas affected by an anxious pain sufferer's cognitive style:

1. Labeling of bodily sensations (pain related or other).
2. Appraisal of new situations.
3. Appraisal of potential threats.
4. Appraisal of oneself.
5. Beliefs about one's ability to effect change in a situation (Eccelston, 1997).

People who catastrophize as a thought strategy tend to relapse more often and have a more persistent pain experience (Rosenthiel & Keefe, 1983; Vlaeyen et al., 1995)—for example, a person who thinks "I cannot possibly live with this pain! I am going to end up in a wheelchair unable to take care of myself and no one will want to have anything to do with me! I will never be able to work again and I will lose my home and my family!" Additional cognitive errors include overgeneralization, negative (degrading) personalization, and selective abstraction to the negative. The patient's thought patterns influence behaviors, which in turn influence thought patterns and behavior in a negative cognitive cycle.

PAIN MANAGEMENT

Pain management is exactly what it says: pain *management*. Patients often come to therapy expecting to be "fixed" and can become quite upset when they discover that they are expected to "manage" their pain, not obliterate it. Most pain management programs include an integrated team approach to improving pain tolerability through physical, emotional, cognitive, and social skill training. Behavioral interventions may include regular exercise, physical therapy, pharmacotherapy, hypnotherapy, or progressive guided-imagery relaxation mastery, acupuncture, behavioral experiments, and biofeedback. These techniques are described in more detail below.

Pharmacotherapy Options

This chapter would be incomplete without a basic review of the most commonly used medications to treat individuals with combined pain and psychological problems. Although no single treatment is a "magic bullet," the adept prescriber evaluates each individual symptomatic presentation and chooses a category of medication that is most likely to help more than one problem in order to simplify the person's treatment regime. For example, a patient who has a history of anxiety disorder and now has a chronic pain condition with resultant depression may be best suited for a selective serotonin reuptake inhibitor (SSRI) given that this category of medication is useful for both depression and anxiety. This is important as conditions of anxiety and depression itself can exacerbate physical pain (Sareen, Cox, Clara, & Asmundson, 2005). Regardless of the agent chosen, the patient should be counseled to understand that the medication will not be effective if he/she is not also using other skills and behaviors for pain management, especially psychotherapy. Specific types and causes of pain may respond better to one category of pain medication than to another.

Recent developments concerning the understanding of pain transmission as it relates to comorbid mood disorders has led to the use of medications that target neurobiological activation systems such as the serotonin and norepinephrine receptor systems (Bailey, 2003; Sareen et al., 2005). In addition, individual responses differ with most pain medication. For example, individuals suffering from neuropathic pain have enjoyed the greatest benefit from tricyclic antidepressants (TCAs) until the more recent development of serotonin–norepinephrine reuptake inhibitors (SNRIs) (Coluzzi & Mattia, 2005). This evidence supports the hypothesis that a balanced inhibition of noradrenaline and serotonin reuptake is more effective in relieving pain. There are currently two choices of SNRIs: duloxetine and venlafaxine. In an open clinical trial, 26 individuals suffering from fibromyalgia responded more robustly to mirtazepine possibly due to its selective blockade of $5\text{-}HT_2$ and $5\text{-}HT_3$ receptors (Samborski, Lezanska-Szpera, & Rybakowski, 2004). TCAs have been used most extensively for visceral pain disorders such as IBS; however, pharmacological therapeutics that modulate the biological amines (serotonin, norepinephrine, dopamine and catecholamines) both peripherally and within the central nervous system may offer more effective therapies for these disorders (Crowell et al., 2004). Finally, another category of medication, the gamma-aminobutyric acid (GABA) receptor agonists and antagonists such as benzodiazepines and anticonvulsants (e.g., gabapentin and pregabalin) may mediate symptoms associated with chronic pain, epilepsy, and schizophrenia (Enna & Bowery, 2004). This, together with results from other types of studies, indicates the potential therapeutic value of developing drugs capable of selectively activating, inhibiting, or modulating $GABA_B$ receptor function.

Chronic pain also has the component of "breakthrough" pain with those pharmacological agents that have shorter half-lives than those with half-lives that are greater than 12 hours. Severe flares of pain that "break through" the medication are perceived as one more stressor that the person has no sense of control over, again increasing the cognitive/emotional responses to pain. Episodic breakthrough pain is often controlled with longer-acting opiate receptor agonists such as methadone, buprenophine, and oxycontin. Methadone was originally developed as an analgesic for individuals with chronic pain conditions due to its long half-life (up to 12 hours). A long half-life minimizes the "ebbs and flows" of pain relief associated with shorter-acting opiate pain relievers such as morphine (Lynch, 2005). Buprenorphine is a partial opiate receptor agonist with a longer half-life than most opiate pain relievers. These unique properties make it extremely useful in those individuals who are at risk for accidental (or intentional) overdose as it has a "ceiling" effect that prevents complications in even extremely high doses (except in those cases when the individual is also taking a benzodiazepine) (Malinoff, Barkin, & Wilson, 2005; Muriel, Failde, Mico, Neira, & Sanchez-Magro, 2005). Finally, fentanyl (Fentanyl) transdermal patches allow for a continuous exposure to opiate-based analgesia (Kornick, Santiago-Palma, Moryl, Payne, & Obbens, 2003).

Categories of medications used to treat pain include the following:

- *Analgesics* such as acetaminophen (Tylenol) and tramadol (Ultram) can relieve pain but do not have the anti-inflammatory effects of nonsteroidal anti-inflammatory drugs (NSAIDs).

- *Nonsteroidal anti-inflammatory drugs (NSAIDs)*. Aspirin, ibuprofen (Motrin, Nuprin, Advil), naproxen (Naprosyn), and celecoxib (Celebrex) are examples of nonsteroidal anti-inflammatory drugs (NSAIDs) used to reduce inflammation and relieve pain. Long-term use of analgesics and NSAIDs may cause stomach ulcers as well as kidney and liver problems.

- *Muscle relaxants* such as cyclobenzaprine (Flexeril), and baclofen (Liorisol) can be used to treat pain associated with muscle spasms and spasticity.

- *Anticonvulsants* such as phenytoin (Dilantin) and carbamazepine (Tegretol), gabapentin (Neurontin), and topiramate (Topamax) can be used to relieve neuropathic pain such as that found in diabetic neuropathies, trigeminal neuralgia, painful paresthaesia (e.g., subsequent to Guillian Barre or multiple schlerosis episodes), and migraine pain. Lamotrigine (Lamictal) and gabapentin have antimanic and antidepressant properties but also carry potentially serious side effects.

- *Steroids* can be used to reduce the swelling and inflammation of the nerves. They are taken orally (as a Medrol dose pack) in a tapering dosage over a 5-day period. They have the advantage of providing pain relief within a 24-hour period. Steroid injections may be prescribed if the pain is severe. Steroid medications are known to induce manic episodes and sometimes depression with prolonged use.

- *Narcotics* (opioids) are very powerful pain relievers that actually deaden a person's perception of pain. They are used for a short period (2 to 4 weeks) after an acute injury or surgery. Common narcotics include codeine (Tylenol 3), meperidine (Demerol), propoxyphene (Darvocet), hydrocodone (Vicodin), and oxycodone (Percocet, Oxycontin). Sumatriptan (Imitrex) and naratriptan (Amerge) are used to relieve migraine headaches. Narcotic medications cause impaired mental function, drowsiness, nausea, constipation, and sometimes addiction.

TABLE 9.1. Antidepressant and Anticonvulsant Pain Augmentation Agents

Selective serotonin reuptake inhibitors (SSRIs)	Serotonin–norepinephrine reuptake inhibitor(s) (SNRIs)	Tricyclics and tetracyclics	Anticonvulsants
Citalopram (Celexa)	Venlafaxine (Effexor)	Amitripyline (Elavil)	Gabapentine (Neurontin)
Escitalopram (Lexapro)	Duloxetine (Cymbalta)	Doxepine (Sinequan)	Topiramate (Topamax)
Fluoxetine (Prozac)		Imipramine (Tofranil)	Pregabalin (Lyrica)
Fluvoxamine (Luvox)	(serotonin–norepinephrine modulator)	Clomipramine (Anafranil)	
Paroxetine (Paxil)	Mirtazapine (Remeron)	Amoxapine (Asendin)	
Sertraline (Zoloft)		Maprotiline (Ludiomil)	
	(dopamine–norepinephrine reuptake inhibitor) Bupropion (Wellbutrin; Zyban)	Nortriptyline (Pamelor)	

Note. U.S. trade names are in parentheses.

Table 9.1 lists commonly used medications in for chronic pain management.

Behavioral Interventions

Pain Diary

The pain diary allows for both the patient and the therapist to track behaviors, interventions, responses to interventions, and emotional variables regarding the individual's pain experience. The pain diary can be used in conjunction with the Dysfunctional Thought Record (DTR) to track dysfunctional thought patterns associated with pain levels, pain locations, situations and activities, coping measures, and medication use. The therapist and patient can then use these data to explore cognitive restructuring possibilities (White, 2001).

Relaxation and Guided Imagery Training

The benefits of relaxation training include generalized lower arousal levels, improved body awareness and muscle relaxation, and distraction with pain replacement images. Lewandowski, Good, and Draucker (2005) demonstrated that verbal descriptions of pain change with the use of a guided imagery technique. The researchers used 210 pain descriptions obtained across five time points. Data were analyzed using content analysis. Six categories emerged from the data: pain is never-ending, pain is relative, pain is explainable, pain is torment, pain is restrictive, and pain is changeable. For participants in the treatment group, pain became changeable. The meaning of pain as never-ending was a prominent theme for participants before randomization to treatment and control groups. It remained a strong theme for participants in the control group but did not resurface for participants in the treatment group (Lewandowski et al., 2005).

Sleep

Sleep disturbances of less than 7 to 8 hours in individuals with pain disorders creates a negative reciprocal relationship. Pain disturbs sleep, sleep deprivation leads to fatigue (both mental and physical), the development of myofascial trigger points, increased pain perception, and potentially, depression (Roehrs & Roth, 2005). The body restores and repairs during the sleep process; without restful sleep the individual continuously loses the ability to recover from painful processes.

Dietary Factors

Harmful health habits such as smoking, drinking alcohol, and illicit substance use increase pain and may interfere with prescribed medication. Diets deficient in fruits and vegetables and containing excessive amounts of meat, refined grain products, and sugar can have numerous adverse biochemical effects, all of which create a pro-inflammatory state and predispose the body to degenerative diseases. These effects may be associated with the amounts of omega-3 fatty acids. It appears that an inadequate intake of fruits and vegetables can result in a suboptimal intake of antioxidants and phytochemicals and an imbalanced intake of essential fatty acids (Perez, Ware, Chevalier, Gougeon, & Shir, 2005; Seaman, 2002).

Maintaining Healthy Height/Weight Ratios

The increasing incidence of obesity has had a tremendous impact on the physical, psychological, social, and economic health of our nation with important long-term implications for the development of future social and health care policies. Clinically severe obesity is a chronic disabling disease that results in significantly decreased health status in seven of the eight areas measured with a 36-item health report questionnaire prior to gastric bypass surgery. Preoperatively, patients with clinically severe obesity scored significantly lower in all areas except role activities than the national "normal" population. Disability scores resolved with successful weight reduction. In some areas, function even surpasses the national "normal" population (Choban, Onyejekwe, Burge, & Flancbaum, 1999). Other factors measured included emotional factors, physical activities, role activities, physical factors, general mental health, general health perceptions, social functioning and bodily pain, and vitality.

Pacing Principles

Pacing refers to the need to regulate and control the frequency, intensity, and duration of energy-expending activities. Pain conditions deplete energy stores as a baseline. If the individual overexerts him/herself, he/she risks exhaustion, pain increases, and even injury occurs. Individuals with chronic pain conditions tend to use the cognitive distortion of "all-or-nothing" thinking when it comes to physical exertion. "When I feel better I want to catch up on all of the activities I have been missing." Often overexertion is related to an individual's change in role as a result of developing a pain syndrome. They may want to give others the perception that they are "still who they always were," maintain friends and fun activities, and keep up with family during "play times." As a result of overdoing it the person has an increased amount of pain, decreased energy, and feelings of helplessness and hopelessness that "he/she will never be normal again." Therefore it is critical that activities that the individual is planning to engage in are evaluated realistically and "paced" to limit harm while allowing for as close to a normal living experience as possible.

Exercise/Physical Therapy

Gentle stretching and mild exercise improves overall muscle tone and control. Muscles that are underused and weak are more susceptible to pain than toned, flexible muscles. Physical therapists can prescribe a sequence of exercises to strengthen muscles that support the spine, limit muscle spasms, and prevent further injury. Stretching exercises help muscles to stay flexible. Inactivity leads to increased pain due to muscle atrophy. Immobile muscles lose approximately one-third of their size and power over a 6–8-week period. In fact, exercise has been determined to be the first-line treatment for patients suffering from fibromyalgia disorder. Fibromyalgia is an often misunderstood condition that has no definable or demonstrable cause. Pain is usually widespread with tender points in at least 11 of 18 known region of the body (low cervical, trapezius, gluteal, knee, etc.). Patients have been diagnosed with rheumatoid conditions related to sleep disturbances in the past; however, primary or idiopathic fibromyalgia syndromes are now considered unique musculoskeletal disorders.

Homework and Reading

Homework and reading are critical components in the cognitive-behavioral therapy setting as they allow for therapy to continue outside the therapy office (Kazantzis & Lampropoulos, 2002a, 2002b). Homework assignments include the use of DTRs, activity schedules, pain diaries, and behavioral experiments, to name a few. Homework is reviewed at the beginning of each therapy session and is evaluated regarding successes, noncompletion, partial successes, and opportunities for additional interventions. I use the workbook *Managing Pain before It Manages You* (Caudill, 2001) as an adjunct to therapy. This particular workbook is easy to read and has supportive information for the therapist and the patient and includes preprinted worksheets for the patient to complete. It includes explanations about pain generation, control, and numerous cognitive and behavioral exercises/techniques for the person to complete over the course of the therapy.

Cognitive Interventions

Thought Monitoring

Thought monitoring is useful in educating patients to distinguish between thought and feelings. For example, the patient who uses *dichotomous (all-or-nothing)* thinking is able to evaluate this style and the specific components of his/her thoughts, feelings, and behavioral outcomes that he/she is using. The patient is able to capture the thoughts that precede the "automatic" responses to pain that he/she has come to accept as factual. The therapist can then assist the patient to identify the specific cognitive distortions that may intensify his/her own personal pain experience. Once identified, these cognitive distortions may then be altered or eliminated along with the resultant maladaptive patterns of behavior that increase the experience of suffering and therefore increases pain.

The following is an example of thought monitoring:

Event: Getting out of bed in the morning.
Thought: "It hurts so bad to get out of bed that I would rather lie here all day."
Feeling: Anxiety and depression 80%.
Behavior outcome: Stayed in bed until late for work.

Types of Cognitive Distortions

DICHOTOMOUS, OR ALL-OR-NOTHING, THINKING

This type of cognitive distortion tends to be fear or anxiety based in people suffering from chronic pain conditions. They see few if any shades of gray in their pain and life experiences. Many patients report that they have "good and bad" days or "severe disabling pain or regular pain." They also become systematically trained to scan for potential peaks (as opposed to valleys) in their pain levels focusing on minute signals or triggers that may indicate they are about to experience catastrophic pain. The evaluation of only "good" or "bad" days leads to the perception that an entire day is "bad" if they experience a peak in pain perception. In addition all events, behaviors, and functions are usually labeled "terrible" or avoided altogether on "bad" days. Once this pattern takes hold it usually exacerbates another style of distorted thinking called *disqualifying the positive* (Eimer & Freeman, 1998).

DISQUALIFYING THE POSITIVE

Patients who have developed the "all-or-none" style often use this additional style in order to maintain and justify the conclusions that they have drawn and act on. They may discount the fact that they enjoyed a movie or a visit from a friend or were able to attend a party because "It was only *one* time! Things are *never* like that for long!" Another common manifestation of this type of cognitive distortion style is its use to justify avoidance behaviors. For example, "I may have *attended* the party, but I paid for it for the entire next day—I hurt so bad I couldn't even get out of bed! So what's the use of even going to anything anymore!"

SELECTIVE ABSTRACTION

Persons experiencing chronic pain may tend to become preoccupied with their pain experience to the point that little else matters. They constantly review their pain in order to avoid potential aggravations that may intensify the pain. As a result they begin to *expect* more pain. One patient described feeling severely anxious when she planned to drive her car anywhere because she "knew that she would have horrible pain as soon as she got out of the car—IF she could get out of the car." The fact that she drove almost daily and did in fact get out of the car for her appointments and for work indicated selective conditioning of her physical responses.

PAIN-BASED EMOTIONAL REASONING

Pain-based emotional reasoning (PBER) ignores important evidence that may lessen motivation based on negative expectations. For example, a patient complains that "my husband doesn't understand how much pain I am in or he would never ask me to have dinner ready for him when he gets home!" Pain may be perceived as unfair and misunderstood, leading the person to "up the ante" by becoming angry or demanding when others do not defer to him/her because he/she is suffering so much. This process may lead a person to *act* worse than he/she feels in order to reinforce to others that he/she is in pain and cannot be expected ever to recover or have a normal life.

CATASTROPHIZING

Catastrophizing is defined as the tendency to interpret events as much more negative than they are in reality, to the point of erupting into a panic state, or expecting negative consequences to be out of proportion to the reality (Eimer & Freeman, 1998). In some cases a person's catastrophic expectation may lead to suicidal ideation or physical violence toward others. It is therefore one of the most critical cognitive distortion styles to interrupt in therapy.

Case Study

Linda was a 48-year-old mother of three who was diagnosed with fibromyalgia (described above) 4 years after her third back surgery, including two spinal fusions. This patient was usually tearful in her sessions, describing her life as "over" and that she had "nothing" to look forward to each day except more pain. "I can't even help my 6-year-old get himself ready for school in the morning! I am useless as a mother!" She would take the experience of having severe morning pain to the extremes of devaluing her importance as a wife, mother, and friend to the point that she felt worthless, hopeless, and angry. Her expectations that she would "never" have a normal life or be a "good" mother brought new episodes of tears along with the announcement "I have nothing to live for! I'm a cripple—I wish I had the guts to just take all of my medicine and die!" This announcement may seem, on the surface, to be hysterical ravings or attempts to gain sympathy, but the research has shown that people with chronic disabling pain are much more likely to commit suicide than other groups of patients without disabling pain (Fishbain, 1996). Given this information the therapist is actually faced with a potential crisis situation that requires serious attention.

THERAPIST: Are you suicidal?

LINDA: Well, of course I am! Wouldn't you be?

THERAPIST: You said that you have nothing to live for and that you are a cripple. Yet you have also told me how much you enjoy your children, especially in the evenings when you read to them.

LINDA: That is only about 1 hour a day out of 24 hours! I just can't take it anymore!

THERAPIST: Are you saying that because you are in pain that you are useless as a mother?

LINDA: No. Of course I know I am useful as a mother. I just can't be the kind of mother I should be!

THERAPIST: You mean that you know you are useful as a mother, you just want to be able to do more than you are doing now.

LINDA: Yes, that's what I mean. I won't be able to be the kind of mother my children need.

THERAPIST: What kind of a mother will your children need?

LINDA: I have to be able to go to their games, help them with their homework and go to the things in their lives that are important to them. I know I can do that.

THERAPIST: You can't go to their school or help them with homework.

LINDA: I see what you are doing. I am able to do those things—I just wish it didn't hurt so much to do it.

THERAPIST: If you could rate yourself on a continuum of "completely useful = 100" and "useless = 0" where would you put yourself today?

LINDA: I guess I am about a 60.

THERAPIST: Would you be willing to explore ways to get you to a 65 or 70?

LINDA: I guess so. Every little bit helps.

THERAPIST: Are you still feeling suicidal?

LINDA: No, I'm not. I guess I really wound myself up there (laughs slightly).

THERAPIST: Would you be willing to keep me informed if that feeling comes back again?

LINDA: Yes, I would. I guess I just really need someone to calm me down when I get so overwhelmed. I guess that should be something else we should work on, isn't it?

The therapist hears Linda state "I have nothing to live for!" and determines that an evaluation of the seriousness of her statement must be dealt with before intervening with her anxiety and anger. Patients who come in to therapy exhibiting high levels of agitation, anxiety, and anger often produce equal levels of anxiety and agitation in the therapist due to the noxious presentation. The therapist must first put aside his/her own automatic responses to an agitated individual and look at the underlying cause of upset. It is quickly determined through direct questioning that Linda is expressing serious suicidal ideation and possible intent. Knowing that suicidal ideation is often the result of feeling hopeless, helpless, and frustrated the therapist needs to quickly interrupt her catastrophic thinking and negative cognitive escalation. Reassuring Linda would most likely not be helpful given the perfusion of symptoms that she is experiencing both emotionally and physically. In fact, reassuring her that she will be all right, or that she has reasons to live, or that others need her may further escalate her negativity as she tries to convince the therapist that she is in a great deal of distress. The therapist chooses instead to guide her through the implications of her catastrophizing by breaking the "all-or-nothing" attribution that she has voiced ("I am useless!") by using the scaling technique. This technique takes the dichotomous viewpoint and breaks it up along a continuum of possibilities. Once Linda is able to see that her conclusion of "uselessness" is in fact an exaggeration of her actual situation she deescalates and develops a sense of hope for improvement. The therapist ends the interaction by normalizing the feelings Linda had regarding suicidal ideation by inviting her to bring these thoughts to future therapy sessions and contracts with Linda to make them explicit when she is experiencing them.

Medical/Surgical Procedures

It is important for a therapist working with patients who are experiencing a chronic pain condition to have general knowledge about current medical procedures available for pain management. The very short list of procedures and definitions that follows is by no means complete; however, it explains the more common procedures that a person may undergo in his/her treatments for pain relief.

Epidural Steroid Injections

This procedure, usually performed under fluoroscopic X-ray, involves a series of steroid/analgesia injections into the epidural space of the spine to reduce the swelling and inflammation of the nerves. About 50% of patients will notice relief after an epidural injection. This intervention provides temporary relief that is often enough of a break for the patient to "regroup" and strengthen other healthy coping behaviors. Epidural injections are usually done in a series of three, at 2-week intervals up to three times a year (Rowlingson, 2005).

Facet Injections

Facet injections are similar to epidural injections but target low back pain due to inflammation or irritation of the facet joints. They are also conducted under fluoroscopy (X-ray) to outline the spinal structures while a needle is inserted through skin and muscles to specific sensory nerves located in the facet joints. A combination of anesthetic and steroids are injected into the facet joint to decrease swelling, inflammation, and irritation (Ramamurthy, 2005).

Acupuncture

Acupuncture is an ancient treatment for a variety of physical illnesses. It involves the introduction of very fine needles into specific points of the body that correlate with the illness. Recent research using fMRI has shown that acupuncture produces decreased activity in the nucleus accumbens, amygdale, hippocampus, ventral tegmentum, anterior cingulate gyrus, caudate putamen, temporal pole, and insula (Leung, 2005). In addition, it has been found that more than 70% of acupuncture points correlate with myofascial trigger points (Melzack, Stillwell, & Fox, 1977).

Radiofrequency Ablation

Radiofrequency ablation is a process of targeted destruction of nerves that carry the pain signal to the brain (Panchal, 2005). This procedure is conducted under the same conditions as facet joint or epidural injections, except that instead of introducing medications the needle is actually burning the nerve with electrical stimulation to the targeted nerve (Panchal, 2005).

Peripheral Nerve Stimulation and Spinal Cord Stimulation

These procedures involve the surgical implantation of electronic stimulators directly onto the nerves that are generating pain (Schon, 2005). Electronic nerve stimulation is a highly invasive technique that involves a surgical incision and permanent placement of the implantation device. It is therefore reserved for those patients who have not achieved adequate benefit from less invasive procedures (Schon, 2005).

Narcotic Pain Medication: Addiction or Undertreatment?

Physiological forces may also thwart attempts to control chronic pain conditions. The stimulating or modulating neurophysiological system pathways produce both euphoria (opiate based) and pain modulation (Sagen & Proudfit, 1985; Woolf, 1992). In a person with persistent pain conditions there is an increased responsiveness of spinal cord neurons and excitation of the central nervous system (CNS) resulting in a hypersensitized state of pain perception and hyperexcitability in the spinal cord neurons (Curatolo et al., 2001). Persistent irritation to these neurons stimulates a release of glutamate and nitric oxide which researchers have hypothesized may contribute to long-term neuroplastic changes in pain transmission (Meller & Gebhart, 1993; Neugebauer, Weidong, Bird, Bhave, & Gereau, 2003). This hyperexcitability coupled with glutamate-induced injury may result in dramatic permanent changes in the reaction of the CNS to sensory inputs—in other words, pain that is highly exaggerated in quality and quantity as well as resistant to usual treatment methods (Abrams, 2000; Koob & LeMoal, 2001). Compounds that produce analgesia as well as intensely pleasurable feelings are self-reinforcing (i.e., the drugs produce an effect that the user wants to experience repeatedly). Clinical confusion occurs in a chronic pain situation with long-term administration of opiates when development of tolerance, withdrawal, and hyperalgesia occurs, which may in fact mimic substance misuse syndromes.

Opiate pain relievers increase cell firing and stimulate dopamine (DA) release in the nucleus accumbens (NA) by decreasing presynaptic GABA release on the dopaminergic cells (Portenoy & Payne, 1992). The DA response in the NA is perceived as a "rush" of well-being that is highly rewarding and reinforcing (Portenoy & Payne, 1992). The gray matter adjacent to the third ventricle along with myriad other limbic structures are highly responsive to opiates (Fields & Basbaum, 1999; Morgan, Heinricher, & Fields, 1992). Prolonged activation of pain receptors in these areas increases second-order responses, overrides analgesic effect, and produces hyperalgesia, manifesting as decreased tolerance to pain or increased neuroadaptive tolerance of the opiate (Colpaert et al., 2001). In other words, it appears as if the person is now "hooked" on the narcotic pain reliever.

Understanding the nuances involved in physiological dependence, or neuroadaptive processes of the brain to specific drugs such as opiate, is critical. First and foremost, physiological dependence is the expected response to repeated opiate administration. This process includes both tolerance to effects of a drug and physical withdrawal symptoms to discontinuation of drug.

Case Study

Bill is a 36-year-old single farmer who was injured in a motor vehicle accident when the ambulance in which he was riding was struck by an oncoming truck during a routine trip. Subsequent to the accident Bill developed severe back, neck, and shoulder pain resulting from several herniated discs and entrapped spinal nerves. Despite multiple surgical interventions including spinal fusion and epidural and facet joint injections Bill remains unresponsive to treatment. Bill has been referred by his pain management specialist for evaluation of failed pharmacological interventions to help him with his pain. He is currently using a fentanyl patch (50 µg every 3 days), gabapentin (1200 mg a day), and Vicodin (acetaminophen/hydrocodone combination) two 500mg/5mg tablets every 4 hours. The pain management specialist was concerned that Bill was "overusing" his pain medication and possibly exaggerating his pain. He based this conclusion on Bill's escalating frustration during his treatment visits and his requests for either more medication or "something stronger."

The first session with Bill included a review of his preinjury activities and behaviors in addition to an agreement to allow the therapist to obtain his medical records and have regular contact with his health care providers, immediate family members, and pharmacist. Bill was agreeable to "anything that would help" even though he felt personally "insulted" that he had been sent to a "shrink." It was noted that Bill stood approximately 6'7" tall with a thin body type. He described his preinjury activities as working as an emergency medical technician on an ambulance on the weekends and running his farm during the week. Bill was responsible for several hundred head of cattle, which required him to ride a horse twice daily to check on them and to herd them either to a pasture or back to the barn. In addition he had 350 acres of land that was planted in grain and hay to feed his livestock. Bill was also required to lift 50-pound sacks of grain into feeding troughs during the colder months and to assist his animals physically when they gave birth to new calves. Bill was very proud of the fact that he maintained his farm alone and was very successful, enabling him to build a four-bedroom home for himself and a smaller home for his parents.

Bill's description of his premorbid activity was not consistent with someone who intended to malinger or exaggerate his physical symptoms. In fact, he was much more at risk for overexerting himself and now allowing for recovery time for his injuries due to his massive physical workload. This information, in addition to his physical stature, was taken into account when evaluating Bill's complaints that he was undermedicated.

BILL: I can take a lot of pain. I have to in order to take care of my animals, but this is ridiculous! And no one believes me!

THERAPIST: What do you mean, no one believes you?

BILL: Those doctors who say I am making this up and sent me to a shrink because it's all in my head!

THERAPIST: What have you been told about your pain medication?

BILL: That I am on the highest doses and if I am still hurting they can't explain it.

THERAPIST: (*Reviews medications, response patterns, and expectations with Bill.*)

BILL: The mornings are the worst! I can't even get out of bed!

THERAPIST: Is there anything that makes the pain better?

BILL: Only if I lie on the couch all day—then who will take care of my animals?

THERAPIST: Is there anything else that helps the pain?

BILL: Sometimes sitting in a hot bath—I feel like a sissy!

THERAPIST: Do you ever use any other medication or drug to help with the pain?

BILL: No, the doctors told me not to mess with the pills because they might not work right.

THERAPIST: What about alcohol?

BILL: To tell the truth I have had a beer or two almost every night even though they told me not to. It's the only way to get to sleep. But it only lasts about 3 hours then I'm up again hurting like crazy!

At this point the therapist is considering the possibility that Bill is suffering from "breakthrough" pain as a result of pain levels dropping during the times in between oral dosing of medication. He is also sleep deprived, which is likely to increase his pain levels, lower his frustration tolerance, and decrease his energy. There is also a possibility that due to Bill's large stature, the dose of 50 µg of fentanyl is under the metabolic window for his body size and type. In other words, Bill is metabolizing his medication too rapidly for it to be fully effective.

THERAPIST: Would you be interested in ways to help yourself improve the effects of the pain medications that you are taking?

BILL: What do you mean?

THERAPIST: We can use certain training techniques to work with your thoughts and your activities to help the medication instead of fight it.

BILL: I am all for anything that would help at this point.

THERAPIST: Let's start with some relaxation training techniques that you can use while you are resting to help your muscles relax. That will help them heal more effectively.

BILL: OK. I don't have any problem with learning something new as long as it helps.

The therapist, with Bill's permission, contacted the patient's pharmacy and family to verify Bill's story. A review of Bill's pharmacy records confirmed that he was filling his medication as ordered and had not attempted to fill any "lost" prescriptions. Bill's family confirmed his reports regarding his preinjury activity levels and his pride in being a hard worker. The therapist then contacted the pain management specialist and discussed her concerns that Bill might be undermedicated based on his preinjury behavior, his pain level reports, and his physical stature. The therapist recommended a longer-acting oral medication that would last through the night to assist Bill in sleeping. In addition, the pain specialist added gabapentin to reduce neuropathic pain transmission and venlafaxine to augment the opiate pain relievers and decrease his depressive symptoms and his fentanyl patch was increased to 75 µg every 3 days.

Bill's symptoms showed a marked decrease with the change in medication along with relaxation training. He continued to overexert himself, but it was determined that he had limited his activities as much as possible given his responsibilities for his farm management. Once Bill's level of pain and frustration were under control he was more amenable to additional techniques to help him cope with the significant changes in his professional roles. Given that the hallmark of problematic substance misuse is loss of control over one's use of the substance, it was determined that Bill did not meet any of the criteria of substance dependence. He did not demonstrate loss of control (e.g., intent to stop without ability to stop) or deliberate adjunctive use of other chemicals in addition to his pain relievers for purposes of mood alteration. If it had been determined that Bill was using his medications to help him sleep, or refilling his prescriptions too often with intent to alter his mood, or had lied about his preinjury activity levels, the therapist would have reinforced compliance to the current regime of therapy as opposed to advocating for improved pain control.

CONCLUSION

Patients who experience severe, disabling chronic pain often experience psychological disruptions that include panic, depression, and possibly suicidal or violent thoughts. The therapist working with this group of patients is often witness to disruptive emotional behaviors such as panic and anger as well as argumentative, catastrophic behavior. Socializing the patient to the cognitive therapy treatment program improves the likelihood that he/she will be able to respond positively should one of these episodes threaten his/her, or others', safety. The therapist helps patients to identify the cognitive distortions that limit their ability to respond and attend to physical treatments as well as decrease their enjoyment of life outside their pain experience. Therapists should have a basic working knowledge of the physical interventions their patients are likely to experience in order to support their patients during these processes and prepare them for the experience if needed. In addition, it is important to separate those symptoms that indicate exaggerated psychological suffering as opposed to extreme physical suffering. Having a good working knowledge about medication management options and potential problems with controlled medication symptoms is also critical. Patients who feel they are undertreated or misunderstood are more likely to discontinue use of therapeutic interventions and/or experience catastrophic feelings when overwhelmed.

The therapist needs to maintain a full list of all medications that an individual is taking in addition to maintaining lines of communication with other health care providers and family members to ensure that the individual is using this intervention appropriately. It is very easy to develop a negative response to this population of patients and to jump to conclusions that lack of response to treatment may be the fault of the patient. A thorough understanding of assessment processes, ongoing monitoring, and medical/pharmacological interventions are imperative.

REFERENCES

Abrams, S. E. (2000). Pain pathways and mechanisms. In S. E. Abram & J. D. Haddox (Eds.), *The pain clinic manual* (2nd ed, pp. 20–32). Philadelphia: Lippincott Williams & Wilkins.

American Pain Society. (1999). *Chronic pain in America: Roadblocks to relief.* Retrieved December 5, 2005, from *www.painfoundation.org/page.asp?file=Library/PainSurveys.htm.*

Bailey, K. P. (2003). Physical symptoms comorbid with depression and the new antidepressant duloxetine. *Journal of Psychosocial Nursing and Mental Health Services, 41*(12), 13–18.

Bergner, M., Bobbitt, R. A., Carter, W. B., & Gilson, B. S. (1981). The Sickness Impact Profile: Development and final revision of a health status measure. *Medical Care, 19*(8), 787–805.

Bruns, D., & Disorbio, M. (2000). Hostility and violent ideation: Physical rehabilitation patient and community samples. *Pain Medicine, 1,* 131–139.

Caudill, M. A. (2001). *Managing pain before it manages you* (rev. ed.). New York: Guilford Press.

Choban, P. S., Onyejekwe, J., Burge, J. C., & Flancbaum, L. (1999). A health status assessment of the impact of weight loss following Roux-en-Y gastric bypass for clinically severe obesity. *Journal of the American College of Surgeons, 188*(5), 491–497.

Colpaert, F. C., Tarayre, J. P., Alliaga, M., Bruins, L. A., Attal, N., & Koek, W. (2001). Opiate self-administration as a measure of chronic nociceptive pain in arthritic rats. *Pain, 91,* 33–45.

Coluzzi, F., & Mattia, C. (2005). Mechanism-based treatment in chronic neuropathic pain: The role of antidepressants. *Current Pharmaceutical Design, 11*(23), 2945–2960.

Coughlan, G. M., Ridout, K. L., Williams, A. C. D., & Richardson, P. H. (1995). Attrition from pain management programme. *British Journal of Clinical Psychology, 34,* 471–479.

Craig, A. D., & Bushnell, M. C. (1994). The thermal grill illusion: unmasking the burn of cold pain. *Science, 265*(5169), 252–255.

Crowell, M. D., Jones, M. P., Harris, L. A., Dineen, T. N., Schettler, V. A., & Olden, K. W. (2004). Antidepressants in the treatment of irritable bowel syndrome and visceral pain syndromes. *Current Opinion in Investigational Drugs, 5*(7), 736–742.

Curatolo, M., Peterson-Felix, S., Arendt-Nielson, L., Giani, C., Zbinden, A. M., & Radanov, B. P. (2001). Central hypersensitivity in chronic pain after whiplash injury. *Clinical Journal of Pain, 17,* 306–315.

De Vellis, B. M. E. (1993). Depression in rheumatological diseases. In S. Newman & M. Shipley (Eds.), *Psychological aspects of rheumatoid disease* (Vol. 7, pp. 241–257). London: Bailliers Clinical Rheumatology.

deCharms, R. C., Maeda, F., Glover, G. H., Ludlow, D., Pauly, J. M., Soneji, D., et al. (2005). Control over brain activation and pain learned by using real-time functional MRI. *Proceedings of the National Academy of Sciences, USA, 102*(51), 18626–18631.

Eccelston, C. (1994). Chronic pain and attention: A cognitive approach. *British Journal of Clinical Psychology, 33,* 535–547.

Eccelston, C. (1997). Pain and thinking. In V. J. Thomas (Ed.), *Pain: Its nature and management* (pp. 35–53). London: Bailliere Tindall.

Eimer, B. N., & Freeman, A. (1998). *Pain management psychotherapy.* New York: Wiley.

Enna, S. J., & Bowery, N. G. (2004). GABA(B) receptor alterations as indicators of physiological and pharmacological function. *Biochemical Pharmacology, 68*(8), 1541–1548.

Fields, H. L., & Basbaum, A. I. (1999). Central nervous system mechanisms of pain modulation. In P. D. Wall & R. Melzack (Eds.), *Textbook of pain* (pp. 89–147). Edinburgh, Scotland: Churchill Livingstone.

Fishbain, D. A. (1996). Current research on chronic pain and suicide. *American Journal of Public Health, 86,* 1320–1321.

Fishbain, D. A., Cutler, R., Rosomoff, H. L., & Rosomoff, R. S. (2000). Risk for violent behavior in patients with chronic pain: Evaluation and management in the pain facility setting. *Pain Medicine, 1,* 140–155.

Fishman, S. (2004). The role of the pain psychologist. Retrieved December 1, 2005, from *www.painfoundation.org/page.asp?file=QandA/Psychologist.htm*

Gallagher, R. M., & Verma, S. (1999). Managing pain and comorbid depression: A public health challenge. *Seminars in Clinical Neuropsychiatry, 4*(3), 203–220.

Gil, K. M., Abrams, S. E., Phillips, G., & Keefe, F. J. (1989). Sickle cell disease pain: Relations of coping strategies to adjustment. *Journal of Consulting and Clinical Psychology, 57,* 725–731.

Goldberg, D., & Williams, P. (1988). *User's guide to the General Health Questionnaire.* Hampshire, UK: NFER Nelson.

Hamner, M. B., & Robert, S. (2005). Emerging roles for atypical antipsychotics in chronic posttraumatic stress disorder. *Expert Review of Neurotherapeutics, 5*(2), 267–275.

Kazantzis, N., & Lampropoulos, G. K. (2002a). Reflecting on homework in psychotherapy: What can we conclude from research and experience? *Journal of Clinical Psychology, 58*(5), 577–585.

Kazantzis, N., & Lampropoulos, G. K. (2002b). The use of homework in psychotherapy: An introduction. *Journal of Clinical Psychology, 58*(5), 487–488.

Kerns, R. D., Turk, D. C., & Rudy, T. E. (1985). The West Haven–Yale Multidimensional Pain Inventory (WHYMPI). *Pain, 23*(4), 345–356.

Koob, G. F., & LeMoal, M. (2001). Drug addiction, dysregulation of reward and allostasis. *Neuropsychopharmacology, 24*(2), 97–129.

Kornick, C. A., Santiago-Palma, J., Moryl, N., Payne, R., & Obbens, E. A. (2003). Benefit–risk assessment of transdermal fentanyl for the treatment of chronic pain. *Drug Safety, 26*(13), 951–973.

Leung, A. Y. (2005). Acupuncture. In M. S. Wallace & P. S. Staats (Eds.), *Pain medicine and pain management: Just the facts* (pp. 260–265). New York: McGraw-Hill.

Lewandowski, W., Good, M., & Draucker, C. B. (2005). Changes in the meaning of pain with the use of guided imagery. *Pain Management Nursing, 6*(2), 58–67.

Linton, S. J. (1994). Chronic back pain: Integrating psychological and physical therapy—an overview. *Behavioral Medicine, 20*(3), 101–104.

Lynch, M. E. (2005). A review of the use of methadone for the treatment of chronic noncancer pain. *Pain Research and Management, 10*(3), 133–144.

Malinoff, H. L., Barkin, R. L., & Wilson, G. (2005). Sublingual buprenorphine is effective in the treatment of chronic pain syndrome. *American Journal of Therapeutics, 12*(5), 379–384.

McCracken, L. M., Zayfert, C., & Gross, R. T. (1992). The Bain Anxiety Symptom Scale: Development and validation of a scale to measure fear of pain. *Pain, 50*(1), 67–73.

Meller, S. T., & Gebhart, G. E. (1993). Nitric Oxide (NO) and nociceptive processing in the spinal cord. *Pain, 52*, 127–136.

Melzack, R., Stillwell, D. M., & Fox, E. J. (1977). Trigger points and acupuncture points for pain: Correlations and implications. *Pain, 3*, 3–23.

Melzack, R., & Wall, P. D. (1965). Pain mechanisms: A new theory. *Science, 150*(699), 971–979.

Morgan, M. M., Heinricher, M. M., & Fields, H. L. (1992). Circuitry linking opioid-sensitive nociceptive modulatory systems in periaqueductal gray and spinal cord with rostral ventromedial medulla. *Neuroscience, 57*, 411–418.

Muriel, C., Failde, I., Mico, J. A., Neira, M., & Sanchez-Magro, I. (2005). Effectiveness and tolerability of the buprenorphine transdermal system in patients with moderate to severe chronic pain: A multicenter, open-label, uncontrolled, prospective, observational clinical study. *Clinical Therapeutics, 27*(4), 451–462.

Neugebauer, V., Weidong, L., Bird, G. C., Bhave, G., & Gereau, R. W. (2003). Synaptic plasticity in the amygdala in a model of arthritic pain: Differential roles of metabotropic glutamate receptors 1 and 2. *Journal of Neuroscience, 23*(1), 52–63.

Nicholas, M. K. (1989). *Self-efficacy in chronic pain.* Edinburgh, Scotland: St. Andrews University.

Panchal, S. J. (2005). Radiofrequency ablation. In M. S. Wallace & P. S. Staats (Eds.), *Pain medicine and pain management: Just the facts* (pp. 309–314). New York: McGraw-Hill.

Perez, J., Ware, M. A., Chevalier, S., Gougeon, R., & Shir, Y. (2005). Dietary omega-3 fatty acids may be associated with increased neuropathic pain in nerve-injured rats. *Anesthesia and Analgesia, 101*(2), 444–448.

Portenoy, R. K., & Payne, R. (1992). Acute and chronic pain. In J. H. Lowinson, P. Ruiz, R. B. Millman & J. G. Langrod (Eds.), *Substance abuse: A comprehensive textbook* (2nd ed., pp. 691–721). Philadelphia: Lippincott Williams & Wilkins.

Ramamurthy, S. (2005). Facet joint blocks. In M. S. Wallace & P. S. Staats (Eds.), *Pain medicine and pain management: Just the facts* (p. 295). New York: McGraw-Hill.

Roehrs, T., & Roth, T. (2005). Sleep and pain: Interaction of two vital functions. *Seminars in Neurology, 25*(1), 106–116.

Rosenthiel, A. K., & Keefe, F. J. (1983). The use of coping strategies in chronic low back pain patients: Relationship to patient characteristics and current adjustment. *Pain, 17*, 33–44.

Rowlingson, J. C. (2005). Epidural steroid injections. In M. S. Wallace & P. S. Staats (Eds.), *Pain medicine and pain management: Just the facts* (pp. 289–294). New York: McGraw-Hill.

Sagen, J., & Proudfit, H. K. (1985). Evidence for pain modulation by pre- and post-synaptic noradrenergic receptors in the medulla oblongata. *Brain Research, 331*, 285–293.

Samborski, W., Lezanska-Szpera, M., & Rybakowski, J. K. (2004). Effects of antidepressant mirtazapine on fibromyalgia symptoms. *Roczniki Akademii Medycznej w Bialymstoku, 49*, 265–269.

Sareen, J., Cox, B. J., Clara, I., & Asmundson, G. J. (2005). The relationship between anxiety disorders and physical disorders in the U.S. National Comorbidity Survey. *Depression and Anxiety, 21*(4), 193–202.

Schon, L. C. (2005). Peripheral nerve stimulation. In M. S. Wallace & P. S. Staats (Eds.), *Pain medicine and pain management: Just the facts* (pp. 315–317). New York: McGraw-Hill.

Seaman, D. R. (2002). The diet-induced proinflammatory state: A cause of chronic pain and other degenerative diseases? *Journal Manipulative and Physiological Therapeutics, 25*(3), 168–179.

Strahl, C., Kleinknecht, R. A., & Dinnel, D. L. (2000). The role of pain anxiety, coping, and pain self-efficacy in rheumatoid arthritis patient functioning. *Behavior Research and Therapy, 38*(9), 863–873.

Thomas, V. J. (2005). Cognitive behavioural therapy in the management of chronic pain. In S. M. Freeman & A. Freeman (Eds.), *Cognitive behavior therapy in nursing practice* (pp. 145–166). New York: Springer.

Vlaeyen, J. W. S., Geurts, S. M., Koler-Snijders, A. M. J., Boeren, R. G. B., & van Eck, H. (1995). *Fear of movement in chronic low back pain and its relation to performance.*

Wasan, A. D., Wootton, J., & Jamison, R. N. (2005). Dealing with difficult patients in your pain practice. *Regional Anesthesia and Pain Medicine, 30*(2), 184–192.

White, C. A. (2001). Chronic pain. In C. A. White (Ed.), *Cognitive behaviour therapy for chronic medical problems* (pp. 123–146). New York: Wiley.

Williams, D. A., & Thorn, B. E. (1989). An empirical assessment of pain beliefs. *Pain, 36*(3), 351–358.

Wolf, N. (1990). *The beauty myth.* New York: Harper Perennial.

Woolf, C. J. (1992). Excitability changes in central neurons following peripheral damage: Role of central sensitization in the pathogenesis of pain. In W. Willis (Ed.), *Hyperalgesia and allodynia* (pp. 221–243). New York: Raven Press.

SUGGESTED READINGS

Caudill, M. A. (2001). *Managing pain before it manages you* (rev. ed.). New York: Guilford Press.

Eimer, B. N., & Freeman, A. (1998). *Pain management psychotherapy.* New York: Wiley.

Thorn, B. E. (2004). *Cognitive therapy for chronic pain: A step-by-step guide.* New York: Guilford Press.

Wallace, M. S., & Staats, P. S. (Eds.), *Pain medicine and pain management: Just the facts.* New York: McGraw-Hill.

Winterowd, C., Beck, A. T., & Gurener, D. (2003). *Cognitive therapy with chronic pain patients.* New York: Springer.

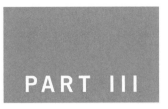

PART III

Child and Family Crises

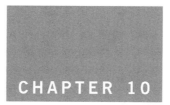

CHAPTER 10

Child Sexual Abuse

Anne Hope Heflin
Esther Deblinger

*C*hild sexual abuse (CSA) is a public health problem that affects children in all ethnic, racial, educational, and socioeconomic groups (Sedlak & Broadhurst, 1996; Wyatt & Peters, 1986). Unfortunately, most graduate programs in mental health disciplines offer little or no formal training in how to recognize, evaluate, and intervene in cases of child sexual abuse. Because of this lack of training, mental health professionals often do not respond in the most effective way to the crisis precipitated by a child's disclosure of sexual abuse. Thus they may miss a crucial opportunity to influence the response of the family as well as the system of professionals involved with the child in ways that facilitate a positive outcome for the child.

This chapter is written to provide professionals with some of the information needed to respond effectively to the crisis of a CSA disclosure. In the first portion of the chapter, information is provided regarding the phenomenon of CSA, professional responses to abuse, recognition and reporting of abuse, and the subsequent investigations. In the next part of the chapter, a guide to practice is offered, which provides suggestions for the clinician faced with assisting the child and his/her family through the crisis of a CSA disclosure. Finally, the third section of the chapter provides a case study that illustrates the process of responding to clients who are in the midst of the crisis of a disclosure of CSA.

PREVALENCE

Although it is widely agreed that sexual abuse is a significant societal problem, it is difficult to ascertain how many children are affected by sexual abuse in the United States. This difficulty occurs because many cases go unreported to mental health, social service, and law enforcement professionals; definitive medical evidence of abuse is typically lacking; and there are no psychological symptoms characteristic of and specific to sexual abuse (London, Bruck, Ceci, & Shuman, 2005). However, a number of attempts have been made to clarify the prevalence of CSA. Perhaps, most notably, a series of federally funded national incidence studies have been pursued to identify the frequency of CSA in the United States. Most recently, the Third National Incidence Study of Child Abuse and Neglect (NIS-3) provided estimates of the incidence of child abuse and neglect in the United States during 1993. The study relied on reports from child protective services as well as from professionals in 166 public schools and daycare centers, hospitals, public health departments, and law enforcement agencies (Sedlak & Broadhurst, 1996). The findings of this study indicated that approximately 300,200 children (4.5 per 1,000) in the United States experienced sexual abuse during 1993. This incidence rate had more than doubled since the Second National Incidence Study, which was conducted in 1986. However, these figures undoubtedly still underestimated the actual rates of CSA. The study did not include cases of sexual abuse perpetrated by noncaretakers. Furthermore, the study did not include the many cases of CSA of which professionals are not aware. The Fourth National Incidence Study of Child Abuse and Neglect is currently ongoing, with data being collected between September 2005 and May 2006 (Administration for Children and Families, U.S. Department of Health and Human Services, n.d.). The project is scheduled for completion in February 2008.

More accurate statistics concerning the lifetime prevalence rates of CSA may be gleaned from retrospective surveys of adult community samples. For example, Finkelhor, Hotaling, Lewis, and Smith (1990) conducted a national telephone survey and found that 27% of adult females and 16% of adult males surveyed suffered contact sexual victimization before the age of 18. Similarly, Elliott and Briere (1992) mailed a questionnaire to a stratified random sample of professional women throughout the United States and found that 26.9% of women reported experiencing sexual abuse prior to the age of 16. Boney-McCoy and Finkelhor (1995) looked at prevalence rates in a nationally representative sample of youth between the ages of 10 and 16 in the United States. During telephone interviews, 15.3% of the females and 5.9% of the males in that age group reported that they had experienced sexual assault. The discrepancy between the incidence rates reported by professionals during a given year and the lifetime prevalence rates reported retrospectively by CSA victims highlights the need for increased recognition and reporting of suspected cases of CSA. These steps are critical both to prevent further victimization and to lessen the long-term impact of CSA.

IMPACT

The psychosocial impact of CSA is widely variable (Saywitz, Mannarino, Berliner, & Cohen, 2000). Investigations have demonstrated that CSA survivors seem to be affected by their abusive experiences in different ways and to different degrees (Kendall-Tackett, Williams, & Finkelhor, 1993). Some survivors appear to suffer minimal or no apparent effects; others develop severe social and or psychiatric problems including behavior problems (such as aggression or sexualized behaviors during childhood), substance abuse, sexual dysfunction during adulthood, major depression, suicidal tendencies, and fears (Beitchman et al., 1992; Boney-McCoy & Finkelhor, 1995; Briere & Elliott, 1994; Kendall-Tackett et al., 1993; McLeer, Deblinger, Henry, & Orvaschel, 1992; Neumann, Housekamp, Pollock, & Briere, 1996). Although research has not found evidence for a specific, cohesive post-sexual abuse syndrome (Beitchman et al., 1992; Kendall-Tackett et al., 1993), studies do indicate that more than 50% of sexually abused children exhibit symptoms of posttraumatic stress disorder (PTSD) while 32–48% of clinical samples of sexually abused children meet full criteria for the diagnosis (Ackerman, Newton, McPherson, Jones, & Dykman, 1998; Famularo, Kinscherff, & Fenton, 1992; McLeer et al., 1992; Saywitz et al., 2000).

Studies also have demonstrated that certain patterns of cognitions—such as self-blame for negative events, feelings of being different from peers, lower interpersonal trust, belief that the world is a dangerous place, maladaptive attitudes toward sexuality (including both a preoccupation with and an aversion to sexuality), and negative body image—are more common among children who have been sexually abused than among those who have not (Cohen, Deblinger, Maedel, & Stauffer, 1999; Heflin, Mears, Deblinger, & Steer, 1997; Mannarino & Cohen, 1996; Noll, Trickett, & Putman, 2003; Owens, Chard, 2001).

Numerous researchers have attempted to identify factors that might explain the differential effects of CSA. Although the findings have been somewhat inconsistent, several variables have been associated repeatedly with more severe reactions. Sexual abuse perpetrated by a person who is in a close relationship with the child appears to result in more severe postabuse symptomatology than abuse by someone in a more distant relationship with the child (Beitchman et al., 1992; Briere & Runtz, 1988; Kendall-Tackett et al., 1993; Noll et al., 2003; Wyatt & Newcomb, 1990). However, closeness has not been defined in any consistent way. Often, it is determined by degree of kinship, although it might be more appropriate to measure the degree of emotional connection between the child and the perpetrator (Kendall-Tackett et al., 1993). The number of perpetrators also appears to mediate the effects of abuse, with experiences with more than one perpetrator being associated with increased levels of psychological distress (Steel, Sanna, Hammond, Whipple, & Cross, 2004). The threat of force or the use of force in CSA also has been associated with more negative outcomes (Beitchman et al., 1992; Briere & Elliott, 1994; Kendall-Tackett et al., 1993; Russell, 1986; Steel et al., 2004). In addition, more invasive or intimate sexual contact has been linked to more traumatic reactions (Beitchman et al., 1992; Kendall-Tackett et al., 1993; Peters, 1988; Tufts New England Medical Center, 1984). Again, though, the invasiveness of the abuse has been operationalized in a variety of ways, making it difficult to compare the findings of some studies. The most common means of measuring invasiveness is to categorize the abuse according to whether it involved penetration (which might be vaginal, anal, or oral). There also is some suggestion that greater duration and higher frequency of abuse may be associated with increased postabuse symptomatology (Kendall-Tackett et al., 1993; Steel et al., 2004; Steel, Wilson, Cross, & Whipple, 1996). However, isolated violent sexual assaults are also associated with high levels of postabuse symptoms, making it difficult to identify simple, linear relationships between duration and frequency of abuse and subsequent symptoms (Beitchman et al., 1992). Unfortunately, although the information described above is useful in identifying abuse-related variables that may influence the child's postabuse adjustment, these abuse-related variables are inherent and immutable aspects of the abuse and, therefore, cannot be targets for intervention (Conte & Schuerman, 1987).

Another class of variables that may mediate the outcome of sexual abuse experiences and also may be amenable to intervention is cognitive attributions regarding the abuse. For example, negative attributional style, abuse-specific internal attributions, feelings of powerlessness, stigmatization, and shame have been associated with higher levels of psychopathology and distress, including PTSD symptoms, depression, and low self-esteem (Feiring & Taska, 2005; Feiring, Taska, & Chen, 2002; Feiring, Taska, & Lewis, 2002; Kallstrom-Fuqua, Weston, & Marshall, 2004). Furthermore, these relationships have been found to persist over time. A pessimistic attributional style and high levels of shame at the time of abuse discovery have been associated with depression and lowered self-esteem 1 year later (Feiring, Taska, & Lewis, 2002). High levels of shame have been associated with clinically significant levels of intrusive memories 6 years postabuse discovery (Feiring & Taska, 2005). Similarly, internalization of childhood abuse has been found to be associated with psychological distress in adulthood (Steel et al., 2004). A sense of powerlessness and stigmatization has been associated with women's psychological distress in adulthood (Kallstrom-Fuqua et al., 2004). The relationships between these cognitive variables and negative outcomes have been consistent even after the effects of abuse-related variables have been controlled (Feiring, Taska, & Chen, 2002; Feiring, Taska, & Lewis, 2002; Kallstrom-Fuqua et al., 2004). Thus, interventions that focus on the child's cognitive processing of the abuse would seem to be a productive focus of treatment.

Variables associated with the nonoffending parents have also been identified as moderating variables that may be amenable to therapeutic interventions. Specifically, support provided by nonoffending parents to children who have suffered sexual abuse has been identified as a moderating variable that may be amenable to change. The findings of a series of investigations, in fact, show that children's postabuse adjustment may be influenced significantly by the level of support they receive from nonoffending adults following disclosure of the abuse (Conte & Schuerman, 1987; Everson, Hunter, Runyon, Edelson, & Coulter, 1989; Feiring, Taska, & Lewis, 1998; Friedrich, Luecke,

Beilke, & Place, 1992; Spaccarelli & Fuchs, 1997). Indeed, Everson et al. (1989) found that children's postabuse adjustment was more closely linked to maternal support than to the nature or duration of abuse or to the child's relationship to the offender. Given evidence suggesting that as many as one-third of nonoffending guardians vacillate in their support of the abused child following disclosure (Bolen & Lamb, 2004), clinicians have both an opportunity and a responsibility to help those parents or guardians process their own reactions to the disclosure so that they can be available to support their child in the most effective manner possible.

Recent evidence also indicates that maternal levels of psychiatric symptoms or distress may be linked to children's postabuse outcomes (Deblinger, Steer, & Lippmann, 1999; Deblinger, Taub, Maedel, Lippmann, & Stauffer, 1997; Runyon, Hunter, & Everson, 1992). Runyon et al. (1992) reported that in addition to support variables, maternal psychiatric symptoms appeared to contribute significantly to the prediction of sexually abused children's adjustment difficulties. Deblinger et al. (1999) found that mother's severity of depression was positively related to children's PTSD symptoms and parent-reported internalizing behaviors.

Researchers have extended the examination of the influence of parental support and emotional distress to the outcome of treatment for children who have been sexually abused. Friedrich et al. (1992) found that initial levels of maternal support and depression were significantly related to the outcome of therapy with sexually abused boys. Similarly, Cohen and Mannarino (1996) found that parental emotional distress was significantly related to the presence of both internalizing symptoms and behavior problems among sexually abused preschool children at the end of treatment, regardless of whether the children received cognitive-behavioral treatment or nondirective supportive therapy.

More general assessments of family functioning also indicate that the overall quality of family relationships may be associated with the adjustment of sexually abused children. For example, Friedrich, Urquiza, and Beilke (1986) found that increased family conflict and less cohesive family functioning were related to greater behavioral symptoms in sexually abused children. Similarly, Oates, O'Toole, Lynch, Stern, and Cooney (1994) found that family functioning was a critical variable influencing the adjustment of CSA victims. Kouyoumdjian, Perry, and Hansen (2005) found that parents and teachers have negative expectations about the outcomes for sexually abused children and suggest that these expectations may negatively influence the children's recovery. Friedrich et al. (1992) found that a high degree of family conflict was associated with a negative outcome of therapy with sexually abused boys. Finally, preliminary evidence indicates that the type of parenting style utilized may be related to the symptoms exhibited by children who have been sexually abused. Deblinger et al. (1999) found that in a sample of 100 children who had been sexually abused, those who perceived their mothers' parenting style to be rejecting reported increased levels of depressive symptomatology. In addition, the perceived use of guilt and anxiety-provoking parenting methods was associated with higher levels of PTSD symptoms and parent-reported externalizing behavior problems.

In summary, these findings suggest that nonoffending parents play a crucial role in influencing their children's postabuse adjustment as well as their response to therapy. Indeed, the nonoffending parents may be their children's greatest potential "natural resource." Thus one of the most effective ways in which mental health professionals can assist sexually abused children may be by helping their nonoffending parents to overcome those psychosocial difficulties that impede their ability to be therapeutic and supportive to their children.

PROFESSIONAL RESPONSE

Although there have been enormous advances in the last several decades in our recognition of and response to CSA, many professionals continue to find themselves ill prepared for the events precipitated by a child's disclosure of sexual abuse. Frequently such a disclosure creates a crisis for the child and his/her family, which requires an appropriate and effective response from the clinician. Although a child's disclosure may set off a significant period of psychological turmoil, it also represents a new beginning free from the secrecy and shame associated with the sexual abuse. Moreover, during such a crisis, the child and his/her family may be more amenable to outside help, providing the therapist with a unique opportunity to stimulate positive growth and change. Given the widespread prevalence and the highly disruptive impact of CSA, it is essential for all human services professionals to be prepared to respond to a suspicion or disclosure of CSA. Unfortunately, few graduate programs offer formal training in the area of child abuse. Thus many clinicians find themselves poorly prepared to assist a child during such a crisis. In addition to the lack of appropriate training regarding sexual abuse, professionals may experience personal discomfort regarding the issue, which can compromise their response to the situation. As a result, many well-meaning professionals may be unprepared to identify or inquire about such childhood trauma. They may also find it difficult to respond calmly and effectively to a spontaneous disclosure. Thus, in addition to obtaining formal training regarding CSA, the clinician preparing to offer crisis intervention may need to explore his/her professional attitudes and personal feelings regarding this disturbing problem. Professional attitudes that may interfere with recognition and effective intervention in cases of CSA may stem from personal biases as well as common misconceptions. Perhaps the most fundamental bias may be reflected in personal perceptions regarding the prevalence of CSA. Clearly, individuals who continue to view CSA as a rare phenomenon, despite the prevalence data reported earlier, are less likely to recognize or inquire about this childhood trauma. Because many survivors of sexual abuse do not spontaneously report CSA as a presenting complaint (Femina, Yeager, & Lewis, 1990; London et al., 2005), clinicians who do not routinely screen for such trauma are less likely to identify victimization in their clients. In fact, the findings of two investigations demonstrated that when clinicians were given specific instructions to inquire directly about CSA, the rates of sexual abuse reports increased elevenfold for adult psychiatric patients (Briere & Zaidi, 1989) and fourfold for child psychiatric patients (Lanktree, Briere, & Zaidi, 1991). These findings strongly suggest that direct inquiry is essential to (1) the identification of CSA victims, (2) the formulation of appropriate diagnoses and treatment plans, and (3) the possible prevention of further victimization.

Social biases also can interfere with effective recognition, reporting, and intervention in CSA cases. Kelley (1990), for example, found that such biases influence the practices and attitudes of professionals in the field. Specifically, many professionals demonstrated more tolerance and recommended less severe punishments for offenders with high social status. In addition, they considered the effects of the sexual abuse to be more severe when the offender represented a lower social status. Suspected cases of CSA should be evaluated and treated equally regardless of the alleged offender's social and demographic characteristics. This may be accomplished only if clinicians make active efforts to acknowledge and counter their personal biases and prejudices. Sex offenders are not easily identifiable and they do not generally fit the "dirty old man" or "perverted stranger" stereotypes. Rather, many offenders are trusted individuals who appear to be highly regarded in their communities, successful in their work, and particularly engaging with children.

There is also evidence that gender bias may influence professional and personal attitudes toward CSA victims. Lab, Feigenbaum, and De Silva (2000) reported that psychologists, psychiatrists, and nurses at a large teaching hospital rarely inquired about sexual abuse in males and had extremely variable knowledge of prevalence rates of sexual abuse among boys. The findings of several investigations suggest a tendency to minimize the impact of CSA on male victims as opposed to female victims (Eisenberg, Owens, & Dewey, 1987; Kelley, 1990). Furthermore, Kelley (1990) found that professionals tended to recommend less severe punishment for offenders who sexually abused boys. In addition, Stauffer and Deblinger (1996) found that mothers of sexually abused boys were less likely to participate in therapy than mothers of victimized girls, perhaps due to their underestimation of the impact of CSA on boys. To date, however, the empirical evidence that exists generally has not demonstrated that CSA is any less traumatic for boys than for girls (Beitchman et al., 1992; Boney-McCoy & Finkelhor, 1995; Jumper, 1995; Kendall-Tackett et al., 1993).

Biases and misconceptions concerning nonoffending mothers of children who have been sexually abused also appear to be widespread. The early clinical literature regarding CSA often depicted mothers in quite negative ways, implicating them as being indirectly responsible for the sexual abuse of their children based on a pattern of denial and collusion (Cormier, Kennedy, & Sangowicz, 1962; Sarles, 1975). However, there is little, if any, empirical data to support that depiction. In fact, the majority of mothers appear to believe and support their children following disclosures of CSA (Deblinger, Stauffer, & Landsberg, 1994; Sirles & Franke, 1989). One recent study by Bolen and Lamb (2004) reported that approximately one-third of nonoffending guardians respond with vacillation in their support of their sexually abused child. These authors suggest that the ambivalence in support most often reflects the conflict in the guardian's feelings for the child and the perpetrator. Furthermore, they suggest that such ambivalence should be viewed as a normal response when the costs of disclosure are very high and the disclosure is a traumatic event for the nonoffending guardian as well as for the child. Nonoffending parents experiencing such conflicts require sensitive and supportive care to help them process their own responses to the disclosure in order to maximize their availability to their child.

Mothers who have their own histories of CSA often have been the subject of particular concern from clinicians. Some clinicians have been concerned that mothers who have such a personal history will be unable to acknowledge and respond appropriately to their child's experience of sexual abuse. On the other hand, other clinicians have suggested that mothers with a personal history of abuse may be predisposed to suspect sexual abuse, even when the evidence does not support such concerns. Several studies have explored the relationships between mothers' personal histories of CSA and maternal levels of emotional distress following their child's disclosure of sexual abuse as well as maternal responses to the child's disclosure (Deblinger et al., 1994; Hiebert-Murphy, 1998; Timmons-Mitchell, Chandler-Holz, & Semple, 1996). The findings of the studies generally do indicate that mothers who have a personal history of child sexual abuse tend to experience greater levels of emotional distress when confronted with their child's abuse experience than do mothers without such a personal history of abuse (Deblinger et al., 1994; Hiebert-Murphy, 1998; Timmons-Mitchell et al., 1996). However, a personal history of sexual abuse does not appear to be related to the mother's belief in her child's disclosure or to her support for the child (Deblinger et al., 1994). These findings underscore the need to design interventions that allow nonoffending parents to assist a child during a crisis of CSA and that also help the parents cope successfully with their own emotional distress.

There is also a common misconception that mothers frequently raise false allegations of CSA to get back at ex-spouses during divorce and custody disputes (Humphreys, 1997). Actually, sexually abused children may be particularly motivated to disclose sexual abuse during separation proceedings due to (1) increased feelings of safety, (2) reduced control by the perpetrator, (3) increased time and enhanced communication with the nonoffending parent, and (4) fear of unsupervised visits with the perpetrator. Interestingly, findings of an empirical investigation revealed that CSA allegations arising during custody disputes were just as likely to be substantiated as sexual abuse allegations in the general population (Thoennes & Tjaden, 1990). However, allegations brought during divorce proceedings often appear to require a greater degree of evidence before they are considered seriously compared with allegations of CSA brought outside divorce proceedings (Humphreys, 1997). Disclosures made during divorce proceedings deserve the same professional response and rigorous investigation afforded to children who disclose abuse under other circumstances. Although false allegations do occur, it is inappropriate for clinicians to assume that disclosures made during custody disputes are less valid than others.

Of course, there are many other biases and misconceptions that can interfere with the appropriate management of suspected cases of CSA. To maintain as much objectivity as possible, it is important that professionals in the field keep abreast of the empirical literature and periodically explore and examine their professional attitudes and potential biases. Such exploration is likely to lead to more effective and responsible practice by enhancing one's awareness of and sensitivity to factors that may inappropriately influence professional responses.

RECOGNITION

Many articles in the clinical literature list signs and symptoms of sexual abuse. However, symptoms that are unique to sexual abuse, such as anogenital injury, sexually transmitted diseases, or evidence of seminal fluids, generally are not observed and are rarely present at the time of the child's disclosure (Bays & Chadwick, 1993; London et al., 2005). On the other hand, many children who have experienced sexual abuse do exhibit fears, regression, withdrawal, behavioral problems, and school difficulties. However, these problems also are exhibited by children who have suffered other childhood traumas or family difficulties. In fact, studies comparing children who have been sexually abused to other psychiatrically disturbed, nonabused children demonstrate few differences (Friedrich, Beilke, & Luecke, 1988; Goldston, Turnquist, & Knutson, 1989). Based on their review of the literature, Kendall-Tackett et al. (1993) suggest that children who have been sexually abused may be no more symptomatic than other clinical, nonabused, children except in their levels of PTSD symptoms and sexualized behaviors. Even PTSD symptoms do not consistently differentiate these children from other nonabused children, as PTSD is not specific to sexual abuse. In fact, any number of traumatic childhood experiences may lead to this disorder. However, the type and quality of the PTSD symptoms exhibited by a child may offer clues regarding the nature of the underlying trauma. Thus sexually abused children may be more likely to exhibit unusual and persistent fears in response to sexual abuse reminders such as bathing or undressing or displays of physical affection. For example, one might carefully evaluate the possibility of sexual abuse for a child who insists on wearing several layers of clothing to bed each night. The behavioral symptom that is most likely to differentiate sexually abused from non–sexually abused children is sexually inappropriate and sexually abusive behaviors (Deblinger, McLeer, Atkins, Ralphe, & Foa, 1989; Friedrich, 1993; Kendall-Tackett et al., 1993; Kolko, Moser, & Weldy, 1988). Children exhibit a range of normal sexual behaviors that tend to reflect age-appropriate sexual curiosity and exploration. However, sexual knowledge inappropriate to the child's age and sexual behaviors that are imitative of adult sexual activity (i.e., oral, anal, and vaginal intercourse) should be considered suggestive of sexual abuse and further explored. Still, it is important for clinicians to recognize that such behaviors are not always the consequence of CSA. Indeed, there are alternative explanations for such behaviors and symptoms that must be considered, including accidental exposure to adult sexual activity or pornography. In summary, the presence of sexualized fears and behaviors should encourage the exploration of underlying sexual abuse in the context of a comprehensive psychological evaluation but should not be viewed as unequivocally indicative of a sexually abusive experience.

Although the behaviors and symptoms described previously may raise suspicions concerning sexual abuse, ultimately a child's disclosure is the most essential piece of evidence in cases of alleged CSA. However, a recent review of the literature suggests that only approximately one-third of adults who experienced CSA retrospectively reported that they disclosed their abuse during their childhood (London et al., 2005). Numerous factors motivate children to remain silent about their abusive experiences.

Children may be verbally or physically threatened into secrecy by their perpetrators; others may remain silent out of embarrassment, shame, or fear that no one will believe them. Some children may maintain the secret in order to avoid family disruption or to protect the perpetrator from imprisonment. Indeed, some studies have documented that children who experience intrafamilial abuse are less likely to disclose or exhibit a greater delay in disclosure than children who experience extrafamilial abuse (Goodman-Brown, Edelstein, Goodman, Jones, & Gordon, 2003; Hanson, Resnick, Saunders, Kilpatrick, & Best, 1999; Smith et al., 2000), although this finding is not consistently reported (London et al., 2005).

When children do disclose their abuse, the disclosure is often delayed (Goodman-Brown et al., 2003; London et al., 2005), with boys appearing to be more reluctant to disclose than girls (DeVoe & Faller, 1999; Goodman-Brown et al., 2003; Gries, Goh, & Cavanaugh, 1996; Stroud, Martens, & Barker, 2000). Studies examining the process of disclosure have historically suggested that the disclosure process commonly is a complex mixture of denials, acknowledgments or revelations, and recantations (Nagel, Putnam, & Noll, 1997; Sorenson & Snow, 1991); however, recent evidence indicates that denials and recantations may be much less common than originally suggested (London et al., 2005). One factor that may influence a child's willingness to disclose sexual abuse is the presence of supportive caretakers. Lawson and Chaffin (1992) found that among children with confirmed cases of sexually transmitted diseases, 63% of those with supportive caretakers (who acknowledged that abuse was a possibility) disclosed, whereas 17% of those with nonsupportive caretakers disclosed.

When studies have focused on children with clearly substantiated experiences of abuse, it has been found that most children do disclose their abuse when interviewed about it directly by a professional (London et al., 2005). This finding suggests that it is critical that professionals involved with these children be knowledgeable regarding current practices in interviewing children whom they suspect have been sexually abused.

REPORTING

All states have laws that require human services professionals to report suspected CSA to the appropriate child protection authorities. The statutes in most states further indicate that any person making such a report in "good faith" will be immune from any civil or criminal liability, whereas professionals who knowingly fail to report suspected CSA will be subject to a penalty in the form of a fine and/or imprisonment. While the states' laws stipulate that reports are mandated on the basis of reasonable suspicions, not concrete evidence, it is well documented that many professionals fail to report suspected cases (Kalichman, Craig, & Follingstad, 1988; Swoboda, Elwork, Sales, & Levine, 1978). Indeed, the Third National Incidence Study (Sedlak & Broadhurst, 1996) reported that child protective services only investigated 42% of the cases of sexual abuse that were identified by professionals. The 58% of cases that were not investigated include both cases in which professionals failed to make a needed report as well as cases in which the child protection agency screened out the case before an investigation was initiated.

Empirical investigations indicate that professionals who fail to report suspected abuse frequently offer the following explanations: (1) lack of certainty that the alleged abuse had occurred, (2) concerns regarding the disruption of the therapeutic process, (3) lack of confidence in the child protection system, and (4) belief that the suspected abuse was not ongoing (Kalichman et al., 1988). Although these concerns are reasonable, they do not mitigate one's responsibility to report suspected abuse. Indeed, mandated reporters such as clinicians cannot ignore the opportunity as well as the responsibility to engage the child protection agency in an effort to assist the child. Flango (1991) found that allegations from mandated reporters were substantiated 40–64% of the time, whereas those made by anonymous reporters were validated 3–25% of the time, suggesting that the allegations described by mandated reporters may be particularly valuable in eliciting assistance for the child. The clinician should make the required report and then allow the child protective agency as well as any law enforcement agencies involved to conduct the investigation. The clinician typically is not responsible for investigating past or present abuse and indeed usually is not able to adequately investigate possible abuse while also ensuring the safety of any children exposed to the alleged perpetrator. Clinicians, therefore, must rely on the child protection and law enforcement agencies in their communities to address these concerns.

MULTIDISCIPLINARY COLLABORATION

When CSA is suspected, a report initiates an investigation that requires the involvement of professionals from many different disciplines, including child protective services, law enforcement, medicine, and mental health. The multidisciplinary response to an allegation of CSA involves a number of different components. The order in which the various processes occur will vary depending on the needs of the child and the policies of the agencies involved. Ideally, the child protection and the law enforcement agencies collaborate in investigating possible abuse. In some locales, multidisciplinary teams work together as formal units, with common work facilities. These facilities are often called child advocacy centers. In other locations, the agencies cooperate in joint investigations in less formal ways, without pooling their resources. Finally, in some locations the agencies work fairly independently, which sometimes has the unfortunate consequence of adding to the child's trauma by requiring multiple interviews. These interviews also may lead to conflicting evidence, which may be challenged by the defense in court (Pence & Wilson, 1994). Thus, whenever possible, it is useful to advocate for the coordination of services by the various agencies involved.

Investigation by the Child Protection Agency

When the child protection agency investigates an allegation of sexual abuse, its purpose is to determine whether sexual abuse actually occurred, so that they can intervene, if necessary, to ensure the child's safety and well-being (Sgroi, Porter, & Blick, 1982). Such an investigation may begin under the auspices of a crisis unit or, in less urgent cases, with the assignment of a specific intake worker. Typically the investigation consists of a series of interviews with the child, the alleged perpetrator, the person to whom the child first disclosed the abuse (if such a disclosure has been made), and other persons involved in the situation. Depending on the results of that initial investigation, the child protection agency may formulate a variety of plans ranging from placing the child in foster care (if the presence of the alleged perpetrator in the home jeopardizes the child's safety) to monitoring the situation to closing the case. At the time of the investigation, the child protection agency may also make a referral to a mental health professional for a psychological evaluation and or psychotherapy.

Investigation by Law Enforcement Officials

In many cases, law enforcement officials also will launch an investigation into the allegations of sexual abuse. The general purpose of that investigation is to determine whether the alleged perpetrator has violated any laws and, thus, whether he/she should be prosecuted (Sgroi et al., 1982). Again, the nature of the investigation by law enforcement officials depends in part on the urgency of the situation. If the alleged abuse is ongoing and the child is currently at risk, the local police may intervene immediately. In other cases, when the allegations are focused on previous events, the police or the local prosecutor's office may initiate an investigation without immediate intervention. The specific procedures used in those interviews vary from area to area. In some offices, anatomically correct dolls or drawings may be used to facilitate the child's interview. In many offices, the interviews are videotaped or audiotaped for possible use later in the legal process.

Medical Examination

Another phase of the multidisciplinary response to an allegation of CSA is the medical examination. In almost all cases of CSA, it is appropriate for the child to receive a thorough medical examination, preferably by a pediatrician or gynecologist (if the victim is a late adolescent) experienced in issues of CSA. This examination is of value for a variety of reasons. First, the examination should be done to diagnose and treat physical injuries and sexually transmitted diseases resulting from the alleged sexual abuse. Second, the examination allows the doctor to answer any worries or concerns that the child might have as a result of the alleged sexual contact. Most often the sexual abuse does not result in any residual physical damage or health problems. Thus, the examination can establish concretely that there are no problems resulting from the abuse, and the physician can provide reassurance that the child's body is healthy and intact. If a child or adolescent is aware of any residual problems that do exist, he/she may benefit by learning the facts about what those difficulties are and how they will be addressed. Third, medical findings that substantiate the allegations of sexual abuse can be important in the legal prosecution of the case. Although it is important that the child receive a medical examination, rarely does that examination need to be scheduled immediately. In most cases, the sexual abuse has been ongoing and the most recent episode may have occurred some time ago. In such situations, an urgent trip to a local hospital emergency room is not indicated. Instead, it would be more appropriate to have the child seen by a physician skilled in the assessment of alleged sexual abuse, if possible, as soon as the physician's schedule permits. In a few cases, there is a more urgent need for an examination. For example, a medical examination should be pursued immediately if the child clearly is suffering physical problems resulting from the abuse. Similarly, if the child reports that an episode of abuse occurred during the previous 72 hours, the medical examination should be conducted immediately as it may yield important forensic medical evidence (e.g., semen) (American Academy of Pediatrics, 1991).

The procedures used in the medical examination vary somewhat depending on the specific needs of the child and the practice of the physician. Most often the child receives a head-to-toe examination, which allows the physician to complete a full health assessment while looking for any extragenital indications of trauma (Finkel & DeJong, 1992). The child's genital and anal areas will be inspected for any evidence of acute or chronic trauma (Finkel & DeJong, 1992). That examination may be completed with the use of a colposcope, an instrument that provides light, magnification, and the capacity to obtain photographic or video documentation. During the examination, the physician collects oral, vaginal, and rectal cultures as indicated by history. Depending on the types of sexual activities alleged, blood samples may be collected. In addition, a test for pregnancy may be completed for postmenarchal girls.

Psychological Evaluation

An additional component sometimes included in the multidisciplinary response to a CSA allegation is a psychological evaluation. In some communities, mental health professionals conduct the initial interviews with suspected victims of CSA as members of the investigating team. In other communities, a psychological evaluation may only be requested when the findings of the initial investigation by child protection or law enforcement are inconclusive.

The purposes of such an evaluation are to gather history about the alleged sexual activity, assess the credibility of the allegations, and assess the child's emotional and behavioral status, both currently and historically. A variety of techniques may be used during this evaluation, including interviews with the child, his/her parents, and other significant persons in the child's life; the use of anatomically correct dolls or drawings; objective and projective assessment instruments; and structured play sessions. When possible, this evaluation should be completed by a mental health professional skilled in pursuing such evaluations, as the evaluation may be a crucial component in criminal or family court proceedings. *The evaluation should be conducted by a professional who has not been seeing the child in therapy previously.* This allows the evaluating professional to offer an unbiased and objective opinion and preserves the confidentiality of the ongoing therapeutic relationship. Based on the findings, the evaluator will likely offer treatment recommendations. If the findings indicate that the child has been sexually abused, at least a brief course of therapy is likely to be recommended to help the child process his/her thoughts and feelings about the abusive experience. Research also suggests that when a child has suffered sexual abuse, it is important to actively involve the nonoffending parent(s) in treatment, particularly when the child presents with depressive symptomatology or acting-out behavior problems (Deblinger, Lippmann, & Steer, 1996).

GUIDE TO PRACTICE

Based on the foregoing information regarding the phenomenon of CSA and the investigatory process, the following guide to practice offers suggestions regarding how a clinician might most effectively assist a child and his/her family through the crisis precipitated by disclosure of CSA.

Reporting the Abuse

As described earlier, when CSA is suspected, the professional has a legal responsibility to ascertain that a report is made to the appropriate authorities. While responding to the client in a calm and supportive way, the professional should communicate decisively that the necessary report must be made. Often clients are relieved to make that report in order to have some action taken regarding the sexual abuse. In some cases, however, clients may be reluctant to make such a report because of fear of the alleged perpetrator, love for the perpetrator, hesitancy to disrupt the family, fear that child protective services will assume custody of the child, embarrassment, or shame. If the client expresses such reluctance, the clinician may empathize with his/her concerns but also should state that filing such a report is not optional. Further, the therapist may encourage the client by saying that filing the necessary report is the first step toward resolving this difficult situation for everyone involved. Typically it is most appropriate to make the necessary telephone call reporting the alleged abuse from the professional's office. In that way, the clinician is afforded the opportunity to support the client(s) while verifying that the report has been made. The most appropriate person to place that initial telephone call may vary from situation to situation. Typically, the investigating professionals will need to speak with the person to whom the child made the initial disclosure of sexual abuse. Thus in cases in which the child initially disclosed to the clinician, the clinician him/herself should make the telephone call to report the abuse allegations. In other situations, the child will have made an initial disclosure to a nonoffending parent, who will then need to provide investigating professionals with information regarding that disclosure. However, in either case there appears to be some merit to having the professional place the telephone call, if only to introduce the parent and inform the investigating professionals that a report of alleged abuse is forthcoming. As was indicated previously, there is some indication that reports of CSA are more likely to be substantiated when made by professionals than when made by the general public. For example, 47.6% of the reports of child abuse and neglect made by health professionals in New Jersey were substantiated in 1988, compared with a substantiation rate of 38% for all reports filed (New Jersey Governor's Task Force on Child Abuse and Neglect, 1990).

All mental health professionals should be familiar with their state's laws governing the reporting of suspected child abuse. The ways in which child abuse is defined and the requirements in terms of the timing and agencies to which these reports may differ somewhat across the states. Initial reports of suspected child abuse are most often made to child protection agencies. During business hours, that report can be filed by calling the local office of the child protection agency. In many states, a toll-free number can be used to make such a report during evenings and weekends. That agency may then determine whether a report needs to be filed with the law enforcement agency as well and if necessary may initiate that report. In such cases, an investigation of the allegations may be conducted jointly by the child protection agency and the law enforcement agency. Child abuse reporting laws may not necessarily apply in cases in which the perpetrator was not functioning in a caretaking capacity (i.e., an adolescent raped on a date). In those situations, the child protection agency may not have the authority to investigate. However, law enforcement officials could pursue the investigation. Depending on the practices of the local community, the report of such incidents may be filed by the child's parents or legal guardians with the area police department or with the local prosecutor's office. Professionals should acquaint themselves with the policies of their professions and the practices of their communities so that they can provide accurate information, referrals, and support to clients facing this type of crisis. In some instances, clinicians may find it useful to contact the child protection agency to determine whether the concerns regarding possible child maltreatment are sufficient to warrant a child abuse investigation. Finally, given the complexity of this field, at times it may be helpful for the mental health professional to consult an attorney familiar with the laws pertaining to child abuse and mental health practice.

Responding to the Child's Initial Disclosure

While making sure that the report has been made to the appropriate agency, the clinician simultaneously must focus attention on helping the child and the child's family cope with this crisis. If the child makes the initial disclosure to the clinician, the professional should respond to the child in a calm and supportive manner. For example, the clinician might respond to the child's disclosure by saying, "I'm really glad you told me about that. Sometimes it is hard to talk about experiences like that and I think you were really brave to tell me." Although the clinician should not discourage the child from sharing any information about the abusive experience, the clinician need not attempt to gather detailed and specific information regarding the abuse from the child. As was described earlier, unless specifically trained for this purpose and requested to do so, the clinician is not responsible for conducting the evaluation of the abuse allegations. If the clinician hearing the initial disclosure does wish to ask a few questions to clarify the child's experience, those questions should be phrased in a general and nonleading way, in an attempt to elicit a free narrative account. For example, the clinician might simply ask, "Can you tell me more about that?" It is important not to ask questions in leading ways that may suggest responses to the child. Furthermore, it is preferable to avoid asking closed-end questions that can be answered with a simple yes or no. If a child misinterprets such a question and unintentionally responds erroneously, it may create confusion and weaken the credibility of the rest of his/her disclosure. The child's disclosure is most credible and meaningful when it is provided in the child's own words, without a great deal of prompting from an interviewer. In general, unless the clinician has been trained specifically in how to appropriately interview a child regarding a disclosure of sexual abuse, the investigatory questioning is better left to the professionals from child protective services or law enforcement agencies, or to a mental health clinician skilled in the assessment of children's allegations of sexual abuse. In any situation in which a child does make a disclosure about sexual abuse to the clinician or provides new details about the abuse, the clinician should keep careful records of both what the child said and any questions or comments offered by the clinician. These records may be critical in helping the clinician recall exactly what was said and may be incorporated in a report that might eventually be submitted to the court as evidence.

It is important to inform the child that other people will need to be told about this experience. For example, in initiating a discussion of the need to make a report to child protective services, initially the clinician might say, "We're going to need to talk with some other people so that we can help you with this." In addition, if the child has not disclosed to his/her nonoffending parent(s), the child may be told that the nonoffending parent(s) should be informed about the disclosure so that they can assist the child during the investigation. With children who are particularly anxious about their nonoffending parent's response, the clinician should offer whatever support he or she can provide. For example, it may be appropriate to suggest, "I would be glad to be here with you while you tell your mom, if you would like." In cases in which the clinician shares the child's concerns about the nonoffending parent's initial response to this information, it may even be helpful for the clinician to offer to talk with the parent privately about the child's disclosure before asking the child and parent to discuss the issue. In that way, the therapist provides the parent(s) with the opportunity to process their emotional distress regarding this disclosure privately in order to facilitate their ability to respond to the child in the most effective way possible. In most cases, however, it may be helpful to provide an opportunity for the parent and child to talk about the child's disclosure briefly together, with the clinician facilitating that discussion, in order to help them begin to learn how to communicate effectively about this experience. In the event that the nonoffending parent is overtly unsupportive and disbelieving of the child's disclosure, it would be inadvisable to ask the parent and child to discuss the disclosure together, as it would expose the child to that disbelief and might provide pressure that would influence the child's further disclosure of details regarding the alleged abuse. In situations in which it is not clear whether it would be helpful to include the nonoffending parent in a discussion of the disclosure, it may be useful to talk with the investigating personnel from the child protection agency or the law enforcement agencies to be certain that such a discussion would not hinder their investigation.

In general, it is most appropriate to wait until the child has been interviewed by investigatory professionals before involving the child in therapeutic or educational activities specific to the issue of sexual abuse. It is most useful if the investigating professionals are able to elicit the child's disclosure without it being altered significantly by information the child has obtained from a therapist. However, it is important to note that simply by having the clinician respond to the child's initial disclosure in a calm, supportive, and accepting way the child is learning that it is safe to talk about this experience, that he/she is believed, and that people still accept the child without blame or criticism.

Education about the Investigatory Process

Another way in which the professional can assist both the nonoffending parents and the child is to educate them so that they know what to anticipate after the disclosure is made. The clinician may explain to the clients the typical process of investigations conducted by the child protection agency and law enforcement agencies. Because the procedures in those investigations vary from one community to another, clinicians should educate themselves about the investigatory procedures followed in their community. If the professional has questions about the procedures at the time of the investigation, he/she should ask the investigators to clarify what will happen next. Simply having the clinician take the initiative in gathering some of that information may give the clients a sense of support.

Some clients have significant concern about the child protection agency becoming involved in the life of their family. These concerns may be based on a variety of different issues. At the most extreme, parents and children may be worried that the child protection agency will remove the child from the care of the nonoffending parent. Other clients may be angry about what they perceive as an implication that they are inadequate parents who require the intervention of the child protection agency. Yet another basis for frustration may be the perception of parents that the child protection agency is unnecessarily intruding in their lives and in their decision-making role as parents. Although it is important not to offer false reassurance to clients, it may be possible to dispel some unnecessary anxiety simply by providing accurate information about the role of the child protection agency. For example, the clinician might describe the child protection agency's role as intervening when necessary to provide for the safety and well-being of children. The clinician might further describe how the child will benefit most if parents can view the professionals from the child protection agency as allies in their efforts to protect their child. It is important that if at all possible, the clinician should encourage the parent(s) to work in a cooperative way with the child protection professionals and to avoid any adversarial relationships.

Clients also frequently have significant anxiety about the legal process. For example, they may question: Will the alleged perpetrator be arrested? When will that happen? Will the case go to trial? When will that happen? Will my child have to testify? Typically the professional will not be able to answer most of these questions right away. However, he/she can educate clients regarding the variety of courses the legal process can take, depending on the practices specific to that community or state. It also may be possible to facilitate contact between clients and other professionals who may be better able to respond to legal questions. For example, in many communities a victim witness advocate is available to assist victims of crime. That person may be invaluable in assisting clients through the legal system. It also is important to inform clients that although the first interview with law enforcement officials may occur shortly after the initial disclosure, the rest of the legal process often proceeds slowly, with many delays. Thus, it is rarely useful to focus the child's attention initially on the legal process as that focus may unnecessarily heighten the child's anxiety.

Another aspect of the investigatory process that may be anxiety provoking for clients is the medical examination. It is important to discuss the medical examination in a calm, matter-of-fact way, so that it is not presented as a threatening experience. When talking with nonoffending parents it is useful to highlight the benefits of an examination. For example, the examination provides the opportunity to treat any physical complications from the sexual abuse, to educate the child about his/her body, to offer reassurance that the child's body is intact, or to educate the child appropriately about any medical problems he/she is experiencing (Sgroi et al., 1982). It is difficult to predict for clients exactly what procedures will be involved in the medical examination without being familiar with the practices of the examining physician. Thus, in most cases, the referring clinician may simply provide the child with some general information such as, "The doctor will check you from head to toe to make sure that you are okay." Then just prior to the actual examination, a professional familiar with the particular physician (such as a nurse or counselor in the physician's office, or the physician him or herself) should provide the child with more detailed information about what to anticipate during the examination.

Finally, the clinician will need to provide clients with some education regarding the psychological evaluation that may be done following a disclosure of CSA. When talking with nonoffending parents, the clinician may explain that the evaluation is needed to help clarify the sexual abuse allegations and to assess the impact of the alleged abuse on the child's psychosocial functioning. Furthermore, the evaluator will attempt to determine how the child is coping with the crisis precipitated by the disclosure and may make some recommendations for treatment. When discussing the psychological evaluation with the child, the clinician may simply tell the child that he/she will be going to see a person who will help the child talk about his/her thoughts and feelings. It is important not to be too leading in preparing the child to discuss the abuse allegations. For example, it would be inappropriate for the referring professional to say, "You can tell this doctor all about how the perpetrator touched you and you touched him."

Acting as an Advocate for the Child

As clients move through the investigatory process, the professional needs to be comfortable assuming an advocacy role for the child. The child and his/her nonoffending parent(s) will be negotiating unfamiliar systems and agencies and may be overwhelmed by all the processes involved in the investigation of CSA. They may benefit greatly from having a professional available as a source of support and information regarding the systems involved. Furthermore, the clinician may assist them significantly by serving as the child's advocate among all the investigating professionals and agencies involved. Although it is certainly the intent of virtually all the professionals involved in the investigation of CSA to assist the child, in reality the child's needs occasionally may get lost in systems overloaded with too many cases and too few resources. Thus, having an advocate within the system who can speak to the child's needs can be invaluable.

Preliminary Therapeutic Interventions with the Child

Once the child has been interviewed by the investigating professionals, it may be useful to engage the child in some preliminary therapeutic work regarding the sexual abuse and the subsequent disclosure. If unsure whether or not such therapeutic work would interfere with an ongoing investigation, the clinician might discuss the issue with the investigating professionals, with the client's consent. A thorough discussion of a complete treatment plan for victims of CSA is beyond the scope of this chapter. (Comprehensive descriptions of a treatment approach for sexually abused children that has received empirical support is provided by Deblinger and Heflin [1996] and by Cohen, Mannarino, and Deblinger [2006].) This chapter, however, offers some guidelines for crisis management for clinicians who are already working with children and parents at the time of disclosure. Even if the clinician working with the child during this time is not the therapist who ultimately provides a full course of therapy regarding the sexual abuse, the therapeutic interventions offered during this crisis may yield significant benefits.

Therapist as Role Model

Most children are acutely sensitive to the reactions of other people when they learn of the sexual abuse. Indeed, children often avoid discussing the abuse because they anticipate negative responses. Thus a clinician working with a child at the time of disclosure has both an opportunity and a responsibility to model for the child how to communicate effectively regarding the abuse. The therapist should communicate both verbally and behaviorally that he or she is available to talk about any of the child's thoughts, questions, or concerns regarding the abuse. Although many adults are uncomfortable hearing a child describe a sexually abusive experience and seeing a child experience significant emotional distress, it is crucial that the clinician not model avoidance for the child. A clinician who avoids discussions of the sexual abuse communicates to the child that those discussions are not appropriate. A child may interpret such avoidance in many different negative ways—for example, that the abuse is shameful, that it is too horrible to discuss, or that the child was responsible for the abuse. If the clinician models avoidance, the child is likely to cope with the abuse in a similar way. Such a behavior pattern will only make later therapeutic work more difficult. Although it is important for the clinician to model openness and a willingness to discuss the sexual abuse, at this point it is not appropriate to push a child to discuss the experience unless the clinician has committed to providing a full course of treatment around this issue. The difficult work of confronting painful thoughts and memories associated with the sexual abuse is best pursued in the context of an ongoing therapeutic relationship.

Education Regarding CSA

In addition to serving as a model for the child, the clinician working with a child in the midst of the crisis of disclosure has the opportunity to provide some basic education regarding CSA. Again, it is important to wait to provide this education until after the child has been interviewed by the investigating professionals, so that the information does not influence the child's disclosure. In providing the education, it is usually helpful to provide some basic facts such as a definition of CSA, its prevalence, who is affected, who is responsible, why it occurs, and how children feel who have been abused. Often it is useful initially to elicit from the child his or her own responses to those questions. In that way it may be possible to identify any misconceptions that the child has so that they may be corrected. For example, if when asked why CSA occurs, a girl responds that it occurs because the child was dressed in inappropriately revealing clothing, the clinician has the opportunity to educate the child in a way that could have significant therapeutic effect. In explaining that CSA occurs because the perpetrator has a problem with being sexually attracted to young children and has nothing to do with any style of dress or behavior exhibited by the girl, the clinician may afford the child significant relief and diminished distress. In general, the clinician can describe how children may be confused by such an experience and have thoughts and emotions regarding the experience that adults would not necessarily anticipate. Thus, it is important that the child talk about his/her thoughts and feelings so that the professional can help the child correct any erroneous thoughts and can help the child cope with any emotional distress he/she is experiencing.

Preliminary Therapeutic Interventions with Parents

Similarly, the professional should attempt to serve as a source of support and a therapeutic agent for the nonoffending parents. Unfortunately, parents' needs are not always recognized. When the parents' needs are ignored, professionals lose a valuable opportunity to intervene in ways that ultimately could benefit the child significantly. As discussed earlier in this chapter, a number of studies have demonstrated that children's postabuse adjustment may be related to the ways that their nonoffending parents cope with the crisis of CSA (Conte & Schuerman, 1987; Deblinger et al., 1999; Deblinger et al., 1997; Everson et al., 1989; Spaccarelli & Fuchs, 1997). Thus, any interventions that help the parent(s) cope with this crisis probably will benefit the child as well.

Parents as Role Models

It is important to inform parents that they will serve as models for their child with respect to how he/she should respond to the sexual abuse. Thus the parents' responses to the sexual abuse may be very influential in determining how their child copes with this situation. The clinician should encourage the parents to remain as calm and supportive of the child as possible. The parents should avoid any tendencies to overreact and catastrophize the situation, as that type of response is likely to heighten the child's anxiety. Similarly, parents should be encouraged to be open to any discussions of the abuse that the child may initiate. Parents should be cautioned not to model avoidance, in the same way that clinicians should be careful about that issue. On the other hand, parents should also be discouraged from pushing a child to provide details regarding the abuse, unless the child initiates those conversations. A well-intentioned parent may inadvertently ask the child leading questions or respond to the child's disclosure in a way that inhibits further discussion. Thus, it is more appropriate if the parent waits to pursue detailed abuse-related conversations with the child until he/she can do so with the guidance of a therapist who is pursuing a course of treatment with the child specifically focused on the abuse allegations.

Cognitive Coping Strategies

While working with the parents during the crisis of the disclosure, the clinician also may offer the parents a variety of coping strategies to assist them in effectively managing their own emotional responses. One such strategy involves providing a combination of education regarding CSA and cognitive coping skills training. Often parents have misconceptions about sexual abuse that serve to intensify their own emotional distress. The clinician can educate the parents in a way that dispels some of those misconceptions. Moreover, the clinician can teach the parents how to use that new information to dispute their own dysfunctional and distressing thoughts. For example, parents may feel very guilty for not recognizing "the signs" that indicated that the alleged perpetrator was a sexual offender. The first step in helping the parents cope more effectively with those feelings is to educate the parents about the fact that there is no typical psychological or physical profile of a sexual offender and thus there are no specific signs that can be recognized. Subsequently, the clinician can help the parents practice replacing their erroneous and dysfunctional thoughts with more accurate and effective thoughts. In this example, a parent might replace the thought, "It's all my fault because I should have been able to tell what kind of pervert that coach is," with "Even professionals usually cannot recognize sex offenders because there is no consistent psychological profile, so there was no way I could have anticipated this." This combination of education and cognitive coping skills may help significantly to reduce the parent's feelings of guilt. This same combination of techniques may be used effectively to help parents cope with other distressing emotions such as anger, sadness, anxiety, and fear. In teaching parents how to use these skills, it is important to elicit from them which distressing emotions they are experiencing and what thoughts are underlying those emotions. Only by focusing on their specific dysfunctional thoughts and effectively replacing them will the client experience significant symptom relief.

Psychotherapy

Following the CSA investigation, it is usually important for the child to participate in psychotherapy focused specifically on helping him/her cope with the experience of sexual abuse. When the child already has been participating in psychotherapy regarding other issues, a decision must be made as to whether the child should continue with the previous clinician or see a new therapist to deal with this specific issue. One obvious advantage to continuing with the previous therapist is that a trusting relationship already may have been established. Although that is an important factor, it is only one of several factors that must be considered. Another important consideration is the current clinician's level of comfort and expertise in dealing with the issue of CSA. Such expertise and personal comfort are important in conducting successful therapy and probably should outweigh the issue of a previously established relationship. However, in many communities it may be difficult to find clinicians with true expertise in the field of CSA. In such situations, one must rely on the therapist's own judgment as to his/her level of comfort in dealing with these issues. Another issue to be considered in deciding whether to continue working with the current therapist is that clinician's relationship with family members. It must be clear to the child that the clinician helping him/her cope with the sexual abuse experience is truly an advocate for that child. Thus, if the clinician previously has had a working relationship with another family member, which might make the child doubt the therapist's commitment to the child, that clinician may not be the best choice to continue work with the child at this time. For example, if the therapist's previous work with the child has included work with a parent or sibling later accused of being the sexual abuse perpetrator, or with a parent who is unsupportive and disbelieving of the child, it would be more helpful for the child to form a new therapeutic relationship that is not complicated with those previous relationships. In addition, it seems to be preferable, at least initially, for the child to be seen by an individual therapist rather than a family therapist whose allegiances and objectives may be confusing for the child. Eventually, it may be very useful to have some therapy sessions involving multiple members of the family to discuss the impact of the abuse on all members of the family. However, to move into that type of work prematurely may inappropriately minimize the impact of the experience on the child who was actually abused.

Therapy may be offered in individual or group formats to assist children as well as their nonoffending parents in coping with the emotional and behavioral reactions commonly associated with CSA. Some children and parents may prefer to work in individual therapy initially and then move into a group therapy program once they have made progress in dealing with their individual issues. In a group setting, clients enjoy benefits such as receiving support from other group members, realizing that CSA is a relatively common and shared experience, sharing effective coping strategies, and having opportunities both to learn from the modeling of other group members who are coping well with their abusive experiences and to serve as models themselves for members who are not as far along in the adjustment process.

There are many treatment approaches described in the clinical literature that may be helpful to children and their families in the aftermath of CSA (Friedrich, 1994; Gil, 1991; James, 1989). However, recent reviews of the child sexual abuse treatment outcome literature find that trauma-focused cognitive-behavioral treatment (CBT) has the most empirical support for its effectiveness in treating PTSD and re-lated difficulties with this population of children (American Academy of Child and Adolescent Psychiatry, 1998; Putnam, 2003; Saunders, Berliner, & Hanson, 2003; *modelprograms.samhsa.gov*). Research, in fact, has documented the benefits of this model in both individual and group formats (i.e., Cohen, Deblinger, Mannarino, & Steer, 2004; Cohen & Mannarino, 1996, 1998; Deblinger et al., 1996; Deblinger, Stauffer, & Steer, 2001). More detailed descriptions of the model are available in book form (Cohen, Mannarino, & Deblinger, 2006; Deblinger & Heflin, 1996) as well as via the Internet at *www.musc.edu/tfcbt*.

CASE STUDY

The following case study illustrates how a clinician might help a nonoffending parent and his/her children cope with the crisis that may be precipitated by a disclosure of CSA. Diane, a 32-year-old mother, contacted a counselor in order to obtain help for her 5-year-old daughter, Lisa, and her 2-year-old son, Michael. She reported that she had been having great difficulty managing her children's behavior ever since she and her husband had separated approximately 6 months earlier. Diane indicated that her husband, Tom, was the disciplinarian in the family. Although she maintained physical custody of the children, Tom frequently visited during the week and took the children for overnight visits every other weekend without fail. Diane hesitantly acknowledged that she and her husband had some problems with domestic violence. Although she admitted that the children had been exposed to some of the violence, Diane denied their exposure to any other childhood traumas. Diane described the children's emo-tional and behavioral difficulties, noting that the children behaved better for their father and seemed to enjoy his attention and playfulness. The counselor asked Diane to complete a child behavior checklist for each of her children. Although Diane had expressed concerns about managing her son's temper tantrums, her responses to the child behavior checklist revealed that his overall behavior fell within the normal range. However, the child behavior profile for her 5-year-old daughter showed significant ele-vations with respect to somatic complaints and sexualized behaviors. When Diane was asked to describe the sexualized behaviors in greater detail, she reported that her daughter frequently masturbated in public and had been caught several times playing with her brother's penis with her hands and her mouth. Diane reported that she han-dled the incidents poorly; she yelled at Lisa and sent her to her room for punishment.

When asked if she talked to Lisa about the incidents, Diane indicated that Lisa refused to talk about it. However, she recalled that on one occasion Lisa tearfully complained that her daddy let her play with his "peepee." Diane explained that she considered the possibility of sexual abuse, but she feared that she might be overreacting. In response to questioning, Diane reported that to her knowledge, her daughter had never been exposed to any type of adult sexual activity or pornography. The counselor indicated to Diane that she was not overreacting and, in fact, the information she provided indeed raised concern. The counselor further explained that as a mental health professional, she was legally responsible to report a suspicion of sexual abuse so that an investigation could be initiated. This did not mean that Lisa had been sexually abused but that the possibility needed to be fully explored by a team of trained professionals. Diane reacted with shock, dismay, and self-blame. She insisted that although she and her husband had their differences, he always seemed to be a caring and involved father. She could not imagine that he would sexually abuse their daughter. At the same time, she blamed herself, fearing that she was responsible due to her inability to satisfy her husband sexually. While acknowledging Diane's feelings, the counselor corrected her misconceptions, offering some basic information about CSA. She explained to Diane that there is no evidence that a father will choose to sexually abuse his daughter out of frustration regarding his sexual relationship with his wife. The counselor also explained the components of the CSA investigation. She informed Diane that the initial report would be made to the child protection agency. However, if the agency determined that an investigation was warranted, a joint investigation with a law enforcement agency would likely be conducted.

Subsequently, the counselor placed the call to the child protection agency while Diane was in the office. The counselor identified herself to the child protection worker and briefly described the behaviors Lisa had exhibited as well as her statement regarding her father. Then, Diane spoke on the phone to the child protection worker and provided further information about Lisa's behaviors. Because Lisa would not be seeing her father for several days, the child protection worker scheduled an appointment to meet with Diane, Lisa, and Michael the following day. The child protection worker added that she anticipated that an investigator from the county prosecutor's office would observe the interview with Lisa from behind a one-way mirror. After the telephone call was completed, Diane was obviously shaken. When the counselor asked exactly what her concerns were, Diane reported that she could not believe that this was happening, that she never wanted her husband to go to jail. The counselor explained that it was too early to try to guess what the outcome of the investigation would be. She further explained that the reason the investigator would be observing the interview is to try to minimize the number of interviews Lisa would have to experience. She explained that the decision to prosecute a case of alleged sexual abuse is complicated and that the investigator's presence does not indicate that that decision has been made yet.

Diane also expressed concern about how to prepare Lisa for the interview, questioning, "What should I tell her?" The counselor cautioned Diane against trying to prepare Lisa in any formal way. She reassured Diane that the investigating professionals would be skilled in working with children and would want to elicit any information Lisa had to share in a spontaneous way. The counselor and Diane discussed what Diane might tell Lisa about the appointment the next day. Diane requested that the counselor help her talk with Lisa about it, so they asked Lisa to join them in the office. When Lisa joined them, the counselor and Diane explained to her that just as she had met with the counselor today, she would be meeting with another person tomorrow at a different office. They explained that she would be talking with a social worker whose job it is to help kids. Lisa did not seem disturbed by that explanation; rather, she appeared to accept it without significant concern. After they spoke with Lisa for a few minutes, Lisa returned to the playroom next door, where her brother was playing. The counselor then explained to Diane that she would like to continue to provide support and advocacy for Diane and her children during the course of the investigation. She also offered the mother some coping assistance as well as guidelines for responding to her daughter's questions and behavioral reactions. For example, she encouraged Diane to call her or to talk with a trusted friend about her own emotional responses to this situation but cautioned her strongly against discussing the situation at a time when the children could overhear her. Diane expressed concern about how she should handle it if Lisa began talking about any instance of sexual abuse. The counselor suggested that she should allow Lisa to discuss anything, as long as Lisa brought it up spontaneously. It was explained that Diane could be a tremendous source of support to her daughter by simply listening to what her daughter had to say rather than questioning her in any way. However, she discouraged Diane from questioning Lisa about any type of sexual contact, explaining that at this point, it is important not to influence Lisa's disclosure of information in any way. At the end of the session, the counselor and Diane agreed to meet weekly for several sessions to help Diane and her children cope with the immediate crisis. During these sessions, they agreed to formulate a plan for treatment with the current counselor or, if necessary, with a counselor who had more expertise in the area of CSA.

CONCLUSION

Given the widespread prevalence of CSA, all mental health professionals should be prepared to identify and appropriately intervene on behalf of suspected child victims. This chapter provides basic information that may assist clinicians in recognizing and reporting suspected CSA. In addition to outlining reporting requirements, the chapter describes the components of the multidisciplinary investigation that generally ensues once a report is made. Guidelines are also offered for responding to the emotional reactions and coping needs of the child and his/her nonoffending parent(s) in the immediate aftermath of a CSA disclosure. By providing support and advocacy, the mental health professional may critically influence the investigatory process while also reducing the stress experienced by the child and his/her family during this crisis period.

REFERENCES

Ackerman, P., Newton, J., McPherson, W. B., Jones, J., & Dykman, R. (1998). Prevalence of posttraumatic stress disorder and other psychiatric diagnoses in three groups of abused children (sexual, physical, and both). *Child Abuse and Neglect, 22*(8), 759–774.

Administration for Children and Families, U.S. Department of Health and Human Services. (n.d.). NIS-4 description. Retrieved January 3, 2006, from *www.nis4.org/nis4.asp*

American Academy of Child and Adolescent Psychiatry. (1998). Practice parameters for the assessment and treatment of children and adolescents with PTSD. *Journal of the American Academy of Child and Adolescent Psychiatry, 37*(Suppl.), 4S–26S.

American Academy of Pediatrics. (1991). Guidelines for the evaluation of sexual abuse in children. *Pediatrics, 87*(2), 254–260.

Bays, J., & Chadwick, D. (1993). Medical diagnosis of the sexually abused child. *Child Abuse and Neglect, 17*, 91–110.

Beitchman, J. H., Zucker, K. J., Hood, J. E., DaCosta, G. A., Akman, D., & Cassavia, E. (1992). A review of the long-term effects of child sexual abuse. *Child Abuse and Neglect, 16*, 101–118.

Bolen, R. M., & Lamb, J. L. (2004). Ambivalence of nonoffending guardians after sexual abuse disclosure. *Journal of Interpersonal Violence, 19*(2), 185–211.

Boney-McCoy, S., & Finkelhor, D. (1995). Psychosocial sequelae of violent victimization in a national youth sample. *Journal of Consulting and Clinical Psychology, 63*(5), 726–736.

Briere, J. N., & Elliott, D. M. (1994). Immediate and long-term impacts of child sexual abuse. *The Future of Children, 4*(2), 54–69.

Briere, J., & Runtz, N. (1988). Symptomatology associated with childhood sexual victimization in a nonclinical adult sample. *Child Abuse and Neglect, 12*, 51–59.

Briere, J., & Zaidi, L. Y. (1989). Sexual abuse histories and sequelae in female psychiatric emergency room patients. *American Journal of Psychiatry, 146*, 1602–1606.

Cohen, J. A., Deblinger, E., Maedel, A. B., & Stauffer, L. B. (1999). Examining sex-related thoughts and feelings of sexually abused and nonabused children. *Journal of Interpersonal Violence, 14*(7), 701–712.

Cohen, J. A., Deblinger, E., Mannarino, A. P., & Steer, R. A. (2004). A multisite, randomized controlled trial for children with sexual abuse-related PTSD symptoms. *Journal of the American Academy of Child and Adolescent Psychiatry, 43*(4), 393–402.

Cohen, J. A., & Mannarino, A. P. (1996). Factors that mediate treatment outcome of sexually abused preschool children. *Journal of the American Academy of Child and Adolescent Psychiatry, 34*(10), 1402–1410.

Cohen, J. A., & Mannarino, A. P. (1998). Factors that mediate treatment outcome of sexually abused preschool children: Six- and 12-month follow-up. *Journal of the American Academy of Child and Adolescent Psychiatry, 37*(1), 44–51.

Cohen, J. A., Mannarino, A. P., & Deblinger, E. (2006). *Treating trauma and traumatic grief in children and adolescents: A clinician's guide.* New York. Guilford Press.

Conte, J. R., & Schuerman, J. (1987). Factors associated with an increased impact of child sexual abuse. *Child Abuse and Neglect, 11*, 201–211.

Cormier, B. M., Kennedy, M., & Sangowicz, J. (1962). Psychodynamics of father–daughter incest. *Canadian Psychiatric Association Journal, 1*, 203–217.

Deblinger, E., & Heflin, A. H. (1996). *Treating sexually abused children and their nonoffending parents: A cognitive-behavioral approach.* Thousand Oaks, CA: Sage.

Deblinger, E., Lippmann, J., & Steer, R. (1996). Sexually abused children suffering posttraumatic stress symptoms: Initial treatment outcome findings. *Child Maltreatment, 1*(4), 310–321.

Deblinger, E., McLeer, S., Atkins, M., Ralphe, D., & Foa, E. (1989). Posttraumatic stress in sexually abused, physically abused, and nonabused children. *Child Abuse and Neglect, 13*, 403–408.

Deblinger, E., Stauffer, L., & Landsberg, C. (1994). The impact of a history of child sexual abuse on maternal response to allegations of sexual abuse concerning her child. *Journal of Child Sexual Abuse, 3*(3), 67–75.

Deblinger, E., Stauffer, L., & Steer, R. A. (2001). Comparative efficacies of supportive and cognitive behavioral group therapies for young children who have been sexually abused and their nonoffending mothers. *Child Maltreatment, 6*(4), 332–343.

Deblinger, E., Steer, R., & Lippmann, J. (1999). Maternal factors associated with sexually abused children's psychosocial adjustment. *Child Maltreatment, 4*(1), 13–20.

Deblinger, E., Taub, B., Maedel, A., Lippmann, J., & Stauffer, L. (1997). Psychosocial factors predicting parent reported symptomatology in sexually abused children. *Journal of Child Sexual Abuse, 6*, 35–49.

DeVoe, E. R., & Faller, K. C. (1999). The characteristics of disclosure among children who may have been sexually abused. *Child Maltreatment, 4*, 217–227.

Eisenberg, N., Owens, R. G., & Dewey, M. E. (1987). Attitudes of health professionals to child sexual abuse and incest. *Child Abuse and Neglect, 11*, 109–116.

Elliott, D. M., & Briere, J. (1992). Sexual abuse trauma among professional women: Validating the Trauma Symptom Checklist–40 (TSC-40). *Child Abuse and Neglect, 16*(3), 391–398.

Everson, M. D., Hunter, W. M., Runyon, D. K., Edelson, G. A., & Coulter, M. L. (1989). Maternal support following disclosure of incest. *American Journal of Orthopsychiatry, 59*(2), 197–207.

Famularo, R., Kinscherff, R., & Fenton, T. (1992). Psychiatric diagnoses of maltreated children: Preliminary findings. *Journal of the American Academy of Child and Adolescent Psychiatry, 31*, 863–867.

Feiring, C., & Taska, L. (2005). The persistence of shame following sexual abuse: A longitudinal look at risk and recovery. *Child Maltreatment: Journal of the American Professional Society on the Abuse of Children, 10*(4), 337–349.

Feiring, C., Taska, L., & Chen, K. (2002). Trying to understand why horrible things happen: Attribution, shame, and symptom development following sexual abuse. *Child Maltreatment: Journal of the American Professional Society on the Abuse of Children, 7*(1), 26–41.

Feiring, C., Taska, L., & Lewis, M. (1998). Social support and children's and adolescents' adaptation to sexual abuse. *Journal of Interpersonal Violence, 13*, 240–260.

Feiring, C., Taska, L., & Lewis, M. (2002). Adjustment following sexual abuse discovery: The role of shame and attributional style. *Developmental Psychology, 38*(1), 79–92.

Femina, D. D., Yeager, C. A., & Lewis, D. O. (1990). Child abuse: Adolescent records vs. adult recall. *Child Abuse and Neglect, 14*, 227–231.

Finkel, M. A., & DeJong, A. R. (1992). Medical findings in child sexual abuse. In R. M. Reece (Ed.), *Child abuse: Medical diagnosis and management* (pp. 185–247). Philadelphia: Lea & Febiger.

Finkelhor, D., Hotaling, G., Lewis, I., & Smith, C. (1990). Sexual abuse in a national survey of men and women: Prevalence, characteristics, and risk factors. *Child Abuse and Neglect, 14*, 19–28.

Flango, V. E. (1991). Can central registries improve substantiation rates in child abuse cases? *Child Abuse and Neglect, 15*, 408–415.

Friedrich, W. N. (1993). Sexual victimization and sexual behavior in children: A review of the recent literature. *Child Abuse and Neglect, 17*(1), 59–66.

Friedrich, W. N. (1994). Individual psychotherapy for child abuse victims. *Child and Adolescent Psychiatric Clinics of North America, 3*(4), 797–812.

Friedrich, W. N., Beilke, R. L., & Luecke, W. J. (1988). Behavior problems in young sexually abused boys: A comparison study. *Journal of Interpersonal Violence, 2*, 21–28.

Friedrich, W. N., Luecke, W. J., Beilke, R. L., & Place, V. (1992). Psychotherapy outcome of sexually abused boys: An agency study. *Journal of Interpersonal Violence, 7*(3), 396–409.

Friedrich, W. N., Urquiza, A. J., & Beilke, R. (1986). Behavioral problems in sexually abused young children. *Journal of Pediatric Psychology, 11*(1), 47–57.

Gil, E. (1991). *The healing power of play: Working with abused children.* New York: Guilford Press.

Goldston, D. B., Turnquist, D. C., & Knutson, J. F. (1989). Presenting problems of sexually abused girls receiving psychiatric services. *Journal of Abnormal Psychology, 98,* 314–317.

Gonzalez, L. S., Waterman, J., Kelly, R. J., McCord, J., & Oliveri, M. K. (1993). Children's patterns of disclosures and recantations of sexual and ritualistic abuse allegations in psychotherapy. *Child Abuse and Neglect, 17,* 281–189.

Goodman-Brown, T., Edelstein, R. S., Goodman, G. S., Jones, D. P., & Gordon, D. S. (2003). Why children tell: A model of children's disclosure of sexual abuse. *Child Abuse and Neglect, 27*(5), 525–540.

Gries, L. T., Goh, D. S., & Cavanaugh, J. (1996). Factors associated with disclosure during child sexual abuse assessment. *Journal of Child Sexual Abuse, 5,* 1–20.

Hanson, R. F., Resnick, H. S., Saunders, B. E., Kilpatrick, D. G., & Best, C. (1999). Factors related to the reporting of childhood rape. *Child Abuse and Neglect, 23,* 559–569.

Heflin, A. H., Mears, C., Deblinger, E., & Steer, R. (1997, June). *A comparison of body images and views of sexuality between sexually abused and nonabused girls.* Paper presented at the annual meeting of the American Professional Society on the Abuse of Children, Miami, FL.

Hiebert-Murphy, D. (1998). Emotional distress among mothers whose children have been sexually abused: The role of a history of child sexual abuse, social support, and coping. *Child Abuse and Neglect, 22*(5), 423–435

Humphreys, C. (1997). Child sexual abuse allegations in the context of divorce: Issues for mothers. *British Journal of Social Work, 27,* 529–544.

James, B. (1989). *Treating traumatized children: New insights and creative interventions.* New York: The Free Press.

Jumper, S. A. (1995). A meta-analysis of the relationship of child sexual abuse to adult psychological adjustment. *Child Abuse and Neglect, 19*(6), 715–728.

Kalichman, S. C., Craig, M. E., & Follingstad, D. R. (1988). Mental health professionals and suspected cases of child abuse: An investigation of factors influencing reporting. *Community Mental Health Journal, 23*(1), 43–51.

Kallstrom-Fuqua, A. C., Weston, R., & Marshall, L. L. (2004). Childhood and adolescent sexual abuse of community women: Mediated effects on psychological distress and social relationships. *Journal of Consulting and Clinical Psychology, 72*(6), 980–992.

Kelley, S. J. (1990). Responsibilities and management strategies in child sexual abuse: A comparison of child protective workers, nurses and police officers. *Child Welfare, 69*(l), 43–51.

Kendall-Tackett, K. A., Williams, L. M., & Finkelhor, D. (1993). Impact of sexual abuse on children: A review and synthesis of recent empirical studies. *Psychological Bulletin, 113*(1), 164–180.

Kolko, D. J., Moser, J. T., & Weldy, S. R. (1988). Behavioral emotional indicators of sexual abuse in child psychiatric inpatients: A controlled comparison with physical abuse. *Child Abuse and Neglect, 12,* 529–541.

Kouyoumdjian, H., Perry, A. R., & Hansen, D. J. (2005). The role of adult expectations on the recovery of sexually abused children. *Aggression and Violent Behavior, 10*(4), 475–489.

Lab, D., Feigenbaum, J., & De Silva, P. (2000). Mental health professionals' attitudes and practices towards male childhood sexual abuse. *Child Abuse and Neglect, 24*(3), 391–409.

Lanktree, C., Briere, J., & Zaidi, L. Y. (1991). Incidence and impact in a child outpatient sample: The role of direct inquiry. *Child Abuse and Neglect, 15,* 447–453.

Lawson, L., & Chaffin, M. (1992). False negatives in sexual abuse disclosure interviews: Incidence and influence of caretaker's belief in abuse in cases of accidental abuse discovery and diagnosis of STD. *Journal of Interpersonal Violence, 7*, 532–542.

London, K., Bruck, M., Ceci, S., & Shuman, D. (2005). Disclosure of child sexual abuse: What does the research tell us about the ways that children tell? *Psychology, Public Policy, and Law, 11*(1), 194–226.

Mannarino, A. P., & Cohen, J. A. (1996). Abuse-related attributions and perceptions, general attributions, and locus of control in sexually abused girls. *Journal of Interpersonal Violence, 11*(2), 162–180.

McLeer, S. V., Deblinger, E., Henry, D., & Orvaschel, H. (1992). Sexually abused children at high risk for post-traumatic stress disorder. *Journal of the American Academy of Adolescent and Child Psychiatry, 1*(5), 875–879.

Nagel, D. E., Putnam, F. W., & Noll, J. G. (1997). Disclosure patterns of sexual abuse and psychological functioning at a 1-year follow-up. *Child Abuse and Neglect, 21*(2), 137–147.

Neumann, D. A., Housekamp, B. M., Pollock, B. M., & Briere, J. (1996). The long-term sequelae of childhood sexual abuse in women: A meta-analytic review. *Child Maltreatment, 1*(1), 6–16.

New Jersey Governor's Task Force on Child Abuse and Neglect. (1990). *Report on New Jersey's child protection system*. Unpublished report.

Noll, J. G., Trickett, P. K., & Putnam, F. W. (2003). A prospective investigation of the impact of childhood sexual abuse on the development of sexuality. *Journal of Consulting and Clinical Psychology, 71*(3), 575–586.

Oates, R. K., O'Toole, B. I., Lynch, D. L., Stern, A., & Cooney, G. (1994). Stability and change in outcomes for sexually abused children. *Journal of the American Academy of Child and Adolescent Psychiatry, 33*(7), 945–953.

Owens, G. P., & Chard, K. M. (2001). Cognitive distortions among women reporting childhood sexual abuse. *Journal of Interpersonal Violence, 16*(2), 178–191.

Peters, S. D. (1988). Child sexual abuse and later psychological problems. In G. E. Wyatt & G. J. Powell (Eds.), *The lasting effects of child sexual abuse*. Newbury Park, CA: Sage.

Putnam, F. W. (2003). Ten-year research update review: Child sexual abuse. *Journal of the American Academy of Child and Adolescent Psychiatry, 42*(3), 269–278.

Runyon, D. K., Hunter, W. M., & Everson, M. D. (1992). *Maternal support for child victims of sexual abuse: Determinants and implications*. Final report for the National Center for Child Abuse and Neglect. Washington, DC: U.S. Department of Health and Human Services.

Russell, D. (1986). *The secret trauma: Incest in the lives of girls and women*. New York: Basic Books.

Sarles, R. M. (1975). Incest. *Pediatric Clinics of North America, 22*, 633–642.

Saunders, B. E., Berliner, L., & Hanson, R. F. (Eds.). (2003, January 15). *Child physical and sexual abuse: Guidelines for treatment (final report)*. Charleston, SC: National Crime Victims Research and Treatment Center.

Saywitz, K. J., Mannarino, A. P., Berliner, L., & Cohen, J. A. (2000). Treatment for sexually abused children and adolescents. *American Psychologist, 55*(9), 1040–1049.

Sedlak, A. J., & Broadhurst, D. D. (1996). *Third national incidence study of child abuse and neglect: Final report*. Washington, DC: U.S. Department of Health and Human Services.

Sgroi, S. M., Porter, F. S., & Blick, L. C. (1982). Validation of child sexual abuse. In S. M. Sgroi (Ed.), *Handbook of clinical intervention in child sexual abuse* (pp. 39–79). Lexington, MA: Lexington Books.

Sirles, E., & Franke, P. (1989). Factors influencing mothers' reactions to intrafamily sexual abuse. *Child Abuse and Neglect, 13*, 165–170.

Smith, D., Letourneau, E. J., Saunders, B. E., Kilpatrick, D. G., Resnick, H. S., & Best, C. L. (2000). Delay in disclosure of childhood rape: Results from a national survey. *Child Abuse and Neglect, 24*, 273–287.

Sorensen, T., & Snow, B. (1991). How children tell: The process of disclosure in child sexual abuse. *Child Welfare*, 70(1), 3–15.

Spaccarelli, S., & Fuchs, C. (1997). Variability in symptom expression among sexually abused girls: Developing multivariate models. *Journal of Clinical Child Psychology*, 26(1), 24–35.

Stauffer, L. B., & Deblinger, E. (1996). Cognitive behavioral groups for nonoffending mothers and their young sexually abused children: A preliminary treatment outcome study. *Child Maltreatment*, 1(1), 65–76.

Steel, J., Sanna, L., Hammond, B., Whipple, J., & Cross, H. (2004). Psychological sequalae of childhood sexual abuse: Abuse-related characteristics, coping strategies, and attributional style. *Child Abuse and Neglect*, 28(7), 785–801.

Steel, J. L., Wilson, G., Cross, H., & Whipple, J. (1996). Mediating factors in the development of psychopathology in victims of childhood sexual abuse. *Sexual Abuse: A Journal of Research and Treatment*, 8(4), 291–316.

Stroud, D., Martens, S. L., & Barker, J. (2000). Criminal investigation of child sexual abuse: A comparison of cases referred to the prosecutor to those not referred. *Child Abuse and Neglect*, 24, 689–700.

Swoboda, J., Elwork, A., Sales, B., & Levine, D. (1978). Knowledge of and compliance with privileged communication and child abuse reporting laws. *Professional Psychology*, 9, 448–458.

Thoennes, N., & Tjaden, P. (1990). The extent, nature and validity of sexual abuse allegations in custody/visitation disputes. *Child Abuse and Neglect*, 14, 151.

Timmons-Mitchell, J., Chandler-Holtz, D., & Semple, W. E. (1996). Post-traumatic stress symptoms in mothers following children's reports of sexual abuse: An exploratory study. *American Journal of Orthopsychiatry*, 66(3), 463–467.

Tufts New England Medical Center. (1984). *Sexually exploited children: Service and research project. Final report for the Office of Juvenile Justice and Delinquency Prevention.* Washington, DC: U.S. Department of Justice.

Wyatt, G. E., & Newcomb, M. (1990). Internal and external mediators of women's sexual abuse in childhood. *Journal of Consulting and Clinical Psychology*, 58(6), 758–767.

Wyatt, G. E., & Peters, S. D. (1986). Methodological considerations in research on the prevalence of child sexual abuse. *Child Abuse and Neglect*, 10, 241–251.

SUGGESTED READINGS

Berliner, L., & Elliott, D. M. (1996). Sexual abuse of children. In J. Briere, L. Berliner, J. A. Bulkley, C. Jenny, & T. Reid (Eds.), *The APSAC handbook on child maltreatment* (pp. 51–71). Thousand Oaks, CA: Sage.

Deblinger, E., & Heflin, A. H. (1996). *Treating sexually abused children and their nonoffending parents: A cognitive behavioral approach.* Thousand Oaks, CA: Sage.

Pence, D. M., & Wilson, C. A. (1994). Reporting and investigating child sexual abuse. *The Future of Children*, 4(2), 70–83.

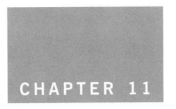

CHAPTER 11

Spousal Abuse

L. Kevin Hamberger
Amy Holtzworth-Munroe

Marital violence is a serious problem in the United States. Data from the recent National Violence Against Women Survey (Tjaden & Thoennes, 2000) indicate that, in their lifetime, 22.1% of women experience physical violence, 7.7% are raped by their intimate partner, and 4.8% are stalked. Partner violence often begins early in a relationship. For example, in one study, over one-third of couples who were planning to marry reported the occurrence of relationship aggression (O'Leary et al., 1989). In addition, O'Leary, Vivian, and Malone (1992) observed that while only about 6% of women seeking marital therapy identified violence as a presenting problem, when directly asked about domestic violence via a structured domestic violence inventory, between 44% and 53% were found to be victims of partner violence.

Without intervention, relationship violence often continues. In a longitudinal study of newly married couples, if a partner had been violent at one point in time, there was a 46–72% probability that he/she would also be violent at the next follow-up assessment (O'Leary et al., 1989). Furthermore, more than 76% of men who were violent during premarital engagement also perpetrated violence during one or more of the three assessment periods over 30 months, and almost 62% were severely violent during one or more of the three assessment periods (Lorber & O'Leary, 2004). Other longitudinal studies have reported similar findings (Feld & Straus, 1989; Quigley & Leonard, 1996). These data support retrospective, anecdotal reports indicating that, for many couples, violence not only continues but also escalates in frequency and severity over time (e.g., Pagelow, 1984).

The potential costs of marital violence are high. Marital violence always carries a risk of physical injury (Kyriacou et al., 1999), homicide (Dannenberg et al., 1995), or suicide (Stark & Flitcraft, 1995). In addition, partner violence is related to relationship distress (e.g., O'Leary et al., 1989) and has been found to predict marital dissolution (Rogge & Bradbury, 1999). Comprehensive reviews of the psychological impact of partner violence demonstrated that individual victims suffer many psychological problems, including depression, alcohol abuse, and posttraumatic stress disorder (Hamberger & Phelan, 2004; Holtzworth-Munroe, Smutzler, & Sandin, 1997). Perpetrators also exhibit a variety of psychological problems (Gleason, 1997; Holtzworth-Munroe, Bates, Smutzler, & Sandin, 1997), ranging from depression and anger (Feldbau-Kohn, Heyman, & O'Leary, 1998; Vivian & Langhinrischen-Rohling, 1994) to alcohol problems and personality disorder (Hamberger, Lohr, Bonge, & Tolin, 1996). In addition, child abuse and other negative effects on the children of such relationships (e.g., Edleson, 2000; Holtzworth-Munroe, Smutzler, & Sandin, 1997) are notable.

Although females report rates of assault perpetration comparable to males (Archer, 2000; Hamberger, 2005), there are a number of reasons to focus on male violence. Most important, men are more likely to injure their partners than are women (Archer, 2000; Hamberger, 2005). Research demonstrates that women are more likely than men to require medical care, to take time off from work, and to spend more time in bed due to illness as a consequence of a physical attack from a partner (e.g., Cantos, Neidig, & O'Leary, 1994; Stets & Straus, 1990). Men's violence also results in more psychological problems than does women's, including stress, depression, and psychosomatic symptoms (Cascardi, Langhinrichsen, & Vivian, 1992; Vivian & Langhinrischen-Rohling, 1994). In addition, emerging data indicate that women's violence tends to be self-defensive or retaliatory, whereas men's violence is more often motivated by its instrumental value (i.e., to control or punish the wife; Hamberger, 2005; Hamberger et al., 1997). The interested reader should refer to Holtzworth-Munroe, Smutzler, and Bates (1997) and Hamberger (2005) for comprehensive reviews of the differential consequences of partner violence for men and women. Therefore, given the serious consequences of husband violence, our primary focus is male-to-female violence.

Given the prevalence of partner violence, the likelihood that it will continue or escalate once initiated, and the resulting negative consequences, the occurrence of partner violence offers many opportunities for cognitive-behavioral crisis management interventions. In this chapter, we discuss three main areas of crisis management in the treatment of partner violence: (1) understanding and intervening in the general crisis, broadly defined, of ongoing (or past) violence in a relationship; (2) the immediate, acute crisis involved when a perpetrator or victim calls for help in a situation with imminent potential for violence; and (3) the crisis created when a therapist is directly confronted by an angry, agitated perpetrator.

THE CRISIS OF PARTNER VIOLENCE

In a broad sense, relationships in which one partner batters the other always constitute a crisis state. This is not to imply that perpetrators constantly batter their wives (although this is true in some cases). However, we consider even relationships with relatively infrequent violence and in which violence is currently not occurring to be in a state of crisis. To understand this point, one must understand the dynamics of battering and the enduring effects of violence on the perpetrator and victim.

Effects of Violence on the Victim

Partner violence affects many aspects of a victim's life. As reviewed earlier, battered women have been found to suffer from psychological and health problems. Even during periods when there is no physical violence, battered women are often "on edge" due to the offender's ongoing use of psychological terror tactics. Pence (1989) has outlined some of these tactics. Some are obviously abusive, such as threats of violence, constant name-calling, and lengthy verbal tirades. In contrast, others (e.g., criticizing the wife's appearance or complaining that she talks with her mother too much) appear relatively subtle and mundane and function to undermine the woman's sense of self and agency (Marshall, 1999). Indeed, in nonviolent relationships, such behaviors are hurtful and irritating but do not have the same impact as they do for battered women. For battered women, such tactics have often accompanied violence; they have been paired with physical violence (the unconditioned stimulus) and its effects (i.e., fear, pain, and injury—the unconditioned response) such that these nonphysical behaviors become conditioned stimuli resulting in conditioned fear responses (Hamberger & Lohr, 1989).

In addition to the stress of psychological abuse, an ongoing stressor for battered women is the cognitive "rules" they have learned from a variety of sources, including societal messages, formal and informal "helpers," and the batterer (Barnett, Miller-Perrin, & Perrin, 2005; Dutton, 1992; Goodman & Fallon, 1995). Such cognitions may include attributions of responsibility for the violence ("It's my fault; I made him hit me") and for keeping the relationship together ("It's a woman's responsibility to keep the family together"), and assumptions about her inability to survive outside the violent relationship ("I can't make it without him"). These cognitions may increase the psychological stress (e.g., depression or anxiety) of victims. In addition to intrapsychic factors, battered women frequently face many situational barriers that lead to futility and entrapment in violent relationships, including being physically prevented from leaving or calling the police and being threatened with violence if such attempts are made (Barnett et al., 2005; Fleury, Sullivan, Bybee, & Davidson, 1998). Battered women are reluctant to disclose the violence to health care providers out of fear that once disclosed, they will have no control over the information and could face retribution from the perpetrator if he becomes aware of the disclosure (Gielen et al., 2000).

Thus, even between acute battering episodes, battered women can be conceptualized as being in a relatively constant state of stress. They are always vigilant for the signs of impending attack, constantly engaging in violence-avoidant behaviors, and are vigilant about protecting the information about their situations. However, they are never actually able to control their partner's behavior and are constantly at risk for further abuse.

Effects of Violence on the Perpetrator

Partner violence also affects the male offender. As outlined by Hamberger and Lohr (1989), battering behavior has functional value. Although many offenders report feeling remorse and sorrow following a battering incident, violence is often reinforced either through negative (e.g., the victim stopping some behavior perceived as noxious by the offender) or positive (e.g., tension release or the acquisition of sexual gratification) reinforcement. This reinforcement increases the probability of further violence. Through such processes, various attributional patterns are also reinforced. For example, relative to nonviolent men, violent husbands attribute more hostile intent to nonviolent, negative wife behavior (Holtzworth-Munroe & Hutchinson, 1993; Tonizzo, Howells, Day, Reidpath, & Froyland, 2000). Such attributions may make it easier for men to view their violence as justified retaliation against a "hostile" wife (Holtzworth-Munroe & Hutchinson, 1993). In addition, domestically violent men often avoid the negative consequences of their behavior by externalizing responsibility for the violence (e.g., "She caused all the trouble"); minimizing their aggression ("We had a little spat"); and denying their behavior ("I never hit her, she bruises easily"). Waltz, Babcock, Jacobson, and Gottman (1991) found a positive correlation between batterers' minimization and victims' reports of psychological abuse. Thus, the cognitions of violent husbands increase the risk of continued abusive behaviors.

Whereas the victim/partner is constantly "on edge" due to threats to her actual safety, the offender is on edge due to perceived threats to his sense of authority in his relationship. He often views the world as a dangerous, threatening place against which he must take extraordinary steps, including violence, to maintain a sense of integrity and keep his partner "in line" (Sonkin & Dutton, 2003; Hamberger et al., 1997). As a result, the batterer is often depressed and anxious. However, due to his defensiveness, he may be unaware of his destructive behavior patterns or their impact on his partner.

Effects of Violence on the Relationship

The impact of ongoing violence on the relationship of an offender and a victim is likely to be profound. Partner violence is related to relationship distress (e.g., Langhinrischen-Rohling, Schlee, Monson, Ehrensaft, & Heyman, 1998) and marital dissolution (Rogge & Bradbury, 1999), and is repeated and chronic. For example, in a survey of battered women Avni (1991) reported that duration of violence ranged from 2 to 30 years, and the first occurrence of violence took place within the first month of marriage. Thus, even without an *acute* episode of violence, it is appropriate to conceptualize intervention in such relationships as crisis management. By confronting the overall crisis of partner violence, the therapist can take steps to prevent further, possibly more severe, violence and injury from taking place.

MANAGEMENT OF THE PARTNER VIOLENCE CRISIS

There is no specific "technique" for managing the crisis of partner violence, but a number of useful guidelines have been developed. Although many of these guidelines have emerged from the medical literature on interventions with battered women in emergency and outpatient settings (American College of Emergency Physicians, 1995;

National Medical Association, 1995; Ambuel, Hamberger, & Lahti, 1997; Hamberger & Phelan, 2004), they are sufficiently flexible to apply in mental health settings as well.

The fundamental tools required for managing the crisis of partner violence are (1) willingness to ask clients about partner violence as part of routine screening and assessment; (2) adequate knowledge of local services for battered women and battering men; (3) a clear moral (but not moralistic) position that violence toward one's partner is wrong, unacceptable, and the sole responsibility of the perpetrator; and (4) willingness to collaborate with the perpetrator, the victim, or both to enhance safety and stop the violence.

The Battered Woman

Inquiry

As noted previously, battered women do not easily volunteer their plight (Plichta, Duncan, & Plichta, 1996). In fact, they frequently go to great lengths to avoid disclosure (Gerbert et al., 1996). Prior help seeking may have resulted in inappropriate or indifferent responses that implied that the violence was not serious and blamed the victim for her plight rather than assigning responsibility for the violence to the offender (Barnett et al., 2005; Hamberger, Ambuel, Marbella, & Donze, 1998).

Given the victim's reticence, inquiry should proceed at a gradual pace, beginning with general questions about relationship conflict and gradually proceeding to questions about verbal and physical abuse. For example, one line of questioning might be: "When you and your partner argue, how does he act when he becomes angry? Does he ever call you names? During arguments, are you ever afraid for your safety? Sometimes, when men get angry with their partner, they become physical and may push or shove. Has that ever happened to you? What other types of physical aggression has your partner used when he's been angry or otherwise upset? Have you ever been injured by your partner's aggression?" O'Leary et al. (1992) found that among marital therapy clients, direct questioning about abuse resulted in higher identification rates than relying on client self-disclosure. Feldhaus et al. (1997) found that a single, direct question—"Have you been hit, kicked, punched, or otherwise hurt by someone within the past year? If so, by whom?"—was nearly as sensitive and specific as the Conflict Tactics Scale (Straus, 1979) in detecting partner violence victims in an emergency department.

Danger Assessment

Assessment and prediction of violence and danger in the field of partner violence is controversial. On the one hand, Hart (1994) argues that battered women have informed the field of many aspects of perpetrator behavior that can lead to decision making about potential danger in given cases. On the other hand, Gondolf (1994) argues that many commonsense risk markers such as gun ownership, previous severe violence, prior police contact, and alcohol and drug abuse have not been shown empirically to predict domestic homicide. Gondolf and Hart both suggest that the situation and behaviors of batterers and victims should be carefully monitored on an ongoing basis, and appropriate action should be taken to protect potential victims when risk markers are evident. Once violence has been reported, one should gather in-depth information on violence duration, frequency and severity, maximum severity, changes in frequency and severity, and the impact of violence on the victim.

Browne (1987) has enumerated characteristics that differentiated battered women who killed their partners from those who did not. These included high levels of severe and injurious violence, sexual abuse of the woman by the perpetrator, drug and alcohol intoxication by the perpetrator, perpetrator threats to kill, and suicide attempts by the battered woman. Hart (1991) has offered a list of risk markers for lethality to either partner, including the centrality of the battered woman in the batterer's life, the batterer's sense of ownership of the battered woman, and sudden changes in the batterer's behavior—especially risk taking, such as breaking into an estranged partner's residence.

The battered woman's perceptions of her own safety and prediction of further assaults have also been found to significantly increase prediction of reassault. Heckert and Gondolf (2004) demonstrated that the woman's perception of danger was a better predictor of violence than several paper-and-pencil risk scales, and almost as good as the Danger Assessment Scale (DAS; Campbell, 1986, described later). In addition Weisz, Tolman, and Saunders (2000) found that the woman's prediction of new violence added significantly to the prediction of new violence based on empirically supported risk factors. Further, women who answer affirmatively to a screening question about domestic violence are more than 11 times more likely to experience new violence in the next 4 months than women who do not screen positive (Houry et al., 2004). Hence, it makes considerable clinical and empirical sense to ask women about intimate partner violence and, for those women who reveal the existence of partner violence, to ask follow-up questions about their perceptions of danger and predictability of new violence.

Campbell (1986) developed the DAS to assess potential lethality in violent relationships. The DAS has 15 items that the battered woman answers in a yes/no format. Campbell (1995) has provided extensive information on the validity and reliability of the DAS. Risk is determined by the total number of items for which the respondent provides an affirmative answer. The woman's responses to the DAS can provide a valuable touchstone for discussing her perceptions of danger and the provider's concerns for her safety, leading to safety planning and supportive interventions.

From a practical perspective, expressions of concern about danger should not be contingent upon the presence of a certain number of observed risk markers; the presence of any risk markers should be cause for concern. Such concern should also take the victim's suicidal ideation and risk into consideration. Stark and Flitcraft (1995) report that nearly 30% of women who attempted suicide were in violent relationships at the time.

Responding to the Battered Woman's Report

Because a battered woman will often disclose her victimization only reluctantly, inappropriate or insensitive responses to such disclosures could destroy an opportunity for effective intervention. Therefore, on learning of the occurrence of violence, it is important that the therapist clearly and unequivocally communicate to the woman that (1) her story is believed, (2) she is not responsible for the violence or for stopping it, and (3) her disclosure will remain confidential and will only be released with her informed consent to the extent allowed by law (Ambuel et al., 1997). The violence must be identified as a problem in its own right, not portrayed as part of communication or other marital problems or a deficiency on the victim's part. While it is true that violent relationships often involve many other problems, Sonkin, Martin, and Walker (1985) and Holtzworth-Munroe, Meehan, Rehman, and Marshall (2002) argue that more general marital problems cannot be effectively treated without first stopping the violence and achieving safety for the battered woman. In addition, there is no evidence supporting the notion that victimization is a function of victim psychopathology. Battered women are not masochistic (Kuhl, 1984) and are no more likely than nonbattered women to exhibit other forms of psychopathology, although they may exhibit symptoms suggestive of trauma (Holtzworth-Munroe, Smutzler, & Sandin, 1997).

Safety Planning

Although the therapist must help a battered woman exonerate herself from culpability for her victimization, it is simultaneously important to help her take responsibility for her safety and that of any children (Ambuel et al., 1997; Hamberger et al., 1998). To do so, one must have knowledge of local resources, agencies, and legal options to support the safety needs of battered women. Such resources include informal supports (e.g., family, friends, medical practitioners, and clergy), formal resources (e.g., local battered women's shelters and advocacy programs), and social services systems for assisting in acquisition of housing, financial assistance, and other necessities if a woman leaves her partner. If there is a shelter in the area, it is important to provide the battered woman with the telephone number, along with encouraging her to use its counseling and shelter services. Legal resources and options should be explored. If there is a mandatory arrest law in the area, it should be described. The availability and function, as well as limitations of restraining orders, should be discussed.

Many practical steps can be discussed and tailored to the individual needs and situation of the battered woman. Examples include not arguing with the offender when he comes home intoxicated; identifying, when possible, predictors of dangerous situations; and using these cues to seek safety immediately (Hamberger & Potente, 1996). Developing and rehearsing escape plans from numerous locations within the residence can be important. Storing extra clothing, money, and copies of important papers in easily accessible places in the event of a necessary quick exit is recommended. The possibility of storing important items at a friend's or relative's residence should be explored. To aid in developing and rehearsing a comprehensive, self-relevant safety plan, Hart and Stuehling (1992) have developed a personalized safety plan workbook; the therapist can help the battered woman to use this guide. Through collaboration, the therapist begins to help the battered woman to develop and trust her own problem-solving skills for seeking safety.

Follow-Up

Although it is important to coordinate with other services for battered women, it is also important for the therapist to maintain continuity of care with the client (Ambuel et al., 1997; Hamberger & Ambuel, 1997). First, leaving a batterer to seek safety is a complex process that often requires many attempts before success; frequent follow-up is needed to review and revise safety plans as well as provide support for the battered woman's efforts. Second, follow-up is necessary to monitor safety when a battered woman leaves her violent relationship, as relationship dissolution is often the single most dangerous time for a battered woman. Rasche's (1988) research indicated that a maximum risk of homicide for battered women continues for up to 2 years after leaving the relationship. Research also indicates that continuity of care that includes brief counseling, community-based advocacy, and case management following a shelter stay is related to improved quality of life, self-esteem, greater social support, easier access to community resources, and less violence (Hagan & Postmus, 2003; Sullivan & Bybee, 1999).

Another reason for continued follow-up is to discuss the woman's cognitive-related blocks to escaping a violent relationship (Barnett et al., 2005; Dutton, 1992). For example, cost–benefit analysis may lead the woman to conclude that it is less costly to stay than to leave. In addition, some battered women truly feel that they are to blame for their partner's violence, and others do not believe they could survive on their own, even if they possess resources to do so. These and other cognitions can be explored, challenged, and modified. This exploration works best in a collaborative relationship where the therapist engages in a dialogue with the battered woman, rather than tries to analyze and prescribe (Dutton, 1992).

Documentation

There are important reasons to document violence when it is reported by a client. First, battered women are at high risk for being injured and/or killed, as well as for committing or attempting homicide or suicide. Therefore, it is important to document assessed dangerousness as well as steps taken to reduce risk, protect potential victims, and enhance safety (Ambuel et al., 1997).

Second, because battered women are often isolated and tell few people of their plight, careful documentation of their victimization and its impact may constitute the only official record of the situation. Such information may have limited impact in criminal proceedings but may be helpful in civil proceedings such as custody hearings. Battered women often appear suboptimal as parents, but with documentation, it can be argued that many of the problems of the woman and children are related to her partner's violence, not to a "defect" within her.

Finally, careful documentation validates the battered woman. Without detailed documentation, the battered woman can become simply a diagnosis without a context. Warshaw (1993) has argued that diagnosing a battered woman without documenting her context dehumanizes and isolates her in the same way that her batterer/partner does when he beats her.

The Offender

Assessment and crisis intervention with male offenders are in many ways similar to those for assisting battered women. That is, it is important to ask about violence, assess danger, develop safety/control plans, conduct follow-up, and provide careful documentation. Nevertheless, working with offenders requires different strategies than does working with battered women.

Inquiry

Asking men about their use of violence should proceed at a gradual pace. Hence, the interview techniques described earlier apply to men as well. Of particular importance in working with men is understanding that male batterers typically deny and minimize their violence relative to reports by their female partners (Sugarman & Hotaling, 1997). Thus questions should be structured in a way that facilitates disclosure and minimizes denial. For example, we have found that men are more likely to admit having engaged in specific aggressive actions (e.g., "Have you ever pushed your wife?" "Have you ever slapped your wife?") (see Straus, 1979; Straus, Hamby, Boney-McCoy, & Sugarman, 1996) than to respond affirmatively to global questions that negatively label such actions as "violence" and "abuse" (e.g., "Have you been violent?" "Have you ever abused your wife?").

However, even when a man admits to having used partner violence, he may defensively blame his partner or portray her as the instigator or as being more violent than he is; in these ways, he justifies his violent actions as necessary self-defense. Given the goal of getting the perpetrator to take responsibility for his actions, it is tempting for a therapist to become argumentative when faced with such reasoning. However, we have found that it is helpful to avoid such confrontation, at least initially. It is often more useful to explore collaboratively with the offender several parameters of his use of force. For example, in addition to assessing violence duration, frequency, and severity, one can ask the man more detailed questions about his partner's use of initiated and defensive force against him. Specific actions should be carefully probed, because it is not uncommon to discover that the man's description of his partner's "initiation" of force involves obnoxious, undesired behaviors (e.g., verbal assault) but not physical aggression. If he reports that she has initiated violence, questions can be asked about what percentage of the time each partner initiates the use of force and whether his partner was the first to initiate violence in the relationship. Men in clinical samples usually report initiating violence a greater percentage of time than do their partners and are more likely to have been the first to initiate violence in the relationship (Hamberger, 1997; Hamberger & Guse, 2002; Phelan et al., 2005). Men can be asked to consider this information and reexamine their belief that their violence is self-defensive or "mutual."

With male offenders, the goal is to maximize their sense of responsibility for the violence and for stopping it. Therefore, even if the offender gives credible accounts of his partner's negative behavior, his stressful life, his drinking problem, or his poor childhood, it is important to empathize with his experience but also confront his violence as unjustified.

Assessing Danger

All violence should be considered dangerous, but as described in the section on battered women, certain factors indicate a risk of highly injurious or even lethal violence. If any of these variables are observed, it is important to respond with concern. It must be emphasized to the man that although the primary concern is the woman's safety, he is also at risk for injury and even death. It is thus imperative to develop, with the offender, appropriate plans for maximizing safety for his partner and minimizing the risk of violence.

Safety and Control Planning

The goal of safety and control planning for offenders is to stop their violence to ensure safety for their partner. There are several steps that can be taken toward this goal.

If the therapist has thus far interviewed only the offender, it is important to contact the victim to conduct an independent, corroborative assessment and initiate crisis management and safety planning with her, as outlined earlier. Although it is important to let the offender know that his partner will be contacted, it is also important to inform him that the therapist will meet with her separately and that the information provided by her will not be disclosed to him. These procedures are important for two reasons. First, she must be provided with safety if she is to be asked to discuss her partner's violence; to ask her to report the violence in front of the offender could place her at risk for further violence after the session. Second, an independent report from the partner can provide information on the extent to which the man is minimizing or denying his use of force. Third, meeting separately highlights individual responsibility for stopping the violence and decreasing the possibility of in-session attempts to control his partner.

A stopgap time-out procedure (see Holtzworth-Munroe et al., 2002, for a detailed description of the procedure and its rationale) is an effective step toward achieving safety and control. "Time out" entails a number of steps that culminate in the man taking a "break" from his violence. The man learns to identify internal and external cues that indicate he is becoming angry and his behavior is escalating toward violence. These cues are signals to the man to take a time out; at that point, he tells his partner that he will take a break to "cool down," and he gives her an estimate of how long he will be away. While out of the situation, the man takes appropriate steps to decrease his arousal and probability of engaging in aggressive behaviors (e.g., reevaluate the situation and his escalating behavior pattern and develop strategies to avoid the occurrence of violence). Once cooled down, he returns to his partner. The procedure is repeated as often as necessary to avoid battering. It is important to instruct the man that the sole function of time outs is to avoid becoming violent or abusive. Many men view time outs as "running away" from a problem that will be there when they return. This interpretation must be changed. Although it is true that time-outs do not solve specific relationship conflicts, they can facilitate a safer environment in which the couple can work toward nonviolent resolution of such conflicts. Therapists should also be mindful of potential misuses of time-out techniques. Specifically, a time out can be used to habitually avoid ever listening to the concerns of a partner and thus effectively control her by blocking her communication attempts. Clients need to be cautioned about this potential misuse and encouraged to avoid it.

Another step taken to facilitate safety is motivating the man to enter treatment to end his battering behavior. If violence is discovered in the context of an ongoing therapy relationship, treatment can occur in that context if the therapist is comfortable and experienced in dealing with partner violence. Alternatively, referral to a batterers' treatment program is recommended. In either case, two issues are important to consider. First, any treatment, regardless of format, must hold the perpetrator solely responsible for the violence and for ending it. A number of treatment approaches designed to aid men in ending violence have been developed, including profeminist approaches, conjoint treatment approaches, cognitive-behavioral, and psychodynamic models. The interested reader is referred to Dutton and Sonkin (2003) and Aldarondo and Mederos (2002) for excellent expositions of different treatment models. Second, one must realize that many violent men are extremely reluctant to enter treatment for their violence (Gondolf & Foster, 1991; Hamberger & Hastings, 1986). Murphy and Eckhardt (2005) describe adaptations of motivational interviewing strategies to facilitate abusive men's interest and commitment to entering abuse abatement treatment.

To facilitate safety and violence control, the therapist must collaborate with the batterer to respect any separation his partner has imposed, with or without a court order. Because many violent men are socially and psychologically isolated, relationship separation can be overwhelming, leading to inappropriate, premature efforts to reconcile with their partner or punish her for leaving. Two steps can be taken to help men avoid such contact. First, the therapist can help the man to interpret the separation not as a threat but, rather, as an opportunity for both partners to work on their problems, find safety, and stop violence so that decisions about the relationship can be made in a safe, rational manner. Second, it is helpful to collaborate with the man to identify formal and informal social supports to assist him through this difficult time; these supports could include friends, family members, counselors and, if relevant, 12-step program sponsors and clergy. Miles (1999) has provided guidelines for clergy to follow in working with families struggling with abuse.

In summary, safety planning for battering men differs in at least one fundamental way from that for battered women: With battering men, the goal of safety and control planning is to foster and develop a sense of personal responsibility for stopping the violence and ensuring safety for their partner. If the man does not accept responsibility, the woman will remain at risk and other treatment will be ineffective.

Follow-up

As with battered women, follow-up with the offender is essential. It is also advisable to conduct periodic follow-up with the victim to corroborate the man's report. Follow-up visits with the offender allow for ongoing assessment of the safety/control plan. Stopping violence and giving up control is seldom a one-session phenomenon. Through many visits, a therapeutic alliance is developed to facilitate change. Confrontational, prescriptive approaches may be perceived by the offender as moralistic attacks, resulting in his leaving therapy.

Documentation

Because of the risks of reoffending and homicide, it is important to document the assessment of violence, steps taken to warn and protect potential victims, and other steps taken to ensure safety. Because many offenders come to treatment under a court order, it is important to develop documentation that assists the courts in monitoring the offender's accountability, including noncompliance. Finally, as with battered women, documentation of violence may prove important in civil proceedings such as child custody hearings.

CALLS IN THE NIGHT: ACUTE CRISES

When a therapist works with battered women or male offenders, he/she must understand that in addition to intervening in the more "general" crisis discussed previously, clients will sometimes call outside regular appointment times. Such calls are usually during an acute, extreme crisis situation in which the caller is either very worried that violence could occur or in which an assault has occurred and the caller is distraught, frightened, and possibly hurt. These are difficult calls to take, but the steps taken in such situations can be crucial in stopping or preventing an assault and possibly saving a life. Management of acute crises requires a willingness to listen, collaborate with the caller to define the problem, and develop alternative solutions to achieve safety and avoid violence.

The Battered Woman

When a battered woman calls in crisis, the first priority is to assess her immediate safety and determine whether she or the children have been assaulted. Questions such as "Have you or your kids been assaulted?" and "Is your partner there with you right now? Can he hear you? Is he listening to this conversation? Is it okay for you to talk right now?" help convey the message that her call is taken seriously and her safety is of paramount importance. If the batterer is nearby and she wishes to continue talking, it is helpful to pose closed-end questions so that she is not required to provide details in front of a partner who is agitated and struggling with control. If the batterer is present, at some point it is appropriate to ask the victim about the advisability of speaking with him directly; often, if the offender is present when the woman calls, she is interested in having him participate in the conversation at some point. The specifics of such a conversation are detailed in the next section.

If her partner is not present, try to ascertain whether she knows where he went and whether she expects him back soon. It is also wise to plan with her what will happen should he return while she is the telephone. For example, we have often worked with a woman to develop a plan that called for hanging up at her signal and agreeing that she will call back again when she feels safe.

Once it is determined that it is safe to talk, the therapist should inquire about injuries. If she has been injured, determine whether she would like to go to an emergency room and whether she would like assistance in facilitating the call for emergency services. It is generally believed that health care providers should not "do too much" for battered women and thus further disempower them. In more extreme cases, however, making a call can be helpful, particularly if the choice to do so was made by the client and if medical danger is a possible consequence of inaction. Some states, such as California, Colorado, Kentucky, New Hampshire, New Mexico, and Rhode Island, require health care providers to report suspected cases of partner abuse to authorities (Rodriguez, McLoughlin, Bauer, Paredes, & Grumbach, 1999). Although mandatory reporting of partner abuse is controversial (Hamberger & Phelan, 2004; Rodriguez et al., 1999), it is necessary for mental health professionals to know applicable local and state laws.

Whether or not she has been assaulted, it is important to continue safety planning. If the therapist has previously worked with the woman to develop a safety plan, the task is to help her implement it, including finding a safe place to stay, calling the police, or, if the batterer is on probation, calling his probation officer. If the woman has not previously developed a safety plan, many of the steps discussed earlier will need to be covered.

In addition to assessing the battered woman's safety, it is important to assess her potential for violence against herself (i.e., suicide) or her partner. Suicidal ideation reveals the desperation, hopelessness, and degradation many battered women feel. Sometimes, these extreme feelings lead to plans for retaliatory violence and even homicide. Dealing with such thoughts and feelings is extremely important. Although there is no formula for managing such intense feelings, we have found a number of efforts to be helpful. Basically, a suicidal or assaultive individual needs to hear the therapist's expressions of support. We assume that the individual would not have called had he/she not wanted support and assurance. Therefore, simply telling clients that you do not want them to commit suicide or assault/kill their partner is a good start.

It is also important to assess the seriousness of suicidal or violent ideation. The therapist should differentiate idea from intent, plans, and the availability of means to implement plans. Many people in crisis wish they or their partner were dead but "would never do it" or "have not considered any plan." If a plan is in place, the caller's ability to carry it out must be assessed. For example, if she wants to shoot her partner, it is important to know whether there is a gun at her immediate disposal, whether the gun is loaded or ammunition is easily accessible, and her own subjective assessment of the likelihood that she will attempt to carry out her plan.

If it is judged that the risk of harm to herself or someone else is not imminent, it is still important to discuss the costs and benefits of any such violence. Such discussion could focus on the well-being of the children if she kills herself, on whether it is worth getting arrested and punished for assaulting or killing her partner, and on whether nonviolent alternatives such as shelter safety or restraining orders are preferable.

If the risk of imminent harm is judged to be high, steps must be taken to protect and warn potential victims. For purposes of this discussion, "protection" could mean helping the woman get to a shelter where she can cool down and rethink her situation. In extreme cases, temporary hospitalization may be necessary.

Once a plan of action has been mutually agreed on, it is important to have the caller review what she will do to implement and execute the plan. At this point, a follow-up contact is arranged. Depending on safety considerations, it may be necessary to leave the specific time of contact open and allow the woman to call in when she feels safe. If the therapist commits to initiating the follow-up contact, an exact time should be specified and rigidly adhered to. Follow-ups for acute crises should not exceed 24 hours. It is important to stabilize and resolve matters of safety and lethality quickly so that other related therapy can proceed. Finally, crisis contacts must be documented.

The Male Offender

In general, male offenders are less likely than battered women to call someone when they are in a crisis. On the other hand, if a therapist has established a trusting, collaborative relationship with a violent man and has permitted crisis calls as part of his safety/control plan, the man may call. When a therapist takes a call from a violent man, the therapist must acknowledge the internal barriers he/she overcame to make the call. This can be accomplished by a simple statement, such as "I'm really glad you called. I know it was hard to do. But you've taken an important step in helping yourself." After establishing an alliance with the man to resolve his crisis, it is important to ascertain whether an assault occurred and whether his partner is with him at his location.

If she is present, steps outlined previously can be followed in talking with her. It should be noted, however, that speaking with the therapist is the woman's option, not the perpetrator's. This expectation can be communicated by simply stating, in a matter-of-fact way, "I want to speak with your partner just to reassure myself that she's okay." This communicates to the man that his actions have consequences for his partner's well-being and that her safety is the therapist's overriding concern.

Further discussion with the offender centers around the necessity of avoiding violence or, if violence has occurred, not repeating it. If violence has occurred, it should be neither moralistically condemned nor "understood." Violence must be responded to as wrong and providing evidence that the man must continue (or begin) treatment to stop his violence. If no violence has occurred, the man can be told that the crisis call is a sign of strength because he is responsibly taking steps toward nonviolence. If the therapist is familiar with the caller and has previously conducted safety/control planning, much of the call will focus on reviewing appropriate options from that plan, Examples of such options include spending the night with a friend or relative, avoiding alcohol and drugs, and taking extended time outs. If the woman has left the residence, the batterer should be encouraged to respect her decision and to view her absence as a time out rather than abandonment. The emotional pain he may feel by her absence can be interpreted as a cue for him to continue working on changing his abusive behavior, which led to her leaving in the first place.

As with female callers, danger and judgments of high risk for imminent violence must be addressed. For example, Hamberger received a call from a highly intoxicated client who was distraught over the recent breakup of his relationship; he was talking on the telephone with his shotgun on his lap and threatened suicide after finishing the conversation. While talking to the client, a clinic associate was notified of the situation and asked to call the police. The police arrived while the client was still on the telephone. He surrendered and was taken to a local hospital for emergency psychiatric hospitalization. Following stabilization and release from the hospital, he resumed batterer's treatment and alcohol rehabilitation.

In less severe cases, frequent follow-up contacts should be part of the control plan and should be explicit. To further enhance the concept of self-responsibility, the offender can be assigned the task of making the follow-up call. Thorough documentation of the crisis contact should be completed.

THERAPIST SAFETY ISSUES IN CRISIS MANAGEMENT

Perhaps the most typical questions we are asked are, "Aren't you afraid for your safety?" and "What do you do when a batterer comes after you?" These questions betray a common underlying fear that working with victims and perpetrators of partner violence is a dangerous occupation for the therapist. Collectively, we have worked in the field of partner violence for 39 years. Hamberger has worked full time for more than 20 years, treating and studying domestically violent men. During that time, neither of us has been the subject of physical attack or even a direct threat to our safety. There are presently no published data to determine the uniqueness of our experience. However, informal conversations with colleagues suggest that physical assault of the therapist is rare, and direct threats are infrequent. This is not to suggest that those who work with battered women need not be concerned about attack; even experienced therapists take precautions when working with an offender in crisis.

Acceptance and Listening

Perhaps most important in working with an offender in crisis is to understand and accept his feelings and his struggle for control while remaining clear that his abusive, manipulative, and aggressive behaviors are not acceptable. This is best accomplished through careful listening and engaging him in a dialogue rather than preaching, moralizing, and asserting professional authority in an attempt to control him. The latter strategies will be ineffective and could place the therapist at risk. Because batterers are very power oriented and acutely aware of when others try to control them, efforts to dominate a batterer can result in an escalating power struggle that may end in assault. It is better to help the offender to control his actions by demonstrating to him an acceptance of his negative feelings and a willingness to help him resolve his crisis, even if he does not "get his way."

Case Study

The following is an example of an angry offender. George is a 25-year-old, Anglo offender who was adjudicated for punching Anna, his wife of 3 years, several times in the face, throwing her to the ground and kicking her in the ribs and lower back, pulling her hair, and attempting to strangle her. The incident occurred after George discovered that she had "gone against his orders" and bought a new dress to wear to her niece's first communion. George was directly ordered to abuse abatement treatment by the judge and placed on 2 years' probation. A presentence investigation revealed that George had battered Anna at least two times per year over the course of their marriage and even for 2 years prior to marriage. The violence showed an escalating pattern over time, and the last two episodes included potentially life-threatening violence. According to Anna, and corroborated by collateral sources, George frequently referred to himself as the "boss" and Anna as his "servant," and he frequently ordered her to do even trivial things just to show his dominance. The probation agent who wrote the presentence investigative report also described George as hostile, arrogant, and controlling. On the day of his initial intake for preabuse abatement treatment evaluation, George came 30 minutes late for his appointment and checked in as if nothing were amiss. When the receptionist notified him that he would not be seen that day due to his tardiness, he became irate and verbally abusive to the receptionist in the presence of other patients in the waiting room. The therapist invited him into an office to discuss the matter. As he approached, the client angrily pointed at the therapist's face and demanded to be seen "or else!" Once in the office, with the door left slightly ajar, the client was invited to sit down. The client refused, so both men stood. The client was encouraged to explain the reasons for the anger. He adamantly demanded to be seen because he "showed up" and had not known that he would not be seen just because he was late. The therapist acknowledged the client's anger and the fact that the client might not have known of the program policy that arrivals later than 15 minutes were not seen. Therefore, the therapist offered to allow the client to reschedule another appointment rather than return to court for having missed this session. The client, while still angry, accepted the offer and indicated that he would be on time for future sessions.

Subsequent evaluation, beginning with his next full session when things had settled down from the present emotional intensity, would focus on his experience of having others make choices that he cannot control, as when his partner bought a new dress without his permission or he was told by a receptionist that he would not be seen even though he "showed up." During this exploration, we would be examining schemata related to his sense of entitlement and the functional value of verbal and nonverbal intimidation tactics, both generally and in the context of his intimate relationship to achieve control, dominance, and compliance. This information, together with other cognitive-behavioral assessment of his battering behavior, will form the basis of initial treatment planning and intervention (Hamberger, 2002). Treatment would target his need to be "the boss" and his pattern of expecting that he should always get his way just because he says so. Other treatment targets would include his use of aggressive interpersonal language and nonverbal behaviors with the goal of learning responsible assertive conflict resolution and negotiation skills.

In analyzing this case, the therapist avoided a loud, hostile, and potentially violent confrontation. This was done by removing the client from a public area, collaborating with him to determine the cause of his upset, yet remaining firm about not seeing him for a therapy session that day. The client's anger was viewed as acceptable (even if based on faulty and naive assumptions), as demonstrated by a willingness to talk about it and to find a solution. However, the hostile, aggressive behavior was not reinforced in that the therapist did not counteraggress and calmly refused to see the client for that session. Nevertheless, because the client did show up and may not have known of the tardiness policy, he was offered an alternative to being terminated from the program. Assertion of power, moralizing that the client should have been prompt, and referral back to court could have escalated the tensions and resulted in aggression. Although still unhappy, the client left the situation having accepted the alternative and resolving to be on time in the future.

Other principles for safety management can also be noted in this case. First, the therapist did not completely close the door—only enough to provide basic privacy without becoming isolated. Because the client had blown up in front of other clinic staff, they were aware of his location and could monitor the situation for any disturbances. Further, the slightly open door provided the therapist and the client with a quick exit if necessary. Hence, the environment was structured to minimize feelings of being trapped.

In addition, when the client refused to sit the therapist also chose to stand. Maintaining a parallel physical posture while also maintaining a reasonable distance (about one arm's length) equalized the power distribution. As the goal of crisis management is to reduce threat through collaboration, sharing power in the interaction is essential.

If You Are Assaulted

There is no easy answer to the question of what to do in the case of an actual attack. The domestic violence literature generally does not address the management of aggressive patients, although other readings may be appropriate (e.g., see Wisted & Freeman, 1994). Many procedures developed for use in inpatient settings may not be appropriate in the outpatient context. For example, a therapist could learn various restraint holds and blocking techniques but must also learn the limitations of such self-defensive maneuvers, both in terms of practicality (i.e., How effective are they in any given situation?) and in terms of liability (i.e., How much, if any, force can a health care provider apply to a client, even in self-defense?). Certainly prevention is the preferable approach to managing safety in working with violent offenders. If attacked, however, the therapist is generally encouraged to prosecute. An attorney should be consulted for guidance.

Preventive Actions

As demonstrated in the previous case, a number of steps can be taken to prevent assault, including listening and collaborating with the client, avoiding isolation, and maintaining a safe distance. Some offices can easily be equipped with an electronic "panic button" to notify security of a serious situation. Clients in crisis should be seen only in a professional setting, where other staff and assistance are available.

If a therapist feels uneasy or threatened in a situation, he/she should be concerned about safety outside the clinic setting. The following measures can be taken to avoid hazards outside the clinic:

1. If driving, park in an open, well-lit area and take the least obstructed route to and from the car; avoid shortcuts past bushes or recessed doorways. If possible, have security or another staff person accompany you to the car.
2. When driving, take different routes to and from work; change your routine frequently.
3. If possible, enlist neighbors to monitor and notify you of any unusual activities around your residence.
4. If necessary, secure an unlisted or unpublished telephone number. Install a caller-identification system to identify and document the source of phone calls. If telephone harassment occurs, times and dates should be documented. Arrangements can be made with the telephone company to install a telephone trap to determine the source of harassing calls. Such documentation can provide additional corroborating evidence in the event of prosecution.

CONCLUSION

In summary, there is no one thing a therapist should do to prevent an assault against him/herself or against the client's partner. In some cases, an assault may occur regardless of steps taken. This is because the perpetrator alone is responsible for choosing to be violent. Nevertheless, a number of things can be done to reduce the probability of an assault.

A primary goal is to develop safety/control plans. The key ingredients of such interventions are based on a number of assumptions. First, safety of potential victims is primary. Second, the offender alone is responsible for his violence and for stopping it. Third, the potential victim is responsible for taking steps to secure safety, either through prevention and avoidance strategies or through escape from attack.

Working to end partner violence is difficult. It often requires multiple meetings to develop appropriate problem solutions and resolve crises. Sometimes, despite the hard work, violence still occurs, which makes the work can frustrating and stressful. But when a battered woman finds safety for herself and her children, and when an offender actively stops his offending, the rewards can be profound and the healing can begin.

REFERENCES

Aldarondo, E., & Mederos, F. (Eds.) (2002). *Programs for men who batter: Intervention and prevention strategies in a diverse society.* Kingston, NJ: Civic Research Institute.

Ambuel, B., Hamberger, L. K., & Lahti, J. (1997). The Family Peace Project: A model for training health care professionals to identify, treat, and prevent partner violence. In L. K. Hamberger, S. Burge, A. Graham, & A. Costa (Eds.), *Violence issues for health care educators and providers* (pp. 55–82). Binghamton, NY: Haworth Press.

American College of Emergency Physicians. (1995). Emergency medicine and domestic violence. *Annals of Emergency Medicine, 25,* 442–443.

Archer, J. (2000). Sex differences in aggression between heterosexual partners: A meta-analytic review. *Psychological Bulletin, 126,* 651–680.

Avni, N. (1991). Battered wives: The home as a total institution. *Violence and Victims, 6,* 137–149.

Barnett, O. W., Miller-Perrin, C. L., & Perrin, R. D. (2005). *Family violence across the lifespan: An introduction* (2nd ed.) Thousand Oaks, CA: Sage.

Browne, A. (1987). *When battered women kill.* New York: The Free Press.

Campbell, J. C. (1986). Assessment of risk of homicide for battered women. *Advances in Nursing Science, 8,* 36–51.

Campbell, J. C. (1995). Prediction of homicide of and by battered women. In J. C. Campbell (Ed.), *Assessing dangerousness: Violence by sexual offenders, batterers, and child abusers* (pp. 96–113). Thousand Oaks, CA: Sage.

Cantos, A. L., Neidig, P. H., & O'Leary, K. D. (1994). Injuries of women and men in a treatment program for domestic violence. *Journal of Family Violence, 9,* 113–124.

Cascardi, M., Langhinrischen, J., & Vivian, D. (1992). Marital aggression: Impact, injury, and health correlates for husbands and wives. *Archives of Internal Medicine, 152,* 1178–1194.

Dannenberg, A. L., Carter, D. M., Lawson, H. W., Ashton, D. M., Dorfman, S. F., & Graham, E. H. (1995). Homicide and other injuries as causes of maternal death in New York City, 1987 through 1991. *American Journal of Obstetrics and Gynecology, 172,* 1557–1564.

Dutton, D., & Sonkin, D. J. (Ed.) (2003). *Intimate violence: Contemporary treatment innovations.* New York: Haworth Maltreatment & Trauma Press.

Dutton, M. A. (1992). *Empowering and healing the battered woman.* New York: Springer.

Edleson J. L. (2000). Children's witnessing of adult domestic violence. *Journal of Interpersonal Violence, 14,* 839–870.

Feld, S. L., & Straus, M. A. (1989). Escalation and desistance of wife assault in marriage. *Criminology, 27,* 141–159.

Feldbau-Kohn, S., Heyman, R. E., & O'Leary, K. D. (1998). Major depressive disorder and depressive symptomatology as predictors of husband to wife physical aggression. *Violence and Victims, 13,* 347–360.

Feldhaus, K. M., Koziol-McClain, J., Amsbury, H. L., Norton, I. M., Lowenstein, S. R., &

Abbott, J. T. (1997). Accuracy of 3 brief screening questions for detecting partner Violence in the emergency department. *Journal of the American Medical Association, 277,* 1357–1361.

Fleury, R. E., Sullivan, C. M., Bybee, D., & Davidson, W. S. (1998). "Why don't they just call the cops?" Reasons for differential contact among women with abusive partners. *Violence and Victims, 13,* 333–346.

Gerbert, B., Johnston, K., Caspers, N., Bleecker, T., Woods, A., & Rosenbaum, A. (1996). Experiences of battered women in health care settings: A qualitative study. *Women and Health, 24,* 1–17.

Gielen, A. C., O'Campo, P. J., Campbell, J. C., Schollenberger, J., Woods, A. B., Jones, A. S., et al. (2000). Women's opinions about domestic violence screening and mandatory reporting. *American Journal of Preventive Medicine, 19,* 279–291.

Gleason, W. J. (1997). Psychological and social dysfunctions in battering men: A review. *Aggression and Violent Behavior, 2,* 43–52.

Gondolf, E. W. (1994). Lethality and dangerousness assessments. *Violence Update, 4*(8), 10.

Gondolf, E. W., & Foster, R. (1991). Pre-treatment attrition in batterer programs. *Journal of Family Violence, 6,* 337–350.

Goodman, M. S., & Fallon, B. C. (1995). *Patter changing for abused women: An educational program.* Thousand Oaks, CA: Sage.

Hagan, J. L., & Postmus, J. L. (2003). *Violence against women: Synthesis of research for advocacy organizations* (NIJ98-WT-VX-K001). Washington, DC: National Institute of Justice.

Hamberger, L. K. (1997). Female offenders in domestic violence: A look at actions in context. *Journal of Aggression, Maltreatment, and Trauma, 1,* 117–129.

Hamberger, L. K. (2005). Men's and women's use of intimate partner violence in clinical samples: Toward a gender-sensitive analysis. *Violence and Victims, 20,* 131–151.

Hamberger, L. K., & Ambuel, B. (1997). Training psychology students and professionals to recognize and intervene into partner violence: Borrowing a page from medicine. *Psychotherapy: Theory, Research, Practice and Training, 34,* 375–385.

Hamberger, L. K., Ambuel, B., Marbella, A., & Donze, J. (1998). Physician interaction with battered women: The women's perspective. *Archives of Family Medicine, 7,* 575–582.

Hamberger, L. K., & Guse, C. E. (2002). Men's and women's use of intimate partner violence in clinical samples. *Violence against Women, 8,* 1301–1331.

Hamberger, L. K., & Hastings, J. E. (1986). Characteristics of spouse abusers: Predictors of treatment acceptance. *Journal of Interpersonal Violence, 1,* 363–373.

Hamberger, L. K., & Lohr, J. M. (1989). Proximal causes of spouse abuse: Cognitive and behavioral factors. In P. L. Caesar & L. K. Hamberger (Eds.), *Treating men who batter: Theory, practice and programs* (pp. 53–76). New York: Springer.

Hamberger, L. K., Lohr, J. M., Bonge, D., & Tolin, D. F. (1996). A large sample empirical typology of male spouse abusers and its relationship to dimensions of abuse. *Violence and Victims, 11,* 277–292.

Hamberger, L. K., Lohr, J. M., Bonge, D., & Tolin, D. F. (1997). An empirical classification of motivations for domestic violence. *Violence Against Women, 3,* 401–423.

Hamberger, L. K., & Phelan, M. B. (2004). *Domestic violence screening and intervention in medical and mental healthcare settings.* New York: Springer.

Hamberger, L. K., & Potente, T. (1996). Counseling heterosexual women arrested for domestic violence: Implications for theory and practice. In L. K. Hamberger & C. Renzetti (Eds.), *Domestic partner abuse* (pp. 53–75). New York: Springer.

Hart, B. (1991, August). *Duties to warn and protect.* Paper presented at the meeting of the American Psychological Association, San Francisco.

Hart, B. (1994). Lethality and dangerousness assessments. *Violence Update, 4,* 7–8.

Hart, B., & Stuehling, J. (1992). *Personalized safety plan.* Unpublished manuscript, Pennsylvania Coalition Against Domestic Violence, Redding, PA.

Heckert, D. A., & Gondolf, E. W. (2004). Battered women's perceptions of risk versus risk factors and instruments in predicting repeat reassault. *Journal of Interpersonal Violence, 19*, 778–800.

Holtzworth-Munroe, A., Bates, L., Smutzler, N., & Sandin, E. (1997). A brief review of the research on husband violence. Part I: Maritally violent versus nonviolent men. *Aggression and Violent Behavior, 2*, 65–99.

Holtzworth-Munroe, A., & Hutchinson, G. (1993). Attributing negative intent to wife behavior: The attributions of maritally violent versus nonviolent men. *Journal of Abnormal Psychology, 102*, 20–21.

Holtzworth-Munroe, A., Meehan, J. C., Rehman, U., & Marshall, A. D. (2002). Intimate partner violence: An introduction for couple therapists. In A. S. Gurman & N. S. Jacobson (Eds.), *Clinical handbook of couple therapy* (3rd ed., pp. 441–465). New York: Guilford Press.

Holtzworth-Munroe, A., Smutzler, N., & Bates, L. (1997). A brief review of the research on husband violence. Part III: Sociodemographic factors, relationship factors, and differing consequences of husband and wife violence. *Aggression and Violent Behavior, 2*, 285–307.

Holtzworth-Munroe, A., Smutzler, N., & Sandin, B. (1997). A brief review of the research on husband violence. Part II: The psychological effects of husband violence on battered women and their children. *Aggression and Violent Behavior, 2*, 179–213.

Houry, D., Feldhous, K., Peery, B., Abbott, J., Lowenstein, S. R., al-Bataa de Montero, S., et al. (2004). A positive domestic violence screen predicts future domestic violence. *Journal of Interpersonal Violence, 19*, 955–966.

Kuhl, A. F. (1984). Personality traits of abused women: Masochism myth refuted. *Victimology, 9*, 450–462.

Kyriacou, D. N., Anglin, D., Taliaferro, E., Stone, S., Tubb, T., Linden, J. A., et al. (1999). Risk factors for injury to women from domestic violence. *New England Journal of Medicine, 341*, 1892–1898.

Langhinrischen-Rohling, J., Schlee, K. A., Monson, C. M., Ehrensaft, M., & Heyman, R. (1998). What's love got to do with it?: Perceptions of marital positivity in H-to-W aggressive, distressed, and happy marriages. *Journal of Family Violence, 13*, 197–212.

Lorber, M. F., & O'Leary, K. D. (2004). Predictors of persistence of male aggression in early marriage. *Journal of Family Violence, 19*, 329–338.

Marshall, L. L. (1999). Effects of men's subtle and overt psychological abuse on low-income women. *Violence and Victims, 14*, 69–88.

Miles, A. (1999). How to care for both victim and victimizer in an emotionally abusive marriage. *Leadership, 20*, 97–100.

Murphy, C. M., & Eckhardt, C. I. (2005). *Treating the abusive partner: An individualized cognitive-behavioral approach.* New York: Guilford Press.

National Medical Association. (1995). National Medical Association surgical section position paper on violence prevention. *Journal of the American Medical Association, 273*, 1788–1789.

O'Leary, K. D., Barling, J., Arias, I., Rosenbaum, A., Malone, J., & Tyree, A. (1989). Prevalence and stability of physical aggression between spouses: A longitudinal analysis. *Journal of Consulting and Clinical Psychology, 57*, 263–268.

O'Leary, K. D., Vivian, D., & Malone, J. (1992). Assessment of physical aggression against women in marriage: The need for multimodal assessment. *Behavioral Assessment, 14*, 5–14.

Pagelow, M. D. (1984). *Family violence.* New York: Praeger.

Pence, E. (1989). Batterer programs: Shifting from community collusion to community confrontation. In P. L. Caesar & L. K. Hamberger (Eds.), *Treating men who batter: Theory, practice and programs* (pp. 24–50). New York: Springer.

Phelan, M. B., Hamberger, L. K., Guse, C. E., Edwards, S., Walczak, S., & Zosel, A. (2005).

Domestic violence among male and female patients seeking emergency medical services. *Violence and Victims, 20,* 187–206.

Plichta, S. B., Duncan, M. M., & Plichta, L. (1996). Spouse abuse, patient–physician communication, and patient satisfaction. *American Journal of Preventive Medicine, 12,* 297–303.

Quigley, B. M., & Leonard, K. E. (1996). Desistance of husband aggression in the early years of marriage. *Violence and Victims, 11,* 355–370.

Rasche, C. (1988, November). *Domestic murder-suicide: Characteristics and comparisons to nonsuicidal intimate partner killings.* Paper presented at the meeting of the American Society of Criminology, Chicago.

Rodriguez, M. A., McLoughlin, E., Bauer, H. M., Paredes, V., & Grumbach, K. (1999). Mandatory reporting of intimate partner violence to police: Views of physicians in California. *American Journal of Public Health, 89,* 575–578.

Rogge, R. D., & Bradbury, T. N (1999). Till violence does us part: The differing roles of communication and aggression in predicting adverse marital outcomes. *Journal of Consulting and Clinical Psychology, 67,* 340–351.

Sonkin, D. J., & Dutton, D. (2003). Treating assaultive men from an attachment perspective. *Journal of Aggression, Maltreatment, and Trauma, 7,* 105–134.

Sonkin, D. J., Martin, D., & Walker, L. E. (1985). *The male batterer: A treatment approach.* New York: Springer.

Stark, E., & Flitcraft, A. (1995). Killing the beast within: Woman battering and female suicidality. *International Journal of Health Services, 25,* 43–64.

Stets, J. E., & Straus, M. A. (1990). Gender differences in reporting marital violence and its medical and psychological consequences. In M. A. Straus, & R. J. Gelles (Eds.), *Physical violence in American families* (pp. 151–165). New Brunswick, NJ: Transactions.

Straus, M. A. (1979). Measuring intrafamily conflict and violence: The Conflict Tactics (CT) Scales. *Journal of Marriage and the Family, 4,* 75–88.

Straus, M. A., Hamby, S. L., Boney-McCoy, S., & Sugarman, D. B. (1996). The revised Conflict Tactics Scales (CTS2): Development and preliminary psychometric data. *Journal of Family Issues, 17,* 283–316.

Sugarman, D. B., & Hotaling, G. T. (1997). Intimate violence and social desirability: A meta-analytic review. *Journal of Interpersonal Violence, 12,* 775–290.

Sullivan, C. M., & Bybee, D. I (1999). Reducing violence using community-based advocacy for women with abusive partners. *Journal of Consulting and Clinical Psychology, 67,* 43–53.

Tjaden, P., & Thoennes, N. (2000). Prevalence and consequences of male-to-female and female-to-male intimate partner violence as measured by the National Violence Against Women Survey. *Violence Against Women, 6,* 142–161.

Tonizzo, S., Howells, K., Day, A., Reidpath, D., & Froyland, I. (2000). Attributions of negative partner behavior by men who physically abuse their partners. *Journal of Family Violence, 15,* 155–167.

Vivian, D., & Langhinrichsen-Rohling, J. (1994). Are bi-directionally violent couples mutually victimized? A gender-sensitive comparison. *Violence and Victims, 9,* 107–124.

Waltz, J., Babcock, C., Jacobson, N. S., & Gottman, J. (1991, November). *Husband and wife reports of interspousal violence: Sex differences in minimization.* Paper presented at the meeting of the Association for the Advancement of Behavior Therapy, New York.

Warshaw, C. (1993). Domestic violence: Challenges to medical practice. *Journal of Women's Health, 2,* 73–79.

Weisz, A. N., Tolman, R. M., & Saunders, D. G. (2000). Assessing the risk of severe domestic violence: The importance of survivors' predictions. *Journal of Interpersonal Violence, 15,* 75–90.

Wistedt, B., & Freeman, A. (1994). Aggressive patients. In F. M. Dattilio & A. Freeman (Eds.), *Cogitive-behavioral strategies in crisis intervention* (pp. 345–361). New York: Guilford Press.

SUGGESTED READINGS

Aldarondo, E., & Mederos, F. (Eds.). (2002). *Programs for men who batter: Intervention and prevention strategies in a diverse society.* Kingston, NJ: Civic Research Institute.

Dutton, D., & Sonkin, D. J. (Ed.). (2003). *Intimate violence: Contemporary treatment innovations.* New York: Haworth Maltreatment & Trauma Press.

Hamberger, L. K. (1996). Group treatment of men who batter their female partners. *In Session, 2,* 49–62.

Hamberger, L. K. (2002). The Men's Group Program—A community-based, cognitive-behavioral profeminist intervention program. In E. Aldarondo & F. Mederos (Eds.), *Programs for men who batter: Intervention and prevention strategies in a diverse society* (pp. 7-1–7-44). Kingston, NJ: Civic Research Institute.

Holtzworth-Munroe, A., Meehan, J. C., Rehman, U., & Marshall, A. D. (2002). Intimate partner violence: An introduction for couple therapists. In A. S. Gurman & N. S. Jacobson (Eds.), *Clinical handbook of couple therapy* (3rd ed., pp. 441–465). New York: Guilford Press.

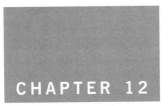

CHAPTER 12

Couple Problems

Stephen E. Schlesinger
Norman B. Epstein

*C*lose, mutually supportive couple relationships have been found to be among the best buffers against the negative impact of life stressors (Cutrona, 1996). Conversely, however, couple relationship problems are among the major life stresses that have been shown to be associated with the development of psychological disorders such as depression and anxiety (Daiuto, Baucom, Epstein, & Dutton, 1998; Beach, 2001), as well as physical health problems (Burman & Margolin, 1992; Wickrama, Lorenz, Conger, & Elder, 1997). Conflict between partners commonly is a chronic state characterized by repetitive behavioral patterns of aversive mutual exchanges, demand–withdraw sequences, or mutual avoidance (Christensen, 1988; Epstein & Baucom, 2002; Epstein, Baucom, & Rankin, 1993). However, many couples experience acute escalations of conflict and other problems that can result in a crisis state, in which the couple's usual ways of coping with stressors are inadequate for dealing with the present circumstances. As the couple's coping abilities are overwhelmed, their normal functioning as a couple and as individuals deteriorates, threatening the well-being of the partners and the stability of their relationship. Unfortunately, it is common for couples to wait until they experience such a severe disruption in their relationships before they seek professional help.

Many aspects of intervention for couple relationship crises overlap significantly with cognitive-behavioral procedures that are used with couples engaged in more chronic patterns of conflict. However, there are some unique aspects of a crisis state that require specific crisis intervention strategies. Consequently, it is important that clinicians who work with distressed couples be skilled in the assessment and treatment of relationship crises. Often, therapists must intervene quickly to stabilize a couple's disequilibrium before the partners are able to focus on changing more chronic problematic conditions in their relationship. Without prompt intervention, there is significant danger that the functioning of the couple will deteriorate quickly, with risks for negative outcomes such as abusive behavior or separation. This chapter provides a description of how crisis theory can be integrated into a cognitive-behavioral approach to the treatment of distressed couples. After we outline couple crisis assessment and intervention procedures, we present a case example illustrating this approach.

FAMILY CRISIS THEORY

Hill's (1949, 1958) ABCX model has had a major impact on theoretical and empirical work concerning the development and resolution of crises in family relationships. More recent models such as McCubbin and Patterson's (1983) double ABCX model, McCubbin and McCubbin's (1989) typology model, Karney and Bradbury's (1995) vulnerability–stress–adaptation model, and Epstein and Baucom's (2002) adaptation model of couple functioning have expanded on Hill's original conceptualization, but the basic components of the ABCX model have remained central in understanding couple and family responses to life stresses. As described by Epstein and Baucom (2002) all these models are based on an assumption that a relationship is not a static entity but, rather, develops over time as its members adapt to changes in various circumstances such as external life situations and individual development of each person. The success of a relationship, in terms meeting the needs of its members and making them happy, depends on how well the couple adapts to changing circumstances.

The ABCX model and its derivatives make an important distinction between *stressful life events* that place pressure on members of a relationship to adapt and the *crisis state of disorganization* that results when the couple's or family's attempts to cope with the impinging stressors fail. The model also delineates two major types of factors that influence how well the family members cope with stressors and therefore determine whether a crisis state develops: the *resources* available to the family and the family members' *perceptions* or *appraisals* of the stressors and their abilities to cope with them. The components in couple and family stress and coping models are consistent with psychological theories of individual coping (e.g., Lazarus & Folkman, 1984) which focus on cognitive and behavioral strategies for managing stressful life events. As described below, some forms of coping effectively reduce the impact of stressors whereas other responses are either ineffective or even exacerbate negative effects of stressors. The following is a description of the components of the ABCX family crisis model, including the stressors, the coping factors of resources and perception/appraisal, and the potential resulting crisis state of disorganized functioning. We note how elaborations of crisis theory address the components of stressors/demands, resources and perception/appraisal in relationship functioning.

Stressors or Demands

The "A" component of the ABCX model includes a variety of stressors that place pressure on the couple or family system for change in the members' relatively stable interaction patterns, as well as in the individual members' typical response patterns. Epstein and Baucom (2002) propose using the term *demands* instead of stressors because the latter commonly connotes events that people experience as negative, whereas the former suggests that pressure can result from events that are desirable as well as those that people consider unpleasant. Thus, an individual may consider a promotion at work to be highly desirable, but it places a number of demands on him/her, such as increased responsibility and work hours.

At the individual level, stressors or demands can impinge on a person's behavioral routines. For example, Mel reported that for over 10 years he had a comfortable and fairly satisfying routine in his middle-management position in an electronics firm. However, when the company "reorganized" and he was laid off, Mel's familiar daily patterns were disrupted and he was faced with looking for a new job. These changes affected not only his daily behaviors but also the topics he thought about and the emotions he felt during a typical day. Furthermore, the stressor of the job loss influenced Mel's individual functioning, as well as the functioning of his relationship with his wife, Beverly. For example, the couple's conversations shifted from the usual sharing of daily experiences with work, family, and friends to a relatively narrow focus on the negative impact of unemployment (e.g., worries about paying bills). Consequently, clinicians who work with distressed couples need to identify the ways in which stressors affect functioning at both the individual and dyadic levels.

Stressors or demands are events that vary along a number of dimensions, such as (1) whether they are internal to the relationship (e.g., an individual partner's characteristic such as substance abuse or a couple's negative dyadic patterns such as chronic mutual nagging) or external (e.g., a storm that destroys the family's home); (2) the suddenness of their onset; (3) whether they are predictable and expected; (4) their degree of ambiguity (e.g., a family member is missing in action during wartime; (5) their severity; (6) their duration; (7) the degree to which the family members choose to be exposed to the stressor (e.g., choosing to move to another city); and (8) how many family members are affected directly (Boss, 2002; McCubbin & Patterson, 1983). These dimensions of stressors can affect how the individuals respond to them; for example, a couple that chose to have a child and now are experiencing stressors associated with having a newborn may conclude, "We don't have any right to be upset, because we chose this."

The presence of a stressor is likely to involve pressure for the members of a family to make changes in important aspects of their relationships, including their goals, roles, and established patterns of interacting with each other. It is not the stressor event itself that creates the pressure for adaptation but, rather, the "hardships" associated with the stressor (McCubbin & Patterson, 1983). For example, moving to another city for a job promotion can involve hardships such as selling one's house, finding and buying a new house, leaving friends and family, finding new doctors and other health care specialists, learning one's way around a new city, and so on. Consequently, clinical assessment requires a careful survey of the idiosyncratic hardships that each couple faces when experiencing a particular stressor.

Furthermore, although any one stressor or demand may not strain the coping abilities of an individual or couple, a series of stressors may pile up, providing a significant cumulative impact (McCubbin & McCubbin, 1989). As noted earlier, a crisis state of disequilibrium can occur when a pileup of stressors exceeds the couple's coping ability. Therefore, for prevention and treatment of crises in couple relationships it is important to identify the range of stressors (and their associated hardships) the couple has experienced over a period of time.

Many stressors affecting couple relationships are normative in that they are parts of common, predictable developmental changes in the family and its members. Among the normative transitions frequently facing couples are marriage, childbirth and parenthood, occupational stages such as promotions and retirement, and deaths of aging family members (Epstein & Baucom, 2002; McCubbin & Figley, 1983; Wright, Nelson, & Georgen, 1994). However, there can be significant variations in normative stages of a couple's relationship development, based on factors such as sexual orientation, culture, race, social class, the partners' gender role beliefs, and the presence or absence of children (Carter & McGoldrick, 1999). Changes in partners' experiences of love in their intimate relationships, including inevitable shifts from the emotional "high" of initial romantic love to companionate love (deep attachment and friendly affection), also can be sources of considerable stress (Coleman, 1988).

Other stressors facing couples (e.g., diagnosis of serious illness or disability in a child, unemployment, death of a loved one) are nonnormative and even catastrophic in that they occur without warning, often are threatening to individual and family well-being, and induce a sense of helplessness (Epstein & Baucom, 2002; Figley, 1983). The degree to which members of a couple perceive themselves to be helpless in coping with unexpected, catastrophic stressors can influence the likelihood of their entering a crisis state.

Stressors or demands disturb the status quo or steady state of functioning in a couple in that they disturb the partners' predictable routines and present obstacles that must be overcome. However, as described earlier, they are not necessarily negative influences. In fact, normal couple and family development involves various desirable changes, such as shifts in family roles as children become more competent and independent of their parents. Family systems theorists have described how healthy family relationships strike a balance between maintaining stability and facilitating growth within and among family members (Leslie, 1988). Therefore, the goal of crisis intervention is not attempt to minimize stressors in people's lives but rather to assist individuals, couples, and families in coping effectively with pressures stemming from positive and negative life events. Successful coping with demands can strengthen a couple's relationship by increasing a sense of intimacy between partners and developing their shared confidence that they can solve problems as a team (Epstein & Baucom, 2002).

Resources

A couple's ability to cope with stressful life events is influenced by a variety of resources (the "B" component of the ABCX model) that may be available to them as individuals and as a couple. There are three major categories of resources relevant for coping with stressors: (1) the personal resources of each individual; (2) resources of the couple; and (3) resources provided by the environment outside the couple. Examples of individual resources include health, intelligence, education, problem-solving skills, job skills, finances, and psychological characteristics such as self-esteem and a sense of mastery (Boss, 2002; McCubbin & Patterson, 1983). Effective coping depends on not only the availability of resources but also the manner in which individuals use their available resources. Research findings indicate that even though coping styles that involve avoiding stressors (e.g., denial and distracting oneself) may provide some short-term relief, they result in poorer long-term adaptation than coping strategies that involve direct attention to using resources for resolving hardships associated with stressors (Snyder, 1999; Suls & Fletcher, 1985).

Resources within a couple's relationship include collaborative problem-solving skills, the degree to which the relationship is characterized by cohesiveness and mutual support, effective communication skills, and adaptability in altering relationship roles and patterns in order to cope with stressors (Epstein & Baucom, 2002; Walsh, 1998). There is considerable empirical evidence that couples in which the partners provide each other forms of support (e.g., emotional support, information, and direct aid in problem solving) experience higher levels of individual well-being and relationship satisfaction (Carels & Baucom, 1999; Cutrona, 1996; Pasch, Bradbury, & Sullivan, 1997). A stable shared belief that the couple or family is strong and can actively exercise control over life events is another relationship resource that is a key component of resilience (Dattilio, 1997; McCubbin & McCubbin, 1989; Schwebel & Fine, 1994; Walsh, 1998). Overall, couples can use their relationship resources either to cope directly with stressors they face or as mechanisms for identifying and accessing resources in their environment. For example, a couple experiencing stress from a tight budget can use their problem-solving skills to brainstorm ways to reduce expenses on their own, or to seek help from community resources such as low-fee money management counselors. Environmental resources are not restricted to direct interactions with other people; they can include archival sources of information, such as books and the Internet.

Social support in a couple's environment includes a variety of resources that they may obtain from their relationships with extended family, friends, neighbors, and community organizations such as social service agencies, health care services, schools, employers, and religious institutions. A growing body of research has identified social support as a major buffer against negative effects of stress on couples and families (McCubbin & McCubbin, 1989; McKenry & Price, 2005). Among the forms of social support are emotional support, validation, assistance in problem solving, financial aid, and instrumental support with tasks and roles such as child care. Consequently, crisis intervention strategies commonly include efforts to broaden and strengthen the environmental social support networks of individuals and families that are in crisis. How-ever, clinicians who are intervening with couples in crisis need to be aware of cultural differences in clients' openness to seeking or accepting assistance from outside sources of support. McGoldrick, Preto, Hines, and Lee (1991) describe tendencies for mem-bers of different ethnic groups to accept or resist assistance from outsiders, including mental health professionals.

Not only may a couple be at risk for inadequate coping with stressors based on an absence of appropriate resources but they also may be at risk based on the presence of *vulnerability* factors. Couple and family stress researchers (e.g., Epstein & Baucom, 2002; Karney & Bradbury, 1995; McCubbin & McCubbin, 1989) define vulnerabili-ties as relatively stable characteristics that impede individual, couple, and family adaptation to stressors. At an individual level, members of a couple may have vulnera-bilities such as posttraumatic stress disorder from past personal traumas, clinical depression, personality disorders (e.g., borderline personality disorder), and neuroti-cism or negative emotional overreactivity (Epstein & Baucom, 2002). At the couple interaction level, vulnerability factors may include partners' tendencies to engage in escalating arguments or mutual avoidance. Some couples respond to past hurts by actively withdrawing from each other, providing some measure of self-protection but interfering both with their levels of intimacy and cohesion and with their ability to work together to cope with life stressors. Thus, the couple's way of coping with con-flict and negative affect in their relationship becomes a vulnerability factor, detracting from their ability to cope with ongoing and future stressors (Epstein & Baucom, 2002). Although the "B" factor in Hill's ABCX model originally focused on the pres-ence or absence of resources that members of a relationship could use to cope with stressors, the identification of individual and couple vulnerability factors in more recent conceptualizations broadens the model in an important way.

Perception and Appraisal of Stressors or Demands

The "C" component of the ABCX model involves the family members' perceptions and appraisals of the stressful events occurring in their lives. Boss (2002) notes that although individual family members may have disparate perceptions of a stressor, powerful shared perceptions can supersede variations in individuals' views; for exam-ple, the members of a family may share a common failure to notice signs that an alco-holic member really has a serious drinking problem. In addition to such selective per-ceptions (Epstein & Baucom, 2002), members of a couple appraise or evaluate stressors or demands in their lives in terms of how dangerous and potent they may be. Individuals also appraise the degree to which they have adequate resources to cope with the stressors. Perceptions and appraisals of life stressors have become important components in models of couple and family coping (Boss, 2002; Epstein & Baucom, 2002; Karney & Bradbury, 1995; McCubbin & McCubbin, 1989).

A number of writers (e.g., Boss, 2002; McCubbin & McCubbin, 1989; Walsh, 1998) have emphasized the implications for positive coping when family members appraise the stressors in their lives as "challenges" that can be overcome through active effort, rather than as uncontrollable events that must be accepted in a fatalistic, passive manner. Boss (2002) notes that although there are circumstances (e.g., when an individual is a prisoner of war) when it may be adaptive for individuals to adopt a passive mode of coping, passivity leads to the maintenance or exacerbation of most problems facing couples and families. She also describes systematic cultural differences in beliefs about mastery versus fatalism regarding life events which are likely to shape a family's attitudes toward problem solving.

Consistent with stress and coping theory (Lazarus & Folkman, 1984), McCubbin and McCubbin (1989) note that when family members are faced with stressors, they tend to identify and weigh the demands inherent in the stressors against their capabilities for meeting those demands. Tension and stress are experienced when it is perceived that the demands of the stressors exceed the couple's or family's resources and coping abilities, regardless of whether the perceptions of the demands and coping abilities are accurate. This view that subjective appraisals mediate individuals' responses to life stressors is highly consistent with the tenets of cognitive-behavioral therapies.

In summary, subjective cognitive factors are viewed as major influences on how family members cope with demands on their relationships. Once a couple has become destabilized and has entered a crisis state, their appraisals of their situation (e.g., whether they view themselves as helpless to change it) are likely to affect their efforts to adapt and reestablish equilibrium. Consequently, the substantial body of cognitive-behavioral theoretical and empirical knowledge about cognitive factors in individual and relationship functioning has much to offer clinicians for assessment and intervention with couples' crises.

The Crisis State

Often couples that are faced with the demands for change posed by life events are able to cope with the stressors by utilizing their resources and perceiving their potential for exercising mastery in the situation. However, when the resources and appraisals do not result in reduction of the pressure from the stressors and their associated hardships, the relationship system's organization and functioning may become destabilized, resulting in a crisis state of disorganization (the "X" in the ABCX model). In a crisis state, roles, typical patterns of interaction, problem solving, and other characteristics that have met the various needs of the partners become immobilized or break down (McCubbin & McCubbin, 1989; McKenry & Price, 2002). The individual partners are likely to experience a variety of cognitive, affective, physiological, and behavioral symptoms that represent notable departures from their typical functioning (Greenstone & Leviton, 2002). Their cognitive functioning is likely to be impaired by indecisiveness, confusion, and a sense of helplessness. Common emotional symptoms of a crisis state are anxiety, irritability, and depression. Among the physiological symptoms commonly experienced are insomnia, decreased appetite, gastrointestinal disturbances, and headaches. Disorganized behavioral responses include unclear communication, disrupted daily routines, general social withdrawal, and clinging to others for help. In addition to the symptoms experienced by individual members, a crisis state also tends to affect the interpersonal patterns within a couple or family. Thus a couple's typical patterns of role enactment, communication, and problem solving tend to deteriorate, and their interactions become more characterized by aversive behavior exchanges and/or withdrawal. This state of disorganization at the individual and relationship levels necessitates changes in the couple or family (e.g., changes in roles and development of new resources) in order to restore stability. Thus a crisis state can provide an opportunity for growth in the couple or family and the achievement of a higher level of functioning. However, a crisis also can lead to a dysfunctional outcome in which the functioning of the relationship or its individual members deteriorates (e.g., depression, physical abuse, and chronic alienation between partners). Consequently, crisis intervention with couples focuses on maximizing constructive adaptation through active intervention with the couple's resources and appraisals.

COGNITIVE-BEHAVIORAL COUPLE THERAPY AND THE ABCX MODEL

The ABCX model of stress and coping in couple and family relationships is a useful framework for guiding cognitive-behavioral assessment and intervention with couples in crisis. Although cognitive-behavioral couple therapy (Baucom & Epstein, 1990; Dattilio, Epstein, & Baucom, 1998; Dattilio & Padesky, 1990; Epstein & Baucom, 2002; Epstein, Baucom, & Daiuto, 1997; Rathus & Sanderson, 1999; Schlesinger & Epstein, 1986) commonly is used with couples that have experienced chronic marital conflict and distress, its goals and procedures are well suited for addressing relationship factors that contribute to the disorganized functioning of a crisis state. The following is a description of cognitive-behavioral interventions that can alter the types and intensity of relationship stressors, a couple's utilization of their resources for coping with stressors, and the partners' appraisals of the stressors and resources.

Assessment for Cognitive-Behavioral Crisis Intervention

Among the major stressors or demands commonly contributing to couples' distress are (1) physical and interpersonal environmental stressors external to the couple's relationship, which place demands on the functioning of the dyad and its two members; (2) stressful aspects of the partners' own interactions with each other; and (3) characteristics of the individual partners (Epstein & Baucom, 2002). As described earlier, external environmental stressors may include normative events (e.g., birth of a child and job problems) or unexpected nonnormative events (e.g., unemployment, injury, and illness). Common stressors in couple dyadic interaction include aversive verbal communication (e.g., criticism, escalating exchanges of insults, and threats of divorce), behavioral withdrawal, and physical abuse. These interpersonal patterns may have preexisted any environmental stressors that the couple has experienced, or they may have developed as dysfunctional responses to particular stressors. For example, a couple may have always relied on criticism and other forms of aversive control to try to influence each other, or a new pattern of mutual criticism may have developed as the partners increasingly have been frustrated by their child's oppositional behavior. Stressors involving the personal characteristics of the individual partners can include personality traits (e.g., an insecure attachment style and a high level of competitive motivation), temperament (e.g., a generally high activity level), and psychopathology (e.g., depression and anxiety disorders) (Epstein & Baucom, 2002).

To plan appropriate interventions to reduce a couple's stressors, the clinician conducts an assessment of the couple's presenting problems and the degree to which the partners are distressed by each type of stressor. Cognitive-behavioral crisis intervention assessment is similar to traditional cognitive-behavioral assessment of couples (Baucom & Epstein, 1990; Epstein & Baucom, 2002; Rathus & Sanderson, 1999) in that the clinician places the presenting problems in context by interviewing the couple jointly about the history of their relationship. In particular, attention is paid to the timeline of when various stressors occurred and how the couple coped with them. This assessment identifies a possible pileup of stressors, as well as the couple's use of available resources. The joint interview also can be used to identify vulnerability factors in the dyad (e.g., vague communication) and the individual partners (e.g., depression). Based on the partners' reports and on observation of the couple's interactions during the interview, the clinician can identify any of the couple's behavioral patterns that need immediate attention to ameliorate the crisis state. Consistent with general crisis intervention practices (e.g., Greenstone & Leviton, 2002), the initial assessment session concludes with the clinician giving the couple feedback to help them understand the disconcerting crisis state they are experiencing and initiating some behavioral changes to produce some quick relief. The feedback includes a summary of the information that the clinician collected about the factors in the ABCX model (stressors, resources, vulnerabilities, perceptions) that seem to have contributed to the crisis state. Providing this kind of conceptualization can reassure clients and decrease their sense of helplessness about their problems; such feedback commonly is used in cognitive therapy (e.g., Beck, Rush, Shaw, & Emery, 1979). The therapist coaches the couple in prioritizing interventions that can most quickly reduce their stress level at least somewhat and increase their sense of control over their lives. Although interventions to improve the couple's use of resources and to increase realistic perception and appraisal of stressors are important, often it is most effective to begin with efforts to reduce specific stressors.

Cognitive-Behavioral Interventions to Reduce Stressors

The following are some behavioral interventions that can be used to produce relief from stressors involved in the couple's own behavioral patterns, as well as those from their physical and interpersonal environment. We usually focus initially on any stressful aversive patterns between the partners, because these tend to detract from the couple's ability to work as a team in solving problems. Epstein and Baucom (2002) have differentiated between *primary distress*, which is caused by various unresolved issues that a couple faces, and *secondary distress*, which is a result of the couple's dysfunctional way of responding to each other about their unresolved issues. In other words, the couple's way of trying to resolve problems in their relationship itself becomes a problem, or in crisis theory terms the attempted solution becomes a significant stressor. Consequently, early interventions commonly focus on improving the couple's communication and joint problem-solving process.

One approach to decreasing aversive behavioral interactions and increasing positive interactions is to have each spouse report the occurrence of specific positive, neutral, and negative partner behaviors. Although partners could be asked to keep detailed logs of such behaviors, extensive logs may be too cumbersome and stressful for people in a crisis state. Consequently, therapists can identify major aversive behavioral patterns through their interviews and direct observations of the couple, as described earlier. The therapist, using the principle of "guided behavior change" that involves coaching partners to exchange types of behavior that do not require learning new skills (Epstein & Baucom, 2002), then collaborates with the couple in devising an agreement for each partner to take some responsibility to increase positive behaviors and decrease negative behaviors involved in the aversive pattern during the next week (Baucom & Epstein, 1990; Epstein & Baucom, 2002). Thus, the couple is coached in devising a behavioral contract in which each spouse agrees to make specific behavior changes that the other person has requested. Detailed guidelines for constructing behavioral contracts with varying degree of structure (e.g., formal quid pro quo contracts vs. informal agreements that each person will enact particular behaviors) are presented by Baucom and Epstein (1990), Epstein and Baucom (2002), Jacobson and Margolin (1979), and Stuart (1980). For a couple whose negative exchanges are taxing their coping abilities, shifts in frequencies of positive and negative behavior can produce a notable reduction in experienced stress.

However, to motivate highly distressed couples to make such behavioral changes, it often is necessary for the therapist to provide a convincing rationale. Especially when spouses are angry with each other, it is important to discuss with them how their present reciprocation of negative behavior is maintaining their high level of stress. The therapist also might coach each spouse in listing the advantages and disadvantages of venting anger toward the partner, with the goal of demonstrating that the costs of such behavior (e.g., eliciting defensiveness and retaliation from the partner) are significant, relative to the rewards (e.g., temporarily gaining compliance from the partner) (Neidig & Friedman, 1984). Guided behavior change also can focus on increasing particular forms of positive interaction, such as mutual social support (Epstein & Baucom, 2002). The therapist provides a brief didactic presentation about forms of support that a person might provide for a partner (e.g., empathic listening, affection, and mutual brainstorming of solutions to a problem) (Cutrona, 1996), has each member of the couple discuss the types of support he/she prefers, and coaches the couple in devising an agreement to engage in the types of support that each person desires during the coming week.

Another procedure for reducing stress by increasing the percentage of pleasant versus stressful interactions between spouses is to have them schedule leisure activities together (Baucom & Epstein, 1990). Because distressed couples often have avoided spending time together and anticipate that shared time will lead to unpleasant interactions, it is important that the therapist coach them in thinking of activities that both people are likely to enjoy and in structuring the time with ground rules for controlling aversive behavior (e.g., an explicit agreement to focus on the pleasurable activity and to avoid talking about their relationship).

In contrast to guided behavior change techniques that involve encouraging partners to exchange types of behavior that tend to be in their repertoires already, therapists can teach the partners specific skills that reduce negative interaction and increase positive interaction when the couple deals with stressors. Training in expressive and listening skills (Baucom & Epstein, 1990; Epstein & Baucom, 2002; Markman, Stanley, & Blumberg, 1994; Rathus & Sanderson, 1999) accomplishes the dual stress-reducing goals of helping couples focus and pace their communication better and short-circuiting the cycle of reciprocal defensiveness that venting often creates. The goal of these interventions is to focus each spouse's attention on the benefits he/she can accrue if the existing negative interaction pattern is changed. In general, spouses are taught to identify and reduce specific forms of negative messages (e.g., interruptions, fault finding, and focusing on the past) and to replace those with alternatives such as positive requests for behavior change (e.g., "I would appreciate it if you would work on the budget as we had discussed last month"). Neidig and Friedman (1984) help sensitize spouses to various negative forms of communication by providing them with a "Dirty Fighting Techniques Handout," which lists 27 common problematic behaviors (e.g., cross-complaining and blaming) and describes how these exacerbate conflict and distress.

Communication skills training involves specific instructions for more constructive verbal and nonverbal communication (Baucom & Epstein, 1990; Epstein & Baucom, 2002; Jacobson & Margolin, 1979; Neidig & Friedman, 1984; Rathus & Sanderson, 1999). The instructions may be through verbal descriptions, written materials, videotape examples, or modeling by the therapist. Some of the more common guidelines for sending constructive messages are (1) using "I" statements, (2) expressing thoughts and emotions clearly and specifically, (3) communicating empathy for the partner's position, (4) acknowledging the subjectivity of one's own thoughts and emotions, (5) acknowledging any positives in the situation, and (6) using nonverbal behavior (e.g., eye contact, facial expressions, and gestures) that convey interest and openness. As is described below, these forms of communication also are important for building a couple's resources for coping with stress, but in themselves the behaviors reduce the stressors exchanged during a couple's daily interactions.

Cognitive-Behavioral Interventions for Building Stress-Buffering Resources

Whether the stressors impinging upon a couple originate inside their relationship or outside, a crisis state of disorganization can be prevented or managed to the degree that the couple has a variety of effective stress-buffering resources. Communication skills, problem-solving skills, and enhancement of mutual social support are among the most important resources that can be strengthened through cognitive-behavioral interventions.

First, a couple's ability to work collaboratively to identify and resolve sources of stress in their lives depends on their capacity to exchange information effectively. Some couples communicate in imprecise and confusing ways, resulting in misunderstandings and undesired actions. A couple can be helped to improve and use their expressive and listening skills as a relationship resource through educational, behaviorally oriented procedures that involve specific instructions, modeling of effective behavior, and extensive rehearsal of new skills by the couple (Baucom & Epstein, 1990; Epstein & Baucom, 2002; Guerney, 1977; Rathus & Sanderson, 1999). Spouses are instructed in taking turns operating in the modes of expresser and empathic listener. As the expresser, the individual is to follow guidelines such as stating views as subjective, making brief and specific statements, and communicating empathy for the partner's feelings and how one's statements may affect him/her. In the mode of empathic listener, the individual is to focus on verbally and nonverbally communicating attention to the expresser's messages, taking the expresser's perspective and empathizing with his/her thoughts and feelings, and reflecting back (i.e., summarizing and restating) the expresser's thoughts and feelings. To practice effective empathic listening, one must avoid various distracting and intrusive behaviors such as expressing one's own opinions and offering solutions. Similar expressive and listening skills have been used in premarital programs designed to prevent the development of relationship problems (Markman et al., 1994).

Another form of communication training that can assist couples in working collaboratively rather than as distressed adversaries is assertiveness training (Alberti & Emmons, 1986; Epstein, 1981; Neidig & Friedman, 1984). Spouses are assisted in differentiating among assertive, aggressive (including passive–aggressive) and submissive forms of behavior and are coached as they rehearse more assertive behavior in their couple interactions. Assertive behaviors include making direct but noncoercive requests of a partner, refusing a partner's request in a nonaggressive manner, and both giving and receiving direct positive messages (e.g., compliments). As a resource for coping with stressors affecting the couple's relationship, assertiveness skills provide the spouses with an important component of constructive negotiation and problem solving rather than escalation of conflict and hostility. Whereas assertively stating preferences does not necessarily lead to agreement on a solution to a relationship problem, the relative absence of coercive aggression is likely to add to a collaborative atmosphere that may instill some hope in the spouses that they can work together to manage stressors.

Training in problem-solving skills can provide another important resource for couples who are faced with life stressors. Whereas expressiveness and listening skills allow spouses to exchange information about their thoughts and emotions concerning their personal experiences, problem solving is a specific kind of communication in which spouses are most effective when they take a cognitive approach to identifying workable solutions to issues. In fact, cognitive-behavioral couple therapists coach couples in telling each other when they prefer to communicate for the purpose of express-ing feelings versus when they want to work on solving a specific problem (Baucom & Epstein, 1990; Epstein & Baucom, 2002).

When partners have agreed to engage in problem solving, there is a common set of steps that they are taught to follow, including (1) defining the problem in specific behavioral terms, (2) generating a set of possible solutions, (3) evaluating the advan-tages and disadvantages of each solution, and then selecting a feasible solution, and (4) implementing the chosen solution and evaluating its effectiveness. For detailed descrip-tions of problem-solving steps, with some variations in how the steps are broken down, see Baucom and Epstein (1990), Epstein and Baucom (2002), and Jacobson and Margolin (1979), as well as the case example in this chapter.

It is common for distressed partners who use good problem-solving skills in other settings (e.g., at work) to fail to use them as a resource for reducing stressors in their home life. Consequently, even though some couples may have a deficit in their *use* of skills rather than in their repertoire of skills, coaching couples in problem-solving steps usually is a productive approach to helping them manage stressors in an active man-ner. When a therapist observes that partners appear to have good problem-solving skills but *choose* not to use them with each other, the therapist must identify and address sources of their noncompliance (e.g., refusal to act positively toward a partner who behaved in a hurtful manner in the past). Intervening with instances of noncom-pliance typically involves assessment and modification of cognitive factors, which are discussed below.

Couples can be coached in using the expressive, listening, and problem-solving communication skills described above as resources for addressing stressors in their external environment, within their couple interactions, and resulting from the charac-teristics of the individual partners. As in our case example, a couple faced with pres-sures from competing demands of their roles involving work, childrearing, and caretaking of elderly parents can problem-solve ways to manage their time, share the various chores and caretaking responsibilities, and set aside some leisure time together. Similarly, a couple that has stressful arguments over their different preferences for lei-sure activities can problem-solve about equitable decisions for their shared time. Finally, a couple in which one member experiences debilitating symptoms of depres-sion can problem-solve ways that the nondepressed partner can behave most helpfully toward the depressed person.

Many couples that are experiencing a pileup of life stressors benefit from assis-tance with time and resource management skills. Therapists may coach a couple in list-ing and prioritizing tasks that demand their attention and energy, scheduling blocks of time to be devoted to one task at a time. The couple also may be assisted in dividing tasks, achieving a distribution of responsibilities that is acceptable to both parties. Of course, for some couples perceived inequities in responsibilities are major sources of distress and conflict, and the resolution of such differences may require problem-solving and cognitive interventions addressing the partners' gender role beliefs.

As described earlier, guided behavior change interventions can be used to increase the degree to which each person serves as a resource for the other by providing various forms of social support (Epstein & Baucom, 2002). Brief didactic presentations by the therapist on different ways of providing support to one's partner serve as psychoeducation for many individuals who have limited conceptions of what kinds of behavior can be supportive. Often individuals assume that what they themselves find supportive will feel supportive to their partner as well, but when their assumption is inaccurate the partner may be frustrated and criticize the giver. Expressive and listening skills can be used to foster mutual understanding of each partner's preferences for types of support, and a couple can be encouraged to let each other know what is and is not helpful when attempts at support are made.

Cognitive-Behavioral Interventions for Addressing Cognitive Appraisals of Relationship Stressors

As noted earlier, the "C" component of the ABCX family crisis model involves cognitive processing of life stressors (McKenry & Price, 2005). A cognitive-behavioral approach provides a variety of assessment and intervention procedures for addressing these cognitive factors which can produce or exacerbate stress in couples' relationships. The following discussion considers the relevance for crisis intervention of five major types of cognition that have been implicated in marital conflict and distress: selective perception, attributions, expectancies, assumptions, and standards (Baucom & Epstein, 1990; Epstein & Baucom, 1993, 2002).

Selective perception (labeled "selective abstraction" by Beck et al., 1979) involves biases in the aspects of couple interaction that each partner notices. There is considerable empirical evidence (cf. Epstein & Baucom, 1993) that distressed partners have low rates of agreement about the occurrence of even concrete behaviors during a 24-hour period, and couple therapists (e.g., Jacobson & Margolin, 1979) have described how distressed couples commonly exhibit "negative tracking" in which they notice negatives and overlook positives occurring in their relationships. Furthermore, distressed partners commonly perceive linear causality in their interactions (e.g., "I withdraw from him because he nags and pursues me"), rather than circular processes of mutual influence (Baucom & Epstein, 1990; Epstein & Baucom, 2002). Such adversarial processes of blame expose couples to what Gottman (1994) has termed the "Four Horsemen of the Apocalypse" in marriage. This "cascade," or sequence of behaviors—criticism, contempt, defensiveness, and withdrawal—places the couple on a course toward dissolving their relationship.

To broaden partners' perceptions of relationship events, cognitive-behavioral couple therapists use a variety of interventions, such as (1) having each person keep logs of daily positive and negative partner behaviors and (2) drawing the couple's attention to behavioral sequences and circular causality in their interactions, through verbal feedback and videotape playback of interactions during therapy sessions (Epstein & Baucom, 2002). The goals of these interventions are to reduce the sense of hopelessness that often results from perceiving consistent negatives in one's relationship and to reduce the blaming involved in linear explanations of events.

Attributions are inferences that an individual makes about causes of events that he/she observes. A considerable body of research has indicated that members of distressed couples are more likely than members of nondistressed couples to attribute negative partner behaviors to stable, global traits and negative intent and to view the behaviors as blameworthy (cf. Baucom & Epstein, 1990; Bradbury & Fincham, 1990; Epstein & Baucom, 1993, 2002). In contrast, members of distressed couples tend to discount positive partner behaviors as due to specific, unstable causes (i.e., factors on which one cannot rely). Furthermore, negative attributions have been found to predict subsequent negative partner interaction during problem-solving discussions (e.g., Bradbury & Fincham, 1992; Fincham & Bradbury, 1988). To the extent that partners' attributions contribute to distress (anger, depression, anxiety) and conflict behavior or helplessness responses, they are likely to exacerbate the level of stress and lead to a crisis state. Consequently, it is important for couple therapists to assist partners in examining the validity of their attributions, differentiating between accurate ones that may call for specific behavior change efforts and those that are distorted. Approaches to testing one's attributions include (1) counteracting a trait attribution by identifying any past situations in which a partner behaved differently, (2) altering an attribution of negative partner intent by obtaining direct feedback from the partner about his/her intentions, and (3) coaching an individual in generating and evaluating the plausibility of alternative attributions concerning causes of an upsetting partner behavior (Baucom & Epstein, 1990; Epstein & Baucom, 2002). When the evidence suggests that an attribution is accurate (e.g., when a partner indeed intended to inflict hurt through sarcastic remarks), the therapist may shift the focus to behavioral interventions such as training the partner in more constructive ways of communicating anger.

Expectancies are the predictions that individuals make about the probabilities that particular events will occur in the future, under particular conditions. Whether accurate or inaccurate, these inferences are likely to influence the individual's emotional and behavioral responses. For example, an individual who anticipates verbal attacks from a partner whenever he/she expresses disagreement with the partner (even when the partner would not have behaved in that manner) may experience anxiety at the thought of disagreeing and then avoid direct communication. Other individuals engage in "preemptive attacks" in order to protect themselves from anticipated aggression from their partners. In terms of the cognitive factors in the ABCX crisis model, negative expectancies can exacerbate stress, because the anticipated stressors can be equally or even more distressing than the actual events. Consequently, it is important for the couple therapist to assess each person's expectancies about stressors or demands affecting the couple, including external environmental stressors (e.g., caregiving burdens), stressors in the couple's interactions (e.g., anticipated couple arguments marked by aversive exchanges), and stressors associated with an individual's characteristics (e.g., a partner's anticipated panic attacks when away from home). Then the couple can be coached in examining the evidence for the predictions, using past experiences in similar situations, considering different kinds of outcomes that have occurred or might occur, and exploring specific actions that the partners could take in order to produce a different outcome (e.g., using new communication skills to discuss disagreements) (Epstein & Baucom, 2002).

Assumptions and *standards* are two forms of cognitive schemata or relatively stable internal representations that an individual has for categorizing things and events, as well as for understanding relationships among them (Fletcher & Fitness, 1996; Holmes, 2000). Cognitive theorists propose that these schemata are formed through an individual's life experiences, including exposure to family relationships as a child. In terms of couples' relationship cognitions, *assumptions* are beliefs about human nature and the way two people relate to each other in an intimate relationship (e.g., whether partners are able to change a relationship once they have established particular interaction patterns), and *standards* are beliefs about the characteristics that intimate partners and their relationships "should" have (Baucom & Epstein, 1990; Epstein & Baucom, 2002). There is evidence that when partners hold extreme assumptions and standards (Epstein & Eidelson, 1981; Eidelson & Epstein, 1982), or when they report that their standards are not met to their satisfaction within their relationship (Baucom, Epstein, Rankin, & Burnett, 1996), they experience greater relationship distress. Couples' assumptions and standards also have been found to be associated with the quality of their current communication and with future marital dissolution (e.g., Bradbury & Fincham, 1993; Gordon, Baucom, Epstein, Burnett, & Rankin, 1999; Kurdek, 1993).

As noted by Boss (2002), family members who accept stressors as uncontrollable (an assumption) are more likely to take a passive approach to coping with their stressors, and several authors (Dattilio, 1997; Holmes, 2000; McCubbin & McCubbin, 1989; Schwebel & Fine, 1994) have described a number of relatively stable "family schemata" that influence appraisals of specific relationship events. Therefore, the cognitive-behavioral approaches for modifying distressed partners' extreme or unrealistic assumptions and standards are highly relevant for addressing the "C" (perception, appraisal) component of the ABCX model.

Members of a couple can be assisted in exploring how their assumptions and standards were shaped by their life experiences, and they can examine whether such schemata that were realistic or appropriate earlier in their lives "fit" their present relationship circumstances. They also can be coached in identifying the advantages and disadvantages of applying their standards to their current relationship. For example, an individual who grew up in a verbally abusive family and now believes that partners should not express any anger toward each other may decide that the disadvantages of this standard (e.g., disappointments and disagreements are not resolved) outweigh its advantages (e.g., daily life is tranquil). Therapists can help couples "rewrite" extreme standards and assumptions, devising more moderate views that still are consistent with each person's basic values (see Baucom & Epstein, 1990; Epstein & Baucom, 2002, for more detailed descriptions of intervention procedures). Then therapists can help partners devise experiments in which they try living according to the revised standards and assumptions. Thus the negative impact of life stressors on a couple's relationship can be reduced by modifying the partners' assumptions and standards that are antithetical to effective problem solving or that themselves produce stress when the couple's relationship fails to match these internalized frames of reference.

Given that relationship distress is associated with the degree to which individuals are satisfied with how their standards are being met in their relationships (Baucom et al., 1996), another relevant cognitive-behavioral intervention is coaching a couple in using problem-solving skills to find better ways to meet both persons' standards. The use of problem-solving skills to maximize mutual satisfaction with relationship standards addresses the "B" or resource component of the ABCX crisis model.

Thus, the goals of a cognitive-behavioral approach to crisis intervention with couples are to (1) reduce the number and intensity of stressors impinging upon the couple's coping capacities, including stressors associated with the couple's own negative ways of interacting with each other, (2) broaden and strengthen their resources for coping with stressors arising both outside their relationship and in their own interactions, and (3) modify extreme or distorted cognitions (or discrepancies in partners' cognitions) that exacerbate the impact of stressors or impede the couple's use of stress-managing resources. The active, structured characteristics of cognitive-behavioral couple therapy are well-suited to intervening when these factors threaten to destabilize a couple's relationship, and for helping couples already in crisis to regain stability.

CASE STUDY

The following case example describes a common set of stressors that can negatively affect couples that are attempting to cope with multiple competing demands from jobs, raising their children, and helping aging parents whose health and independence are rapidly declining. Price (2005) cites statistics showing the rapidly increasing number of households involved in caregiving for elderly family members, as well as the extensive demands on caregivers' personal resources and negative impacts on their physical and psychological well-being and family relationships. Being a caregiver not only creates role conflicts within the family; it also involves stress from attempting to balance caregiving activities with responsibilities from one's job (Hepburn & Barling, 1996). This case reflects the common situation in which women are the primary caregivers, but the entire family system is faced with making accommodations. Although caregiving relations often become long-term patterns in a family, the potential exists for the development of a crisis if the stressors begin to overwhelm the coping abilities of the family members.

Mary (age 37) and Dave (age 38) have been married for 15 years and have two children, a daughter, Sarah, age 13, and a son, Tom, age 11. Within their nuclear family Mary and Dave have experienced a variety of normative demands from their jobs and raising two children, but on the whole they have been able to cope well. However, recently significant problems with Mary's parents' health have added a substantial amount of stress. Mary's 65-year-old mother, Samantha, suffered a stroke and required rehabilitation after a brief hospitalization. The rehabilitation provided an 80% recovery, leaving Samantha with lingering memory, concentration, and muscular coordination problems, as well as generalized impaired left-side functioning. In addition, Mary's 70-year-old father, John, retired from his long-term career as a dentist several years ago because of disabling hypertension and early-stage emphysema. Samantha had been his primary caretaker before her stroke.

Neither Samantha nor John required the services of a nursing home, but each needed more assistance with various activities of daily living and general mobility than they could provide for themselves. They had a good network of friends and had been socially active all their adult lives. However, they could not rely on their friends for the level of care they required. In light of the dynamics of Samantha's and John's family, it fell to Mary to coordinate her parents' care, albeit from afar. Mary's parents live in a city 800 miles distant from her and Dave's home. Mary is the middle of three children. Tom, her older brother, traditionally had been the one from whom their parents sought advice and assistance, because he lived in the next town, but he made it clear that with the parents' more severe problems he would be neither a caregiver nor a coordinator of caregiving services. Mary's younger sister, Barbara, lives overseas with her husband and their three children. Consequently, Mary took on the responsibility of her parents' new medical, emotional, and practical needs occasioned by the deteriorating states of their health. In addition to maintaining her own job and attempting to contribute to caring for the couple's children and home, she traveled to her parents' home on average four times a year and spent several hours each week at home overseeing their finances, maintaining oversight of their care and caregivers, and talking on the phone with her parents about their concerns.

Several issues had arisen in the couple's relationship as a result of Mary's increased involvement with her parents' affairs. These issues concerned the allocation of Mary's time and emotional energy, expenses related to her role as her parents' guardian, a consequent shift in the allocation of responsibilities for the home and children, and a change in the interactions and emotional connection between Mary and Dave. By the time the couple sought help from a therapist, they were experiencing decreased time together and expressions of affection, as well as periodic arguments that often resulted in their keeping a distance from each other.

Assessment

When this couple came for help, it was clear from the initial signs that their family life was headed toward a state of disequilibrium which, if unchecked, would likely lead to a dangerous negative spiral that could significantly damage the marriage. Dave had several concerns about Mary's absences, both when she was away visiting her parents and when she was physically present but distracted by her responsibilities to her parents. The children also had voiced some complaints to both parents about their limited access to Mary. Mary's health was starting to show signs of the strain that she was feeling from the multiple demands on her, and her employer was beginning to raise some concerns about her performance. Although the circumstances of multiple competing life demands facing this couple created an acute state of distress, they likely were developing into a pattern that Mary and Dave would have to deal with over the long term. This family members' awareness of the potential chronic nature of the stresses in their lives was itself a source of additional stress for them. It was important to assess the elements disrupting the couple's marriage and the family and to intervene quickly to prevent further deterioration in the relationships.

The therapist inquired at length into the elements of distress that each partner experienced. From Dave's perspective, Mary's responsibilities for her parents meant that she was less available to him and the children, because of her travels and more consistently due to her distraction from monitoring and supervising her parents' affairs when she was at home. Dave perceived himself as shouldering an inequitable proportion of the couple's child-care and home-care responsibilities. Mary described herself as being overwhelmed by trying to meet all the perceived demands on her and said that she was doing as much as she could. Dave's negative evaluations of her seemed to her to be unfeeling complaints about her deficiencies.

In addition, Dave resented the fact that he had to be more responsible for the family's finances. Mary was unable to take a share of the bill-paying responsibilities, partly because of time constraints and partly because she was not earning as much as she had. Mary had used her vacation time and sick time during periods when she had to be away from work, so she had needed to take occasional unpaid leave to care for her parents. Her view was that she had worked very hard to balance work and personal responsibilities in order to preserve her job and meet her two families' needs, and that Dave had overlooked the Herculean efforts she had put forth to keep everyone happy and satisfied. Mary considered Dave's expectations for her to be unreasonable. Dave's reactions were influenced by his standard that a couple's relationship should come before all else in their lives.

Dave reported that he felt lonelier as Mary became more involved with her parents' needs. He remembered past times in the relationship when Mary and he would make time for each other, even after the children came along. What had appeared previously to him as a robust effort by both of them to nurture their marriage now seemed to be his solitary effort to care for the relationship. Mary could not understand his loneliness because it seemed to her that she had created the best balance she could under the circumstances, and Dave's observations seemed to her to be a set of impossible demands stemming from his lack of understanding—and his unwillingness to understand—the full nature of her emotional and practical struggles.

Clearly, this couple's distress stemmed from a pileup of stressors, the "A" in Hill's (1949, 1958) ABCX model of stress and coping, which overwhelmed their ability to adapt and thrive. Some were internal stressors occurring within and between the partners, and others were external stressors, occurring outside both the family unit and their control. There also was evidence that the partners' perceptions and appraisals of the stressors (the "C" component of the ABCX model) added to their negative impact on the couple. Mary was able to articulate several sources of stress. She believed that she *should* want to take over the care of her parents, because that is what a "good daughter" would want to do (a standard), but she also was aware that she did not want to do it. She also believed that her brother and sister should help with their parents' care, but they had declined to help (a problem with resources, the "B" component of the model) and she felt powerless to engage them in sharing the load. Furthermore, it was difficult for her to mobilize resources for her parents in their local community because of a combination of cost in the face of their own and her limited finances, her physical distance from them, the unreliability of people and organizations providing care for them, her uninvolved siblings' second-guessing of her decisions and actions, and the difficulty inherent in monitoring care from afar. In addition, her parents increasingly resisted accepting needed services that in their minds indicated their diminishing independence. Finally, resources that Mary put in place for her parents seemed to work only as long as her parents' physical status did not change. However, the trend in their health was toward deterioration, and Mary was faced with an ongoing struggle to update resources as those conditions changed.

Mary's employer was another source of stress for the couple. Although initially supportive of her need to take time away from work to care for her parents, more recently her supervisor had been questioning her absences, and it was clear that both her absences from work and her distraction while at on the job were taking a noticeable toll on her performance. Although she did not believe that the situation imminently endangered her job, she predicted that it had great potential to lower her job performance evaluations and at the very least would result in no raise in salary this year. This frightened Dave even more than it disturbed Mary, because he began to view the whole situation—their marriage, family, finances, and their future—beginning to cascade out of control (his negative appraisal and expectancy).

The therapist also discussed with Mary the grief process that she was experiencing as her parents' health conditions deteriorated. Slowly but surely Mary had to accommodate herself to the certainty that she, as well as Dave and their children, were gradually and irretrievably losing the people that her parents had been, and that she would have to give up any hopes for the future she had hoped to have with them. She began to experience anticipatory grief about their ultimate deaths. Her grief responses were compounded by her upcoming task of discussing end-of-life matters with her parents, including the formation of their wishes into living wills and durable powers of attorney for health care.

The therapist next examined with the couple the resources available to them to help cope with their stressors. Dave and Mary were able to identify some resources, such as their history of having good problem-solving skills and having worked well as a team when they faced other life stressors in the past. However, it appeared that the couple was overlooking some other potentially helpful resources that existed in the community. The discussion of alternative resources shifted the work from the assessment phase to intervention.

Intervention

The therapist discussed with Mary and Dave some resources that they appeared to have overlooked. For example, they perceived finances to be a big stumbling block, because Mary's parents were drawing down their own savings to cover living expenses, and Mary's brother and sister contributed meager amounts to their parents' care, in part because they did not believe their parents needed as much care as Mary thought they did. This disagreement among the siblings was rooted in the long-standing relationships within Mary's family of origin, which is addressed later when we discuss interventions.

Guided by the therapist, the couple brainstormed about other resources that could supplement what the parents could provide for themselves financially. The therapist's knowledge of various community resources was invaluable in broadening the couple's awareness of available options. Medical costs could be defrayed by Medicare, and maybe by Medicare disability benefits. If resources ran out, the state's Medicaid program could be a resource. Meals on Wheels in their community could provide daily hot and nourishing meals until Mary's parents could cook for themselves again. A senior companion service could provide help in the house with administration of medication, bathing, getting in and out of bed, visiting the doctor, cleaning the home, and shopping for food and household necessities. A visiting nurse could help with in-home medical care and monitoring, and the physical therapist and occupational therapist who had worked with Samantha during her rehabilitation could come to the home to continue her care. A medical alert system could provide a means for Mary's parents to signal for help in the case of a fall or other emergency. Finally, a consultation could be arranged with the local senior citizen center to refit her parents' home with aids (e.g., bars on their toilet and bathtub) to make it safer for two increasingly infirm people. Identifying a range of resources helped Mary feel more optimistic that she could keep her parents living as independently as possible for as long as possible, in their own home.

The therapist then focused with Dave and Mary on religious and social resources that might help with Mary's parents' care. Samantha's and John's religious community had a program in which congregants visited ill and disabled people in their homes if needed. Their clergyman took an active interest in them and visited them when they could not make it to services. Furthermore, Mary's parents had many friends who visited them and with whom Mary could establish contact to help monitor her mom and dad from afar.

It is important for people in a crisis to be able to identify concrete resources that they can use in their efforts to resolve the crisis. As the therapist helped Mary and Dave pinpoint the resources available to Mary in her struggle to balance the variety of responsibilities she had, it provided some comfort for the couple that Mary would be able to handle the acute situation with her parents. It also reduced their distress to consider how the available resources would be helpful as the parents' conditions worsened over time chronically.

Next, the therapist focused on interventions to prevent the disequilibrium that existed in the couple's own relationship from spiraling negatively toward dissolution both of their marriage and their ability to be effective parents together. It was important to reduce the *secondary distress* that had developed as a result of the couple's ineffective and aversive ways of interacting with each other regarding the stressors involving Mary's parents. The interventions addressed several aspects of available resources and the partners' cognitions regarding their circumstances.

Dave believed that Mary's brother and sister ought to help with the increasing amounts of care that her parents required, and he attributed Mary's inability to engage her siblings in an equitable share of the load to Mary having made a conscious choice to put her family ahead of theirs on her personal list of priorities. He wanted Mary to spend less time and energy on planning and implementing strategies for her parents' care and more time with him and their children. It was Dave's negative attribution about Mary's predicament as due to her own volition that made him angry and resentful toward her.

Dave's negative attribution about Mary's unassertiveness with her siblings illustrated one of the contributions that cognitions made to the couple's stress level. Each partner felt victimized, Dave by Mary's divided attention and Mary by her attempts to serve everyone's needs. However, neither person fully understood the experiences to which the other was reacting behaviorally and emotionally. Consequently, the therapist used both cognitive and behavioral interventions to increase mutual empathy between the partners and decrease inaccurate attributions.

One of the cognitive interventions was to ask Dave to consider other possible explanations for Mary's failure to enlist her siblings in sharing the caregiving burdens with her, other than his attribution about her selfish motivation. Dave was able to describe various situations in the past in which Mary had demonstrated that she considered him and their children to be high priorities in her life. This review led him to consider that Mary's current behavior toward her siblings was inconsistent with her overall pattern, so some factor other than a lack of commitment to him and their children could be operating.

A key behavioral intervention that the therapist used to counteract the partners' negative attributions about each other involved teaching them to use more effective communication skills for expression and listening. He taught them how to express themselves accurately and succinctly, and how to listen empathically to each other. As they started to slow their communication down and to focus it, Dave was able to see how Mary was trying to take care of their family in addition to her parents. Mary was able to appreciate the broader impact on those around her of the many things she tried to do simultaneously. She had had no idea of the confusing and depressing picture it created for Dave when he saw her taking on what seemed to him to be an unending series of unplanned and ever more taxing responsibilities. Each had thought that what he/she was observing, concluding, and reacting to was "obvious" to the other.

The therapist turned next to Mary's difficulty resisting the damaging effects of her family of origin's shared schemata and behavior patterns. For example, her parents voiced their anger at Mary for "interfering" in their lives. A family schema involved denying or minimizing bad news. The parents had traditionally turned to Mary's brother, Tom, for advice, and he told them that their current situation was not nearly as bad as Mary had said the doctors believed, and that they did not need all the auxiliary services Mary was trying to arrange. Consequently, he and their sister, Barbara, joined with their parents in second-guessing Mary's zealousness. Although they did not physically interfere with the arrangements she made, Mary reacted intensely to their criticism of her efforts. The therapist worked with Mary to increase her tolerance of their criticism by recognizing the family schema and its negative impact when a serious problem such as her parents' situation occurred. The therapist coached Mary, in Dave's presence, in challenging the validity of her family members' beliefs and in reminding herself of her goals and the progress that she was making toward those goals. The therapist helped Dave become her coach initially in the effort to refocus her attention on their criticism. Similarly, the therapist helped Dave increase his tolerance of Mary's reactions to her family, which allowed her to vent some of her frustration to Dave instead of trying to ignore it internally. Once Dave reattributed Mary's venting as a stress reducer rather than as an exacerbation of the couple's distress, he became an active participant in what had been previously a grating and resentful experience for him.

Next, the therapist tackled the couple's tendency to attack each other's personal standards. Using the expresser and empathic listener communication techniques they had practiced earlier, Dave and Mary learned to draw out each other's ideas rather than try to prove each other wrong. Once they knew that their beliefs would be heard and understood, Mary and Dave were able to talk much more productively about, and to accommodate, their differences (e.g., regarding the amount of time and effort one should expend with extended family relationships versus one's nuclear family) rather than try to prevail against each other.

The intervention then focused on teaching the couple an organized approach to problem-solving communication, to reduce stressors in their lives. This involved a stepwise process of identifying a problem fully, breaking it into its components, brainstorming approaches to each component, choosing a promising approach, trying it out, evaluating its effectiveness, and modifying the process if it did not work. Dave and Mary were able to use this organized approach to meet a number of challenges. For example, they tackled the challenge of creating time dedicated to their family and to each other. They were able to collaborate on a plan for Mary to talk to her brother and sister about their contributions to their parents' care so, at a minimum, they would be less obstructive. They also were able to talk productively about the extent to which Mary would spend their money and family resources on her parents' care. One source of stress, however, remained unalterable. The couple came to accept that although Mary would try to minimize the number of days away from her work, the financial penalty for work days devoted to her parents' needs was unavoidable.

As a specialized form of problem solving, the therapist coached the couple in devising time management strategies to balance competing demands on their time and energy (jobs, marriage, their family, making arrangements for Mary's parents' care). It was important for them to learn to protect time for themselves, both practically (a schedule) and individually (reducing internal preoccupation and distraction when they are together). Making self-care a priority was vital, in part because it was difficult for Mary to accept the idea that she had to take good care of herself if she wanted to be a good caretaker of others over the long run. The therapist presented psychoeducational material, including an article from a popular magazine, explaining how the risks of burnout increase substantially if caretakers ignore their own needs.

Rebuilding the emotional intimacy that had weakened between Mary and Dave was the next focus of intervention. Initially, the couple cited real obstacles to their devoting more time to each other. The therapist stressed an alternative view, that rekindling their emotional connection could provide sustenance for them (i.e., a resource that buffers stress) while Mary took care of her parents. In addition, the emotional connection would help Mary and Dave maintain their own family's health. To this end, the therapist guided the couple through creating a shared life vision (a new shared schema), taking specific actions that drew them together, learning to balance time they spent together with time they spent apart, getting close when they were in different moods, practicing ways of providing support for each other, and using communication and problem-solving skills to identify and resolve power struggles.

CONCLUSION

Couple relationships can be sources of great satisfaction and mutual emotional support for their members, but they also are at significant risk for dysfunction and dissolution. Stressors originating both within a relationship (characteristics of the dyad and the individual partners) and from external sources (children, extended family, jobs, etc.) have the potential to destabilize and damage a couple's functioning. Family crisis theory provides a framework for understanding and intervening with acute disruptions in couples' relationships in response to internal and external stressors, and it is easily integrated with cognitive-behavioral couple therapy. The action-oriented, present-oriented, structured, and time-limited characteristics of crisis assessment and intervention are highly compatible with a cognitive-behavioral approach.

Working within a crisis intervention framework broadens the therapist's scope beyond the couple's dyadic interactions to assess and intervene with larger system levels influencing the couple. Such system levels include the nuclear family, extended family, friends, neighbors, institutions such as schools, religious organizations and the workplace, and overarching influences such as local and national economic conditions. A crisis-theory-based approach also balances interventions to reduce negative impacts of current stressors on a couple's equilibrium with strategies for increasing the couple's resilience for coping with future stressors. Building resilience involves both decreasing vulnerability factors such as deficits in communication and problem-solving skills and increasing the couple's access and use of available resources within and outside their relationship. In turn, family crisis theory provides a model but no specific clinical approaches for intervention, but cognitive-behavioral couple therapy offers a wealth of specific assessment and treatment techniques for addressing the behavioral, cognitive, and emotional aspects of couple responses to life stressors. This chapter has described the use of cognitive-behavioral crisis intervention for couples and has illustrated its flexibility for intervening with a range of relationship problems. Crisis intervention should be a standard component of training for clinicians who work with distressed couples.

REFERENCES

Alberti, R. E., & Emmons, M. L. (1986). *Your perfect right: A guide to assertive living* (5th ed.). San Luis Obispo, CA: Impact.

Baucom, D. H., & Epstein, N. (1990). *Cognitive-behavioral marital therapy.* New York: Brunner/Mazel.

Baucom, D. H., Epstein, N., Rankin, L. A., & Burnett, C. K. (1996). Assessing relationship standards: The Inventory of Specific Relationship Standards. *Journal of Family Psychology, 10,* 72–88.

Beach, S. R. H. (Ed.). (2001). *Marital and family processes in depression: A scientific foundation for clinical practice.* Washington, DC: American Psychological Association.

Beck, A. T., Rush, A. J., Shaw, B. F., & Emery, G. (1979). *Cognitive therapy of depression.* New York: Guilford Press.

Boss, P. (2002). *Family stress management: A contextual approach* (2nd ed.). Thousand Oaks, CA: Sage.

Bradbury, T. N., & Fincham, F. D. (1990). Attributions in marriage: Review and critique. *Psychological Bulletin, 107,* 3–33.

Bradbury, T. N., & Fincham, F. D. (1992). Attributions and behavior in marital interaction. *Journal of Personality and Social Psychology, 63,* 613–628.

Bradbury, T. N., & Fincham, F. D. (1993). Assessing dysfunctional cognition in marriage: A reconsideration of the Relationship Belief Inventory. *Psychological Assessment, 5,* 92–101.

Burman, B., & Margolin, G. (1992). Analysis of the association between marital relationships and health problems: An interactional perspective. *Psychological Bulletin, 112,* 39–63.

Carels, R. A., & Baucom, D. H. (1999). Support in marriage: Factors associated with on-line perceptions of support helpfulness. *Journal of Family Psychology, 13*(2), 131–144.

Carter, B., & McGoldrick, M. (Eds.). (1999). *The expanded family life cycle: Individual, family, and social perspectives.* Boston: Allyn & Bacon.

Christensen, A. (1988). Dysfunctional interaction patterns in couples. In P. Noller & M. A. Fitzpatrick (Eds.), *Perspectives on marital interaction* (pp. 31–52). Clevedon, UK: Multilingual Matters.

Coleman, J. C. (1988). *Intimate relationships, marriage, and family* (2nd ed.). New York: Macmillan.

Cutrona, C. E. (1996). *Social support in couples: Marriage as a resource in times of stress.* Thousand Oaks, CA: Sage.

Daiuto, A. D., Baucom, D. H., Epstein, N., & Dutton, S. S. (1998). The application of behavioral couples therapy to the assessment and treatment of agoraphobia: Implications of empirical research. *Clinical Psychology Review, 18,* 663–687.

Dattilio, F. M. (1997). Family therapy. In R. Leahy (Ed.), *Practicing cognitive therapy: A guide to interventions* (pp. 409–450). Northvale, NJ: Aronson.

Dattilio, F. M., Epstein, N., & Baucom, D. H. (1998). An introduction to cognitive-behavioral therapy with couples and families. In F. M. Dattilio (Ed.), *Case studies in couple and family therapy: Systemic & cognitive perspectives* (pp. 1–36). New York: Guilford Press.

Dattilio, F. M., & Padesky, C. A. (1990). *Cognitive therapy with couples.* Sarasota, FL: Professional Resource Exchange.

Eidelson, R. J., & Epstein, N. (1982). Cognition and relationship maladjustment: Development of a measure of dysfunctional relationship beliefs. *Journal of Consulting and Clinical Psychology, 50,* 715–720.

Epstein, N. (1981). Assertiveness training in marital treatment. In G. P. Sholevar (Ed.), *Handbook of marriage and marital therapy* (pp. 287–302). New York: Spectrum.

Epstein, N., & Baucom, D. H. (1993). Cognitive factors in marital disturbance. In K. S. Dobson & P. C. Kendall (Eds.), *Psychopathology and cognition* (pp. 351–385). San Diego: Academic Press.

Epstein, N. B., & Baucom, D. H. (2002). *Enhanced cognitive-behavioral therapy for couples: A contextual approach.* Washington, DC: American Psychological Association.

Epstein, N., Baucom, D. H., & Daiuto, A. (1997). Cognitive-behavioral couples therapy. In W. K. Halford & H. J. Markman (Eds.), *Clinical handbook of marriage and couples intervention* (pp. 415–449). Chichester, UK: Wiley.

Epstein, N., Baucom, D. H., & Rankin, L. A. (1993). Treatment of marital conflict: A cognitive-behavioral approach. *Clinical Psychology Review, 13,* 45–57.

Epstein, N., & Eidelson, R. J. (1981). Unrealistic beliefs of clinical couples: Their relationship to expectations, goals and satisfaction. *American Journal of Family Therapy, 9*(4), 13–22.

Figley, C. R. (1983). Catastrophes: An overview of family reactions. In C. R. Figley & H. I. McCubbin (Eds.), *Stress and the family: Vol. II. Coping with catastrophe* (pp. 3–20). New York: Brunner/Mazel.

Fincham, F. D., & Bradbury, T. N. (1988). The impact of attributions in marriage: An experimental analysis. *Journal of Social and Clinical Psychology, 7*, 147–162.

Fletcher, G. O., & Fitness, J. (Eds.) (1996). *Knowledge structures in close relationships: A social psychological approach.* Mahwah, NJ: Erlbaum.

Gordon, K. C., Baucom, D. H., Epstein, N., Burnett, C. K., & Rankin, L. A. (1999). The interaction between marital standards and communication patterns: How does it contribute to marital adjustment? *Journal of Marital and Family Therapy, 25*, 211–223.

Gottman, J. M. (1994). *What predicts divorce? The relationship between marital processes and marital outcomes.* Hillsdale, NJ: Erlbaum.

Greenstone, J. L., & Leviton, S. C. (2002). *Elements of crisis intervention: Crises and how to respond to them.* Pacific Grove, CA: Brooks/Cole.

Guerney, B. G., Jr. (1977). *Relationship enhancement.* San Francisco: Jossey-Bass.

Hepburn, C. G., & Barling, J. (1996). Eldercare responsibilities, interrole conflict, and employee absence: A daily study. *Journal of Occupational Health Psychology, 1*, 311–318.

Hill, R. (1949). *Families under stress.* New York: Harper & Row.

Hill, R. (1958). Generic features of families under stress. *Social Casework, 49*, 139–150.

Holmes, J. G. (2000). Social relationships: The nature and function of relational schemas. *European Journal of Social Psychology, 30*, 447–495.

Jacobson, N. S., & Margolin, G. (1979). *Marital therapy: Strategies based on social learning and behavior exchange principles.* New York: Brunner/Mazel.

Karney, B. R., & Bradbury, T. N. (1995). The longitudinal course of marital quality and stability: A review of theory, method, and research. *Psychological Bulletin, 118*, 3–34.

Kurdek, L. A. (1993). Predicting marital dissolution: A 5-year prospective longitudinal study of newlywed couples. *Journal of Personality and Social Psychology, 64*, 221–242.

Lazarus, R. S., & Folkman, S. (1984). *Stress, appraisal, and coping.* New York: Springer.

Leslie, L. A. (1988). Cognitive-behavioral and systems models of family therapy: How compatible are they? In N. Epstein, S. E. Schlesinger, & W. Dryden (Eds.), *Cognitive-behavioral therapy with families* (pp. 49–83). New York: Brunner/Mazel.

Markman, H. J., Stanley, S., & Blumberg, S. (1994). *Fighting for your marriage.* San Francisco: Jossey-Bass.

McCubbin, H. I., & Figley, C. R. (Eds.). (1983). *Stress and the family: Vol. 1: Coping with normative transitions.* New York: Brunner/Mazel.

McCubbin, H. I., & Patterson, J. M. (1983). Family transitions: Adaptation to stress. In H. I. McCubbin & C. R. Figley, (Eds.), *Stress and the family: Vol. 1. Coping with normative transitions* (pp. 5–25). New York: Brunner/Mazel.

McCubbin, M. A., & McCubbin, H. I. (1989). Theoretical orientations to family stress and coping. In C. R. Figley (Ed.), *Treating stress in families* (pp. 3–43). New York: Brunner/Mazel.

McGoldrick, M., Preto, N. G., Hines, P. M., & Lee, E. (1991). Ethnicity and family therapy. In A. S. Gurman & D. P. Kniskern (Eds.), *Handbook of family therapy* (Vol. II, pp. 546–582). New York: Brunner/Mazel.

McKenry, P. C., & Price, S. J. (Eds.). (2005). *Families and change: Coping with stressful events* (3rd ed.). Thousand Oaks, CA: Sage.

Neidig, P. H., & Friedman, D. H. (1984). *Spouse abuse: A treatment program for couples.* Champaign, IL: Research Press.

Pasch, L. A., Bradbury, T. N., & Sullivan, K. T. (1997). Social support in marriage: An analysis of intraindividual and interpersonal components. In G. R. Pierce, B. Lakey, I. G. Sarason,

& B. R. Sarason (Eds.), *Sourcebook of theory and research on social support and personality* (pp. 229–256). New York: Plenum Press.

Price, C. A. (2005). Aging families and stress. In P. C. McKenry & S. J. Price (Eds.), *Families and change: Coping with stressful events and transitions* (3rd ed., pp. 49–73). Thousand Oaks, CA: Sage.

Rathus, J. H., & Sanderson, W. C. (1999). *Marital distress: Cognitive-behavioral interventions for couples.* Northvale, NJ: Aronson.

Schwebel, A. I., & Fine, M. A. (1994). *Understanding and helping families: A cognitive-behavioral approach.* Hillsdale, NJ: Erlbaum.

Schlesinger, S. E., & Epstein, N. (1986). Cognitive-behavioral techniques in marital therapy. In P. Keller & L. Ritt (Eds.), *Innovations in clinical practice: A source book* (Vol. 5, pp. 137–155). Sarasota, FL: Professional Resource Exchange.

Snyder, C. R. (1999). *Coping: The psychology of what works.* New York: Oxford University Press.

Stuart, R. B. (1980). *Helping couples change: A social learning approach to marital therapy.* New York: Guilford Press.

Suls, J., & Fletcher, B. (1985). The relative efficacy of avoidant and nonavoidant coping strategies: A meta-analysis. *Health Psychology, 4,* 249–288.

Walsh, F. (1998). *Strengthening family resilience.* New York: Guilford Press.

Wickrama, K. A. S., Lorenz, F. O., Conger, R. D., & Elder, G. H., Jr. (1997). Marital quality and physical illness: A latent growth curve analysis. *Journal of Marriage and the Family, 59,* 143–155.

Wright, D. W., Nelson, B. S., & Georgen, K. E. (1994). Marital problems. In P. C. McKenry & S. J. Price (Eds.), *Families and change: Coping with stressful events* (pp. 40–65). Thousand Oaks, CA: Sage.

SUGGESTED READINGS

Baucom, D. H., & Epstein, N. (1990). *Cognitive behavioral marital therapy.* New York: Brunner/Mazel.

Carter, B., & McGoldrick, M. (Eds.). (1999). *The expanded family life cycle: Individual, family, and social perspectives.* Boston: Allyn & Bacon.

Dattilio, F. M., & Padesky, C. A. (1990). *Cognitive therapy with couples.* Sarasota, FL: Professional Resource Exchange.

Epstein, N. B., & Baucom, D. H. (2002). *Enhanced cognitive-behavioral therapy for couples: A contextual approach.* Washington, DC: American Psychological Association.

Figley, C. R. (1989). *Treating stress in families.* New York: Brunner/Mazel.

McKenry, P. C., & Price, S. J. (Eds.). (2005). *Families and change: Coping with stressful events and transitions* (3rd ed.). Thousand Oaks, CA: Sage.

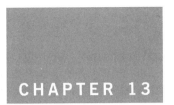

CHAPTER 13

Families in Crisis

Frank M. Dattilio

*I*n comparison to the literature on crisis intervention as a whole, relatively few studies or reports have been devoted to addressing crisis situations within the family context (Crespi & Howe, 2001; Gerrity, 2001; Gold, 1988; Langsley & Kaplan, 1968; Palmer, Glass, & Palmer, 2004; Pittman, 1976; Regehr, 2005; Siskind, 2005). Since the second edition of this book, the literature on cognitive-behavioral approaches to families in crisis has unfortunately remained lean. This may likely be due to the fact that individuals in crisis tend to receive help sooner than families or groups (Roberts, 2005). In recent years, much has been written about the specific application of cognitive-behavioral therapy (CBT) to couples and families (Epstein, Baucom, & Rankin, 1993; Baucom & Epstein, 1990; Dattilio, 1989, 1992, 1998b, 1998c, 2005; Dattilio & Padesky, 1990; Dattilio & Epstein, 2003, 2005; Teichman, 1984; Wright & Beck, 1993). While the cognitive approach to couples in crisis is addressed extensively by Schlesinger and Epstein (Chapter 12, this volume), as well as in previous editions of this book, this chapter focuses primarily on crisis in the context of the family setting.

Historically, cognitive therapy, as it applies to families in general, developed as an extension of its application to couples in conflict in the early 1980s (Epstein, 1982). Although Ellis (1977) reports that he adapted his model of rational-emotive therapy (RET) to work with couples as early as the late 1950s, little was written on this topic prior to 1980 (Ellis, 1977, 1978, 1986). The later studies developed as offshoots of the behavioral approach, which first described interventions with couples and families in the late 1960s and early 1970s.

Principles of behavior modification were applied to interactional patterns of family members only subsequent to their successful application to couples in distress

327

(Bandura, 1977; Patterson & Hops, 1972; Stuart, 1969, 1976). This work with couples was followed by several single case studies involving the use of family interventions in treating children's behavior. For the first time, behaviorists recognized family members as a highly influential factor in the child's natural environment. It was therefore decided that the family as a whole should be included directly in the treatment process (Faloon, 1991).

Several years later, a more refined and comprehensive style of intervention with the family unit was described in detail by Patterson, McNeal, Hawkins, and Phelps (1967) and Patterson (1971). Since that time, the professional literature has addressed applications of behavioral therapy to family systems, with a strong emphasis on contingency contracting and negotiation strategies (Gordon & Davidson, 1981; Jacobson & Margolin, 1979; Liberman, 1970; Patterson, 1982, 1985). Its reported applications remain oriented toward families with children who are diagnosed with specific learning and a wide variety of behavioral problems (Sanders & Dadds, 1993).

Since its introduction almost 40 years ago, behavioral family therapy has received only minimal attention from practitioners of marriage and family therapy due to the overshadowing of some of the more popular interventions, although its visibility continues to increase. Because of the overwhelming popularity of such approaches as the strategic, structural, and, more recently, postmodern approaches to family therapy, many practitioners have been influenced primarily by noted theorists such as Minuchin (1974), Bowen (1978), Satir (1967), Madanes (1981), and White and Epston (1990) to the exclusion of more empirically tested interventions. In addition, the behavioral approach may have been perceived in some circles as too rigid and rigorous in methodology to apply to families, and as failing to capture some of the commonly occurring dynamics of a family's interaction (Dattilio, 1998a). Although the landscape has changed some, with the behavioral approach remaining more flexible, the behavior therapies' strength lies more in addressing specific behavioral problems such as poor communication or acting-out behaviors (common among children and adolescents) than in understanding the comprehensive system of family dynamics (Sanders & Dadds, 1993; Goldenberg & Goldenberg, 1991). Specifically, the behavior therapies focus on observable behavior (symptoms) rather than on efforts to establish any intrapsychic or interpersonal causality. Certain targeted behaviors are directly manipulated through external means of reinforcement. Families are also trained to monitor these reinforcements and make modifications where necessary. Also, an ongoing assessment of observable behavior is made in the interest of empirically evaluating the effects of the therapeutic interventions. This is clearly highlighted in an earlier article by Jacobson and Addis (1993), which reviews the outcome studies available in the literature.

Regarding the development of cognitive family therapy, a cognitive approach or cognitive component to behavioral marital therapy subsequently received attention as providing a supplement to behaviorally oriented couple and family therapy (Margolin, Christenson, & Weiss, 1975). In addition to the work of Ellis (1977), an important study by Margolin and Weiss (1978), which suggested the effectiveness of a cognitive component to behavioral marital therapy, sparked further investigation of the use of cognitive techniques with dysfunctional couples (Baucom & Epstein, 1990; Baucom & Lester, 1986; Beck, 1988; Dattilio, 1989, 1990a, 1990b, 1992, 1993a, 1993b; Dattilio & Epstein, 2003, 2005; Dattilio & Padesky, 1990; Doherty, 1981; Ellis, Sichel, Yeager, DiMattia, & DiGuiseppe, 1989; Epstein, 1992; Finchman, Bradbury, & Beach, 1990; Schindler & Vollmer, 1984; Weiss, 1984). This interest in behavioral approaches to couple therapy also led behavioral family therapists to recognize that cognition plays a significant role in the events that mediate family interactions as well (Alexander & Parsons, 1982; Bedrosian, 1983). The important role of cognitive factors not only in determining relationship distress but also in mediating behavioral change has become a topic of increasing interest (Epstein, Schlesinger, & Dryden, 1988; Alexander, 1988; Dattilio, 1993a).

Marital and family therapists began to realize decades ago that cognitive factors were also very important in the alleviation of relationship dysfunction (Dicks, 1953). It has unfortunately taken some time before cognition was formally included as a primary component of treatment (Munson, 1993). Now, even though most practitioners combine cognitive-behavioral techniques, some still remain stalwart to using only a straight behavioral approach (Forgatch & Patterson, 1998).

As research continues on the significance of cognition in couple therapy, so will its integration with other modalities (Bedrosian, 1983; Baucom & Lester, 1986; Dattilio, 1993a, 1994, 1998a; Dattilio & Bevilacqua, 2000).

A COGNITIVE-BEHAVIORAL APPROACH
TO FAMILY THERAPY

Cognitive-behavioral couple therapy grew out of the behavioral approach, first as a supplemental component and later as a more comprehensive system of intervention. The same progression holds true to some degree for cognitive-behavioral family therapy (Dattilio, 1998b). Munson (1993) notes that there are at least 18 distinct subtypes of cognitive therapy used by various practitioners, with the result that it would be impossible to discuss cognitive family therapy broadly in a single chapter. This discussion is therefore limited to those approaches proposed by the rational-emotive theories (Ellis et al., 1989; Ellis, 1978; DiGuiseppe & Zeeve, 1985) and the cognitive-behavioral theories (Beck, 1988; Dattilio, 1993a, 1998a; Epstein et al., 1988; Teichman, 1984, 1992).

The rational-emotive approach to family therapy,[1] as proposed by Ellis (1978), places emphasis on each individual's perception and interpretation of the events that occur in the family environment. The underlying theory assumes that "family members largely create their own world by the phenomenological view they take of what happens to them" (p. 310). The therapy focuses on how particular problems of the family members affect their well-being as a unit. During the process of treatment, family members are treated as individuals, each of whom subscribes to his/her own particular

---

[1] This has been renamed "rational-emotive-behavior therapy" (REBT).

set of beliefs and expectations (Huber, 2000; Huber & Baruth, 1989; Russell & Morrill, 1989). The family therapist helps members realize that illogical beliefs and distortions serve as the foundation for their emotional distress.

The use of the A-B-C theory is introduced. According to this theory, family members blame their problems on certain activating events in the family environment (A) and are taught to probe for irrational beliefs (B), which are then to be logically challenged by each family member and finally debated and disputed (C). The goal is to modify the beliefs and expectations to fit a more rational basis (Ellis, 1978). The role of the therapist, then, is to teach the family unit in an active and directive manner that the causes of emotional problems lie in irrational beliefs. By changing these self-defeating ideas, family members may improve the overall quality of the family relationship (Ellis, 1978).

Some of the more modern adaptations of the REBT approach to families have evolved into recognizing the family as a system. As Charles Huber (2000) writes:

> Although the term family appears in its name primarily as a means of distinguishing REFT [rational-emotive family therapy] from traditional REBT, family as a unit of focus in REFT is synonymous with system. Thus, the primary unit of focus in REFT is the particular system under consideration, be it an individual, a couple, or a family. (p. 72)

The cognitive-behavioral approach, which balances the emphases on cognition and behavior, takes a bit more of an expansive and inclusive approach by focusing in greater depth on family interaction patterns and by remaining consistent with elements derived from a systems perspective (Epstein et al., 1988; Leslie, 1988; Watts, 2001). In fact, cognitive-behavioral family therapy (CBFT) is conducted against the backdrop of systems theory and relies heavily on a systemic approach (Dattilio, 2005). Within this framework family relationships, cognitions, emotions, and behavior are viewed as exerting a mutual influence, so that a cognitive inference can evoke emotion and behavior, and emotion and behavior can likewise influence cognition. Teichman (1992) describes in detail the reciprocal model of family interaction, proposing that cognitions, feelings, behaviors, and environmental feedbacks are in constant reciprocal process among themselves and sometimes maintain the dysfunction of the family unit. For a more detailed explanation of this concept, see Dattilio (1998a, 2005).

Consistent and compatible with systems theory, CBFT includes the premise that members of a family simultaneously influence and are influenced by each other. Consequently, a behavior of one family member leads to behaviors, cognitions, and emotions in other members, which, in turn, elicit cognitions, behaviors, and emotions in response in the former member (Epstein & Schlesinger, 1996). As this cycle continues, the volatility of the family dynamic escalates, rendering family members vulnerable to a negative spiral of conflict. As the number of family members involved increases, so does the complexity of the dynamic, adding more fuel to the escalation process. Epstein and Schlesinger (1991, 1996) cite four ways in which family members' cognitions, behaviors, and emotions may interact and build to a volatile climax. Each serves as stimulus or combinations of stimuli during family interactions that often become ingrained in family patterns and permanent styles of interaction.

1. The individual's own cognitions, behaviors, and emotion regarding family interaction (e.g., the person who notices him/herself withdrawing from the rest of the family).
2. The actions of individual family members toward the individual.
3. The combined (and not always consistent) reactions that several members have toward the individual.
4. The characteristics of the relationships among other family members (e.g., noticing that two other family members usually are supportive of each other's opinion).

Cognitive therapy, as set forth by Beck (1976), places a heavy emphasis on schemata or what have otherwise been defined as core beliefs (Beck, Rush, Shaw, & Emery, 1979; DeRubeis & Beck, 1988). As this concept is applied to family treatment, the therapeutic intervention is based on the assumptions with which family members interpret and evaluate one another and the emotions and behaviors that are generated in response to these cognitions. Although cognitive-behavioral theory does not suggest that cognitive processes cause all family behavior, it does stress that cognitive appraisal plays a significant part in the interrelationships existing among events, cognitions, emotions, and behaviors (Epstein et al., 1988; Dattilio, 1998b, 2005). In the cognitive therapy process, restructuring distorted beliefs plays a pivotal role in changing dysfunctional behaviors.

Schemata are also very important in the application of cognitive-behavioral therapy with families (Dattilio, 2005). Just as individuals maintain their own basic schemata about themselves, their world, and their future, they maintain a schema about their family. I believe that heavier emphasis should be placed on examining cognitions among individual family members as well as on what may be termed the *family schemata* (Dattilio, 1993a). These are jointly held beliefs that the family has formed as a result of years of integrated interaction. I suggest that individuals basically maintain two separate sets of schemata about families. These are family schemata related to the parents' family of origin and schemata related to families in general, or what Schwebel and Fine (1994) refer to as personal theory of family life. It is the experiences and perceptions from the family of origin that shape the schemata about both the immediate family and families in general. These schemata have a major impact on how the individual thinks, feels, and behaves within the family setting. Epstein et al. (1988) propose that these schemata are "the longstanding and relatively stable basic assumption that he or she holds about how the world works and his or her place in it" (p. 13). Schwebel and Fine (1994) elaborate on the term *family schemata* as used in the family model by describing it as

> all of the cognitions that individuals hold about their own family life and about family life in general. Included in this set of cognitions are an individual's schema about family life, attributions about why events occur in the family, and beliefs about why events occur in the family, and beliefs about what should exist within the family unit (Baucom & Epstein, 1990). The family schema also contains ideas about how spousal relationships should work, what different types of problems should be expected in marriage and how they

should be handled, what is involved in building and maintaining a healthy family, what responsibilities each family member should have, what consequences should be associated with failure to meet responsibilities or to fulfill roles, and what costs and benefits each individual should expect to have as a consequence of being in a marriage. (p. 50)

Elsewhere (Dattilio, 1993a, 1998b, 2005), I have suggested that the family of origin of each partner in a relationship plays a crucial role in the shaping of the immediate family schema. Beliefs funneled down from the family of origin may be both conscious and unconscious and contribute to a joint schema or blended schema that leads to the development of the current family schema (see Figure 13.1).

This family schema then is disseminated and applied in the rearing of the children, and, when mixed with their individual thoughts and perceptions of their environment and life experiences, contributes to the further development of the family schema.

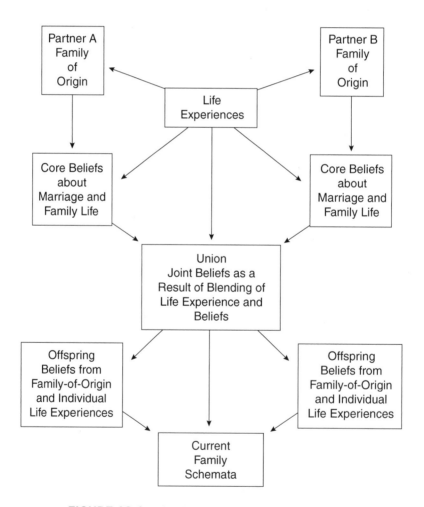

FIGURE 13.1. The development of family schemata.

Family schemata are subject to change as major events occur during the course of family life (e.g., death and divorce), and they also continue to evolve over the course of ordinary day-to-day experience (Dattilio, 2005, 2006).

CRISIS INTERVENTION

Normally, when a family enters into family therapy, the standard procedure is to take a detailed history, which includes gathering information from both parents' families of origin and following a procedure of clinical assessment that may involve individual interviews with family members (Dattilio, 1993a, 1998a; Dattilio & Padesky, 1990). This process may require as many as four to six sessions before the assessment is complete. Crisis situations do not usually afford the therapist the luxury of accumulating such information. Essentially the therapist is obliged to "cut to the chase" by targeting current thoughts and behaviors that are contributing to the family's immediate dysfunction and escalating its crisis. It is important that some family background be gathered, but in such cases the therapist may have to make initial assumptions and interventions in order to stabilize the family as quickly as possible. This, of course, depends on the situation at hand. The focus, once again, must be placed on defusing the immediate crisis. This may involve the use of behavioral strategies up front such as instituting contracts or teaching some emergency problem-solving skills so that the volatility may be reduced. This is analogous to wafting away the smoke in order to determine the extent of the flames, and it paves the way for the identification of individual schemata and later family schemata, at which point the restructuring process may begin.

Schwebel and Fine (1994) outline four assumptions which they state are central to implementing the cognitive-behavioral model with families. Following is a modified version of these assumptions that may also be applied to crisis situations.

Assumption 1

Individuals seek to maintain their environment in order to fulfill their needs and wants. They try to understand their environment and how they can function most effectively in it.[2] "As they gather data about how the family works, they use the information to guide their behaviors and to aid in building and refining family-related cognitions. This process lends itself to the development of their personal theory of family life and family relationships" (Schwebel & Fine, 1994, p. 41). The personal theory shapes how individuals think and perceive and serves as the central organizer to the mass of life events that they are exposed to (internally and externally).

---

[2] I contend that, in addition, family members draw from their own family of origin a model or a frame of how the family system should run. This may at times be a conscious or unconscious process.

Assumption 2

Individual members' cognitions affect virtually every aspect of family life. These are determined by five categories of cognitive variables identified by Baucom, Epstein, Sayers, and Sher (1989):

1. *Selective attention* (which is noticed).
2. *Attributions* (how individuals explain why any given event occurs).
3. *Expectancies* (what individuals predict will occur in the short-, middle or long-term future).
4. *Assumptions* (individuals' perceptions about how the world works).
5. *Standards* (how individuals think the world should be).

Assumption 3

This assumption proposes that certain "obstacles" block healthy family functioning. The roots of these obstacles lie within individual family members' personal theories; specifically the cognitions in the personal theories.

Assumption 4

Members need to become more aware of the family-related cognitions—how these cognitions affect them in certain situations, noting when such cognitions are causing distress and replacing unhealthy ones with healthy ones.

These four assumptions serve as guides for the therapist's intervention with the family, and may be modified to suit the specific situation or the level of crisis at hand. With these assumptions as a philosophical guideline, the therapist attempts to enter the family's world and to help the members, in a collaborative fashion, to identify the areas of dysfunction and to institute the restructuring process.

SUGGESTED STEPS

The strategies used in a crisis setting should be similar to those typically suggested for inpatient units (Miller, Keitner, Epstein, Bishop, & Ryan, 1993) but adapted for the crisis situation:

1. Define the current problem or crisis at hand. Attempt to establish some level of agreement among the family members about the definitions of the problem at hand and the characterization of the family in general.
2. Maintain a definite, directive stance in entering into the family unit and actively introducing change.
3. Attempt to establish some general understanding of the history and family of origin with the parents.

4. Identify schemata derived from the parents' families of origin and determine how these have filtered into the immediate family schema and the expectations of family members.

5. Ascertain automatic thoughts and schemata of family members via Socratic questioning.

6. Introduce the concept of testing automatic thoughts and challenging underlying beliefs of individual family members. Also, make some suggestions for alternative behaviors and the modification of family interactions.

7. Introduce the concept of agreeing to a behavioral contract in an attempt to defuse the current crisis. The time frame should extend from session to session, with a new contract developed at each session.

8. Move toward permanent schema restructuring and behavioral change/enactment.

9. Focus on communication skills and improved problem-solving strategies.

10. Reinforce the implementation of the above-mentioned strategies for future crises. (p. 159)

It is essential to defuse the volatility of a family crisis prior to focusing on permanent schema change. Depending on how well the family learns to deal effectively with crises, their therapy is less likely to be derailed by any other crises that may arise and can focus on permanent change.

The following case study may help demonstrate how this approach is implemented during a crisis situation.

CASE STUDY

Mavis, a young African American female in her early 30s, who was married with three children, was brought into a mental health clinic for an evaluation after the police responded to her home due to a domestic dispute witnessed by neighbors. Mavis was witnessed by several neighbors sustaining a physical beating by her husband, Lenny. Upon being investigated by the police, Mavis was taken to a hospital crisis center where she was first seen by a physician and subsequently by a clinical psychologist.

During the clinical interview, Mavis presented herself as a withdrawn and collected woman, much like many women who have been the victims of physical abuse. Mavis was cooperative but expressed several times during the interview that she did not feel that it was necessary for her to be there. When asked about what had recently occurred between her and her husband that contributed to the police involvement, Mavis explained that her husband had been consuming alcohol earlier in the evening and came home in "one of his moods" and "smacked me around a little bit." This "smacking around" had caused Mavis to incur a broken cheekbone and numerous bruises, all of which occurred in the presence of their three children.

It was at this point that Mavis was convinced to issue a restraining order against her husband and seek alternative housing through a temporary shelter for her and the three children. At first, Mavis was very resistant to agreeing to the restraining order; however, she became convinced after she was informed by the authorities that the child protection agency would definitely remove her children from her care if she did not protect them with a restraining order against her husband.

At this point Mavis was offered individual psychotherapy, which she declined. She did, however, express the desire to become involved in family therapy with her husband and children. It was suspected that this was Mavis's attempt to show the authorities that everything was "OK" and that her family could return to the status quo. It was only after it could be determined that Mavis and the children would remain physically separated from her husband that this family meeting was instituted. Within the week, Mavis's husband, Lenny, contacted this psychologist, stating that he was ready to address his problems and wanted his family back. Lenny was informed that for his family's safety, I would first need to get approval from the court. I also informed him that his wife and children would be residing in an undisclosed location and would meet here with him at a designated time. Lenny also agreed to abide by the restraining order and not have any contact with any of his immediate family members, except during designated family therapy sessions. He was also informed that his wife and children would leave each session 20 minutes prior to his departure for safety reasons.

During the initial family session, Mavis and the three children were brought to my office by the local Office of Children and Families. The children consist of Dafnese, age 13; Katrina, age 11; and Reggie, age 10. Lenny came to the session separately.

At first, the atmosphere was somewhat tense. Everyone was sort of quiet. They acknowledged each other's presence but in a rather sullen way. The youngest girl, Katrina, ran up and hugged her father. It was at that point that I introduced myself to everyone again and informed them of my role. I then attempted to get a handle on what everybody's perceptions were about what had occurred with the incident. My dialogue with this family went as follows:

THERAPIST: Everyone is here tonight because we've been having some problems at home and we want to attempt to straighten them out. Before we try to do that, however, I just want to get a little bit of an impression of what everybody's thoughts are about what happened with the family last week that involved the police.

[Interestingly, as in many cases, Mavis, being the mother and the main victim, was the first to speak up.]

MAVIS: Well, you see, my husband got to drinkin' and things got out of hand and somebody in the neighborhood saw it and called the police and they made us separate.

[All of the children sat very quietly during this period, as did Mavis's husband, Lenny.]

THERAPIST: So, when you say things got a little out of hand, it's my understanding that you actually were pretty seriously hurt?

MAVIS: It ain't all that bad.

THERAPIST: Mavis, let me tell you something. I think you're minimizing things here. You had a broken cheekbone and numerous bruises, enough for you to have to go to the hospital.

[Everyone was silent. The oldest, Dafnese, began to cry.]

THERAPIST: What's going on here? It seems to me like this is something that's been occurring for quite some time.

[It was at that point that Mavis began to speak up.]

MAVIS: Yeah, it happens from time to time, but it ain't no big thing.

THERAPIST: So, why do you allow it to go on? I mean, this isn't right.

[I looked at Lenny for some response—he hung his head.]

MAVIS: Well, you see, it's like this—my husband has a drinking problem because he's under a lot of pressure and sometimes things get out of hand and we say and do the wrong things and he gets a little physical. It doesn't happen that much; we can take care of it.

[I then asked the children what they thought about what mother was saying, all of whom, up to that point, had remained silent. The youngest child, Reggie, age 10, spoke up.]

REGGIE: My dad gets mean sometimes when he drinks and he shouldn't drink, but he does, and when he does, he gets mean.

THERAPIST: Has he ever done this with any of the three of you?

[Everybody shook their head "no" in unison. Lenny subsequently spoke up.]

LENNY: No, I never done nothing like that to the kids, it's just between me and the wife sometimes that things get out of hand and it's not that big of a deal.

THERAPIST: Well, look Lenny, it is that big of a deal, OK? You're a big guy, you could hurt your wife. In fact, you did hurt your wife, and this can't continue to go on.

[I then turned to Mavis and asked her to tell me a little bit about why she thinks this occurs.]

MAVIS: Well, you see, it's like this, I know he's under a lot of pressure and sometimes he drinks, and so he gets a little physical. I can handle it.

[With additional probing, Mavis went on to inform me that it has always been her belief that she should absorb the abuse from her husband because it's her "wifely duty." When an attempt was made to understand how Mavis developed such a belief system, she began to speak of her own family-of-origin experiences.]

It was at this point that I decided to delve into Mavis's family of origin, as I would also do later with her husband Lenny. Often the hallmark of working with families is to try to understand what each parent was exposed to with their respective family of origin. This is a way of getting at some of the core belief systems that both spouses carry about their relationship and their family. What is more, it was also too early in the family therapy process to expect that the children would speak about how they feel or what they think. Obviously, Lenny was also inhibited by the entire process. I felt that, rather than pressure them at this point, I would let the parents talk a little bit and then ease the children in over time. Because Mavis was the more vocal one, I let her begin to speak about her family of origin. It was important that I understood how she developed her schema on relationships and what made it so ingrained.

Mavis went on to describe her family of origin as including her mother, father, three brothers, and three sisters. Her mother was not employed outside the home and her father supported the family financially. Mavis described her mother as being a passive–submissive individual who was very dependent on her husband. Her mother also idolized men and believed that they were the "heads of the household." Mavis's father was a well-mannered man when he was sober; however, he did consume alcohol and, when he did, he would become verbally aggressive and physically abusive to all of the females in the home. When intoxicated, he would also frequently physically abuse Mavis's mother, who, in Mavis's words, "would take the beatings in stride because she loved my father and the family and that it is the role of the mother."

I watched the other family members' faces intensively as Mavis went on to describe this scenario. I could tell, nonverbally, that her daughters, Dafnese and Katrina, were not buying into this because of the smirks on their faces. I then decided to open up the question to the family regarding the belief system about physical abuse. It was at that point that Mavis attempted to speak up about her beliefs. I halted her and directed my question to her husband, Lenny, about what his thoughts were. I deliberately wanted Lenny to speak so that Mavis would not dominate the session.

THERAPIST: Lenny, you've listened a little bit to what your wife had to say about her family of origin. What do you have to say about this whole idea of physical abuse and what your beliefs are?

LENNY: Well, I don't know what I think about it. I'm not an abusive man. When I do drink, I do get to feeling a lot of anger and sometimes I just got to release it.

THERAPIST: But, what are your thoughts about releasing it on your wife and children? I mean, doesn't it bother you that you physically hurt them?

LENNY: I never hurt the children. I never touch the children.

[I look at the children, who agree by nodding their heads that they were not the target of abuse.]

LENNY: But I do admit that sometimes Mavis pushes me to the brink and I get out of control.

THERAPIST: OK, but what is your belief about using physical force? What did you experience in your own family of origin?

LENNY: Well, my father was a drinker, but so was my mother, and they would get into it sometimes pretty bad physically. It wasn't always pretty for us to watch, but, you know, they did the best they could, I guess.

THERAPIST: Well, Lenny, how did you feel about the fact that your parents were physically abusive with each other?

LENNY: I didn't like it, but, you know, it's when people get to drinking that these kind of things happen—and that's life.

THERAPIST: So, you both come from environments where there is abuse and extensive alcohol use, and I guess, in a sense, what you are both saying to me is that this is something that you consider to be normal and should just tolerate.

[It was at this point that Mavis attempted to chime in again.]

MAVIS: You've got to understand that my father had a rough upbringing and he took a lot of whoopings and was also going through the same thing. What's worse, he was sexually molested by his aunt, but never spoke of the abuse to anybody. He didn't sexually abuse any of us, but he did physically abuse us when he drank.

THERAPIST: So, therefore, what's your schema about all of this Mavis?

[I attempted to educate the family about the use of the terms *schema* and *automatic thoughts* in very simple terms due to their low levels of education.]

MAVIS: When the father's under pressure, he needs a release. So, sometimes, you know, he drinks and things get out of hand and we just have to live with it.

[I've already begun to uncover Mavis's schema, which was a rationale for defending her father's behavior, as well as her husband's behavior for the fact that this is just the way people express themselves when they have feelings bottled up. Mavis went on to state, "My daddy could be a good father and provide well for everybody financially and so does Lenny, and I think that he's loyal and that he's got a lot of pressure to deal with and I think that this isn't such a big deal and that it happens sometimes."]

THERAPIST: Let me ask you both something. If we could come up with a different way that you could deal with pressure, rather than drinking and losing your temper, would that be something that you would consider?

[Lenny and Mavis both nodded their heads in acknowledgment. Then Lenny chimed in.]

LENNY: But, it ain't all that easy 'cause, you know, I've been drinking a long time and that's the first thing I do when there's stress in my life.

THERAPIST: Well, what we want to begin to do is to interrupt this system a little bit because it's not working well for you.

[I went on to explain to them about the entire concept of systems theory and that, in this particular case, the family had to become the patient, and we had to work with restructuring the system of the family. I also went on to describe a little bit about how our thinking needs to begin to change and how, sometimes, we base our thinking on distorted beliefs that develop in our childhood and through our upbringing, and that these emanate from schemata and, sometimes, a schema needs to be restructured.]

At this point, I decided that the best role model to use for this case of getting them to think about changing schemata, was to focus on Mavis. I spoke directly about how Mavis's belief was that, despite her father's and husband's drinking, she rationalized taking the beating because both of the men loved their families and, therefore, part of her love in return to her husband was to take the beating in stride (see Figure 13.2).

At this point, I felt that it would be best if I began to work a little bit with Mavis's schema and address some of the issues that would lead to change. It was my impression that this may begin to serve as somewhat of a role model for the rest of the family and then I could move on to work with the father and the children.

THERAPIST: So, Mavis, the schema that emerged from our discussion, which apparently also was reinforced by your own mother, was that "If a man doesn't beat you, he doesn't love you."

MAVIS: That's right.

THERAPIST: Now Mavis, can you tell me a little bit more about this belief system, like how do you reconcile it when you're actually getting hit?

MAVIS: Well, I say to myself I can tolerate the beatings because I'm tough and it's worth it in order to be loved. I don't think he [Lenny] can help himself sometimes because of his problems and this is just the way I do things and my mother did things.

THERAPIST: So, the schema was handed down [intergenerationally transferred] to you, and your marriage and family, by what you were exposed to during your own upbringing, and your mother and father's interaction?

MAVIS: That's right. My daddy would become the same way and we withstood it in the same way that mother did in the past.

[It was at this point that I then asked Mavis very bluntly in front of her husband and children a very important question.]

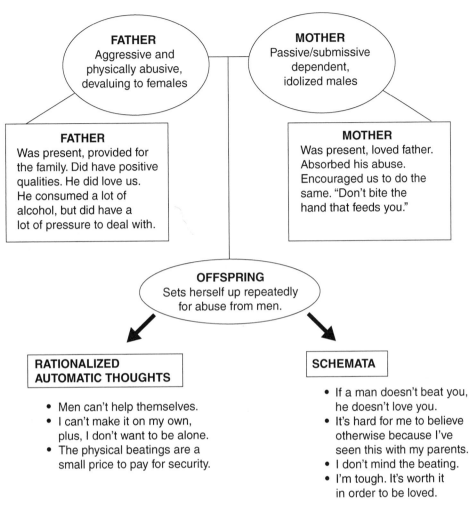

FIGURE 13.2. Schema development from family of origin. Adapted from Dattilio (2006). Copyright 2006 by Springer Science and Business Media. Adapted by permission.

THERAPIST: Mavis, let me ask you this. How do you feel now, in light of this, that you will pass the same kind of behaviors onto your daughters?

MAVIS: (*Looks down and begins to cry.*) I don't know. I don't want this for them.

THERAPIST: But, Mavis, this is what you're doing. You're setting the precedent for this to be handed down intergenerationally if something's not done about it.

[I looked over to Lenny. Lenny was quiet, but each of the children began to cry.]

THERAPIST: What are you thinking about? What's going through your mind?

LENNY: Well, this gets me upset. I don't like to hear about this happening to my daughters.

THERAPIST: But yet, what I mentioned to Mavis is true, you're setting the pace for this to be continued and, maybe, if not for yourself, at least for your family, you should think about changing it.

[Everyone was silent for a while and I just let the silence hang in the air.]

Interestingly, the fact that this behavior had been intergenerationally reinforced with both parties and is now being handed down to the daughters in this family was an important factor to highlight in this case. This was particularly because I was able to use the concept of the welfare of Mavis and Lenny's daughters as the reason for both of them to think about what they were going to hand down to their children. Mavis seemed to be more sensitive about her daughters not being candidates for abuse than she was for herself. The conflict of intervening was obviously significant but also made it very difficult to change because of the strength of momentum of the intergenerational history. It was felt that, in addressing the above schema, which seemed to be rigid and ingrained, it might be best also to consider inviting Mavis's mother, as well as her siblings, into a family-of-origin meeting. Mavis's father had since died due to cirrhosis of the liver in his late 60s, but Mavis's mother was still healthy and she agreed to join a family-of-origin session, along with Mavis's siblings. The goal of this meeting was to establish alternative points of reference for a husband loving his wife and family other than using physical abuse.

I also felt that Mavis was the stronger one in the family and that perhaps this would serve as the foundation for moving forward and helping this family to change. If Mavis would consider change, then the pressure would be on everyone else to change, including Lenny, who needed to go through rehabilitation and discontinue his drinking. Lenny had also mentioned in the initial family session that one of the reasons that he continued with his abusive behaviors is because Mavis tolerated it.

Family-of-Origin Meeting with Mavis

I had Mavis contact her mother and sisters and arrange a group meeting in my office. During our initial meeting, I oriented the family to what I was attempting to accomplish, which was to address the ongoing issue of the physical abuse in the relationships that have occurred intergenerationally with several members of this family. I explained that the law was no longer going to permit Mavis to sustain such beatings and had already begun to intervene with her case by removing the minor children from her care. This paved the way for Mavis to begin to restructure her thinking process and not tolerate such actions or she would otherwise lose her children to the state. I suggested that she and her husband needed to learn new ways of communicating with each other. Mavis's mother corroborated most of what Mavis had explained to me about the dynamics of her family of origin. Mavis's mother went on to reinforce the idea that her own mother had been subjected to a similar type of abuse and maintained a similar thinking style in order to avoid the risks that were involved in not tolerating such abuse, such as being alone. The formal line of thinking for all the women in

Mavis's family was, "the fact that a man is physically abusive means he cares enough for you to beat you. Your role as a female is to absorb these beatings, which stem from the pressures of being the family breadwinner. This gives strength to the family for survival." A further extrapolation was, "If the male cares enough about you to become physical with you, it means that you are important to him. Otherwise, he would abandon you and this would be disastrous because you can't make it on your own" (see Figure 13.3).

This is a very interesting concept, one commonly found among battered women (Hamberger & Holtzworth-Munroe, Chapter 11, this volume). The assumption about a woman's inability to survive outside a violent relationship, along with other intrapsychic factors, has been studied at length in the professional literature (Barnett et al., 2005; Fleury, Sullivan, Bybee, & Davidson, 1988). Such cognitions as those outlined in Figure 13.3 only increase the psychological stress of the battered victim.

I attempted to challenge Mavis's mother's schema by posing the question: "Was there not an alternative, a non-physically abusive way of displaying such love and affection?" This was particularly important now that external pressure was on Mavis,

"If a man doesn't beat you, ————————▶ If he cares enough about you to get physical,
he doesn't love you."   then it means that you are important to him.
                                                                        Otherwise, he'll walk away ⟹ I'm
                                                                        needed in life.

                                                                                        │
                                                                                        ▼

Therapist: Models the challenging ————▶ Can there exist a non-physically painful
of schema content.   alternative to a display of love and affection?

                                                                                        │
                                                                                        ▼

Patient: ———————————————————▶ That's all I know.

                                                                                        │
                                                                                        ▼

Therapist: _____▶ But it doesn't mean that an alternative doesn't
                                                                        exist. Plus, what is the long-term outcome of
                                                                        sustaining ongoing beatings?

                                                                                        │
                                                                                        ▼

Patient: ———————————————————▶ I'm afraid to invest in any other belief.

                                                                                        │
                                                                                        ▼

Therapist: ————————————————▶ What is the risk in trying?

                                                                                        │
                                                                                        ▼

Patient: ———————————————————▶ Being rejected and alone.

Risk = Tremendous loss of identity and security

FIGURE 13.3. Analysis of schema content. Adapted from Dattilio (2006). Copyright 2006 by Springer Science and Business Media. Adapted by permission.

who was part of the current generation, to not tolerate such behavior and to break the established cycle. Mavis and her mother both stated that this was all that they ever knew. They also stated that making a change would involve taking a risk of possibly being rejected and abandoned. In a sense, sustaining the beating guaranteed security in their minds. Consequently, both Mavis and her mother rationalized it by using the automatic thoughts, "I'm tough", "I don't mind", "A beating won't kill you every once in a while." Again, in challenging this schema, the question was raised as to whether or not their offspring would be prepared to face the same type of abuse and how, perhaps, they might not be as tough as Mavis and her mother had been. What is more, it was also important to tap into whether they actually desired to expose them to the same abuse or if an alternative could be identified.

Upon addressing the issue of the loss of identity and security, several steps were introduced to challenge this long-standing schema in an attempt to make some change in terms of the evolutional process.

1. Challenge schemata or beliefs about the potential risk involved.
2. Identify collaboratively the erroneous information that underlies the schema.
3. Accentuate the impact of such beliefs over time.
4. Build skills that will embrace self-concept and self-esteem.
5. Facilitate a sense of empowerment by role modeling and designing cognitive-behavioral homework assignments that will build self-esteem and self-reliance.
6. Underscore the point that people do have a choice as to how they want to be loved and what they are willing to endure.

What was interesting about this case was that in working with Mavis and her mother, as well as her siblings, we were able to develop some joint restructuring about what alternatives might be considered instead of exposing themselves to physical beatings. The direct impetus was the fact that the police intervention, as well as the intervention of other authorities, had already placed pressure on Mavis to make changes. An important element in the work with Mavis was seeing her own mother consider some alternatives to subjecting herself to physical abuse, and observing her mother choosing the option of self-preservation. It is suspected that because Mavis's mother was elderly and more reflective of the past quality of life, she began to view the situation from a different perspective. This was a very powerful component of the change process for Mavis. In addition, Mavis experienced some misgivings about making her children witnesses to the years of abuse from her husband. These concerns were discussed in detail in the family sessions and some enactment was decided on for Mavis to change her thinking.

With some of the schemata restructured and fortified by the family-of-origin visit with Mavis's mother and siblings, I entered into the second family visit with Mavis, Lenny, and the children. Mavis shared her experience with the family-of-origin visit and how she had made a major step in changing her thinking for herself and the family's sake. Mavis made it very clear to Lenny that she was not going to tolerate abuse of any kind any longer because it was not in her, or the family's, best interests. She issued Lenny an ultimatum to enter rehab and become substance free or she could no longer remain in the relationship. Interestingly, the family remained silent through this monologue, at which point Lenny gave a commitment that he would enter into rehabilitation.

Surprisingly, Lenny admitted that he was scared and did not know how he was going to deal with giving up alcohol. We discussed the issue of how he would need to find new mechanisms for dealing with his stress and that this would be part and parcel of the treatment package to which he would be exposed. We also spoke about the addiction process and his own underlying dependency.

Interestingly, the children began to perk up and became involved in the session at the point in which Mavis revealed her decision to change. It was almost as though the children had been waiting for Mavis to make this kind of decision before they started to talk about how they felt. The two older girls expressed how often they were afraid during the incidences in which Lenny was abusive and feared that he would hurt their mother.

We also began to discuss how the adjustment would take place and restructuring the family schema to a life absent of any abuse, be it physical or mental. We further discussed methods for dealing with stress and how to "head stress off at the pass" before allowing it to mount. I underscored the idea that Lenny and Mavis would be very important role models for the children in developing new ways to deal with their stress, which would, ideally, be carried on with the children into the next generation.

Discussion

This is a classic example of how the restructuring of intergenerational schemata may have a significant impact on what offspring sometimes permit themselves to be exposed to because of what was reinforced in their childhood. The power of the schema restructuring process is not only in the challenging of individual schemata but sometimes in the role modeling of a parent's reevaluation of his/her own schemata and choices. The opportunity for Mavis to observe her own mother considering alternatives to abuse served as a significant motivating force for Mavis to do the same. It also served as an endorsement for Mavis to consider restructuring her own schemata about abuse in general and pass on a positive way to deal with this situation to her children. This is not to say that Mavis would not have changed her belief system without seeing her mother do so; however, the shift clearly fortified her decision to modify her thinking, which greatly helped her to deal with this crisis situation. However, Mavis did have to face her greatest fear, which was to be alone and care for her children without the security of her husband's income. This is something that she was encouraged to address in her individual therapy. This change also served as a springboard for Lenny to deal with his own issues, which, up until this point, had remained covert due to Mavis's tolerance and enabling behaviors.

The use of cognitive reconstructing of schemata can be very effective for some ingrained schemata in crisis intervention, but the process of working with the family of origin carries its own unique power. This is particularly the case when dysfunctional schemata have been passed down intergenerationally. In a sense, there is a certain power in numbers, as group therapists will often advocate. The combination of using the power of role models and the insight obtained through generational experience can often be a tool to augment change and, obviously, in this case, began to have an impact on the subsequent generation in the family.

It should also be kept in mind that some schemata may become supported by secondary gain that may develop later on in the developmental process. For example, in the case of Mavis and her family, she may have also been deriving a sense of her own power and control by sustaining the physical abuse from her husband if she later used her battering as a means of manipulating her husband, and even her family, during periods when her husband was maintaining sobriety. She may have used this in a way to instill guilt during these periods, which she could possibly use to her advantage. One might consider this type of secondary gain, especially in a family setting where the female line includes distinct feelings of lack of control and power, as in the case of Mavis. In a case where there is secondary gain, the same type of challenges to schemata can be made by considering possible alternatives. In making Mavis and her family aware of the idea that there may be a secondary gain at play, it would be important to make them aware of this process and how it was affecting the family dynamics. The behavioral follow-through is also an important component in the facilitation of change as the actual enactment of the alternative behavior reifies the change.

Clearly, other issues might become relevant as well, such as the underlying need for some individuals to self-abuse by placing themselves in harm's way. Naturally, this and other issues would also need to be addressed during the course of treatment. In any case, challenging the beliefs and restructuring thinking procedures are resources that may prove effective when dealing with crisis in family situations.

CONCLUSION

In the foregoing case, it was decided to target Mavis because she was perceived by the therapist as being the center of the conflict in this particular crisis. It was my thought that attempting to restructure Mavis's thoughts initially might have a significant impact on the rest of the family members and diffuse the volatility of the situation. Unfortunately, this has its drawbacks and surely would empower Mavis in many ways. Eventually, in subsequent sessions, the focus was placed on having each member restructure his/her thoughts as well as on trying some alternative behaviors as a specific therapeutic exercise. This would balance the system and place equal emphasis on each family member. It would also be suggested that they continue in family therapy for an extended period of time subsequent to the crisis period.

It is important to note that cognitive-behavioral therapy works best with families when it is used against the backdrop of a systems approach (Dattilio, 1998c). It differs from a strict traditional systems approach in that more emphasis is placed on targeting cognitions, particularly belief systems, in order to facilitate change (Dattilio, 2005).

Most important, one of the strengths of the cognitive-behavioral modality of family therapy is that it is readily integrated with other therapeutic modalities and is likely to be utilized more actively in the future, particularly in crisis settings. For the short run, however, it is suggested that cognitive-behavioral strategies be introduced early in order to stabilize the crisis situation, as in the aforementioned case. Clinicians can use cognitive-behavioral strategies effectively as an adjunct to just about any modality of family treatment and are encouraged to do so as a measure of both short- and long-term intervention.

REFERENCES

Alexander, J., & Parsons, B. V. (1982). *Functional family therapy*. Pacific Grove, CA: Brooks/ Cole.

Alexander, P. (1988). The therapeutic implications of family cognitions and constructs. *Journal of Cognitive Psychotherapy*, 2(4), 219–236.

Bandura, A. (1977). *Social learning therapy*. Englewood Cliffs, NJ: Prentice Hall.

Barnett, O. W., Miller-Perrin, C. L., & Perrin, R. D. (2005). *Family violence across the lifespan: An introduction* (2nd ed.). Thousand Oaks, CA: Sage.

Baucom, D. H., & Epstein, N. (1990). *Cognitive-behavioral marital therapy*, New York: Brunner/Mazel.

Baucom, D. H., Epstein, N., Sayers, S., & Sher, T. (1989). The role of cognition in marital relationships: Defunctional, methodological, and conceptual issues. *Journal of Consulting and Clinical Psychology*, 57, 31–38.

Baucom, D. H., & Lester, G. W. (1986). The usefulness of cognitive restructuring as an adjunct to behavioral marital therapy. *Behavior Therapy*, 17, 385–403.

Beck, A. T. (1976). *Cognitive therapy and the emotional disorders*. New York: International Universities Press.

Beck, A. T. (1988). *Love is never enough*. New York: Harper & Row.

Beck, A. T. (1991). Cognitive therapy: A 30 year retrospective. *American Psychologist*, 46(4), 368–375.

Beck, A. T., Rush, J. A., Shaw, B. F., & Emery, G. (1979). *Cognitive therapy of depression*. New York: Guilford Press.

Bedrosian, R. C. (1983). Cognitive therapy in the family system. In A. Freeman (Ed.), *Cognitive therapy with couples and groups* (pp. 95–106). New York: Plenum Press.

Bowen, M. (1978). *Family therapy in clinical practice*. Northvale, NJ: Aronson.

Crespi, T. D., & Howe, E. A. (2001). Facing the family treatment crisis: Changing parameters in marriage and family therapy education. *Family Therapy*, 28(1), 31–38.

Dattilio, F. M. (1989). A guide to cognitive marital therapy. In P. A. Keller & S. R. Heyman (Eds.), *Innovations in clinical practice: A sourcebook* (Vol. 8, pp. 27–42). Sarasota, FL: Professional Resource Exchange.

Dattilio, F. M. (1990a). Cognitive marital therapy: A case study. *Journal of Family Psychotherapy*, 1(1), 15–31.

Dattilio, F. M. (1990b, July). Una guida all teràpia di coppia àd orientàsmente cognitivistà. *Terapia Familiare*, 33, 17–34.

Dattilio, F. M. (1992). Les thérapies cognitives de couple. *Journal de Thérapie Comportmentale et Cognitive*, 2(2), 17–29.

Dattilio, F. M. (1993a). Cognitive techniques with couples and families. *The Family Journal*, 1(1), 51–65.

Dattilio, F. M. (1993b). Un abordaje cognitivo en la terapia de parejas. *Revista Argentina de Clinica Psicologica, 2*(1), 45–57.

Dattilio, F. M. (1994). *Cognitive therapy with couples: The initial phase of treatment* [Videotape]. Sarasota, FL: Professional Resource Press.

Dattilio, F. M. (Ed.). (1998a). *Case studies in couple and family therapy: Systemic and cognitive perspectives.* New York: Guilford Press.

Dattilio, F. M. (1998b). Cognitive-behavior family therapy. In F. M. Dattilio (Ed.), *Case studies in couple and family therapy: Systemic and cognitive perspectives* (pp. 62–84). New York: Guilford Press.

Dattilio, F. M. (1998c, July/August). Finding the fit between cognitive-behavioral and family therapy. *The Family Therapy Networker, 22*(4), 67–73.

Dattilio, F. M. (2005). Restructuring family schemas: A cognitive-behavioral perspective. *Journal of Marital and Family Therapy, 31*(1), 15–30.

Dattilio, F. M., & Bevilaqua, L. J. (Eds.). (2000). *Comparative treatment of relationship dysfunction.* New York: Springer.

Dattilio, F. M., & Epstein, N. N. (2003). Cognitive-behavioral couple and family therapy. In T. Sexton, G. R. Weeks, & M. S. Robbins (Eds.), *The family therapy handbook* (pp. 147–175). New York: Routledge.

Dattilio, F. M., & Epstein, N. B. (2005). The role of cognitive-behavioral interventions in couple and family therapy. *Journal of Marital and Family Therapy, 31*(1), 7–13.

Dattilio, F. M., & Padesky, C. A. (1990). *Cognitive therapy with couples.* Sarasota, FL: Professional Resource Exchange.

DeRubeis, R. J., & Beck, A. T. (1988). Cognitive therapy. In K. S. Dobson (Ed.), *Handbook of cognitive-behavioral therapies* (pp. 349–392). New York: Guilford Press.

DiGiuseppe, R., & Zeeve, C. (1985). Marriage: Rational-emotive couples counseling. In A. Ellis & M. Bernard (Eds.), *Clinical applications of rational-emotive therapy* (pp. 72–95). New York: Springer.

Doherty, W. J. (1981). Cognitive processes in intimate conflict: 1. Extending attribution theory. *American Journal of Family Therapy, 9,* 5–13.

Ellis, A. (1977). The nature of disturbed marital interactions. In A. Ellis & R. Grieger (Eds.), *Handbook of rational-emotive therapy* (pp. 77–92). New York: Springer.

Ellis, A. (1978). Family therapy: A phenomenological and active-directive approach. *Journal of Marriage and Family Counseling, 4*(2), 43–50.

Ellis, A. (1986). Rational-emotive therapy applied to relationship therapy. *Journal of Rational-Emotive Therapy, 12*(2), 4–21.

Ellis, A., Sichel, J. L., Yeager, R. J., DiMattia, D. J., & DiGiuseppe, R. (1989). *Rational-emotive couples therapy.* Needham Heights, MA: Allyn & Bacon.

Epstein, N. (1982). Cognitive therapy with couples. *American Journal of Family Therapy, 10*(1), 5–16.

Epstein, N. (1992). Marital therapy. In A. Freeman & F. M. Dattilio (Eds.), *Comprehensive casebook of cognitive therapy* (pp. 267–275). New York: Plenum Press.

Epstein, N., Baucom, D. H., & Rankin, L. A. (1993). Treatment of marital conflict: A cognitive-behavioral approach. *Clinical Psychology Review, 13,* 45–57.

Epstein, N., & Schlesinger, S. E. (1991). Marital and family problems. In W. Dryden & R. Rentoul (Eds.), *Adult clinical problems: A cognitive-behavioral approach* (pp. 288–317). London: Routledge.

Epstein, N., & Schlesinger, S. E. (1996). Treatment of family problems. In M. Reinecke, F. M. Dattilio, & A. Freeman (Eds.), *Cognitive therapy with children and adolescents: A casebook for clinical practice* (pp. 299–326). New York: Guilford Press.

Epstein, N., Schlesinger, S., & Dryden, W. (1988). Concepts and methods of cognitive behavioral family treatment. In N. Epstein, S. Schlesinger, & W. Dryden (Eds.), *Cognitive-behavior therapy with families.* New York: Brunner/Mazel.

Faloon, I. R. H. (1991). Behavioral family therapy. In A. S. Gurman & D. P. Kniskern (Eds.), *Handbook of family therapy* (pp. 65–95). New York: Brunner/Mazel.

Fincham, F. D., Bradbury, T. N., & Beach, S. R. H. (1990). To arrive where we began: A reappraisal of cognition in marriage and in marital therapy. *Journal of Family Psychology, 4*(2), 167–184.

Fleury, R. E., Sullivan, C. M., Bybee, D., & Davidson, W. S. (1998). "Why don't they just call the cops?": Reasons for differential contact among women with abusive partners. *Violence and Victims, 13,* 333–346.

Forgatch, M. S., & Patterson, G. R. (1998). Behavioral family therapy. In F. M. Dattilio (Ed.), *Case studies in couple and family therapy: Systemic and cognitive perspectives* (pp. 85–107). New York: Guilford Press.

Gerrity, D. A. (2001). A biopsychosocial theory of infertility. *The Family Journal, 9*(2), 151–158.

Gold, J. R. (1988). An integrative psychotherapeutic approach to psychological crises of children and families. *Journal of Integrative and Eclectic Psychotherapy, 7*(2), 135–151.

Goldenberg, I., & Goldenberg, H. (1991). *Family therapy: An overview.* Pacific Grove, CA: Brooks/Cole.

Gordon, S. B., & Davidson, N. (1981). Behavioral parenting training. In A. S. Gurman & D. P. Kniskern (Eds.), *Handbook of family therapy* (pp. 517–577), New York: Brunner/Mazel.

Huber, C. H. (2000). Rational-emotive family therapy: ABC, A'B'C', DE. In J. Carlson & L. Sperry (Eds.), *Brief therapy with individuals and couples* (pp. 71–105). Phoenix, AZ: Zeig, Tucker, and Theisen.

Huber, C. H., & Baruth, L. G. (1989). *Rational-emotive family therapy: A systems perspective.* New York: Springer.

Jacobson, N. S., & Addis, M. E. (1993). Research on couples and couples therapy: What do we know? Where are we going? *Journal of Consulting and Clinical Psychology, 61*(1), 85–93.

Jacobson, N. S., & Margolin, G. (1979). *Marital therapy: Strategies based on social learning and behavior exchange principles.* New York: Brunner/Mazel.

Langsley, D. G., & Kaplan, D. M. (1968). *The treatment of families in crisis.* New York: Grune & Stratton.

Leslie, L. A. (1988). Cognitive-behavioral and systems models of family therapy: How compatible are they? In N. Epstein, S. E. Schlesinger, & W. Dryden (Eds.), *Cognitive-behavioral therapy with families* (pp. 49–83). New York: Brunner/Mazel.

Liberman, R. P. (1970). Behavioral approaches to couple and family therapy. *American Journal of Orthopsychiatry, 40,* 106–118.

Madanes, C. (1981). *Strategic family therapy.* San Francisco: Jossey-Bass.

Margolin, G., Christenson, A., & Weiss, R. L. (1975). Contracts, cognition and change: A behavioral approach to marriage therapy. *Counseling Psychologist, 5,* 15–25.

Margolin, G., & Weiss, R. L. (1978). Comparative evaluation of therapeutic components associated with behavioral marital treatments. *Journal of Consulting and Clinical Psychology, 46,* 1476–1486.

Miller, I. W., Keitner, G. I., Epstein, N. B., Bishop, D. S., & Ryan, C. E. (1993). Inpatient family therapy, Part A. In J. H. Wright, M. E. Thase, A. T. Beck, & J. W. Ludgate (Eds.), *Cognitive therapy with inpatients: Developing a cognitive milieu* (pp. 154–190). New York: Guilford Press.

Minuchin, S. (1974). *Families and family therapy.* Cambridge, MA: Harvard University Press.

Munson, C. E. (1993). Cognitive family therapy. In D. K. Granvold (Ed.), *Cognitive and behavioral treatment: Methods and applications* (pp. 202–221). Pacific Grove, CA: Brooks/Cole.

Patterson, G. R. (1971). *Families: Applications of social learning to life.* Champaign, IL: Research Press.

Patterson, G. R. (1982). *Coercive family processes: A social learning approach* (Vol. 3). Eugene, OR: Castalia.

Patterson, G. R. (1985). Beyond technology: The next stage in developing an empirical base for parent training. In L. L'Abate (Ed.), *Handbook of family psychology and therapy* (Vol. 2, pp. 237–262). Homewood, IL: Dorsey Press.

Patterson, G. R., & Hops, H. (1972). Coercion, a game for two: Intervention techniques for marital conflict. In R. E. Urich & P. Mounjoy (Eds.), *The experimental analysis of social behavior* (pp. 424–440). New York: Appleton.

Patterson, G. R., McNeal, S., Hawkins, N., & Phelps, R. (1967). Reprogramming the social environment. *Journal of Child Psychology and Psychiatry, 8,* 181–195.

Pittman, F. S. (1976). Brief guide to office counseling: Counseling incestuous families. *Medical Aspects of Human Sexuality, 10,* 54–58.

Regehr, C. (2005). Crisis support for families of emergency responders. In A. R. Roberts (Ed.), *Crisis intervention handbook: Assessment treatment and research* (3rd ed., pp. 246–261). New York: Oxford University Press.

Russell, T., & Morrill, C. M. (1989). Adding a systematic touch to rational-emotive therapy for families. *Journal of Mental Health Counseling, 11*(2), 184–192.

Sanders, M. R., & Dadds, M. R. (1993). *Behavioral family intervention.* Needham Heights, MA: Allyn & Bacon.

Satir, V. (1967). *Conjoint family therapy.* Palo Alto, CA: Science and Behavioral Books.

Schindler, L., & Vollmer, M. (1984). Cognitive perspectives in behavioral marital therapy: Some proposals for bridging theory, research and practice. In K. Hahlwag & N. S. Jacobson (Eds.), *Marital interaction: Analysis and modification* (pp. 146–162). New York: Guilford Press.

Schwebel, A. I., & Fine, M. A. (1994). *Understanding and helping families: A cognitive behavioral approach.* Hillsdale, NJ: Erlbaum.

Siskind, D. (2005). Psychotherapy with children and parents during divorce. In P. Hymowitz (Ed.), *A handbook of divorce and custody: Forensic, developmental and clinical perspectives* (pp. 331–341). Hillside, NJ: Analytic Press.

Stuart, R. B. (1969). Operant-interpersonal treatment of marital discord. *Journal of Consulting and Clinical Psychology, 33,* 675–682.

Stuart, R. B. (1976). Operant interpersonal treatment for marital discord. In D. H. L. Olsen (Ed.), *Treating relationships* (pp. 675–682). Lake Mills, IA: Graphic Press.

Teichman, Y. (1984). Cognitive family therapy. *British Journal of Cognitive Psychotherapy, 2*(1), 1–10.

Teichman, Y. (1992). Family treatment with an acting-out adolescent. In A. Freeman & F. M. Dattilio (Eds.), *Comprehensive casebook of cognitive therapy* (pp. 331–346). New York: Plenum Press.

Watts, R. (2001). Integrating cognitive and systemic perspectives: An interview with Frank M. Dattilio. *The Family Journal, 9*(4), 422–476.

Weiss, R. L. (1984). Cognitive and strategic interventions in behavioral marital therapy. In K. Hahlwag & N. S. Jacobson (Eds.), *Marital interaction: Analysis and modification* (pp. 337–355). New York: Guilford Press.

White, M., & Epston, D. (1990). *Narrative means to therapeutic ends.* New York: Norton.

Wright, J. H., & Beck, A. T. (1993). Family cognitive therapy with inpatients: Part II. In J. H. Wright, M. E. Thase, A. T. Beck, & J. W. Ludgate (Eds.), *Cognitive therapy with inpatients: Developing a cognitive milieu* (pp. 176–190). New York: Guilford Press.

SUGGESTED READINGS

Dattilio, F. M. (Ed.). (1998a). *Case studies in couple and family therapy: Systemic and cognitive perspectives.* New York: Guilford Press.

Dattilio, F. M. (1998b). Cognitive-behavioral family therapy. In F. M. Dattilio (Ed.), *Case stud-*

ies in couple and family therapy: Systemic and cognitive perspectives (pp. 62–84). New York: Guilford Press.

Dattilio, F. M. (2005). Restructuring family schemas: A cognitive-behavioral perspective. *Journal of Marital and Family Therapy, 31*(1), 15–30.

Dattilio, F. M., & Padesky, C. A. (1990). *Cognitive therapy with couples.* Sarasota, FL: Professional Resource Exchange.

Schwebel, A. I., & Fine, M. A. (1994). *Understanding and helping families: A cognitive behavioral approach.* Hillsdale, NJ: Erlbaum.

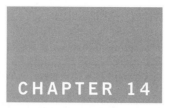

CHAPTER 14

Anger and Aggression in Children and Adolescents

Arthur Freeman
Stephen Timchack

*T*he fabled confrontation between the schoolyard bully and the weaker and frightened victim is the stuff of moral teaching tales. In the wished-for ending, the victim has finally had his/her fill of ongoing victimization and asserts him/herself, verbally or physically, and bloodies the bully's nose. The bully cries and runs away, thereby showing him/herself to be made of bluster and bluff and the former victim is now the hero. In the last several years, however, another ending has become too common. The individual who perceives him/herself to be a victim of teasing, physical bullying, emotional stress, verbal abuse, or exclusion by others comes to school with a weapon and kills the tormentor and any others who are nearby, often "finishing" the job by killing him/herself.

To the victim of bullying, the bully employs a set of behaviors that have been associated by the victim with previous occurrences of pain, embarrassment, damage to property, harm to family, or some other social or physical hardship (generally speaking, a set of worsening conditions) which the victim does not want to experience again. These consequences are not necessarily personal experiences but may have been acquired from other children, movies, or television. For example, as others witness a peer being bullied, the casually observing peer is likely to learn to acquiesce quickly when confronted by a bully, as it is the quickest way to terminate, or at times avoid, a potentially harmful consequence. The successful bully, either child or adult, learns the effective combination of behaviors (physical force, verbal pressures, social influences,

352

and the use of contingency) through a sequence of trial-and-error learning. Once the bully has established a sequence of behaviors that has evoked the desired response in the victim(s), the bully has added an efficient, effective, and less effortful class of behavior to his/her repertoire. However, the bully must learn that not all victims will respond the same way. Therefore, the successful bully must shape and generalize his/her aggressive behavior to fit the changing demands of various victims and various social environments. Also, the generalized form of the bullying behavior goes far in the way of social learning. Bullying can become a very refined and complex repertoire of human behavior. It does not necessarily connote a physically aggressive response, although the successful bully will intermittently follow through on the application of the force. Rather, bullying suggests a more efficient and more effortless form of physical aggression. The bully places the victim under a set of "if–then" contingencies which may involve the social contingency of blackmail or extortion, threatening the welfare of friend or loved one, the destruction of personal property, or the ultimate threat of physical violence to get the victim to act in a desired fashion. According to an operant paradigm of behavior, bullying behavior is common because it is a function of effective consequences for both the bully and the victim. The bully is positively reinforced by receiving some form of social, tangible, or sensory reinforcement, whereas the victim is negatively reinforced by engaging in behavior (giving in to the bully) that avoids punishment or escapes from a harmful set of contingencies. After repeated trials of this "giving-in behavior" the victim may begin to develop an attribution of helplessness, a condition where responding or not responding produces an undesirable effect.

Displays of human aggression, in some form or fashion, can be observed in many areas of daily life. These aggressive displays may be overt and result in the content of the six o'clock news, or they may be more private and insidious as in child or spousal abuse. These aggressive actions may take the form of subtle facial expressions aimed at intimidating or disapproving the actions of another, verbal arguments peppered with antagonistic swear words designed to create emotional injury, the physical bullying behavior on the playground, or in "road rage" or other forms of aggressive driving. They have come to be commonplace in our society and continue to generate several fundamental but troubling questions. At what point are these acts considered problematic, pathological, or dangerous to others? At what point do these aggressive behaviors cross the line into damaging or illegal acts? Is there an acceptable level of aggression that can be sustained in civilized society, in a romantic relationship, or within the classroom? At what point do these aggressive behaviors move from intrusive or annoying to horrific and thereby constitute a crisis for the individual, the family, or the society? Is aggression simply within our biological nature, is it a learned repertoire of operant behaviors, or are certain types of people more prone to act aggressively because of a temperamental disposition or a particular personality style which developed in childhood? Finally, has aggression in our everyday life reached the point of a crisis? If a tendency for aggression exists because of a particular excess of personality, can we then draw relationships between aggression in childhood and the later development of psychopathology? If this is the case, what levels of childhood aggression are considered within normal limits, and which levels of childhood aggression suggest a predisposition to psychopathology? The answers to these questions are often complex and fraught with many confounding variables.

When we witness human acts of physical violence, rape, bullying, robbery, or war we quickly assign various colloquial labels derogating the behavior of humans as animal-like, primitive, or barbaric. When it comes to the matter of child and adolescent aggression, which actually may be observed less frequently over the course of later adolescent development (Cairns & Cairns, 2000), there appears to be significant and alarming concern to understand why some children act in such a fearless and remorseless manner. For instance, the Columbine school shooting tragedy stands as an example of how some children lack the ability to feel sorrow, experience remorse, process consequences or potential consequences, or function under extreme social distress and isolation. In the aftermath of the Columbine tragedy, there has been speculation on the causes for the actions of these two adolescents who horrified the world by their savage and random violence. If a child does not feel remorse, lacks fear, or is unaware, uncaring, or unaffected by the possible consequence(s) of his/her actions, there may be little that can control the child. Developmental psychologists suggest that childhood aggression and defiance are common and developmentally appropriate behaviors at certain ages. As the child matures, it is important to identify the markers that define a child as deviant, an aggressive delinquent, or a youth in crisis.

Prior to attendance in some organized system such as nursery school, toddler playgroups, or school, childhood behavior may be far more private and viewed only by parents, caretakers, or siblings. In fact, the child's aggressive behavior may be mitigated by the closer attention available in the smaller setting of the home. It may also appear to be lessened by virtue of having learned more adaptive and efficient strategies of how to get what he/she wants from parents or caretakers. Once the child enters the school system, the classroom setting may make it far more difficult to control a child's aggression. The child may rather quickly come to the notice of school personnel, be in trouble in school, be involved with the criminal justice system, or be frustrated and pressured by his/her social environment. For example, Roger was a 6-year-old boy attending kindergarten at a public school. He was an only child of a demanding and rigid mother and a rather passive and uninvolved father. His parents were called in for a conference with the teacher regarding Roger's aggressive behavior toward other children and toward the teacher. The aggression took the form of tantrums, which involved screaming and throwing things, destruction of other children's work, and spitting at the teacher when he did not get his way. Mrs. L. became increasingly angry as the teacher detailed what Roger did in class to the other children. Mrs. L. finally said, "Then just give him what he wants. I am not sending him to school for him to be frustrated!"

Once involved in the school system a child may move from designations of "active," "angry," "demanding," or "controlling" to diagnoses such as conduct disorder (CD), oppositional defiant disorder (ODD), attention-deficit/hyperactivity disorder (ADHD), bipolar disorder (BPD), or intermittent explosive disorder (IED) or the criteria for a variety of potential personality or behavioral disorders. With any diagnosis of this nature, the child is on a developmental trajectory that is alarming and requires intervention.

Again, we are faced with questions. Is the child's "personality" to blame for creating angry, hostile, and aggressive thoughts that energize antisocial behavior, is his/her nervous system configured in a way which makes him/her more likely to use aggression as a major tool for coping, are his/her thoughts regarding obtaining gratification and satisfaction the operant issue, or finally, did the environment create and shape the aggressive responding of the child. As noted, some levels of aggression in children are expected, as the developing child has simply not had the time to learn and experience the range and variety of social consequences and to thereby modify his/her aggressive behavior. In addition, cognitive theorists such as Piaget speculate that executive functions including the development of logic, abstract thought, and higher cognitive abilities such as moral reasoning and social judgment do not occur until much later in childhood or adolescence (Miller, 2002). However, in the case of the teenage assailants at Columbine, it was reasonable to believe that they had the necessary cognitive capacities to consider more prosocial and adaptive behaviors to accomplish their goals of "getting even" with those whom they perceived as deserving of killing. However, their behavioral repertoire and cognitive strategies were apparently grossly limited and they likely never would have become the national symbols of violence had they adopted more prosocial behaviors. These could have including informing the administration of their humiliation and identifying those who had teased or injured them. Alternatively, even less prosocial behaviors may have been more acceptable in this situation, including blackmail, spreading rumors, or even fighting. Simply stated, the assailants involved in the Columbine school shooting tragedy were children in crisis. The severity and apparent depth of the behavioral and emotional identifiers went unnoticed because the nature of their crime was a secret, the behaviors went unnoticed, or the casual indifference of society to teenage threats, hostility, or secrecy were not genuinely identified as risk factors.

While aggression in children, as well as some adults, often may produce unpleasant emotional side effects, the violence and physical force a child uses to obtain a desired outcome creates an inherent quick source of satisfaction and consumes less emotional effort than bargaining or compromise. Also, aggression can serve as a default response if an individual lacks other suitable skills for dealing with complex and difficult social situations (Short & Simeonson, 1986). The simple efficiency and expediency of aggression, initially, is far easier to engage and produces more immediate results when compared with other socially acceptable behaviors such as asking, sharing, or turn taking.

This is especially true if a child has not been taught, or had modeled the appropriate adaptive behaviors, or has been shown how to adaptively respond or has received no reinforcement for doing so. Essentially, the prosocial behavior has never entered the child's functional repertoire. However, as the child matures, a learning process is expected to unfold. Many cultures around the world expect that civilized people resolve differences without violence, and the use of physical force is used only after diplomacy has repeatedly failed. But how do we explain and understand the child, and eventual adult, who repeatedly uses violence, verbal threats, or intimidation as an initial response that precludes diplomacy? It would be limiting to try to find a single reason for angry and aggressive behavior. It is determined by many factors, including being born with certain personality traits that predispose them to act aggressively plus neurological and biological factors (the genotype), a culture that has shaped aggressive responding or subgroup demands that encourage and reinforce aggressive behavior and make aggression seem like the best alternative response (the sociotype). For example, a question asked on the Wechsler Intelligence Scale for Children relates to what the child would consider the best alternative behavior if a child much smaller than him starts a fight. The expectation is that the child will know that fighting with a smaller child is wrong and inappropriate. However, in many cultures allowing someone smaller than oneself to take advantage of and physically abuse one labels the recipient of the initial aggression as an easy mark, a coward, and someone who can be taken advantage of easily. It would then seem appropriate for the child who is being hit to respond that he would punch the smaller child in the face, thereby sending out the message to the world that he cannot be easily bothered by such individuals and any further attacks will be met with immediate counterattack.

DEFINING AGGRESSION

For ease and conciseness of discussion, aggression will be discussed as either reactive aggression or proactive aggression. *Reactive aggression* refers to aggression that is generated out of anger, originates out of frustration, and is reactive to a threat or provocation (Connor, Steingard, Cunningham, Anderson, & Melloni, 2004). Reactive aggression has it origins in the frustration–aggression model, which suggests that individuals become frustrated when they are prevented from achieving a goal, and as a result, the probability of aggression becomes more likely as a way of "getting even" with the perceived offender. The goal seems to be to injure the person who is the object of the aggression. This view, originally developed by Dollard, Doob, Miller, Mowrer, and Sears (1939), suggests that this sequence of anger–aggression is natural and predictable. Kendrick, Neuberg, and Cialdini (1999) termed this *emotional aggression*.

Instrumental aggression or proactive aggression (Kendrick et al., 1999) occurs when the aggression is designed for some personal gain (e.g., taking something from another child without injuring the child). In *proactive aggression*, a deliberate coercive strategy is used to attain a goal or control the environment in some desired way (Connor et al., 2004). An example for innate and functional aggression comes from Aronson, Wilson, and Akert (2005), as they explain instrumental aggression as a form of aggression which is commonly demonstrated as a means–end behavior. Instrumental aggression is used when physical pain is not the end goal; rather, another reason was the impetus for the aggressive acts. For example, a child is interested in securing a preferred item (a toy) from another child and may not want to wait her turn to play with the toy. As a consequence, she engages in an instrumental aggressive act, possibly a physical action such as a push. This is not meant to hurt the other child but to accomplish some other goal, usually the attainment of the desired tangible item. This modeled and reinforced behavior may become the preferred and successful coping strategy for the individual to get what she has decided she wants/needs/chooses.

Bandura and Walters (1963) emphasized the role of imitation and reinforcement in the acquisition and maintenance of aggressive behavior in children and adolescents. This social-learning perspective posits that the modeling of aggressive models would lead to aggressive behavior on the part of the child. Ideally, the child would relinquish aggression as he/she becomes more socialized, or learns new modes of expressing it (e.g., competitiveness, achievement-striving, self-reliance, or success seeking). In our success- and performance-oriented culture it may not be the meek who inherit the earth.

Cathartic aggression is based on the psychoanalytic notion that increased anxiety comes about when the individual has unmet needs. This heightened anxiety is then discharged through the aggression, thus bringing the individual into a greater state of comfort. According to this model, the direct expression of aggression should then bring about a diminution of such behavior, that is, aggressive behavior will be self-extinguishing. This hypothesis has received little empirical support. In fact, a permissive approach to aggression leads to a lowering of the inhibitions regarding aggressive expressions, thereby leading to increases in aggressive behavior.

Explaining human aggression in terms of dominance hierarchy, territorial maintenance, and survival may seem outdated and unnecessary, perhaps even startling in the context of a highly complex and technological society. It would seem more acceptable in less "civilized" or technological societies. The drives to meet and satisfy physiological needs such as thirst, hunger, and sleep have strong, undeniable, biological processes that are linked to specific behaviors aimed at maintaining the body's or the species' survival or state of homeostasis.

In the wake of Columbine, some public school systems have instituted zero-tolerance policies for violence or acts of aggression that occur in the classroom or while the student is on school property. Having such a policy would, ideally, force the child or adolescent to develop other behaviors that are physically different but functionally equivalent to the original form. Instead of a child kicking or punching a classmate who has taken his/her handheld video game, the victim would work within the established system and resort to telling the teacher, or he/she can engage in any of a range of behaviors that secretly sabotage his aggressor to gain ultimate access to the desired item or simply to get even. While the demands of the school environment and the implementation of programs and interventions are being designed to reduce aggressive and antisocial actions, a zero-tolerance policy for aggressive behavior in school-age children may actually serve to shape and promote more subtle (though ostensibly more prosocial) forms of antisocial behavior. Moreover, if a child becomes frustrated by his/her inability to achieve a goal, express a behavior, or have any influence on the environment under these particular programs, the likelihood for an aggressive response is more probable, given that a child has little or no concern for consequences.

For example, watch any pair of 2- or 3-year-old children playing together. If one takes the toy of another an argument or fight may ensue. It is within this interaction that the influence of parenting, frustration level, and socialization can typically be observed. Although the desire to aggress was engaged, the influence of an evolved functional equivalent alternative response may serve to abort an initial aggressive response. Understanding which child will push, pull hair, punch, or use weapons to resolve the conflict becomes a key strategy in designing interventions. Although in the older child or adolescent, the behavior may not be as physically observable, initially, the frustration he/she may feel for having a goal blocked, wish denied, or being provoked or humiliated remains central to energizing an aggressive response. Again, understanding and identifying the adolescent in crisis becomes a key strategy for intervention.

Another issue that compounds the problem of aggressive behavior in children is the lack of fear a child may display. Aggression and fear are not mutually exclusive categories but are designed to work in reciprocity one with the other. When a child feels bullied by a perceived stronger classmate who takes his video game, the victim child should feel a certain level of fear and apprehension toward the aggressor. The level of fear that builds within the child energizes a variety of potential responses. If the victim child may feel that he/she is not able to physically subdue the aggressor, the victim child may engage in any number of evolved behaviors that include threatening, blackmail, or other socially mediated contingencies which are ultimately designed to have the aggressor relinquish the desired item without the use of physical force. If the use of threatening with socially mediated contingencies is effective, the victim child has just reinforced the evolved adaptive response to be used when faced with similar situations in the future. If the socially mediated contingencies do not work, the child is more likely to revert to prior behaviors which have achieved previous goals—namely, aggression.

TEMPERAMENT

Temperament can be defined as an infant's individual and stylistic differences which are closely related to the ultimate development of his/her personality. Tolerance for frustration, adaptability to a changing environment, sociability, and intelligence are often some of the central descriptors used when recounting temperament. Discussing the influence temperament has on the development of a child provides a more comprehensive review of potential biological variables for the understanding of childhood aggression. The early works of Thomas and Chess (1977) provided nine dimensions of temperament which continue to be widely used in the field of child development. Activity, approach, adaptability, distractibility, persistence, mood, intensity of behavior, threshold to stimulation, and rythmicity are the original dimensions used to assess child temperament. These nine dimensions, or behavioral characteristics with strong biological origins, provide the individual child with a particular range of responses when confronted with novel situations. An infant's approach to novel stimuli and adaptability to those stimuli describe the youngster's reaction and comfort level around an ambiguous item or situation. Also, these two dimensions predict how an individual may respond and adapt to a changing environment. Distractibility and persistence are perhaps more complex dimensions which refer to the infant's ability to attend and complete a task in the face of distracting stimuli. Thomas and Chess (1977) suggest that all dimensions of temperament have strong biological roots and persist, in some capacity, throughout the lifespan as personality traits. Furthermore, these dimensions will shape the experiences by which a child navigates and perceives his/her world, while also providing a range of individual anchor points, which serve as markers for potential responses and functioning in a changing environment.

EXPRESSIONS OF ANGER AND AGGRESSION

Webster-Stratton and Herbert (1994) list a number of aggressive child-related behaviors. Each type may be conceptualized differently in regard to the focus, object, nature, and frequency of the aggressive behavior. Each may therefore require a different set of interventions.

1. *Aggression against parents.* The parents feel victimized and possibly tyrannized by the child. They may be reluctant to intervene in the child's behavior, waiting instead for the child to "calm down." They may even ignore the behavior believing that it is of little consequence, that all children act this way, or, that if they discipline the child and keep the child from expressing him/herself there will be even greater consequences in the child being stifled and limited and thereby losing creativity.

2. *Aggression against siblings.* The child is violent with siblings to the point of hurting or damaging the sibling. It may even reach the point of a danger of permanent damage or death (e.g., holding a pillow over the face of a sibling or holding a sibling underwater in a pool or tub). Parents often respond by punishment, keeping the children apart, being watchful of the victimized child, and attempting intense observation of the aggressive child and keeping the sibling out of the child's reach.

3. *Aggression against pets.* The child has been seen or suspected of harming pets, either his/her own or those of neighbors. The child may kick, strangle, poison, tease, or hit animals with sticks or stones. When confronted such children may deny their actions, justify their actions, or attempt to reframe their actions as "play."

4. *Aggression toward other children.* This may take place at their home, in the park, in the schoolyard, or in other public places. It may involve taking toys or possessions of other children, breaking their possessions, or threatening them with weapons. This behavior is often modeled after the behavior of adults in the child's family. Kevin, age 13, was referred for therapy because of his threatening behavior in school. In meeting with Kevin's parents, Kevin's father stated that, "Kevin gets his temper from me." There was, in the father's admission, little remorse and more than a little pride.

5. *Damaging the family home.* The child may threaten or actually damage or destroy parts of the home. This might include fire setting or breaking walls, windows,

and furniture. It may also include more minor acts of vandalism such as ripping wallpaper or curtains or destroying carpet and walls.

6. *Vandalism that is damaging in school, church, homes of others, or recreational settings.* The child, either alone or in concert with another individual or group, breaks into a setting and physically damages the structure. This may range from breaking window, graffiti, or setting fires to destroying a structure or setting. For example, going into a cemetery and breaking and knocking over grave markers may be an act of violence with or without religious significance. In the latter case, it may be considered a "hate crime."

7. *General or specific noncompliance and defiance.* The child does not comply with the requests of parents and teachers. In this expression the child is labeled "stubborn," or oppositional, possibly passive–aggressive.

8. *Sleep problems.* The child is resistant to going to bed without difficulties. The child will prefer to play and wake others by his/her actions. Not sleeping may cause such children to come into conflict with parents and caretakers. The poor sleep hygiene then leads to resistance to waking and getting ready for school or sleepiness and problems at school. This child may, in fact, suffer from nightmares or sleep terrors.

9. *Eating problems and dining behavior.* The child becomes a "picky" or "finicky" eater, demanding special foods or preparations that are different from others in the family. There may also misbehavior at the dinner table that could include taking the foods of others, throwing food, or adulterating the food of others.

10. *Transitions and poor coping and adaptability.* The child has great difficulty handling any change in his/her routine, no matter how apparently small it is. There may be difficulty if dinner is late, the table is not set a certain way, or toys are not left in a particular pattern. Vacations that call for sleeping in a different bed or a different sleeping arrangement may bring about aggressive temper outbursts.

11. *Fears and talk of suicide.* Parents are concerned about the child's speaking not simply about death or dying but more about killing him/herself. Such statements may take the form of threats which allow to get his/her way in various family situations.

12. *Hyperactivity, distractibility, high intensity.* The child has a very high rate of activity and appears to be "charged up," "wound up," or "hyper." This hyperresponsive behavior may be threatening to self or to others. The expression of the activity is usually aggressive.

13. *Risk taking.* Related to the foregoing, the child does not appear to have fear or concerns for the consequences even of life-threatening behaviors (e.g., playing on railroad tracks, or playing with guns and explosives).

14. *Variable temperament.* The child demonstrates polar behaviors, at times being sweet, charming, cooperative, social, and good-natured. At other times the child becomes the "evil twin" who is dangerous, angry, hurtful, antisocial, damaging, and uncooperative.

15. *Negative impact on the marital relationship.* The child consumes a major part of the time, energy, and resources of the parents. There may also be direct attempts by

the child to intervene between the parents (e.g., demanding to sleep in their bed or verbal assaults on one or both parents and family members).

16. *Negative impact on the family.* Similar to the foregoing, parents and caretakers cannot spend time, energy, or resources on siblings without the aggressive child demanding their attention and concern.

17. *Negative impact on the broader family system.* The child creates tension with grandparents, neighbors, aunts, and uncles. This may take the form of system members avoiding the family or avoiding the aggressive child.

18. *Sexually aggressive behavior.* The child may seek or demand sexual behaviors from others. This might take the form of rape, forcing oral sex, fondling, or touching.

19. *Publicly disruptive.* The child cannot be taken to a public venue without the threat of verbal aggression, physically aggressive behaviors toward parents, or demands and threats related to demands for the purchase of some object.

20. *Substance use.* The child uses substances that may be disinhibiting and may make it more likely that the child acts in an aggressive manner. It might create circumstances that the place the child in danger or legal difficulty.

21. *Self-harm and self-aggression.* The child is self-injurious in both purposeful and nonpurposeful ways. Aggression may take the form of physical damage, extended and significant substance use, or self-denigration.

These behaviors may occur in an almost endless set of combinations and permutations across both the type of aggression and the level of aggression being mild, moderate, or severe. The aggressive behavior of some children and adolescents may cause significant and severe personal discomfort and dysfunction. Such children do not like being aggressive; they may feel guilt, may be upset by being ostracized, may be unhappy with the negative consequences they experience but do not have (or use) more adaptive prosocial behaviors.

For other children, the aggressive behavior is egosyntonic and the "distress," if any, comes from others (family, peers, school, or church). These children see no problem in being aggressive, they do not see any need to change their behavior and consider the negative consequences inappropriate or born of jealousy or anger on the part of others.

For still others, the aggressive style is, at this point, functional. Few individuals in the child's life are distressed. More positive euphemisms are sometimes used to describe the child's aggressive behavior (e.g., he or she is "a go-getter"). The aggression may be mild, moderate, or severe. Mild manifestation of aggression may (or may not) be noticed, may (or may not) be functional, may often be seen as a personal style, without prejudice, and thus "problems," if any, will depend on the parents, teachers, and school personnel.

Moderate manifestation of aggression has likely been noticed; *often* the pattern is dysfunctional and seen as an impaired personal "style, and severity and impact of the resulting aggression depend on the parents, teachers, and school personnel.

Severe manifestations of aggression have frequently come to the notice of school personnel; the child has impaired function (moderate to severe), or the aggressive behavior causes significant conflict that may be supported or enabled by the family.

CONSIDERATIONS FOR TREATMENT

The aggressive child typically maintains a number of beliefs that guide his/her behavior. These frequently include, but are not limited to, the following beliefs (or combinations and derivatives; adapted from Beck, Freeman, Davis, & Associates, 2004):

- *Justification*—"Wanting something (or wanting to avoid something) justifies my actions."
- *Thinking is believing*—"My thoughts and feelings are completely accurate, simply because they occur to me."
- *Personal infallibility*—"I always make good choices."
- *Feelings make facts*—"I know I have a right to act in the way that I do because I feel right about what I do."
- *Impotence of others*—"The views or actions of others are irrelevant to my decisions, unless they can directly control my immediate consequences."
- *Low-impact consequences*—"If there are limited or undesirable consequences they will not matter to me."
- *Narcissism*—"I am more special than all others."
- *Lack of empathy*—"I do not have to worry about the feelings of others."
- *Lack of societal focus*—"Rules are for fools."
- *Lack of (or flawed) information*—"There are many places in the world where my behavior is acceptable.

It would be naive for the therapist to assume that the aggressive child is coming to therapy with the intent of changing. Often such children are sent for therapy as an alternative to a range of far more serious interventions, including incarceration. Further, because the aggressive behavior has likely been reinforced by others or by the society in rewarding the individual for his/her aggressive actions, change is limited.

Reviewing the cognitive, behavioral, and societal/cultural or environmental determinants of aggression will allow for a more detailed case conceptualization. The more detailed the conceptualization, the better the opportunity for successful treatment. The treatment conceptualization must meet three criteria:

1. Does it explain the child's past behavior?
2. Does it make sense of the child's present behavior?
3. Does it predict future behavior?

If the treatment conceptualization cannot meet this test, it must be revised until it does. It must be recognized that an aggressive child may be hard to treat inasmuch as the aggressive behavior may be powerfully reinforced, over a long period of time, with the reinforcement coming from often powerful, influential, and/or credible sources in the child's life. A number of factors must be taken into account in structuring a realistic treatment protocol. For change to occur, the child (and his/her parents or caretakers) must see some value in behaving in a less aggressive manner. If the child does not perceive a value and purpose in being different, there may be little reason to change. This is reflected in the motivation of the child and his/her parents to participate in therapy.

The child and parents must be at a level to understand and enable the therapeutic process. This includes such variables as level of intellectual functioning, stage of cognitive integration, level of moral development, and verbal ability and style. We cannot assume that children and adolescents can understand the abstraction of empathy. Nor can we assume that their adult parents are any better able to use abstractions and generalizations. Treatment, therefore, must focus on very concrete and simple goals, ideas, and interventions. In a similar vein, the child and parents must be able to sit still, listen, concentrate, focus, and integrate diverse pieces.

In some cases, the referral problem will have a negative impact on the course of the therapy. The child, adolescent, or parent/caretakers may be verbally challenging or threatening, or behaviorally threatening or damaging to the therapist or the therapist's property. A therapist reported that when she left the clinic where she was completing her internship, she encountered a teenage patient who approached her in the parking lot and said, "Now I know what you drive." She was frightened, thinking that in the future he would wait for her at night, damage her car, or hurt her. She asked a fellow staff member to walk her to her car each evening. She and her supervisor met with the adolescent to discuss his behavior. He stated that he was just walking through the parking lot on his way to the bus and made what he believed to be a rather neutral and nonthreatening statement. He believed that he should not be held responsible for her "misinterpretation" of his meaning or intent.

In general, cognitive-behavioral therapy (CBT) provides the clinician with an approach to therapy which allows for structure and focuses on the composite of related beliefs and behaviors often manifested by persons with difficulties (Beck et al., 2004).

BEHAVIORAL PERSPECTIVE FOR TREATMENT

Aggression may result from frustration due to a skill deficit. Henin, Warman, and Kendall (2002) report that "it is the child's appraisal and expectations of the environment that are believed to mediate the connection between environmental events and anger arousal" (p. 292). Furthermore, they suggest that the treatment of childhood aggression should focus on the instruction of social skills to identify the situations when conflicts are like to arise, how to take perspective, identify problem-solving steps, analyze the options, and consider the consequences of the of the chosen solutions. Specifically, Henin et al. (2002) illustrate a social skills program where the child narrates self-instructions: "Stop and think," "What can I do," "Have I looked at all the possibilities," "I'd better concentrate and focus on think only think of what I'm doing now," "I think it's this one," and "I did a good job" (p. 293). Perhaps the major area of skill deficit is in problem solving. The work of Spivack and Schure (Shure, 1994, 2004; Spivack, 1973; Spivack & Shure, 1977) helps children to develop basic skills for assessing the needs of a situation and then to identify the best possible choice of response, both as a class of response and a specific response.

Although the clinician working with the aggressive child is initially recommended to rule out any evidence of brain insult, toxin exposure, or active disease processes that may better account for the development of aggression, doing so does not provide a comprehensive functional analysis of the child's aggressive behavior. If, however, medical evaluations do reveal significant areas of brain damage central to the role of aggressive behavior, then behavioral treatment strategies will need to be adjunctive to other treatment modalities including medication. In cases such as these, where there is clear and convincing evidence of biological origins of aggression, as in the case of traumatic brain injury, the use of medications becomes a treatment necessity to restore or establish adaptive functioning. Even in these cases, a behavioral analysis is key inasmuch as the child will still have learned a series of behaviors that influence his/her aggressive behavior or style. In cases in which no biological etiology is of concern, the process of functionally analyzing the causes of behavior needs to occur, but some assumptions must first be made. Like his other behavioral counterparts, Durand (1990) suggests that severe behavior problems including aggression should be conceptualized in the following manner: "Behavior problems are not abnormalities. Instead, these responses are reasonable behavioral adaptations necessitated by the abilities of our students and the limitations of their environments (p. 6). Behavior analysis has produced several powerful, empirically supported principles that can be applied to the understanding of a variety of complex human behaviors. For example, the interplay of schedules of reinforcement, extinction, discrimitive stimuli, and establishing operations all exert control over behavior. Accordingly, the behavioral perspective is likely to see the aggression as being under the multiple influences of these behavioral determinants. Also, the laws and principles of behavior apply to the shaping and maintenance of aggressive and antisocial behavior just as they do to virtually any other behavior in the human repertoire. However, to understand the development of aggressive behavior from a functional analytic perspective, reducing labels and diminishing the possibility of other "emotional" causes is necessary for accurate identification of the maintaining variables.

A failure to conform to social norms, repeated lying, defiance, property destruction, abuse of animals, deceitfulness, bullying, physical aggressiveness, irritability, lack of remorse, and irresponsibility are all descriptors used in the explanation for aggressive, angry, or antisocial children—they are, in a loose sense, a response class. Most if not all of these descriptors can be broken down and operationally defined. If we are able to operationalize and quantify the occurrence of behavior, a functional explanation of the behavior is more likely. Nevertheless, when confronted by the behavior of the adolescents involved in the Columbine shooting, there is a strong tendency to employ diagnostic categories or psychiatric labels to classify their behavior. Psychiatric labels are simply a manifestation of classes of behavior that allow psychiatrists and psychologists to better communicate and allow for greater ease in understanding the condition of their patient. An argument may arise when the assignment of a label becomes the cause of the behavior. For example, some may suggest the students at Columbine committed such awful acts of inhumanity due to their CD or antisocial personality. Although the use of these diagnostic labels are helpful in understanding patterns of behavior exhibited by the assailants, it does little to functionally describe environmental forces that may ultimately have shaped their behavior over the course of years. Another example would suggest that a child does not listen to authority because he/she has ODD. While defiance to authority is what the child does, it does not functionally explain the maintaining variables of defiance, such as not being effectively reinforced for compliance. DSM-IV-TR (American Psychiatric Association, 2000) provides descriptions and criteria for the diagnosis of disorders, not necessarily the explanation of their causes or functions. For treatment to be effective, understanding the maintaining variables of the aggression is imperative. If the environmental contingencies that reinforce and maintain the use of aggressive behavior of a child are not discovered, studied, and modified, the maintenance of aggressive behavior is likely to continue or even increase. (Roberts, 2004).

Aggression is more likely to occur if the effect of the behavior produces or improves conditions for the aggressor. Conversely, if aggression produces worsening conditions, namely, it is met with a punishing contingency, the future likelihood of similar aggression is less probable. Take, for example, the "antisocial" aggressive child who uses stealing as a means to obtain a desired snack food by surreptitiously taking the snack of another child. If the child is not caught and provided with a punishing consequence, then the entire response chain is likely to be repeated in the future under similar conditions. So, it can be explained that in the case of stealing snack food, for example, the aggressive or antisocial label is not the reason for the occurrence of the behavior; rather it is the function of past contingencies that maintain the future occurrences of stealing. As children grow and learn the contingencies of their environment, especially those that are most useful, they become more likely to repeat sequences of behavior that helped them obtain, avoid, or escape particular negative events. A child's language is also shaped by the same operant principles used to consequate their repertoire of nonverbal behavior. The use of threats, swear words, and aggressive or angry tones of voice, as well as the complex combination of word pairs, are learned patterns of verbal behavior which ultimately influence patterns of thought. The frequency, manner, and venue in which a child learns to use language as a behavior class that controls the environment often becomes far more efficient than punching, kicking, or other aggressive body responses—usually because it consumes less energy. Skinner (1957) was the first to describe a functional analysis of how language, or what he called verbal behavior, developed. Skinner (1957) also applied the basic behavioral principles to conversation and explained how verbal behavior influences the environment through the speaker–listener relationship. Again, it is not coincidental that adults with aggressive patterns of behavior or who meet the diagnostic criteria for antisocial personality disorder often have children who can meet the same criteria. Because language is learned in an environment usually consisting of various individuals with different styles of speaking and relating to others, like that of other behaviors, the opportunity for generalization of all types of aggressive behavior abound. For instance, if a child sees his father swear at and chastise his mother while he demands dinner, and if his mother complies with the hostile demands, then a simple but powerful three-term contingency learning trial has just occurred. The child, through observation and imitation of his father, may use the same words and tone toward his mother to get a desired response from her or others (e.g., teachers). Furthermore, if the child's mother does not correct this behavior and fulfills the demand in the absence of appropriate prosocial behavior, she could expect more of this behavior in the future. Likewise, if a child learns that screaming obscenities for 7½ minutes at a particular pitch will produce a desired change in his mother's behavior while at the grocery or toy store, and the mother does in fact change her behavior to quiet the child by providing the desired item—a candy bar, for example—then the child's behavior is reinforced and he is likely to emit the behavior again under the same stimulus conditions in the future. If the child has strong reinforcement histories for responding in an aggressive manner, and doing so continues to be functionally valuable, the principles of human behavior would dictate that he would continue to generate responses that are functionally and topographically similar to those of the past. Unless significant assessment of the environmental variables is performed and then interrupted while new alternative responses are taught concomitantly, the future probability of aggressive behavior is likely to become a certainty. For example, Lisa, age 10, would comment publicly on her female teacher's clothes, hair, or makeup (e.g., "That dress makes you look fat," "Your hair looks like your cat slept on it," or "That sweater is a yucky color"). Her teacher was reluctant to do or say anything, fearing further insults.

Jason, a 16-year-old boy, was a member of his high school basketball team. He had been ejected from a game because of a flagrant foul that resulted in a member of the other team being taken to a hospital with a possible concussion. Jason was told that he had to meet with a counselor before being allowed back on the team. The coach called the counselor before the meeting with Jason and tried to make the point that this was simply good basketball. That Jason was just doing what he (the coach) had trained them to do, which was to play hard and to win. Jason's description of the altercation was that Jason was dribbling the ball downcourt when the opposing team member planted himself in Jason's path. Rather than trying to pass or go around the opposition player, Jason increased his speed, lowered his shoulder, and collided with the other player. The other player was knocked over and hit his head. When Jason was asked what happened, he said that the opposing player was bigger and that he (the opposing player) had to learn to get out of Jason's way. "I'm shorter than most of these guys so I have to be more aggressive to keep them out of my way." It makes some sense to suggest that the bullying behavior learned in childhood is carried through into adulthood because it is functional. If it were not, it would have fallen out of our behavioral repertoire.

COGNITIVE PERSPECTIVE FOR TREATMENT

The clinician focuses on three main areas of cognition, which ultimately become the targets of intervention. These include (1) automatic thoughts, (2) schemata, and (3) cognitive distortions. Freeman, Pretzer, Fleming, and Simon, (2004) state: "Automatic thoughts, underlying assumptions, cognitive distortions and the impact of mood on cognition combine to set the stage for a self-perpetuating cycle ... " (p. 6). Howell (1998) illustrates specific treatment strategies for helping the individual with aggression function more effectively. Initially, assisting the client to understand the components of the problem in a psychoeducational process is helpful in beginning the course of therapy. The analysis of triggering events in the environment and the discussion of cognitive processes, as well as behavioral and physiological arousal, should be shared with clients to help establish and understand and the nature of their aggression. The modification of maladaptive schemata and cognitive attribution is another strategy indicated for the treatment of anger and aggression in higher-functioning adolescents. The identification of schemata for anger is explored with the client, and depending on level of functioning, the cognitive restructuring process is engaged. Howell (1998) provides the example of eye contact. That is, sustained eye contact from another does not indicate that the other child may have an aggressive intent, nor should it necessarily be interpreted as negative evaluation, criticism, and other related threats. Such automatic and dysfunctional thoughts are often at the root of how one feels and may ultimately energize an aggressive response. In addition, for the child who possesses the cognitive capacity, exploring the origins of angry schemata will be helpful. This will involve identifying early experiences that predispose the aggressive child to interpret the behavior of another as ridiculing, oppressive, or threatening.

Understanding a child's aggression, anger, or antisocial tendencies involves a discussion of the development of their core schemata. Schemata are an individual's habitual, unspoken, and unrecognized underlying assumptions about events they experience (Freeman et al., 2004). For example, each individual interprets the world quite differently; one's interpretation or experience of the events around him/her is characterized by particular schemata. Schemata for anxiety would include themes of threat, danger, or a fear of failure, while a schema for depression generally includes themes of loss, failure, or deprivation. A schema for anger includes themes of insult, humiliation, or violation of rules (Leahy, 2003, p. 256). Schemata are shaped and created from the various interactions with out parents, siblings, friends, culture, or religion.

The development of aggression and anger is fed by the schemata an individual has internalized throughout the course of his/her life. The schemata serve as a filter for expressive and receptive data. If, for example, the child has a schema that relates to the imminence of attack, the child will adaptively always be on guard. If this is a recognized pattern the child may be labeled "careful" (mild), "suspicious" (moderate), or "paranoid." If a concomitant schema is "When in danger, run like the wind," the child will avoid confrontation whenever possible. If, however, the concomitant schema is "Fight off any potential enemy with every fiber of your being," the child may use preemptive attacks to avoid a feared assault. The schema will then serve as the substrate for the automatic thoughts or cognitive distortions. Novaco and Welsh (1989) have identified a number of the cognitive variables of anger and aggression such as attribution error, false consensus, and anchoring effects. These are just some of the faulty biases that predispose people to episodes of anger and aggression. Furthermore, Beck et al. (2004) suggest that individuals with antisocial personality disorder (ASPD), an adult manifestation that frequently includes anger and aggression, need to develop skills in the areas of perspective taking, impulse control, effective communication, emotional regulation, frustration tolerance, assertiveness, consequential thinking, response delay, and cognitive restructuring (p. 177). In addition, Howell (1998) reports that individuals with anger and aggression appraise events or judge people as aversive, negligent, of or others intentionally committing acts of injustice against them. It is often this bias in assessment or appraisal that is a core focus of therapeutic intervention.

The cognitive therapy can be summarized in the following way: The child's more typical behavior is one of stimulus–response. That is, the child experiences a triggering event and quickly (and possibly thoughtlessly) responds. The goals of a successful set of cognitive interventions would result in the following sequence of behaviors:

Stimulus: The child encounters a stimulus.

Awareness: The child learns to be aware of the stimulus.

Recognition: The child recognizes his/her internal and external reactions to that stimulus.

Problem solving: The child uses problem-solving strategies to mediate between what he/she wants and the consequences of responding in an aggressive mode.

Decision making: The child chooses between alternatives.

Response: The more elements that the child can interpose between the stimulus and the response, the more successful the child will be in avoiding negative consequences (Spivack & Shure, 1977; Spivack, 1973; Shure, 1994, 2004).

TREATMENT FOCUS

There are several possible foci for treatment.

1. The child or adolescent may be seen alone for individual therapy. What must be taken into account is the child's motivation and ability to meet with an adult for rather lengthy periods of time (45–50 minutes) and to engage in a therapeutic alliance.

2. For most children and adolescents we recommend that the individual be seen for multiple half-sessions and the remaining half-session used for seeing the parents or the family. This reduces the stress on the child of being in such close proximity to an adult. It requires that the therapist set an agenda, structure the session, and make maximum use of available time.

3. The parents are seen alone. Many of the problems that are encountered with aggressive children have their origin in the interactions within the family of origin. Unless the aggressive style is monitored and modified at home, if contingencies are not maintained, or the child continues to be reinforced for aggressive behavior by parents and caretakers, little will change. The child and the parents can be seen for full but alternating sessions on a weekly basis.

4. Limited family therapy can be prescribed. The family members may be carefully chosen to include those that may best serve to support change. Psychotic family members (with limited control) may be briefly seen but may do more to disrupt family therapy than support it.

5. System therapy (extended). In this mode, all members of the family system are included, as is reasonable. For example, an older sibling that is away from home would not be required to be at each session.

6. Residential treatment for the entire family is possible, though unlikely due to the cost and availability of resources. A superb model for this mode is used at the Modem Bad Nervsanitorium in Vickersund, Norway. Under government funding, they bring families to their facility, and provide food and a residential setting and paid leave for the parents from their jobs for a month or more. Treatment includes individual therapy, child groups, parent groups, family therapy, family groups, and medication, as needed.

7. The use of intensive outpatient or day treatment options can serve to provide support for the child. This can include both day hospital or night hospital where the child goes to school but is removed from the home for the evenings and sleeps in a residence.

8. For children who have been adjudicated, placement in a secure and locked shelter may be used to remove the child from the general population. At an extreme, and depending on the age of the child, the placement may be in a prison.

9. For children who have severe and significant comorbid problem on Axis I, Axis II, or Axis III, inpatient treatment and pharmacotherapy in a hospital may be indicated.

10. Remove the child from the home because of abuse or imminent danger and place the child in a secure and appropriate foster home or residential setting.

ENVIRONMENTAL INTERVENTIONS

The identification and modification of both short- and long-term triggering events are a focus of therapy. Howell (1998) describes the importance of modifying the triggering stimuli more than the client's response to it. For instance, identifying stimuli that contribute to the aggressive behavior and avoiding the stimuli may be indicated for aggressive young children. Using stimulus control, the child is encouraged to avoid events or people who are likely to trigger anger, aggression, or conflict. Newman (2002) also reports the appropriateness of collaborating with the patient, the family, and the school to arrange the environment so it is less likely or even difficult to be a party to situations wherein the identified aggressive behaviors are more likely to be enacted.

The influence and modification of contextual stressors must be a focus of therapy. Howell (1998) suggests that the modification or reduction of stressors related to the aggressive behavior need to be addressed in therapy due to their potentially provocative role in aggressive responding. Family difficulties and classroom variables including class placement, selecting optimal teacher choices, program placement, particular seating arrangements, task difficulty, and task variation are contextual variables in need of possible modification to reduce the probability of an aggressive response. Although some contextual and ecological stressor cannot be reduced due to other controlling and unchangeable circumstances, such as living in violent and dangerous neighborhoods, the identification and avoidance of these variables is recommended and altered when possible.

CULTURAL, FAMILY, AND SOCIETAL INTERVENTIONS

The family interaction is an interactive system with numerous feedback and feedforward loops. These encompass affect, cognition, behavior, and the environmental stressors. The outcome of these influences is reflected in all the involved elements and initiates endless cycles of new mutual influences.

Traditionally, families have been viewed as being a major source of the child's difficulties. Families of aggressive children have been grouped as one of two types, the first being the overinvolved and "emeshed" family and the second being the underinvolved family. The systemic view is that the borderline child is viewed as manifesting the family's problems by reflecting the disorder and disorganization of the family, thereby adopting the "sick" role. The systemic therapist would thereby see the family system as the focus of the therapeutic work, believing that "Individual symptomology can best be understood and changed within the context of the systemic, repetitive interactions of the family group. Individual symptoms have a functional role for the family, so that a change in the individual is not possible without a concomitant change in the rest of the family and vice versa" (Clarkin, Frances, & Perry, 1986, p. 124).

Cognitive therapists advocate early contact with significant others (Beck, Rush, Shaw, & Emery, 1979; Bedrosian, 1981). Beck and colleagues believe that in the absence of any obvious contraindications, the significant others should be interviewed immediately after the initial interview with the child. Such an interview would yield data regarding the child's personal style, symptoms, and level of functioning; the reactions of those close to the patient; and the nature of their interactions with the patient. This information may help identify sources of distress and alert the therapist, family, and patient to the types of experiences or situations that might trigger impulsive behavior.

Meeting with significant others early in therapy identifies the therapist to the family and allows him/her to gain collateral information and to explain the treatment goals, rationale, and plan, including the role of homework. Early education about the nature of therapy and the nature of the child's problems helps dispel misinformation, erroneous beliefs, and distortions held by significant others. It also offers the therapist a window into the child's life and system. The involvement of the child's social or family network in the therapy involves balancing confidentiality with the need to inform, individual needs versus group expectations, and proximal versus distal goals of treatment. When working with children and adolescents, family involvement is essential. Shapiro (1982, p. 215, cited in Gunderson, 1984) summarizes the importance and benefits of family treatment in working with children and adolescents as follows:

1. Childhood and adolescence itself, and the shared family regression that is recapitulated during these stages, allows for a reworking of earlier conflicts.
2. The adolescent's continuing need for family support during this period.
3. The powerful effects of new experience with his parents on strengthening the adolescent's still flexible character structure.
4. The possibility of reintegration of projected and acted-out conflicts into a modification of parental functioning.

SIGNIFICANT OTHERS AS SOURCES OF DATA

The family members and other individuals who are significant and meaningful to the child (significant others, or SOs) can be important sources of information about the child's life, personal history, medical or psychiatric history, social or developmental history, and the family schema. They may have facts that are not available to the child (e.g., birth history and early childhood development), or they can offer different views of the situations and circumstances reported by the patient, which can provide the therapist with a more balanced view of the child's life. Family members can also offer feedback to the therapist about the therapy and its immediate and longer-term effects on the child.

Family members may deny the seriousness of the behavior and the need for any action, may oppose hospitalization, may punish the child for the behavior by criticizing or withdrawing from the child, or may label the child or other family members as the problem. It is therefore necessary to assess both the strengths and weaknesses of those individuals making up the child's social environment. Such assessment may help the therapist judge the risk of allowing the child to remain in the company of those significant others.

Significant others play a substantial role as the patient's social environment, responding to him/her in ways that support treatment gains. Significant others may assist in therapy to the point of acting as auxiliary therapists, helping the child to identify negative situations or negative cognitions and respond to them. Family and friends may assist the child in carrying out behavioral assignments. They may practice new skills with the patient such as conversational skills (e.g., giving and receiving criticism and issuing invitations) or skills in daily living (e.g., responding to siblings or adults). It is important that significant others provide accurate feedback. In an effort to be encouraging, friends and family may be oversolicitous and their comments may appear patronizing or ingenuous.

The SOs may assist the therapist by acting as change agents and assisting the child in making life changes. As they support positive change in the child's behavior, they may serve to keep the therapeutic changes in process outside the therapist's office. The family members can both generate and assist in the child's compliance with the therapeutic regimen by monitoring and assisting in doing homework, or in taking medication. Families can also identify warning signs of impulsive or aggressive behavior that a therapist may miss.

The SOs can also serve as potential saboteurs of treatment. Gunderson (1984) in discussing parental involvement in treatment of hospitalized adolescents states, "If a hospital does not involve them, they will become actively hostile to treatment. Efforts to exclude the family from involvement heightens the separation anxiety of the family and leads them to withhold support for the individual treatment" (p. 156). In addition, the SO who perceives the therapy or the patient–therapist relationship as threatening, exclusionary, or potentially harmful may work to withdraw the child from treatment, covertly encourage noncompliance, or reinforce or "enable" dysfunctional behaviors (e.g., substance abuse). We can summarize a number of reasons to include families (or SOs) in treatment, based in part on Bedrosian and Bozicas (1992).

1. Family systems can reorganize very quickly in response to a member's psychopathology. This rapid reorganization can have both positive and negative consequences in that it might serve to keep the identified patient (IP) in the same role or, more adaptively, help the IP to function better.

2. The family organization that accompanies individual psychopathology may not necessarily support increased adaptive behavior on the part of the parties involved. If the therapist can be aware of the subtle, and possibly well-meaning, sabotage, the therapist can point it out and work toward limiting the problem.

3. At times, dysfunctional family interactions can exacerbate the identified patient's symptoms, including his/her cognitive distortions. If the family shares the distortions (or schemata), they may work toward making things worse.

4. Symptom relief in the individual patient may increase stress, at least temporarily, on other family members. If the patient changes, and that change puts another family member into the spotlight of the family's dysfunctional system, that member might respond in dysfunctional ways.

5. Having SOs in therapy can allow for psychotherapeutic intervention to focus directly on family dysfunction.

6. The therapist can use a psychoeducational focus in therapy that is taught to all members (e.g., skills training, communication skills, and stress reduction techniques).

7. In situations in which the outcome of therapy is only limited (or no) change, families need to learn how to live with a chronically ill member.

8. "Splitting" between therapist and family, between family members, or between patient and family can be contained and dealt with in the context of the family sessions.

9. Noncompliance with the therapeutic regimen can be dealt with more rapidly when all members have received the same therapeutic message.

As trusted members of the community and authorities on religious teachings, clergy are often consulted by families. Freeman et al. (2004) points to the importance of the therapist understanding the family's religious schema as central to understanding the substrate that generates the impulsivity, aggressiveness, and destructive automatic thoughts. For example, one can easily find passages in scripture about turning the other cheek and also much about "smiting" offenders. For families that hold strong religious beliefs, clergy may have information that is useful to therapists in understanding the particular religious rules with which the child has grown up. The use of the child's SOs can provide the therapist with allies in dealing with the patient. These others can, ideally, provide information, decrease stress at home, and work as cotherapists. Conversely, in a dysfunctional family system, the therapist can offer direction for action and directive statements to help to alter the system.

The child's cultural group and subgroup may maintain schemata that encourage and support aggressive behavior. It must be ascertained as to what level the child and the family endorse these aggressive schemata.

THE USE OF ANGER MANAGEMENT INTERVENTIONS WITH AGGRESSIVE YOUTH

Based upon Novaco's (1977) early work with adults, Feindler and her colleagues (Feindler & Ecton, 1986; Feindler & Kalfus, 1990) developed an approach to treatment that would focus on the emotional arousal often preceding an aggressive outburst. This approach focuses on teaching the child to recognize the progressive increases in arousal, identify triggers for arousal, and develop cognitive and behavioral skills for arousal reduction with direct emphasis on the physiological and cognitive components of anger. The anger management protocols focus on three hypothesized components of the anger experience; physiological responses, cognitive processes, and behavioral responses (Novaco, 1977). The anger management treatment protocols focus on the three hypothesized components of the anger experience: physiological responses, cognitive processes and behavioral responses (Novaco, 1977).

The child is asked to learn to identify and track the most common triggers of his/ her anger by using a self-monitoring assessment called the Hassle Log (Feindler & Ecton, 1986). This involves keeping track and identifying daily occurrences of anger (whether handled well or not). This serves to help the youth to recognize his/her particular patterns of anger loss and control, and to increase awareness of external triggers and internal physiological and cognitive reactions. Finally, several arousal management skills such as deep breathing, imagery, and relaxation are taught to help the youth reduce the accumulated physical tension and to increase the probability that he/she will think through the interpersonal event in a more rational fashion.

The anger management skills were modeled and rehearsed during extensive role playing using scenarios generated from completed Hassle Logs. The role plays are arranged in a hierarchical fashion so that the child experiences graduated exposure to greater levels of provocation and conflict. These can then be matched to the child's skill attainment. Each treatment session included a variety of graded homework assignments designed to have the child practice newly acquired skills and to foster generalization to the natural environment.

Many of the cognitive restructuring strategies have been transformed into games to which participants in group treatment seem quite receptive. Clients are able to learn aspects of problem solving, to develop alternative perspectives, and to generate nonhostile attributions in response to hypothetical conflict situations. Role play with coaching then helps the youth to practice these improved cognitive responses to problem situations in which they themselves are provoked.

SUMMARY

Conceptualizing the aggressive child or adolescent by incorporating the biological, cognitive, and behavioral determinants is an integral step in formulating an appropriate and comprehensive treatment plan. Early identification of the variables that promote and maintain aggression in children is becoming far more important in today's schools, families, and peer groups. These include:

1. Biological factors, which includes the child's genetic makeup and constitutional factors (genotype).
2. Behavioral factors, which include learned factors and the expression of the genotype which could include sensation/excitement seeking, impulse control deficits, poor moral reasoning, problem-solving skill deficits, peer influence, maladaptive social skills, or substance use (phenotype).
3. Family factors, which include parental conflict, expressions of family and individual psychopathology; family substance use; failure to supervise the child; physical, verbal, sexual, or emotion abuse; and harsh, inappropriate, extreme or inconsistent discipline.
4. Cultural factors wherein aggression and direct expressions of anger and frustration are taught, expected, modeled, and reinforced (sociotype).

The various examples of the acts that aggressive children perpetrate seem to be more plentiful today than in years past. While some attribute this to a turbulent and ever-changing culture of angry youth, the problem seems to be worsening and the acts of violence appear to be escalating. The shooting incidents at Columbine High School, or the various "hazing" incidents seen on the nightly news are all indicators of aggressive youth who are in crisis. Understanding the environment pressures under which such aggressive children operate is often the first task in helping them choose more reasonable and prosocial responses. Although only a few of its strategies and recommendations are provided here, CBT provides the clinician with a compendium of tools and resources which may be invaluable in helping angry youth resolve their conflicts and develop more long-term, healthy responses to everyday stressors.

As aggression in children is seemingly becoming more prevalent in schools, families, and peer groups, the need to provide a comprehensive conceptualization which guides an age-appropriate comprehensive treatment plan is becoming increasing critical in the treatment community. With the popularity of aggressive video games demonstrating vulgar episodes of violence and strong themes of sex, as well the increasing popularity of the aggressive and antisocial "hip-hop" culture, the adolescent appetite for aggression, violence, and other antisocial behavior appears to be rapidly increasing. This chapter provided a review of the various dimensions related to the occurrence of childhood and adolescent aggression. A brief review of the evolutionary, cognitive, and temperamental perspective is provided. Importance is placed on identifying youth who are either in crisis or at risk for developing potentially violent behavior, as well as conceptualizing their unique circumstances to develop an effective and comprehensive plan of treatment.

The cognitive, behavioral, and family interventions are key components in a comprehensive treatment program. The use of individual and group work can be useful, with anger management being an important part of the program.

The cost to the individual, the community, and society is too great for us not to take a concentrated focus on treating aggressive and maladaptive children and adolescents.

REFERENCES

American Psychiatric Association. (2000). *Diagnostic and statistical manual of mental disorders* (4th ed., text rev.). Washington, DC: Author.

Aronson, E., Wilson, T. D., & Akert, R. M. (2005). *Social psychology.* (5th ed.). NJ: Pearson/ Prentice Hall.

Bandura, A., & Walters, R. H. (1963). *Social learning and personality development.* New York: Holt, Rinehart & Winston.

Beck, A., Freeman, A., Davis, D., & Associates. (2004). *Cognitive therapy of personality disorders* (2nd ed.). New York: Guilford Press.

Bedrosian, R. C., & Bozicas, G. D. (1994). *Treating family of origin problems: A cognitive approach.* New York: Guilford Press.

Cairns, R. B., & Cairns, B. D. (2000). The natural history and development functions of aggression. In A. J. Sammeroff, M. Lewis, & S. M. Miller (Eds.), *Handbook of developmental psychopathology* (2nd ed., pp. 403–429). New York: Plenum Press.

Clarizio, H. F., & McCoy, G. F. (1970). *Behavior disorders in school-age children.* Scranton, PA: Chandler.

Connor, D. F., Steingard, R. J., Cunningham, J. A., Anderson, J. J., & Melloni, R. H. (2004). Proactive and reactive aggression in referred children and adolescents. *American Journal of Orthopsychiatry, 74*(2), 129–136.

Dollard, J., Doob, J., Miller, N. E., Mowrer, O. H., & Sears, R. R. (1939). *Frustration and aggression.* New Haven, CT: Yale University Press.

Durand, V. M. (1990). *Severe behavior problems: A functional communication training approach.* New York: Guilford Press.

Feindler, E. L., & Ecton, R. B. (1986). *Adolescent anger control.* New York: Elsevier.

Feindler, E. L., & Kalfus, G. R. (Eds.). (1990). *Adolescent behavior therapy handbook.* New York: Springer.

Freeman, A., Pretzer, J., Fleming, B., & Simon, K. (2004). *Clinical applications of cognitive therapy* (2nd ed.). New York: Springer.

Gunderson, J. G. (1984). *Borderline personality disorder.* Washington, DC: American Psychiatric Press.

Henin, A., Warman, M., & Kendall, P. C. (2002). Cognitive behavioural therapy with children and adolescents. In G. Simos (Ed.), *Cognitive behavior therapy: A guide for the practicing clinician* (pp. 275–313). East Sussex, UK: Brunner-Routledge.

Howell, K. (1998). Cognitive behavioural interventions for anger, aggression, and violence. In

N. Tarrier, A. Wells, & G. Haddock (Eds.), *Treating complex cases: The cognitive behavioural therapy approach* (pp. 319–339). West Sussex, UK: Wiley.

Klein, S. B. (2000). *Biological psychology*. New Jersey: Pearson/Prentice Hall.

Leahy, R. L. (2003). *Cognitive therapy techniques: A practitioners guide*. New York: Guilford Press.

Miller, P. H. (2002). *Theories of developmental psychology* (4th ed.). New York: Worth.

Moyer, K. E. (1983). The physiology of motivation: Aggression as a model. In C. J. Scheier & A. M. Rogers (Eds.), *G. Stanley Hall lecture series* (Vol. 3). Washington, DC: American Psychological Association.

Newman, C. (2002). Cognitive therapy of bipolar disorder. In G. Simos (Ed.), *Cognitive behavior therapy: A guide for the practicing clinician* (pp. 71–96). East Sussex, UK: Brunner-Routledge.

Novaco, R. W. (1976). Treatment of chronic anger through cognitive and relaxation controls. *Journal of Consulting and Clinical Psychology, 44*(4), 681.

Novaco, R. W. (1977). Stress inoculation: A cognitive therapy for anger and its application to a case of depression. *Journal of Consulting and Clinical Psychology, 45*(4), 600.

Novaco, R. W., & Welsh, W. N. (1989). Anger disturbances: Cognitive mediation and clinical prescriptions. In K. Howells & C. R. Hollins (Eds.), *Clinical approaches to violence*. Chichester, UK: Wiley

Roberts, A. R. (Ed.). (2004). *Juvenile justice sourcebook: Past, present, and future*. New York: Oxford University Press.

Short, R., & Simeonson, F. T. (1986). Social cognition and aggression in delinquent adolescent males. *Adolescence, 66*, 361–366.

Shure, M. B. (1994). *Raising a thinking child*. New York: Pocket Books.

Shure, M. B. (2004). *Thinking parent, thinking child*. New York: McGraw-Hill.

Spivack, G. (1973). *Social adjustment of young children: A cognitive approach to solving real life problems*. San Francisco: Jossey-Bass.

Spivack, G., & Schure, M. B. (1977). *Problem solving approach to adjustment*. San Francisco: Jossey-Bass.

Skinner, B. F. (1957). *Verbal behavior*. Acton, MA: Copley.

Thomas, A., & Chess, S. (1977). *Temperament and development*. New York: Brunner/Mazel.

Webster-Stratton, C., & Herbert, M. (1994). *Troubled families-problem children: Working with parents, a collaborative process*. Chichester, UK: Wiley.

SUGGESTED READINGS

DiGiuseppe, R., & Tafrate, R. C. (2006). *Understanding anger disorders*. New York: Oxford University Press.

Feindler, E. L. (Ed.). (2006). *Anger-related disorders: A practitioners guide to comparative treatments*. New York: Springer.

Shure, M. B. (1994). *Raising a thinking child*. New York: Pocket Books.

Shure, M. B. (2004). *Thinking parent, thinking child*. New York: McGraw-Hill.

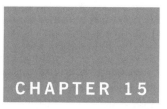

CHAPTER 15

Crisis with Older Adults

Helen M. DeVries
Suzann M. Ogland-Hand

Practitioners face an increasing likelihood of having older adults among their client population, unless they limit their practice solely to children and adolescents. Demographic data tell us that the age 65 and older population will increase at more than triple the rate of the general population during the next few decades. The age 85 and older population will grow even faster during that time period (King, 2005). Few clinicians, however, are prepared by their academic or clinical training to assess and treat this unique population. In fact, it has been estimated that, although almost 70% of psychologists have treated older adults in their practice, fewer than 30% had graduate coursework in geropsychology and fewer than 20% had supervised clinical experiences with this population (Qualls, Segal, Norman, Nierdehe, & Gallagher-Thompson, 2002). Clinicians should have a basic framework for understanding aging and older adults to guide assessment and intervention with this population.

FRAMEWORK FOR UNDERSTANDING AGING AND OLDER ADULTS

Older adults are a diverse population. They experience the same broad array of psychological issues and disorders that affect younger adults. However, differences in education, health status, economic status, and life experiences are often greater in older clients than in younger clients. Gerontologists often break old age into four categories: pre-old (ages 55–65), the "young old" (ages 65–75), the "old" (75–85), and the "oldest old" (age 85+). Current generations of the "young old" and the aging baby-boomer population are healthier and better educated than past cohorts. They are entering old age with more resources and different expectations than those in earlier cohorts. However, the current cohort of older adults, especially those over 70, generally have had little experience with psychotherapy and consequently may be reluctant to seek out psychological services when faced with emotional distress. This failure to access services at an early stage of crisis often means that older adult clients may be quite overwhelmed by the time they present for treatment.

While the majority of older adults do manage to face problems and overcome them effectively, others may need help facing the challenges of aging. Several researchers have noted the increase in stressful life events associated with the process of aging, including biological, psychological, and social factors (Duffy & Iscoe, 1990; Kasl-Godley, Gatz, & Fiske, 1998; Karel, 1997). As the number and frequency of these stressors pile up, the older adult becomes increasingly at risk for psychological crisis. Taxonomies for categorizing life stressors have noted four types of stressful life events: (1) *biological factors* (e.g., physical and sensory disabilities, illness), (2) *physical and environmental factors* (e.g., retirement, loss of income, changes in housing or living conditions), (3) *psychological factors* (e.g., changes in cognitive ability, loss and bereavement), and (4) *social/cultural factors* (e.g., changes in role or expected behavior) (Reese & Smyer, 1983; Nordhus, VandenBos, Berg, & Fromholt, 1998). These stressors may frequently occur simultaneously or in close succession, thus complicating efforts to cope.

Although stressful life events often act as precipitating forces in "crisis" situations, it is the individual's subjective experience of that stress that signals whether a crisis exists. Duffy and Iscoe (1990) argue that crisis experience is related to the way in which life stressors or events are perceived by the individual. Drawing on Seligman's "learned helplessness" model, they define crisis as "the subjective experience of loss of control, helplessness, and perceived inability to cope" (p. 304). Therefore, although many older adults encounter increasing life stressors (death of a spouse, mandatory retirement, etc.), only those who perceive these events as threats or as events beyond their coping abilities will go into crisis. This definition of crisis (the subjective experience of feeling out of control) provides a framework for understanding individual differences in responding to stressful situations and identifying those in crisis.

Psychological crisis, therefore, is not the inevitable outcome of the multiple stressors associated with aging. Rather, the interaction between stressful events and the person's perception of those events predicts outcome. When an individual makes the appraisal that the stressors exceed the resources needed to cope, a crisis situation exists. For each individual, the threshold is different. Yet, when that threshold is crossed, the individual experiences psychological crisis.

Despite the multiple stressors and risk factors confronting older adults, most do adapt and do not exhibit psychiatric symptoms. "Normal" aging is not characterized by pathological reactions or hopelessness and despair. However, coping is a process that must take place over time. Assessing where an individual is in the coping process and identifying those who have exceeded their coping threshold are essential. Differentiating normal patterns of reaction to stressful events from pathological reactions is critical in anticipating and intervening in crisis situations. Of particular importance is the need to identify older adults who are at risk for suicide, the most devastating extreme of psychological crisis.

RISK FOR SUICIDE

Epidemiological evidence indicates that older adults are among the highest-risk groups for suicide and that the ratio of suicide attempts to deaths is almost five times higher for older adults than for the general population (Heisel & Duberstein, 2005). Complicating the identification of suicide risk among the elderly is the finding that older adults are more likely to engage in determined and planned self-destructive acts and to give fewer warnings of suicidal intent (Conwell et al., 1998). Rather than seeking psychological services, suicidal older adults are more likely to consult a primary care physician, who may not be trained to assess suicide risk (Liptzin, 1991). In addition, a growing concern exists about frequently undetected "silent" suicides among older adults who determine to die through self-starvation or noncompliance with essential medical treatment (Simon, 1989).

Age alone, however, is not a sufficient predictor of suicide in late life. Like other forms of psychological crisis, suicide is the consequence of multiple and interacting stressors that exceed the individual's perceived ability to cope. Mood disorders, especially depression, are frequently noted as the principal risk factor for suicide (Blazer, Bachor, & Manton, 1986; Heisel & Duberstein, 2005; Lindesay, 1991; Losee, Parham, Auerbach, & Teitelman, 1988; Richardson, Lowenstein, & Weissberg, 1989). Other commonly identified risk factors include social isolation, losses and physical illness, suicidal ideation or a past history of suicide attempts, psychiatric illness, and access to lethal means (Conwell, 1997; Heisel & Duberstein, 2005). In addition, Blazer (1991) identified seven demographic factors that interact with age to increase risk for suicide: sex, race, marital status, economic status, mental illness, suicide attempts, and biochemical factors. For example, white males who live alone and are recently widowed are at higher risk for suicide than the general population of older adults. As another example, males commit suicide at a significantly higher rate than do females. Thus, the apparent relationship between suicide and age is due almost entirely to the association between suicide and elderly males (Blazer, 1991). Awareness of psychosocial and demographic risk factors that interact with age to increase the possibility of suicidal behavior in an older adult population is a beginning step toward effective assessment and intervention.

FOCUS FOR THE CHAPTER

This chapter focuses on two main components of crisis work with older adults: assessment and cognitive-behavioral therapy (CBT) intervention. The goal is to enable the reader to evaluate whether an older adult is at risk or experiencing a psychological crisis, to provide information and identify measures useful in assessing psychological crisis in this population, to describe cognitive-behavioral strategies for intervening with this group, and to provide case studies illustrating these themes.

ASSESSMENT

Diagnosing psychological crisis in the elderly is difficult. Because of older adults' unfamiliarity not only with seeking psychiatric or psychological services but also with typical psychiatric vocabulary, they present problems in different ways compared with younger adults with similar issues as they enter into mental health settings. In the current cohort of elders, somatic distress is the most common presenting problem and indicator of psychological distress. For example, an 85-year-old woman may be referred to a psychologist's office for evaluation by her physician, and at the first session with the psychologist she may say, "I don't know why I'm here. My doctor told me to see you, which doesn't make sense to me, because my stomach is really my problem." Typically, the older patient has greater comfort and familiarity with seeking treatment for a medical condition than for emotional distress. Alternatively, many older adults prefer to turn to the clergy for help when they experience personal problems (Weaver & Koenig, 1996). Thus, both physicians and clergy need to be sensitive to the possibility of psychological illness. Psychologists working with elders are encouraged to develop relationships with and to educate primary-care physicians and clergy about how and when to refer for mental health services.

Eliciting information regarding stressful life events and the patient's perception of those events is a necessary part of the assessment of psychological well-being. Because feelings of loss of control and inability to cope often trigger catastrophic or crisis reactions, recognizing situations that would increase the risk for these reactions is essential. As older adults face the multiple stressors associated with aging, some will cross the coping threshold and experience psychological crisis. In particular, older adults who present with the following complaints or situations may be at high risk for experiencing psychological crises: depression, complicated bereavement, alcohol or drug abuse, cognitive impairment, chronic or serious illness, and changes in family roles/dynamics or living arrangements. Examination of these multiple domains is critical to the effective assessment of risk for psychological crisis in the elderly.

Depression

The relationship between depression and psychological crisis is particularly strong among the elderly, for whom depression is the most frequently noted functional (nonorganic) mental disorder (Koenig & Blazer, 1992; Losee et al., 1988). Although most older adults acknowledge some depressive symptoms, the majority are not clinically depressed (Gallagher & Thompson, 1983). Research indicates that more women than men are diagnosed with a depressive disorder in early adulthood and old age, whereas more males are severely depressed in late mid-life (ages 55–64) (Leaf et al., 1988). A major depressive episode that occurs for the first time in patients age 60 or older is referred to as late-onset depression. There is some controversy in the literature about whether a first-time episode of major depression in late life might be an early symptom of a dementia process. In addition, it is often difficult to differentiate late-onset depression from a physical or medical condition. For example, depression has been linked to a variety of chronic medical problems, such as endocrine disorders, cancer, and cardiovascular disease (Delano-Wood & Abeles, 2005). Koenig and Blazer (1992), however, suggest that late-onset depression can be associated with situational as well as illness-related biological factors. Distinguishing between biological (e.g., medical condition and dementia process) versus situational factors contributing to depression in older adults clearly has significant treatment implications.

Although many of the symptoms of depression reported by older clients are similar to those found in other age groups, several differences have been noted. As previously mentioned, older adults are more likely to report somatic rather than psychological symptoms and to seek medical services rather than psychiatric services for treatment of depression. In addition, older adults more frequently evidence symptoms of apathy and agitation, as well as increased problems with concentration and memory, and report lower prevalence of dysphoria and ideational symptoms, such as guilt or suicidal ideation (Kasl-Godley, Gatz, & Fiske, 1998; Koenig & Blazer, 1992). Cavanaugh (1990) reports that depressed older adults are more likely to withdraw, confine themselves to bed, and neglect bodily functions than are younger adults.

Standard self-report measures are frequently used as tools to assess symptoms of depression, although accurate diagnoses cannot be made without a thorough clinical interview. Most commonly used are the Beck Depression Inventory (BDI; Beck, Ward, Mendelson, Mock, & Erbaugh, 1961) and the Center for Epidemiological Studies Depression Scale (CES-D; Radloff, 1977). Caution should be exercised in interpreting results, however, as these scales are weighted heavily with physical symptoms that are not always reliable indicators of depression in an older population. The Geriatric Depression Scale (GDS; Yesavage et al., 1983) attempts to remedy this difficulty by focusing primarily on the psychosocial aspects of depression. In general, the BDI is recommended for adults who have at least an eighth-grade reading level who present with psychiatric difficulties, while the GDS is more widely used with less educated elders or medically ill and/or cognitively impaired elders age 55 and older.

Complicated Bereavement

Multiple losses, especially including the loss of a spouse, associated with aging appear to put older adults at greater risk for psychological crisis. Epidemiological data indicate that married people have the lowest suicide rate, while the divorced and widowed have the highest (Blazer, 1991). Studies of bereavement in older spouses have found that most cope well with loss but that the affective and cognitive effects of bereavement may continue for at least 2 to 7 years after the loss (Thompson, Gallagher-Thompson, Futterman, & Peterson, 1991; Lund, 1989). While acknowledging the highly stressful nature of spousal bereavement, Lund (1998) argues that "older adults are quite resilient and find ways to manage the many losses that they experience throughout their lives" (p. 108).

Nevertheless, some older adults lack the resources (external or internal) to effectively weather the bereavement process. The most intense psychological impact appears to occur within the first several months, with gradual improvement over time (Thompson, Gallagher, Cover, Gilewski, & Peterson, 1989). Most at risk for psychological crisis are those who continue to experience high levels of psychological distress 1 to 2 years after the death of their spouse (Thompson, Gallagher-Thompson, et al., 1991). Variables that have been found to correlate with poor adjustment to loss and risk for psychological crisis include low levels of internal resources, such as independence, self-efficacy, and self-esteem (Lund, 1989). Also, older bereaved persons who remain significantly depressed following their spouse's death are particularly vulnerable to other kinds of symptoms (Gilewski, Farberow, Gallagher-Thompson, & Thompson, 1991).

Identifying those who are not adapting or coping adequately with loss is critical to effective crisis assessment. The Inventory of Complicated Grief (ICG) developed by Prigerson et al. (1995) has been shown to be effective in detecting complicated grief in elderly widows and widowers. Research by Breckenridge, Gallagher, Thompson, and Peterson (1986) compared BDI profiles of older bereaved persons with those who were sociodemographically comparable but had not lost a spouse within 5 years of the evaluation. They found that certain symptoms reliably distinguished the two groups, such as frequency of crying, dissatisfaction with self, and various somatic disturbances. Other symptoms, such as guilt and a sense of failure as a person, were uncommon in the normal bereaved group and were, in fact, more typically associated with a significant depressive disorder that warranted treatment in its own right.

Alcohol or Drug Abuse

Older adults are at high risk for deliberate or accidental misuse of drugs or alcohol for many reasons: the high rate of prescribed medication use, increased physiological sensitivity to drug effects, and the danger of interaction effects of multiple medications and/or alcohol. In addition, the use of alcohol to help cope with stressful life events increases the risk of addiction and/or toxic interactions. Data indicate that about 10% of older adults have a notable substance abuse problem (Kemp, Brummel-Smith, & Ramsdell, 1990), although good epidemiological data are hard to find and estimates vary widely across studies. Regardless of age, more men than women (approximately 12 to 1) are diagnosed with a substance abuse problem (Hopson-Walker, 1990). In later life, data indicate that elderly widowers have the highest rate of alcoholism of any group (Freund, 1984).

Detection of alcohol abuse can be difficult. Factors such as the isolation of the older adult, absence of social or work schedules and demands, and the tendency of the older adult to drink at home rather than in public all conspire to mask the problem (Solomon, Manepalli, Ireland, & Mahon, 1993). With the exception of alcohol, substance abuse in older adults involves a different set of substances than those abused by younger adults (Atkinson, Ganzini, & Bernstein, 1992). Specifically, older adults are less likely to use illicit drugs but rather to be at risk for abuse of prescribed or over-the-counter medications. The danger, of course, is that alcohol and/or drug abuse will increase the possibility for depression, illness (including risk for falls and accidents), and cognitive impairment. LeSage and Zwygart-Stauffacher (1988) emphasize that all health care providers should be knowledgeable about common adverse reactions to drugs frequently used by the elderly. To assess the potential for substance abuse in the elderly, at a minimum, the professional must explore the following factors: whether medication use is being coordinated and monitored by a primary physician for interaction effects, whether the older adult is able to manage the administration of multiple medications, and whether alcohol abuse exists. Because alcohol is metabolized differently in the older person, smaller amounts may cause problems. (See Lamy, 1988; Shimp & Ascione, 1988, for fuller discussion of this issue.)

The Michigan Alcoholism Screening Test—Geriatric Version (MAST-G; Blow et al., 1992) was developed as an elderly-specific measure of alcohol abuse and may be useful in evaluating whether a client has a substance abuse problem. Many elderly patients, however, are reluctant or even completely unwilling to be evaluated, and their refusal and/or denial can prevent important information from coming to light. Solomon et al. (1993) recommend honesty and directness in questioning both the patient and others involved in the patient's care, along with careful history taking and a urinary drug screen for all new patients. They believe that even with these measures, some patients may not be able to be adequately evaluated for substance abuse problems.

Cognitive Impairment

Cognitive impairment is not an automatic consequence of "normal" aging. Research has demonstrated that cognitive functions, such as intelligence and memory, remain relatively stable across adulthood, with only selective normative changes with age. When significant cognitive impairments are noted, they are usually the result of a dementing illness, cerebrovascular accident, physical illness, toxic reaction to medication, or depression. Approximately 15% of people over age 65 have some type of dementia (Davies, 1988). Fortunately, many of the conditions leading to cognitive impairment are treatable if they are properly diagnosed. Thus it is important to briefly use a standardized screen with norms when evaluating an elder in a crisis situation (e.g., MMSE, 3MS, or COGNISTAT).

Often, however, older adults experiencing a problem with memory or cognitive functioning assume that the problem is irreversible and become depressed, anxious, frightened, or hopeless about the future. The fear of dementia may prevent their seeking appropriate diagnosis and treatment. A medical exam (to rule out possible underlying illness), neuropsychological testing, functional assessment, and psychosocial history are all useful for establishing a diagnosis of dementia. Appropriate assessment provides information for identifying possible causes for noted impairments, planning intervention strategies, and addressing psychological distress. An additional concern is that dementia and depression can coexist. Undiagnosed and untreated depression in persons with dementia will likely increase their risk for mortality, as well as for behavioral and functional problems (Teri, McKenzie, & LaFazia, 2005).

Comprehensive reviews of the specifics of such assessments have been published in recent years. Three that contain good reviews of measures and information regarding age-appropriate norms include (1) a chapter on neuropsychological assessment of the elderly (Crawford, Venneri, & O'Carroll, 1998), (2) a review of norms for the Mini-Mental State Examination (MMSE) adjusted for age and education (Crum, Anthony, Bassett, & Folstein, 1993), and (3) a special issue of *International Psychogeriatrics* (Miller & Lipowski, 1991), which focuses on assessment of delirium in its various forms and provides excellent information about measures that can be used to assist clinicians in making a differential diagnosis between delirium (which is treatable) and the dementias (which are not). In addition, the clinician should be sensitive to the need for norms appropriate for special populations (e.g., based on such things as education, ethnicity, and health) when evaluating the cognitive status of an older adult (Espino, Lichtenstein, Palmer, & Hazuda, 2001; Fields, Fulop, Sachs, Strain, & Fillit, 1992; Strickland, Longobardi, Alperson, & Andre, 2005). If the outcome of the assessment indicates that some type of dementia, such as Alzheimer's disease, is likely, this can potentially create a crisis for the patient or the family (family crisis is discussed later in this chapter).

Chronic Illness

Approximately 80–85% of the present older adult cohort have some type of chronic illness, such as arthritis, diabetes, hypertension, respiratory problems, and cardiac problems for which there are no cures and that cause at least mild levels of disability (Cavanaugh, 1990; Knight, 2004). For example, epidemiological data indicate that approximately 85% of persons ages 75–79 have osteoarthritis, 59% of persons in their 70s or 80s have chronic obstructive pulmonary disease (COPD), 32% of those over age 75 have some form of heart disease, and 39% of those over the age of 65 have hypertension (Cavanaugh, 1990; Mongan, 1990; Ries, 1990).

Often, the consequence of chronic illness for the person means permanent changes in lifestyle to accommodate restrictive medical schedules and regimens. In addition, many must endure chronic pain and adjust to physical limitations. Data suggest that by age 85, 60% of the population has at least some degree of disability that requires regular, ongoing assistance (Zarit, Davey, Edwards, Femia, & Jarrott, 1998).

The demands imposed by chronic illness or disability are stressful and may strain coping resources and challenge the person's sense of self-worth or control. Assessing the individual's beliefs about changes in body image, competence, and sense of self is critical in identifying those at risk for psychological crisis.

Data suggest that among physically ill older adults, suicidal thoughts are more closely associated with depression than with the illness per se (Lindesay, 1991).

Relatedly, those who hold negative beliefs about themselves and their ability to cope with their illness are likely to develop symptoms of depression. It is these persons who are at greatest risk for psychological crisis. For example, an elder who believes she is "stupid" and attributes difficulties to her lack of ability, when she experiences normal physical problems of aging such as osteoarthritis, may incorrectly attribute her joint pain to her perceived "stupidity," which would significantly contribute to her subsequent depression.

Another risk facing older adults with a chronic illness is the risk for *excess disability*. This term refers to the added impact of a psychological disorder (such as depression or anxiety) which exacerbates the limitations imposed by the medical condition itself. For example, a person with cataracts may become too depressed to seek alternate ways to enjoy reading, such as books on tape or large-print editions (Knight, 2004). Assessment of psychological crisis in the elderly must not ignore the impact of chronic illness on the individual's mental health and coping resources.

Changes in Family Roles/Dynamics or Living Arrangements

Normative changes in family structure occur as the family moves through developmental stages (i.e., no children, preschool children, school-age children, adolescents, launching, and postparental phases). Although much attention has been directed toward the impact of early family transitions, less has been directed toward understanding the dynamics of late-life families. In particular, older adults and their adult children face multiple shifts in relationships that require adjustments to new roles and responsibilities.

Retirement, loss of a spouse, geographic distance from adult children, or physical illness of an elderly parent exemplify ways in which family roles and dynamics may be challenged or require restructuring. While data suggest that many older adults prefer to maintain independence from their children (Brody, Johnsen, Fulcomer, & Lang, 1983; Lee, 1985), financial constraints or a parent's physical frailty/illness may force dependence on adult children as caregivers. While most caregiving is provided by spouses, adult children usually serve as secondary caregivers, or if there is no surviving spouse, as primary caregivers. Pilisuk and Parks (1988) report that approximately 80% of elder care is provided by families, with fewer than 10% relying on formal support services. Females (daughters and daughters-in-law) assume the major share of responsibility for parental caregiving. Complicating this picture is the increase in divorce and remarriage rates that blur family lines and add complexity to the situation.

Intergenerational differences and conflicts are bound to emerge when elderly parents and adult children negotiate new roles and responsibilities. For example, elderly parents may become distraught if forced to become dependent on children or, conversely, if they perceive that their children are not willing or available to care for them (Loebel, Loebel, Dager, & Centerwall, 1991). So, too, adult children may experience depression, resentment, anger, guilt, or burden when confronted with caring for frail or needy parents.

Some of the stresses on the family may be unexpected, such as reappearance of sibling rivalries as adult children are forced to work together to make decisions about parent care. In fact, these types of conflict are often more difficult to manage than the actual parent care itself. In addition, long-term successful marriages can be thrown into chaos when one spouse becomes disabled due to illness or injury, thus disrupting set patterns of functioning. Due to the importance of family support for many elders, assessment of family functioning and dynamics is critical. Specific issues that should be explored include level of caregiver stress, meaning of role reversal to elder and to adult child, and the elder's fears regarding being a burden, "abandonment," and/or long-term care placement. High levels of distress regarding any of these issues put the elder and family at risk for crisis.

Due to the increased stress on families caring for an elderly relative, the clinician should always be careful to assess the risk for elder abuse. Elder abuse includes physical abuse, neglect, and chronic verbal aggression most commonly at the hands of a spouse, adult child, grandchild, or professional caregiver. It occurs at all economic levels and among all age groups in later adulthood. Abuse is much more likely to occur when the older person is experiencing physical, emotional, or cognitive problems (APA Working Group on the Older Adult, 1997). It is important for the mental health professional to question the cause of any physical injuries or bruises. Many states require reporting by health care, social service, or other professionals if abuse is suspected in the home.

COGNITIVE-BEHAVIORAL APPROACHES
TO CRISIS INTERVENTION WITH OLDER ADULTS

One of the most important and consistent findings of recent studies of the efficacy of psychotherapy is that psychotherapy is as effective with older adults as with younger adults in treating depression and other mental disorders (Engels & Vermey, 1997; Gallagher-Thompson, 1992; Gallagher-Thompson, Hanley-Peterson, & Thompson, 1990; Gallagher-Thompson & Thompson, 1996; Scogin & McElreath, 1994; Thompson, Gallagher, & Breckenridge, 1987). In addition, psychotherapy may be particularly helpful to older adults for whom medication is not appropriate or contraindicated because of health problems. Although psychotherapy can be helpful to this population, some modifications and adaptations may be necessary (see Zeiss & Steffen, 1996).

Multiple studies have documented the usefulness of CBT in working with older populations (Gatz et al., 1998; Scogin, Welsh, Hanson, Stump, & Coats, 2005; Teri, Curtis, Gallagher-Thompson, & Thompson, 1994; Thompson & Gallagher-Thompson, 1991. It is assumed that most readers will have familiarity with the basic theory and techniques of CBT. Good overviews of CBT approaches to treatment of older adults are available (DeVries, 2007; Gallagher-Thompson, Lovett, & Rose, 1991; Karel, Ogland-Hand, & Gatz, 2002; Laidlaw, Thompson, Dick-Siskin, & Gallagher-Thompson, 2003; Thompson, 1996; Thompson, Gantz, et al., 1991). The next section focuses on CBT intervention strategies that have been found effective with elders in crisis.

CBT with older adults typically begins with a brief socialization to treatment for the patient, with an emphasis on education about psychotherapy. This socialization is particularly important for older adults, as they typically have little experience with any kind of psychotherapy, and thus do not know what to expect or how to behave. For example, with an older client you might explain that the relationship with the therapist is like "a combination of talking with your primary care physician (to whom you might say, 'I've got this problem with my left knee') and talking with a close friend (where you tell them what you really think about things) . . . so here, we will talk about things that are bothering you, and things that are really important to you and maybe figure out together some different ways of handling situations." Furthermore, older clients might fear the stigma of psychological or psychiatric treatment, thinking that it means that they are "crazy." Here, a little reassurance is usually quite helpful (e.g., "I don't think you're crazy, I think you are just dealing with some difficult things").

When working with an elderly patient in a crisis situation, the socialization period must necessarily be shortened in order that treatment can begin as quickly as possible. Although brief, it should not be glossed over, because misunderstandings at the outset are very common and can impede the development of a therapeutic relationship and treatment.

CBT with an older adult generally consists of "early, middle, and late stages" using a 16- to 20-session model (see Thompson, 1996; Thompson, Gantz, et al., 1991). In crisis intervention work, the initial goal is to stabilize the patient. Therefore, therapy will proceed in a modified fashion. In consultation with other colleagues (most notably, the older adult patient's primary-care physician), a plan should be developed to assess the overall situation, to establish the various currently active diagnoses, and to provide limited cognitive-behavioral therapy until the immediate crisis has passed and further evaluation can be done. In most cases, the immediate crisis situation will be resolved within 1 to 2 weeks, and the patient frequently decides to continue CBT, along with other medical or psychiatric regimens. At that point, the more usual model of short-term CBT would then be followed.

In other instances (which are far less common) a referral needs to be made after the initial period of stabilization is completed. This can occur for several reasons, but most typically occurs when the individual's presenting complaints are so complex that an inpatient hospital stay (either medical or psychiatric) is really needed to sort out various contingencies. In very few instances it may be necessary to refer the patient for other forms of therapy, such as electroconvulsive therapy (ECT), but this may occur with intractably depressed psychotic elders who have a poor history of responding to other forms of treatment.

CASE STUDIES

The following examples illustrate some of the issues that trigger crisis in the older adult and provide assessment and treatment approaches that were useful in addressing the crisis situation. The first case addresses suicide risk and the second case addresses caregiving stress. Although these are only two examples of the kinds of crises that bring older adults in for treatment, they provide a framework for the two tasks of crisis intervention: stabilizing the immediate crisis and providing follow-up support and skills training for more adaptive future functioning.

Case 1: Suicide Risk

Mr. Richard Adams is a 72-year-old widowed European American male whose wife, Nellie, died of heart disease about a year ago. While Nellie had hypertension for years, she had developed congestive heart failure only a few months before her death. Mr. Adams was not psychologically prepared for her death, nor did he feel that he could make the necessary adjustments to live alone after being married for the past 51 years. He had little experience with household management tasks such as cooking and cleaning and was not used to setting up the social calendar. Nellie had done these things, and now that she was gone, his life seemed quite empty and meaningless. He had two grown daughters and their families in town, and he enjoyed their company, but he did not feel that it was appropriate to turn to them often in his time of grief. Instead, he waited for them to visit him and to talk about their absent mother. Only then did he respond in kind. Even then, he found it almost impossible to cry or to be demonstrative with any of his feelings regarding the loss of his wife; it just did not feel like the right thing for a man to do.

Then, 3 months ago, he was diagnosed with Parkinson's disease. As a retired English professor at the local college, he knew two colleagues who developed dementia from Parkinson's disease after having the illness for a number of years. He knew that dementia was not inevitable, but he was frightened of the possibility. He believed that having dementia would make him totally dependent on his daughters, a thought he found intolerable. About 1 month before coming for evaluation with a psychologist at the older adult clinic, Mr. Adams was forced to move out of his home of more than 30 years due to the demolition of the building for new freeway construction. He had moved to a small apartment near his oldest daughter's home. He described this move as the "the last straw." All the changes in his life circumstances left him feeling depressed and hopeless about the future. He had difficulty imaging how to live in the small apartment he was in and had no idea how to build a life without his wife, which his daughters kept pushing him to do. His declining health, although it was not precipitous, made him wary of the future. He thought about using alcohol to block out some of his painful feelings and although he knew that was not going to solve his problems, he was "at his wits' end." By the time his oldest daughter brought him for therapy, Mr. Adams was talking about "ending it all" and seemed to be taking steps to put his affairs in order, as if he were planning to commit suicide in the relatively near future.

The assessment process revealed a BDI score in the "severe" range (score: 25/30), an MMSE score of 29/30 (within the normal range of cognitive functioning for his age and education), a diagnosis of major depressive disorder with questionable alcohol abuse, and a man with few emotional and social resources at the time of the evaluation. He had very negative ideas about his ability to live on his own and about what life held for him. He could not seem to visualize a more positive life for himself in the future, and he was able to acknowledge that he had developed a concrete plan for committing suicide. He kept a gun in the apartment and was a Korean Conflict veteran so he knew how to use the weapon. He felt that the only deterrent to ending his life was the shame that this would bring on his daughters, and if it were not for them, he would commit suicide without hesitation.

Following this assessment, Mr. Adams's primary-care physician was contacted, and she and the psychologist convinced Mr. Adams to agree to a voluntary psychiatric hospitalization. During his 10-day stay on the geropsychiatry unit at the city hospital, he was treated with CBT by the consulting psychologist and was given antidepressant medications by his psychiatrist. The low dosage of Lexapro would not be helpful immediately, but it would likely be beneficial in the long run. He also received milieu therapy and participated in group therapy nearly every day of his inpatient stay.

Some of Mr. Adams's cognitive distortions were similar to those of other inpatients with suicidal ideation, including the belief that suicide would bring an end to his suffering. He saw suicide as a respite or a solution to his problems rather than as an untenable way to deal with his life. For Mr. Adams, as well as for many other widowers and widows (see Worden, 2002), suicide may represent a way to be reunited with the deceased loved one. This belief became apparent after several sessions, when Mr. Adams's intense loneliness and sadness were more apparent. Mr. Adams kept daily thought records so that he and his psychologist could become more aware of his dysfunctional thoughts. He was trained to identify negative automatic thoughts and began to learn how to challenge them. Specifically, the thought record helped to point out that he was not as alone as he thought, as his daughters were very supportive, and that he did not have dementia, only the fear that someday he would develop it. He read information about Parkinson's disease so that he could see for himself that dementia was not an inevitable consequence of the disease.

Mr. Adams also worked very hard to overcome his belief "I can't go on anymore." By challenging his all-or-nothing thinking, he realized that even though he felt overwhelmed, some positive things were going on in his life. For example, he acknowledged that his former home was actually quite large and difficult to maintain, and that while his wife had enjoyed the yardwork, he did not. Moving into a smaller apartment did make the practical housekeeping chores easier for him. He also disclosed that he had previously played golf and had several male friends with whom he had lunch on a fairly regular basis. He was encouraged to contact these men again to let them know of his situation and to see what kind of support they would be willing to provide. This behavioral assignment resulted in a very surprising—to him—outpouring of support from his friends. This, in turn, helped to challenge the thought that suicide was the only solution to his current problems.

Finally, considerable time was spent examining the consequences of a suicidal action. He talked about the strong negative impact that it would have on his daughters and grandchildren and expressed that he would think of himself as "a quitter" if this really were the path he chose. Through some structured reminiscence work, he shared with the therapist many of his prior success experiences in life and began to realize that he had coped with previous difficult situations in a much more adaptive manner. Throughout the course of treatment, he was given a great deal of emotional support, as he clearly felt overwhelmed by the number of negative life circumstances to which he had to adjust.

Following his discharge from the inpatient unit, he was seen for outpatient therapy with the same cognitive-behavioral therapist, twice a week for 1 month, then weekly for approximately 6 months, then biweekly for 6 months, rather than the more typical 16 to 20 sessions, in order to be sure that he was reintegrated into the community. During his course of treatment, he had a total of 40 sessions of individual therapy, with the final 15 being spread out at more than weekly intervals so that he had ample opportunity to practice becoming reengaged with his friends and his social activities. In fact, over the course of treatment, the emphasis shifted from the more cognitive approach to a more behavioral approach, with grief work, gradual reengagement in pleasant activities, and development of friendships. He continued to be seen periodically by his psychiatrist during that time and remained on a low dose of Lexapro. Follow-up 2 years posttreatment indicated that he continued to maintain himself well in his new apartment, and that his health had declined somewhat but not in a major way. At the last follow-up contact 2½ years ago, Mr. Adams was glad to be alive and had found new purpose in life. He said that he was ready to live out the remainder of his days and to die when his creator called him.

Case 2: Family Caregiving Crisis

Sue Benden is a 67-year-old married woman of Latino ethnicity who is the primary caregiver for her 93-year-old mother, Edna Sanchez. Edna is physically frail yet cognitively alert and has lived with Sue and Sue's husband for the past 6 years. Although Mrs. Benden has two older brothers, both live in other states and are not involved in the caretaking responsibilities. Mrs. Benden was referred to the older adult clinic by her priest who was concerned about her significant anger and frustration regarding the care for her mother.

On intake, Mrs. Benden's presenting complaint was feeling overwhelmed with the relentless demands of caregiving and unable to cope any longer. In particular, she voiced frustration that she and her husband were unable to enjoy the type of retirement they had anticipated due to her caregiving responsibilities. She also felt guilty because she knew her duty as a daughter was to care for her mother, especially because her father had died so many years ago. She had not taken a vacation since her mother moved in with them because she could not leave her mother alone.

With prompting, Mrs. Benden voiced feeling hurt by her mother's critical remarks and lack of appreciation and described their interactions as negative and unpleasant. In fact, she had begun avoiding conversations with her mother and limiting interactions to necessary caregiving tasks due to her anger and resentment. She stated that she had "no personal life" and had given up many enjoyable activities as the demands of caregiving increased. She stated she had become a bitter, resentful, unhappy person.

The crisis occurred one day when she found herself becoming enraged while she was assisting her mother on the usual slow and tedious walk from the bedroom to the bathroom. She felt she needed help because such a small thing triggered such a powerful emotional reaction and left her feeling "out of control." She scored 98/100 on the 3MS (within normal range for her age and educational background), and 20/30 on the GDS, signifying moderate–severe depressive symptoms.

A critical component of the assessment process was to determine whether any indications of elder abuse existed, that is, whether her mother was being abused or at risk for abuse. Although Mrs. Benden acknowledged feeling "ready to burst" with frustration at many different times, she denied having acted on these feelings. She was worried she might scream or yell if the stress continued, and she acknowledged occasional thoughts of intentionally hurting her mother, which mortified her. Clearly, the prevention of inappropriate expressions of anger and frustration was an immediate treatment goal. In addition, Mrs. Benden would also benefit from acquiring coping skills that would help her manage the caregiving responsibilities with less resentment and frustration.

Treatment approaches included both cognitive and behavioral components. To help reduce the risk of elder abuse, Mrs. Benden was asked to maintain a record of the thoughts that accompanied the bursts of anger at her mother. Examination of her thought record indicated that most of the negative feelings were associated with thoughts regarding implied criticism from her mother. For example, over the years, Mrs. Sanchez had acquired several small rental properties, which Mrs. Benden was managing for her. When her mother would ask repeatedly whether tasks associated with the rental property had been taken care of, Mrs. Benden would tell herself, "She thinks I'm irresponsible" or "She's treating me like a child." Mrs. Benden learned to challenge these unhelpful thoughts and to generate more helpful ones (e.g., "Mother is feeling helpless and needs reassurance that everything is okay"). Once Mrs. Benden recognized the way her own thoughts were fueling her anger and resentment, she felt empowered to challenge other automatic thoughts and to develop more adaptive alternatives.

The second component of treatment was to help Mrs. Benden increase the pleasant activities in her life, with an initial focus to increase positive interactions between Mrs. Benden and her mother. Mrs. Benden enjoyed writing and frequently used family history as the source of her stories. She was encouraged to reframe her time with her mother as an opportunity to gather stories about her childhood and her mother's childhood as background for her writing. Although initially skeptical about her mother's willingness to share stories with her, Mrs. Benden was pleasantly surprised to find her mother cooperative. She began to tape-record her mother's reminiscences and found that they both began to look forward to sharing memories. Although the caregiving tasks remained demanding, the introduction of a pleasant common activity eased the tension between the two and improved the quality of their interactions.

A longer-term goal of treatment was to help Mrs. Benden get some respite from caregiving by going on a long-wished-for vacation with her husband. The initial task was to challenge her beliefs that she should be the one to care for her mother, that she should never ask any of her family for relief or help, and that none of her family would be willing to help. She acknowledged she had no evidence for these beliefs and agreed to talk with her grown children and older brothers about the need for a short break from caregiving. Once again, she was pleasantly surprised to learn that not only were they appreciative of her caregiving, but they were also aware of her distress and were more than willing to provide temporary relief so she and her husband could take a short vacation.

Mrs. Benden entered into the planning of the vacation with enthusiasm. She even built into the plans an insurance policy that would refund 90% of her money if she had to cut her vacation short due to an emergency with her mother, and she felt pleased with her resourcefulness. The vacation was a great success and provided needed respite from the strain of caregiving. As a consequence, she became more optimistic that she could plan other short caregiving breaks in the future. She also felt more supported by her family.

At a 1-year follow-up, Mrs. Benden reported continued positive coping despite the deteriorating health of her mother and increased caregiving demands. She reported that she was still able to take occasional short "get-aways" of an afternoon or weekend with her husband and no longer felt as though her personal life had disappeared.

CONCLUSION

In summary, this chapter has emphasized the value of cognitive-behavioral techniques and strategies in assessing and treating psychological crisis in older adults. Many older adults face life-altering events, including chronic illness; death of loved ones and friends; and changes in work, living, and financial status. Most cope effectively with these events. However, for some older adults the resources for coping with multiple stressors are not available, and they become overwhelmed. Health care professionals need to be sensitive to the needs of these individuals and to provide services to help them cope with crisis. This chapter has identified factors that put older adults at risk for crisis, described the signs of psychological crisis in the elderly, and provided cognitive-behavioral strategies that would be useful in crisis intervention with the elderly.

ACKNOWLEDGMENT

We gratefully acknowledge the contribution of Dolores Gallagher-Thompson to earlier editions of this chapter.

REFERENCES

APA Working Group on the Older Adult. (1997). *What practitioners should know about working with older adults.* Washington, DC: American Psychological Association.

Atkinson, R., Ganzini, L., & Bernstein, M. (1992). Alcohol and substance-use disorders in the elderly. In J. Birren, R. B. Sloane, & G. Cohen (Eds.), *Handbook of mental health and aging* (2nd ed., pp. 515–555). San Diego: Academic Press.

Beck, A. T., Ward, C. H., Mendelson, M., Mock, J., & Erbaugh, J. (1961). An inventory for measuring depression. *Archives of General Psychiatry, 4,* 561–571.

Blazer, D. (1991). Suicide risk factors in the elderly: An epidemiological study. *Journal of Geriatric Psychiatry, 24,* 175–190.

Blazer, D., Bachar, J., & Manton, K. (1986). Suicide in late life: Review and commentary. *Journal of the American Geriatrics Society, 34,* 513–525.

Blow, F. C., Brower, K. J., Schulenberg, J. E., Demo-Dananberg, L. M., Young, J. P., & Beresford, T. P. (1992). The Michigan Alcoholism Screening Test—Geriatric Version (MAST-G): A new elderly-specific screening instrument. *Alcoholism: Clinical and Experimental Research, 16,* 372.

Breckenridge, J. N., Gallagher, D., Thompson, L. W., & Peterson, J. (1986). Effects of bereavement on self-perceptions of physical health in elderly widows and widowers. *Journal of Gerontology, 39*(3), 309–314.

Brody, E. M., Johnsen, P. T., Fulcomer, M. C., & Lang, A. M. (1983). Women's changing roles and help to elderly partners: Attitudes of three generations of women. *Journal of Gerontology, 38,* 597–607.

Cavanaugh, J. C. (1990). *Adult development and aging.* Belmont, CA: Wadsworth.

Conwell, Y. (1997). Management of suicidal behavior in the elderly. *Psychiatric Clinics of North America, 20*(3), 667–683.

Conwell, Y., Duberstein, P., Cox, D., Herrmann, J., Forbes, N., & Caine, E. (1998). Age differences in behaviors leading to completed suicide. *American Journal of Geriatric Psychiatry, 6*(2), 122–126.

Crawford, J. R., Venneri, A., & O'Carroll, R. E. (1998). Neuropsychological assessment of the elderly. In A. Bellack & M. Hersen (Eds.), *Comprehensive clinical psychology* (Vol. 7, pp. 133–169). New York: Elsevier Science.

Crum, R. M., Anthony, J. C., Bassett, S. S., & Folstein, M. F. (1993). Population-based norms for the Mini-Mental State Examination by age and education level. *Journal of the American Medical Association, 269*(18), 2386–2391.

Davies, P. (1988). Alzheimer's disease and related disorders: An overview. In M. K. Aronson (Ed.), *Understanding Alzheimer's disease* (pp. 3–14). New York: Scribner's.

Delano-Wood, L. & Abeles, N. (2005). Late-life depression: Detection, risk reduction, and somatic intervention. *Clinical Psychology: Science and Practice, 12*(3), 207–217.

DeVries, H. M. (2007). Cognitive-behavioral interventions. *Encyclopedia of gerontology* (2nd ed., pp. 283–291). Oxford, UK: Elsevier.

Duffy, M., & Iscoe, L. (1990). Crisis theory and management: The case of the older person. *Journal of Mental Health Counseling, 12,* 303–313.

Engels, G., & Vermey, M (1997). Efficacy of nonmedical treatments of depression in elders: A quantitative analysis. *Journal of Clinical Geropsychology, 3*(1), 17–35.

Espino, D. V., Lichtenstein, M. J., Palmer, R. F., & Hazuda, H. P. (2001). Ethnic differences in Mini-Mental State Examination (MMSE) scores: Where you live makes a difference. *Journal of the American Geriatrics Society, 49*(5), 538–548.

Fields, S. D., Fulop, G., Sachs, C. J., Strain, J., & Fillit, H. (1992). Usefulness of the Neurobehavioral Cognitive Status Examination in the hospitalized elderly. *International Psychogeriatrics, 4*(1), 93–102.

Gallagher, D., & Thompson, L. W. (1983, August). *Elders' maintenance of treatment benefits following individual psychotherapy for depression: Results of a pilot study and preliminary data from an ongoing replication study.* Paper presented at the annual meeting of the American Psychological Association, Washington, DC.

Gallagher-Thompson, D. (1992). The older adult. In A. Freeman & F. Dattilio (Eds.), *Comprehsive casebook of cognitive therapy* (pp. 193–200). New York: Plenum Press.

Gallagher-Thompson, D., Hanley-Peterson, P., & Thompson, L. (1990). Maintenance of gains versus relapse following brief psychotherapy for depression. *Journal of Consulting and Clinical Psychology, 58,* 371–374.

Gallagher-Thompson, D., Lovett, S., & Rose, J. (1991). Psychotherapeutic interventions for stressed family caregivers. In W. Myers (Ed.), *New techniques in the psychotherapy of older patients* (pp. 61–78). Washington, DC: American Psychiatric Association.

Gallagher-Thompson, D., & Thompson, L. W. (1996). Applying cognitive-behavioral therapy to the psychological problems of later life. In S. H. Zarit & B. G. Knight (Eds.), *A guide to psychotherapy and aging: Effective clinical interventions in a life-stage context* (pp. 61–82). Washington, DC: American Psychological Association.

Gatz, M., Fiske, A., Fox, L. S., Kaskie, B., Kasl-Godley, J. E., McCallum, T. J., et al. (1998). Empirically validated psychological treatments for older adults. *Journal of Mental Health and Aging, 4*(1), 9–46.

Gilewski, M., Farberow, N., Gallagher-Thompson, D., & Thompson, L. (1991). Interaction of depression and bereavement on mental health in the elderly. *Psychology and Aging, 6,* 67–75.

Heisel, M. J., & Duberstein, P. R. (2005). Suicide prevention in older adults. *Clinical Psychology: Science and Practice, 12*(3), 242–259.

Hopson-Walker, S. D. (1990). Substance abuse in older persons with disability: Assessment and treatment. In B. Kemp, K. Brummel-Smith, & J. W. Ramsdell (Eds.), *Geriatric rehabilitation* (pp. 279–293). Austin, TX: PRO-ED.

Karel, M. J. (1997). Aging and depression: Vulnerability and stress across adulthood. *Clinical Psychology Review, 17,* 847–879.

Karel, M. J., Ogland-Hand, S., & Gatz, M. (2002). *Assessing and treating late-life depression: A casebook and resource guide.* New York: Basic Books.

Kasl-Godley, J., Gatz, M., & Fiske, A. (1998). Depression and depressive symptoms in old age. In I. Nordhus, G. VandenBos, S. Berg, & P. Fromholt (Eds.), *Clinical geropsychology* (pp. 211–217). Washington, DC: American Psychological Association.

Kemp, B., Brummel-Smith, K., & Ramsdell, J. W. (1990). *Geriatric rehabilitation.* Austin, TX: PRO-ED.

King, D. A. (2005). Introduction to the special issue. *Clinical Psychology: Science and Practice, 12*(3), 203–206.

Knight, B. (2004). *Psychotherapy with older adults* (3rd ed.). Thousand Oaks, CA: Sage.

Koenig, H., & Blazer, D. (1992). Mood disorders and suicide. In J. Birren, R. B. Sloane, & G. Cohen (Eds.), *Handbook of mental health and aging* (2nd ed., pp. 379–407). San Diego: Academic Press.

Laidlaw, K., Thompson, L., Dick-Siskin, L. L., & Gallagher-Thompson, D. (2003). *Cognitive behaviour therapy with older people.* Chichester, UK: Wiley.

Lamy, P. P. (1988, Summer). Actions of alcohol and drugs in older people. *Generations,* pp. 9–13.

Leaf, P. J., Berkman, C. S., Weissman, M. M., Holzer, C. E., Tischler, G. L., & Myers, J. K. (1988). The epidemiology of late-life depression. In J. A. Brody & G. L. Maddox (Eds.), *Epidemiology and aging: An international perspective* (pp. 117–133). New York: Springer Verlag.

Lee, G. R. (1985). Kinship and social support of the elderly: The case of the United States. *Aging and Society, 5,* 19–38.

LeSage, J., & Zwygart-Stauffacher, M. (1988, Summer). Detection of medication misuse in elders. *Generations, 12*(4), 32–36.

Lindesay, J. (1991). Suicide in the elderly. *International Journal of Geriatric Psychiatry, 6,* 355–361.

Liptzin, B. (1991). The treatment of depression in older suicidal persons. *Journal of Geriatric Psychiatry, 24,* 203–215.

Loebel, J. P., Loebel, J. S., Dager, S., & Centerwall, B. (1991). Anticipation of nursing home placement may be a precipitant of suicide among the elderly. *Journal of the American Geriatrics Society, 39,* 407–408.

Lossee N., Parham, I., Auerbach, S., & Teitelman, (1988). *Crisis intervention with the elderly: Theory, practical issues, and training procedures.* Springfield, IL: Thomas.

Lund, D. A. (Ed.). (1989). *Older bereaved spouses: Research with practical applications.* New York: Hemisphere.

Lund, D. A. (1998). Bereavement. In A. Bellack & M. Hersen (Eds.), *Comprehensive clinical psychology* (Vol. 7, pp. 95–112). New York: Elsevier Science.

Miller, N. E., Lipowski, Z. J., & Lebowitz, B. D. (Eds.). (1991). Advancing age and the syndrome of delirium: Ancient conundrums and modern research advances. *International Psychogeriatrics, 3,* 103–113.

Mongan, E. (1990). Arthritis and osteoporosis. In B. Kemp, K. Brummel-Smith, & J. W. Ramsdell (Eds.), *Geriatric rehabilitation* (pp. 91–105). Austin, TX: PRO-ED.

Nordhus, I. H., VandenBos, G. R., Berg, S., & Fromholt, P. (Eds.). (1998). *Clinical geropsychology.* Washington, DC: American Psychiatric Association.

Pilisuk, M., & Parks, S. H. (1988). Caregiving: Where families need help. *Social Work, 33,* 436–440.

Prigerson, H. G., Maciejewski, C. F., Reynolds, C. F., III, Bierhals, A. J., Newsom, J. T., Fasiczka, A., et al. (1995). Inventory of complicated grief: A scale to measure maladaptive symptoms of loss. *Psychiatry Research, 59,* 65–79.

Qualls, S. H., Segal, D. L., Norman, S., Niederehe, G., & Gallagher-Thompson, D. (2002). Psychologists in practice with older adults: Current patterns, sources of training, and need for continuing education. *Professional Psychology: Research and Practice, 33,* 435–442.

Radloff, L. S. (1977). The CES-D Scale: A self-report depression scale for research in the general population. *Applied Psychological Measurement, 1,* 385.

Reese, H. W., & Smyer, M. A. (1983). The dimensionalization of life events. In E. J. Callahan & K. A. McCluskey (Eds.), *Life-span developmental psychology: Non-normative life events* (pp. 1–33). New York: Academic Press.

Richardson, R., Lowenstein, S., & Weissberg, M. (1989). Coping with the suicidal elderly: A physician's guide. *Geriatrics, 44,* 43–47.

Ries, A. L. (1990). Pulmonary rehabilitation. In B. Kemp, K. Brummel-Smith, & J. W. Ramsdell (Eds.), *Geriatric rehabilitation* (pp. 107–120). Austin, TX: PRO-ED.

Scogin, F., & McElreath, L. (1994). Efficacy of psychosocial treatments for geriatric depression: A quantitative review. *Journal of Consulting and Clinical Psychology, 62,* 69–74.

Scogin, F., Welsh, A. H., Stump, J., & Coates, A. (2005). Evidence-based psychotherapies for depression in older adults. *Clinical Psychology: Science and Practice, 12*(3), 222–237.

Shimp, L. A., & Ascione, F. J. (1988, Summer). Causes of medication misuse & error. *Generations, 12*(4), 17–21.

Solomon, K., Manepalli, J., Ireland, G., & Mahon, G. M. (1993). Alcoholism and prescription drug abuse in the elderly: St. Louis University grand rounds. *Journal of the American Geriatrics Society, 41,* 57–69.

Strickland, T. L., Longobardi, P. G., Alperson, B. L., & Andre, K. (2005). Mini-Mental State and Cognistat performance in an older African American sample. *The Clinical Neuropsychologist, 19*(1), 87–98.

Teri, L., Curtis, J., Gallagher-Thompson, D., & Thompson, L. W. (1994). Cognitive-behavior therapy with depressed older adults. In L. S. Schneider, C. F. Reynolds, B. D. Lebowitz, & A. J. Friedhoff (Eds.), *Diagnosis and treatment of depression in late life: Results of the NIH consensus development conference* (pp. 279–291). Washington, DC: American Psychiatric Press.

Teri, L., McKenzie, G., & LaFazia, D. (2005). Psychosocial treatment of depression in older adults with dementia. *Professional Psychology: Research and Practice, 12*(3), 303–316.

Thompson, L. (1996). Cognitive-behavioral therapy and treatment for late-life depression. *Journal of Clinical Psychiatry, 57,* 29–37.

Thompson, L., Gallagher, D., & Breckenridge, J. (1987). Comparative effectiveness of psychotherapies for depressed elders. *Journal of Consulting and Clinical Psychology, 55,* 385–390.

Thompson, L. W., Gallagher, D., Cover, H., Gilewski, M., & Peterson, J. (1989). Effects of bereavement on symptoms of psychopathology in older men and women. In D. Lund (Ed.), *Older bereaved spouses: Research with practical applications* (pp. 17–24). New York: Hemisphere.

Thompson, L. W., & Gallagher-Thompson, D. (1991, November). *Comparison of desipramine and cognitive/behavioral therapy in the treatment of late-life depression: A progress report.* Paper presented at the annual meeting of the Gerontological Society of America, San Francisco.

Thompson, L. W., Gallagher-Thompson, D., Futterman, A., & Peterson, J. (1991). The effects of late-life spousal bereavement over a thirty-month interval. *Psychology and Aging, 6,* 434–441.

Thompson, L. W., Gantz, F., Florsheim, M., DelMaestro, S., Rodman, J., & Gallagher-Thompson, D. (1991). Cognitive/behavioral therapy for affective disorders in the elderly. In W. Myers (Ed.), *New techniques in the psychotherapy of older patients* (pp. 3–19). Washington, DC: American Psychiatric Association.

Weaver, A., & Koenig, H. (1996). Elderly suicide, mental health professionals, and the clergy: A need for clinical collaboration, training, and research. *Death Studies, 20*(5), 495–508.

Worden, J. W. (2002). *Grief counseling and grief therapy: A handbook for the mental health practitioner* (3rd ed.). New York: Springer.

Yesavage, J. A., Brink, T. L., Rose, T. L., Lum, O., Huang, V., Adey, M., et al. (1983). Development and validation of a geriatric depression scale: A preliminary report. *Journal of Psychiatric Research, 17,* 37–49.

Zarit, S., Davey, A., Edwards, A., Femia, E., & Jarrott, S. (1998). Family caregiving: Research findings and clinical implications. In A. Bellack & M. Hersen (Eds.), *Comprehensive clinical psychology* (Vol. 7, pp. 499–523). New York: Elsevier Science.

Zeiss, A. M., & Steffen, A. (1996). Treatment issues with elderly clients. *Cognitive and Behavioral Practice, 3*(2), 371–389.

SUGGESTED READINGS

Gatz, M., Fiske, A., Fox, L. S., Kaskie, B., Kasl-Godley, J. E., McCallum, T. J., et al. (1998). Empirically validated psychological treatments for older adults. *Journal of Mental Health and Aging, 4*(1), 9–46.

Karel, M. J., Ogland-Hand, S., & Gatz, M. (2002). *Assessing and treating late-life depression: A casebook and resource guide.* New York: Basic Books.

Laidlaw, K., Thompson, L., Dick-Siskin, L., & Gallagher-Thompson, D. (2003). *Cognitive behaviour therapy with older people.* Chichester, UK: Wiley.

Scogin, F., Welsh, A. H., Stump, J., & Coates, A. (2005). Evidence-based psychotherapies for depression in older adults. *Clinical Psychology: Science and Practice, 12*(3), 222–237.

Thompson, L. (1996). Cognitive-behavioral therapy and treatment for late-life depression. *Journal of Clinical Psychiatry, 57,* 29–37.

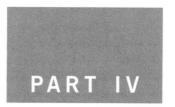

PART IV

Environmental and Situational Crises

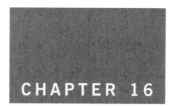

CHAPTER 16

Disaster Trauma

Lata K. McGinn
Carrie B. Spindel

All traumatic events pose a palpable threat to safety. The defining feature of a disaster, however, is that it threatens the safety of an entire community as well as its individual members (Norwood, Ursano, & Fullerton, 2000). Disaster-related trauma affects individuals directly, by their own exposure to the event and its consequences, as well as through the community in which they live, by word of mouth, media coverage, and disruptions in services and events that make up everyday life (Galea et al., 2003). The September 11, 2001, terrorist attacks, one of the most significant disasters of the 21st century, provide a stunning example of the profound political, psychological, and economic effects that may follow a disaster. Thus, society must confront not just the needs of individuals affected by the disaster but those of the community as well.

Disasters include natural environmental events, such as hurricanes, tornadoes, floods, and earthquakes, which often strike without warning and cannot be prevented (Fullerton, Ursano, Norwood, & Halloway, 2003; Norwood et al., 2000). The tsunami spawned by the Indian Ocean earthquake on December 26, 2004, is a striking example. Man-made disasters result from human actions, and include two types: intentional acts such as mass violence and terrorism and nonintentional acts such as accidents. The latter, often categorized as technological disasters, refer to failures of man-made products (Norris, 2001; Norris, et al., 2002). Examples include the accident at the Three Mile Island nuclear power plant in 1979 and the crash of Pan Am flight 759 in 1982. Further, "complex disasters" such as Hurricane Katrina in 2005, where the natural impact of the storm was exacerbated by the breakdown of the levees in New Orleans and the nation's disaster relief system, comprise both natural and man-made elements (Ericsson, n.d.).

POSTDISASTER SYMPTOMATOLOGY

Common Reactions

Community studies suggest that approximately two-thirds of individuals exposed to a trauma will have a normal acute response to stress that will abate over time, suggesting that resilience is the most common outcome of trauma (Yehuda & McFarlane, 1995). A variety of emotional, cognitive, and physical reactions, as well as problems of living, are seen as natural consequences of the adjustments individuals must make following a disaster (van Etten & Taylor, 1998). Common emotional responses may include temporary shock, fear, anxiety, and disbelief. Individuals also respond with anger, sadness, irritability, resentment, guilt, and shame. High levels of arousal often lead to emotional numbness or sleep disturbances (Norwood et al., 2000; Young, Ford, & Watson, 2005). Feeling helplessness is common and individuals may turn to alcohol, tobacco, caffeine, or other substances to help them cope (Norwood et al., 2000).

Disaster survivors often describe a range of cognitive reactions that accompany anxiety, such as confusion, disorientation, indecisiveness, decreased attention span, and memory loss. Furthermore, worry thoughts and thoughts of self-blame, as well as intrusive and unwanted memories of the disaster experience, are commonly described (Young et al., 2005). Somatic complaints include muscle tension and aches, fatigue, restlessness, reduced libido, and appetite changes (Young et al., 2005). The direct impact on the community infrastructure also leads to problems of living, such as financial and occupational stress. Disaster victims may suffer a loss of social support, either due to relocation or conflictual social relationships resulting from increased distrust, irritability, withdrawal, and isolation (Norris, 2002; Young et al., 2005).

Children tend to show similar general responses to disasters. Commonly reported symptoms and behaviors include heightened alertness to danger, confusion, nightmares, and separation fears (Hamblen, 2005; Yule, 2001). More specific responses have been observed among children in different developmental stages. Young children tend to show helplessness, passive behaviors, and regressive symptoms, and they have difficulty discussing the event and identifying their feelings. School-age children often demonstrate repetitive traumatic play, aggressive behavior, anger outbursts, and impairments in concentration and attention span. Finally, adolescents show more depression, social withdrawal, decreased academic functioning, shifts in relationships, self-consciousness, self-concern, and rebellious behavior (Hamblen, 2005; Norwood et al., 2000). Physical symptoms among children include bedwetting, stomachaches, body pains, and changes in appetite (Padesky et al., 2002).

Effects may also vary widely depending on the type of trauma experienced. In their empirical review of disaster research, Norris et al. (2002) found that the highest level of impairment was observed for mass violence (67%), followed by natural disasters (39%) and technological disasters (34%). Research also suggests that the consequences of man-made disasters may persist longer than that for natural disasters (Solomon & Green, 1992). The meaning individuals place on man-made disasters and violence, including maliciousness and human carelessness, may account for some of this difference (Norris et al., 2002).

Disasters also typically affect the community even beyond destruction of the physical landscape and infrastructure. In the aftermath of a trauma, an influx of outsiders, including relief teams, media coverage, or curiosity seekers, can disrupt the culture and natural routine of the community. Depending on how it is provided, outside relief may also be experienced as intrusive and insensitive. At first, it is common for communities to respond with sympathy for victims of a disaster. However, anger may develop for those who are held accountable for failing to take measures that could have prevented the disaster or the extent of its effects (Fullerton et al., 2003; Norwood et al., 2000). This was demonstrated by the heavy criticism of federal authorities and their relief actions in the aftermath of Hurricane Katrina in 2005.

Pathological Reactions to Trauma: Posttraumatic Stress Disorder

Although the impact of a trauma varies greatly depending on the type of disaster, evidence suggests that for most individuals, reactions to disasters and other traumatic events are transient and resolve over time (Fullerton et al., 2003). For example, a long-term prospective study conducted on an entire cohort born in Kauai, Hawaii, found that most individuals exposed to various emotional traumas were largely resilient to its effects (Werner & Smith, 1982).

However, approximately one-third of exposed individuals go on to develop pathological symptoms (Yehuda & McFarlane, 1995). The two trauma-related anxiety disorders included in the *Diagnostic and Statistical Manual of Mental Disorders*, fourth edition, text revision (DSM-IV-TR) include posttraumatic stress disorder (PTSD) and acute stress disorder (ASD) (American Psychiatric Association, 2000). Symptoms of ASD may be diagnosed immediately following a disaster and may last for a minimum of 2 days to a maximum of 4 weeks. If symptoms persist for 4 or more weeks, the individual may be diagnosed with PTSD if criteria are met (American Psychiatric Association, 2000).

While both disorders require exposure to a traumatic event and emphasize the individual's subjective reaction to the trauma, ASD and PTSD have some differences. For PTSD, an individual must experience symptoms from three key areas, including at least one reexperiencing, three avoidance, and two arousal symptoms (American Psychiatric Association, 2000). Difficulty concentrating and an exaggerated startle response appear to be the most commonly reported PTSD symptoms among disaster victims (North et al., 1999). Although similar symptoms are required for the diagnosis of ASD, dissociation is also a required and necessary criterion. Dissociative symptoms include emotional numbness, feeling detached from one's body, difficulty remembering details of the event, and experiencing things in a dream-like fashion (American Psychiatric Association, 2000).

PTSD is one of the most commonly diagnosed anxiety disorders and has a lifetime prevalence of 5–10% in the general population (Ballenger et al., 2000). However, prevalence estimates range from 9.2 to 27.8% depending on the type of trauma, population sample, study methodology and design, and diagnostic criteria used (Breslau et al., 1998; Kessler, Sonnega, Bromet, Hughes, & Nelson, 1995; Kilpatrick, Saunders, Veronen, Best, & Von, 1987). Even within disaster populations, there is wide variability in rates. Rates may vary between 0 and 100% depending on the type of disaster, sample selection, and type of assessments conducted (*Disaster Mental Health Response Handbook*, 2000).

In natural disasters, for example, reports indicate a 4% prevalence rate among victims of torrential rains and mud slides (Canino, Braveo, Rubio-Stipec, & Woodbury, 1990), and a 54% rate following the Ash Wednesday bushfires in Australia (McFarlane, 1986). While definitive prevalence rates in response to the 2004 South Asian tsunami or the 2005 hurricane in New Orleans are not yet available, many projections have been made based on preliminary assessments or based on findings from previous natural disasters. For example, approximately 30% of Tsunami survivors are projected to suffer from posttraumatic stress and depressive disorders (Thailand Center of Excellence for Life Sciences, 2006). An assessment prepared for the Louisiana Office of Mental Health by the Centers for Disease Control and Prevention (CDC) in the wake of Hurricane Katrina, found that 45% of survivors scored "high enough on a PTSD rating scale" to warrant a referral for mental health services (Voelker, 2006, p. 259). As evident in wake of the September 11, 2001, attacks, projected estimates may be helpful for crisis intervention efforts but may differ considerably from true prevalence rates (Galea et al., 2003).

A review conducted by Gidron (2002) suggested that approximately 28% of individuals who experience terrorist attacks develop PTSD (see Gidron, 2002, for a review). However, rates within individual studies vary substantially. For example, Abenhaim, Dab, and Salmi (1992) assessed 254 survivors of terrorist attacks occurring in France between 1982 and 1987 and found a prevalence rate of 18% ranging between 10.5% among uninjured victims and 30.7% among severely injured victims. In another study, 50% of participants ($n = 26$) who survived the November 1987 Enniskillen bombing in Northern Ireland met criteria for PTSD 6 months following the incident (Curran et al., 1990).

Relatively few studies have assessed the rates of PTSD following terrorist attacks in the United States given their limited occurrence. North and colleagues reported that more than one-third (34.3%) of the assessed 1995 Oklahoma City bombing survivors met DSM-III-R criteria for PTSD 6 months following the event (North et al., 1999). By comparison, the prevalence rate of probable PTSD was 7.5% among individuals living in Manhattan, south of 110th street, and 20% among those living in closer proximity to the World Trade Center, 6 weeks following September 11, 2001 (Galea et al., 2002). In another study, Schlenger et al. (2002) reported a probable prevalence rate of 11.2% among those in the New York City area on the day of the attacks compared to a national estimate of 4.3%.

Children may also be at risk for developing severe psychological symptoms following a disaster (Norris, 2001). Common diagnoses include PTSD, major depression, and separation anxiety disorder (Norwood et al., 2000). For example, Hoven, Mandell, and Duarte (2003) found that 10.5% of school children living in New York City met criteria for probable posttraumatic stress disorder six months after the World Trade Center attack.

Even among those who develop PTSD, symptoms generally tend to abate over time. A meta-analysis of 177 trauma studies conducted by Norris (2001) found that symptoms usually peaked within the first year and then declined in prevalence. During the first year after 9/11, Galea et al. (2003) found that the prevalence of probable PTSD declined from 7.5% to 1.2% to 0.6% and only 5.3% of the subjects continued to report even subclinical symptoms 6 months later. In another study, McGinn and Massey (2004) demonstrated that the majority of people reported mild to minimal symptoms of posttraumatic stress, depression, and worry, 3 years after September 11, 2001.

PSTD: A Valid Diagnostic Entity?

Although clinicians and researchers have long recognized the potentially debilitating effects of trauma, given that the bulk of individuals experience posttraumatic symptoms that decline over time without intervention, it is worth questioning whether PTSD is a valid diagnostic entity. In fact, the diagnosis of PTSD has been shrouded with controversy since its introduction in the third edition of the DSM (DSM-III). Initial opponents of the diagnosis expressed concern that PTSD was a political or a social construct rather than a medical one, and that reactions to trauma could be better accounted for by combinations of existing diagnoses (Herbert & Forman, 2006; McNally, 2004). In support, research suggests that traumatic events also lead to other psychological problems including major depression (MDD), generalized anxiety disorder (GAD), panic disorder (PD), and substance use disorders (McGinn & Massey, 2004; Norris et al., 2002). However, these tend to occur most often as comorbid diagnoses, with MDD reported as the most common comorbid disorder (Breslau, Davis, Andreski, & Peterson, 1991; Norris et al., 2002). For example, in a study of Oklahoma City Bombing survivors 6 months after the disaster, North et al. (1999) reported that almost half of the sample met criteria for at least one psychiatric disorder. Among this portion of the sample, more than one-third met criteria for PTSD specific to the bombing, and 63% of these individuals suffered from a comorbid diagnosis.

Although a majority of researchers accept the validity of PTSD and suggest that it is a universal concept with a biological basis (Ballenger et al., 2000; Yehuda & McFarlane, 1997), concerns that PTSD may be a "culture-bound socially constructed idiom of distress" continue to exist and appear to be growing (McNally, 2004, p. 10; Herbert & Sageman, 2004). In support, several accounts suggest that reactions to trauma appear to differ substantially transhistorically and cross-culturally, both of which raise serious questions about the universality of PTSD (Herbert & Sageman, 2004; Silove & Bryant, 2006; Yeomans, Herbert, & Forman, in press; Young, 2004).

Other recent criticisms note specific problems with the DSM formulation of the diagnosis (McNally, 2004; Resick, 2004). For example, some argue that the concept of a traumatic event has become diluted by including the full range of common human stressors rather than limiting traumatic events to those outside the range of common human experience (McNally, 2004). Others recommend that PTSD be reclassified within a category of stress-related disorders and offer a reformulated diagnosis which includes at least one each of the following criteria: the traumatic event, recurrent intrusions, cognitions, emotion/arousal, and escape/avoidance (Resick, 2004).

RISK AND RESILIENCE AMONG DISASTER SURVIVORS: WHO DEVELOPS PTSD?

Although epidemiological studies demonstrate that a minority of individuals who experience trauma develop PTSD (Kessler et al., 1995), these studies also indicate that if symptoms have not remitted after approximately 12 months, there appears to be an increased likelihood that symptoms will persist in both intensity and duration (Cancro, 2004). The probability of developing clinically significant symptoms appears to be at least partially determined by the existence of specific risk and protective factors (Ballenger et al., 2000; Yehuda, 1999). Although the mechanism through which these factors increase the risk is not yet understood (Litz, Gray, Bryant, & Adler, 2002), research suggests that as the number of risk factors increase, so does the probability of psychological impairment (Norris et al., 2002). Therefore, an essential aspect of crisis intervention is identifying individuals who face increased risk of psychological impairment and developing targeted interventions to address their needs.

Individual (Pretrauma) Factors

Many individual factors appear to increase the risk for developing long-term psychological distress after surviving a disaster. There is overwhelming consensus that females are at greater risk for developing PTSD, MDD, and GAD after exposure to a disaster (Norris, 2002; North et al., 1999). In a meta-analysis, females in 93% of the samples studied for gender influence reported being affected more adversely by the disaster than their male counterparts, and for longer durations of time (Norris, 2001). This pattern is consistent among children, adolescents, and adults (Norris et al., 2002; Udwin, Boyle, Yule, Bolton, & O'Ryan, 2000).

Studies indicate that the severity of psychological consequences following a disaster may decline across the lifespan. School-age children have been found to be more severely affected by disasters compared to middle-age adults, while adults appear to suffer more severe pathology and stress compared to older adults (Norris, 2001; Norris et al., 2002). It has been hypothesized that middle-age adults suffer from higher everyday demands due to obligations of work and family, thus putting them at higher risk of increased stress postdisaster (Norris, 2001). Maturity and experience have also been proposed as buffers against the impact of trauma. For example, older adults are more likely to have experienced various types of suffering and loss (i.e., property loss and physical impairments) which may prepare them with more knowledge and skills for coping when an actual trauma is experienced (Norris et al., 2002).

Evidence is mixed on the role of marital status in the development of PTSD following disasters. A review of disaster studies found that women reported increased marital stress after surviving a disaster, and that a husband's symptom severity predicted the wife's symptom severity more strongly than the reverse (Norris, 2001). However, being unmarried increased the probability of being diagnosed with PTSD after the 9/11 attacks (Galea et al., 2003).

Research suggests that a history of psychiatric illness may be one of the strongest individual predictors of postdisaster symptomatology among trauma survivors in general (North et al., 1999; Perkonigg, Kessler, Storz, & Wittchen, 2000) as well as specifically among disaster survivors (Norris et al., 2002; North et al., 1999). Individuals with preexisting anxiety or depressive disorders appear to be particularly at risk (Breslau et al., 1991; Perkonigg et al., 2000). For example, 90% of hotel employees with a prior psychiatric history experienced postdisaster symptoms after a plane crashed into the hotel where they were employed, as compared to 25% of the sample without a prior diagnosis (Smith, North, McCool, & Shea, 1990). In another study, 66% of Oklahoma City bombing survivors who reported at least one predisaster psychiatric condition met criteria for a disorder after the bombing, as compared to 34.3% of the total sample of survivors (North et al., 1999). Finally, mental health difficulties in childhood were significantly associated with developing PTSD in a sample of young adults who had experienced a ship disaster during adolescence. More specifically, those with childhood separation anxiety disorder were more likely to suffer from more symptoms of PTSD (Udwin et al., 2000).

Trauma Factors

Many aspects of the specific trauma experience increase the probability of psychological consequences, including proximity to the disaster, severity of exposure, duration of exposure, and injury during exposure (Norris, 2001; Udwin et al., 2000; Young et al., 2005). Galea et al. (2003) found that geographic proximity to the World Trade Center on 9/11, seeing the attacks in person, being injured in the attacks, and being involved in the rescue effort were significantly associated with probable PTSD. A web-based survey of the U.S. population two months after the 9/11 attacks demonstrated that individuals who were in New York City at the time were almost three times more likely to have probable PTSD compared to those who lived elsewhere in the United States (Schlenger et al., 2002). Among those exposed to the disaster at Mount St. Helens in 1980, individuals with greater exposure (i.e., those who experienced death of a loved one or a significant amount of property loss) were diagnosed significantly more often with PTSD, MDD, and GAD compared to those with less exposure (Shore, Tatum, & Vollmer, 1986). Exposure to particularly gruesome sights also appears to increase the likelihood of distress. For example, seeing blood was one of the two strongest risk factors in the development of PTSD among those surviving the sinking of the ship *The Jupiter* (Rubonis & Bickman, 1991).

Posttrauma Factors

Posttrauma factors also appear to increase the likelihood of developing greater distress. A loss of resources following a disastrous event, in the form of property damage, discontinuation of employment, and financial loss, has been repeatedly associated with greater pathology (Norris, 2001; Young et al., 2005). Reinforcing the unique impact of disasters on the development of symptoms, a study conducted by Phifer and Norris (1989) (as cited in Solomon & Green, 1992) following the 1981 and 1984 floods in Kentucky reported that community destruction led to a longer duration of symptoms than did individual property loss.

Disaster victims may also be more likely to experience a posttrauma decline in social support through death, relocation, or increased stress within relationships. A meta-analysis of disaster studies found that the higher the death rate, the greater the pathology observed among surviving victims. Possible explanations may be the increased distress over the loss of a loved one or, alternatively, the increased threat to one's life experienced when the death toll is high (Rubonis & Bickman, 1991). Relocation can be another factor. Often, in the wake of severe destruction, communities are relocated to safer regions and as a result victims are separated from their original social supports and may have difficulty attaching to new social networks. After Cyclone Tracy devastated a community in the city of Darwin, Australia, researchers found that the people who remained in Darwin fared better during the recovery period compared with those who were relocated to other areas (Gerrity & Steinglass, 2003).

Survivor Reactions to Disaster

Research suggests that survivor reactions to trauma and their way of coping may buffer or, conversely, maintain postdisaster symptoms (Norris, 2001). For example, those who use acceptance rather than denial, self-blame, and avoidance appear to exhibit less posttraumatic stress following a disaster (McGinn & Massey, 2004; Schlenger et al., 2002). Survivor beliefs about coping abilities also appear to be linked to better outcomes than actual coping strategies (Norris, Byrne, Diaz, & Kaniasty, 2005). Based on an empirical review of the literature, Norris (2001) observed that self-efficacy, mastery, perceived control, self-esteem, hope, and optimism were all associated with positive, strong, and consistent mental health.

A Cognitive-Behavioral Model of PTSD

Specific cognitive styles appear to be related to the development and maintenance of PTSD following traumatic events (Dunmore, Clark, & Ehlers, 1999, 2001; Ehlers & Clark, 2000). In general, cognitive models suggest that appraisals relating to impending threat lead to anxiety (Beck, Emery, & Greenberg, 1985; Ehlers & Clark, 2000). To account for the fact that PTSD is the memory of a traumatic event that occurred in the past, Ehlers and Clark (2000) suggest that PTSD occurs when individuals cognitively process the event and/or its sequelae in a manner that creates appraisals of either current or impending threat. The threat may be either external, in which individuals perceive the world as a dangerous place or, more commonly, internal, in which individuals perceive that they are not capable of achieving important life goals (Ehlers & Clark, 2000).

Accordingly, individuals who recover naturally tend to see the trauma as a time-limited event that does not have global, negative implications for the future. By contrast, individuals with persistent PTSD tend to process the traumatic event as having made an indelible, negative change in their lives ("I will never be the same again"). They may overgeneralize the fear from the trauma to normal life events, and thereby perceive normal events as more dangerous than they are in reality (e.g., riding the subway). Such individuals may personalize the event ("I am a magnet for attracting disaster") and overestimate the possibility of experiencing future catastrophic events (Ehlers & Clark, 2000).

Persistent PTSD is also associated with interpretations made by individuals regarding their behavior during the traumatic event ("I should have stayed to help my friend"), their initial PTSD symptoms (e.g., judging normal posttrauma symptoms to be abnormal), the behavior of others in the aftermath of events ("No one is helping me"), and the consequences of the trauma in other life domains ("I can no longer be an effective father") (Ehlers & Clark, 2000).

In addition, Ehlers and Clark (2000) suggest that individuals with persistent PTSD have specific memory impairments, such as poor intentional recall combined with vivid unintentional recall, which suggest difficulties in the way that trauma is encoded in memory. The trauma memory is conceptualized as being poorly elaborated and inadequately integrated into its context in time, place, with prior information and memories, as well as with incoming information. However, such individuals also exhibit stronger associative learning and perceptual priming, which leads to a lowering of the threshold to elicit trauma memories (Ehlers & Clark, 2000).

Ehlers and Clark (2000) describe a reciprocal relationship between the nature of the appraisals and the traumatic memories. They propose that biased, negative appraisals lead to a selective retrieval of information that is consistent with these appraisals, which prevent these appraisals from being modified over time. Conversely, problems with intentional and unintentional memory are appraised negatively ("I am slowly going insane"), with the resulting appraisals leading to a further disorganization of autobiographical memory (Ehlers & Clark, 2000).

Moreover, the model proposes a reciprocal relationship between appraisals and coping strategies used by individuals following the traumatic event. Depending on the nature of the appraisals, a variety of negative emotions may be triggered (e.g., fear, anger, sadness, and guilt), which, in turn, lead to the development of ineffective coping strategies that paradoxically increase PTSD symptoms by preventing changes in the appraisals themselves, as well as by preventing a change in the nature of the trauma memory itself. A variety of maladaptive coping strategies have been identified, including thought suppression, distraction, selective attention to threat cues, safety behaviors, behavioral avoidance of reminders of the trauma, use of substances, dissociation, and rumination (Ehlers & Clark, 2000).

Ehlers and Clark (2000) propose that several thought processes experienced during the traumatic event may influence the subsequent development of biased appraisals and memory impairments and, in turn, lead to persistent symptoms. They suggest that individuals who experience mental defeat, dissociation, and numbness and report feeling confused and overwhelmed by sensory impressions during the traumatic event appear to be more likely to develop biased appraisals over time ("I knew I would never be the same again"), develop chronic PTSD, and respond less well to treatment (Ehlers & Clark, 2000).

Finally, according to this model, characteristics of the traumatic event (e.g., duration and predictability), prior traumatic experiences and beliefs, state factors (e.g., alcohol consumption and degree of arousal), and demographic characteristics (e.g., age and intellectual ability) may contribute to the development of PTSD by interacting with appraisals of the trauma and its sequelae.

Research Supporting the Cognitive Model of PTSD

A growing body of research supports the cognitive model of PTSD. A number of studies demonstrate a link between persistent PTSD and beliefs about PTSD symptoms during the trauma, appraisals about the trauma, and negative judgments about other people's behaviors following the trauma (Ehlers & Clark, 2000). Although initial findings were drawn from cross-sectional studies that examined trauma memories and appraisals retrospectively, recent studies have examined the cognitive model using prospective designs.

For example, in an early study of 92 victims of physical or sexual assault, Dunmore et al. (1999) found that individuals who developed PTSD after a physical or sexual assault reported a greater degree of mental defeat, confusion, mental planning and detachment, and more negative appraisals of their emotions during the assault, as compared to those who did not develop PTSD. Individuals with PTSD also reported more negative appraisals of their symptoms in the month after the assault, were more likely to perceive the reactions of others to be negative, and less likely to perceive their responses to be positive. The PTSD group was also more inclined to believe that the assault had a permanent negative effect on their lives. When investigators controlled for previous history and perceived and objective measures of assault severity, all the cognitive variables, with the exception of mental confusion, accounted for the development of PTSD (Dunmore et al., 1999).

Research also confirms that negative beliefs held before the traumatic event may be associated with the development and maintenance of PTSD (Ali, Dunmore, Clark, & Ehlers, 2002; Dunmore et al., 2001). Ali et al. (2002) found that individuals with PTSD reported more negative preassault beliefs as compared to those without PTSD and those who had never been assaulted. As compared to the other groups, individuals with PTSD also reported more negative appraisals of "victims" before the assault and were more likely to endorse beliefs indicating a lack of trust in others and a negative view of themselves and the world as unsafe (Ali et al., 2002).

It is important to note that, unlike the Dunmore et al. (1999) study, the Ali et al. (2002) study failed to control for risk factors other than gender. Further, given that individuals in the never-assaulted group reported experiencing other types of trauma, it is possible that individuals in this group may have had undiagnosed PTSD (Ali et al., 2002). A more salient limitation is that given the cross-sectional design of both studies, causality cannot be presumed. Finally, the use of retrospective measures, particularly in a population with presumed faulty intentional recall, is less than ideal.

However, later studies using a prospective design have also found support for the cognitive model. Dunmore et al. (2001) demonstrated that cognitive variables predicted PTSD severity 6 and 9 months after a physical or sexual assault, while another study conducted in Northern Ireland following the 1998 bombing in the town of Omagh (Clark, 2000) also found that cognitive factors were most strongly associated with the subsequent development of PTSD. Specifically, negative views of symptoms/self and rumination following the bombing were most predictive of PTSD symptom. Other factors associated to a lesser degree included in order of statistical strength: thought/emotion suppression, the appraisal that one would die during the bombing, presence in the marketplace during the bombing, "unsafe world" beliefs, and the occurrence of an injury during the bombing (Clark, 2000).

In summary, studies conducted so far are consistent with the cognitive conceptualization of symptom maintenance (Ehlers & Clark, 2000) and offer some tentative support for their developmental model of PTSD. However, given the methodological issues inherent in most studies assessing the cognitive model, alternative explanations that are inconsistent with the cognitive model cannot be ruled out as yet. Future studies assessing premorbid cognitive styles are still needed to definitively test the Beckian premise that premorbid cognitive schemata provide a vulnerability for PTSD. Further, given that a prior history of psychiatric illness predicts subsequent PTSD symptoms and research has demonstrated that dysfunctional cognitions covary with mood and anxiety disorders, it is feasible that dysfunctional cognitions simply reflect premorbid psychopathology and thereby represent a methodological artifact. Hence, future studies may need to either partial out coexisting psychopathology or prospectively assess cognitive styles in individuals prior to the development of psychopathology.

DISASTER TRAUMA: IMPLICATIONS FOR INTERVENTION

Acute Crisis Intervention: Immediate Disaster Relief

Postdisaster intervention is multifaceted, ranging from emergency rescue efforts to financial support from governmental agencies to interventions by mental health workers. As evidenced by the ineffective federal, state, and local response to Hurricane

Katrina, a smooth and immediate government response to a disaster is critical in meeting the basic needs of survivors, such as safety and food, thereby preventing or reducing continued traumatization or retraumatization.

In the acute aftermath of a disaster, mental health interventions are typically offered promptly to survivors. Critical incident stress debriefing (CISD), originally developed as a brief intervention for emergency service workers exposed to traumatic stress (Mitchell, 1983; van der Kolk, McFarlane, & Weisaeth, 1996) and subsequently described as psychological debriefing has become a social movement and is used worldwide (Hiley-Young & Gerrity, 1994; Raphael & Meldrum, 1995). The goal of debriefing is to encourage the processing of emotions through ventilation and to normalize reactions to traumatic events (Bisson & Deahl, 1994). It is conducted in a single group session and is recommended to occur within 24 to 72 hours after the event (van der Kolk et al., 1996).

However, given the dearth of empirical evidence and rigorous methodological studies on such treatments, psychological debriefing has come under heavy criticism and is no longer recommended as a treatment for acute trauma (Devilly & Cotton, 2003, 2004). Most research has failed to demonstrate beneficial effects relative to untreated controls, and several studies have found that debriefing may actually *increase* the likelihood of the development of chronic symptoms, including PTSD (Devilly & Cotton, 2003, 2004).

Based on the available evidence, interventions in the immediate aftermath of a trauma should be limited to "immediate restorative and recuperative measures" (e.g., adequate sleep using short-term tranquillizers if necessary) in the "context of supportive, optimistic messages about recovery" (National Institute of Mental Health, 2002, as cited in Herbert & Forman, 2006, p. 9). The overall goal in the acute phase is to provide "psychological first aid," which aims to reduce the initial distress and foster both short- and long-term adaptive functioning through the facilitation of natural emotional processing (National Child Traumatic Stress Network and National Center for PTSD, 2004; Padesky et al., 2002). This is accomplished by relating to victims in an empathic, compassionate fashion, enhancing immediate safety and physical comfort, providing practical assistance for basic and immediate needs such as food and shelter, helping them connect with emergency and social supports, and facilitating further response efforts when necessary (National Child Traumatic Stress Network & National Center for PTSD, 2004). Early sleep and anxiety problems should be symptomatically treated, and if indicated, disaster survivors may require sedation in the acute hours or days following the trauma (Herbert & Sageman, 2004).

At the acute stage of intervention, it is important to educate survivors about normal and expected responses to trauma, such as anxiety, nightmares, and irritability, and that such effects are transient for the vast majority of individuals (Bryant, Moulds, & Nixon, 2003). Given the cognitive risk factors associated with the development of PTSD, every effort should be made to prevent pathological beliefs about the possibility of permanent damage and disability. Critical therapeutic elements appear to be validation of the individual's suffering as real and painful on the one hand yet normal and temporary on the other.

Given findings that the size, vitality, and closeness of social network are strongly related to positive mental health outcomes (Norris, 2001), other critical strategies for acute intervention include ensuring the availability of support networks, including links to emergency and relief agencies. If the community is highly disrupted and traumatized following the disaster, helping relocation efforts and linking survivors to social supports outside the traumatized zone become essential. Although trauma survivors are encouraged to talk to family or friends about their traumatic experiences, their natural inclination, including a reluctance to share experiences, is respected. No therapeutic effort is made to elicit details of experiences and losses from survivors. Instead, individuals are encouraged to become involved in some form of meaningful activity in order to prevent morbid preoccupation with the trauma (Herbert & Sageman, 2004).

Subacute Crisis Intervention: Two Weeks Postdisaster

In the subacute phase of the trauma, the goals of mental health interventions are to continue to optimize survivor's resources and identify those who may be at risk for more severe reactions. This may be done by screening individuals for risk and protective factors and identifying those who are experiencing persistent distress (Shalev et al., 2003). Continued validation of the individual's pain and suffering combined with continued education regarding expected but transient effects of trauma is indicated. Psychosocial support by clinicians, friends, family, and the community continues to be as critical in the weeks following the trauma with a focus toward creating safety and minimizing further threat (Ballenger et al., 2000). Individuals should be encouraged to engage in familiar cultural rituals to acknowledge the traumatic event or to mourn losses arising from the disaster (Herbert & Sageman, 2004).

In addition, providing information and advice against using avoidance and excessive alcohol or drugs as coping mechanisms is critical to preventing the development of maladaptive coping strategies linked to the development of PTSD (Ballenger et al., 2000). The emergence of somatic symptoms must be immediately addressed before they become chronic. Tracking mechanisms must also be established to identify individuals who do not recover and will require formal psychological intervention (Herbert & Sageman, 2004).

For individuals whose stress levels remain high 2 or 3 weeks posttrauma, referrals for psychological or medication treatment should be provided. Emerging research suggests that brief, prevention treatment programs provided within 2 weeks to a month following a traumatic experience may be effective in preventing the development of chronic and severe PTSD symptoms in vulnerable individuals (Bryant et al., 2003; Foa, Hearst-Ikeda, & Perry, 1995). Unlike debriefing programs, these studies target only individuals experiencing clinically significant symptoms at least 2 weeks following the traumatic event.

Foa et al. (1995) conducted a four-session, multicomponent cognitive-behavioral therapy (CBT) program for 10 victims of sexual assault approximately 2 weeks following the assault. All participants met provisional diagnostic criteria for PTSD. Results demonstrated that the group receiving CBT had significantly less severe symptoms 2 months after treatment was completed as compared with a matched, untreated group. Ten percent of the CBT group and 70% of the control group met criteria for PTSD 2 months following the trauma. However, at 5½ months following the trauma, the rates of PTSD were comparable between groups (Foa et al., 1995).

A similar study conducted on 24 survivors of various civilian traumas found that participants treated with CBT had fewer symptoms and lower rates of PTSD at posttreatment, and 6 months following the trauma (Bryant, Harvey, Dang, Sackville, & Basten, 1998). At posttreatment, only 8% of the CBT group met criteria for PTSD, compared to 83% of those who received supportive counseling. Six months following the trauma, 17% of participants who had received CBT met criteria for PTSD as compared with 67% of participants in the control condition (Bryant et al., 1998). These results were subsequently replicated using a larger sample (Bryant, Sackville, Dang, Moulds, & Guthrie, 1999) and were maintained at a 4-year follow-up (Bryant et al., 2003).

Taken together, these studies suggest that early intervention with CBT approximately 2 weeks posttrauma may be beneficial to trauma survivors who exhibit clinical significant posttraumatic stress symptoms. Specifically, results strongly suggest that a multicomponent, short-term cognitive-behavioral treatment offering education about common trauma reactions; breathing and relaxation training; prolonged imaginal exposure to the assault; *in vivo* exposure to feared, but safe, situations; and cognitive restructuring to feared beliefs may be needed to arrest the development of PTSD symptoms and further impairment in clinically symptomatic individuals. Preliminary findings suggest that prolonged imaginal exposure to trauma memories plus cognitive restructuring may be the most critical ingredient in the treatment of acute stress disorder (Bryant et al., 1999).

Although results are promising, no studies have yet evaluated such programs for disaster survivors. In addition, given a lack of comparison to programs providing immediate physical recuperation and normalization of symptoms in the acute aftermath of a trauma, it is unclear whether CBT prevention programs are comparably better in preventing the development of symptoms (Herbert & Sageman, 2004). Arguing in favor of long-term resilience, it is also noteworthy that although the CBT groups maintained gains in all the studies, rates in the control groups also declined at long-term follow-up. In the Foa et al. (1995) study, the CBT and supportive counseling groups exhibited similar rates of PTSD at a 6-month follow-up. In addition, in a follow-up study by Bryant and colleagues rates of PTSD, although still comparably higher in the supportive counseling group (25% vs. 8%), fell by more than half over a 4-year period (56–25%) (Bryant et al., 2003). Hence, clinicians must balance the necessity of intervening early for at-risk individuals against the danger of intervening unnecessarily in cases in which individuals may recover on their own, with enough time and support.

Postcrisis Intervention: Treatment of PTSD 4 Weeks and Beyond

Empirically Supported Treatments

Expert Consensus Guidelines (Foa, Davidson, & Frances, 1999) recommend CBT and antidepressant medications as effective treatments for PTSD. Cognitive-behavioral strategies are recommended over medications in milder cases for all populations whereas CBT or medications, or a combination of the two, are offered as equally viable alternative in more severe or chronic cases. A combination of medications and CBT is recommended over CBT alone only for individuals suffering from comorbid depression and other anxiety conditions (Foa et al., 1999).

Cognitive-Behavioral Therapy

A growing literature supports the effectiveness of cognitive-behavioral treatments for the treatment of PTSD (Ballenger et al., 2000). Several versions of CBT, including exposure therapy, cognitive therapy, and stress-inoculation training, have been described in the literature. Taken together, these strategies target traumatic memories, symptom distress, and impairment in functioning. A meta-analysis of controlled and uncontrolled trials concludes that CBT is effective for the treatment of PTSD, with large observed effect sizes (van Etten & Taylor, 1998). Exposure-based strategies appear to be most effective along with cognitive restructuring of the meaning of the event. CBT programs emphasizing cognitive processing (Resick & Schnicke, 1992, 1993) and prolonged exposure (Foa et al., 1999; Foa & Rothbaum, 1998; Foa, Rothbaum, Riggs, & Murdoch, 1991) appear to be more effective than wait-list control groups (Resick, Nishith, Weaver, Astin, & Feuer, 2002), supportive counseling (Blanchard et al., 2003; Bryan et al., 2003), and non-trauma-focused behavioral interventions such as relaxation training (Marks, Novell, Noshirvani, Livanou, & Thrasher, 1998).

EXPOSURE THERAPY

Exposure therapy is designed to help individuals overcome their tendency to avoid distressing reminders of the trauma. The patient is systematically and repeatedly exposed to thoughts, images, and memories associated with the traumatic experience in imagination until the fear associated with it declines (prolonged imaginal exposure). Exposure is increasingly heightened with the use of present-tense narratives and sensory cues, with the patient ultimately required to vividly relive the traumatic experience with all salient and most fearful details of the event included (Foa et al., 1999). Once patients habituate to the memory of the traumatic event, imaginal and *in vivo* exposure are conducted to target any continued fear and avoidance of situations and events in the individual's current environment that are objectively safe. Although exposure therapy is occasionally used alone, it is typically conducted along with other cognitive-behavioral strategies (Foa, 2000).

A review of the literature shows that exposure therapy demonstrated efficacy in 12 methodologically rigorous trials (Foa, Keane, & Friedman, 2000). Exposure-based therapies have been shown to be effective for various traumatized populations, including victims of combat, accidents, rape, physical assault, and natural disasters (Bryant et al., 1999; Foa et al., 1991; Foa et al., 1999; Marks et al., 1998). Moreover, early dissemination studies indicate support for the generalizability of findings (Ballenger et al., 2000).

COGNITIVE THERAPY

Cognitive therapy is also well established as a treatment for posttraumatic symptoms and is typically used in conjunction with exposure therapy. Following Beck's original cognitive-behavioral model of anxiety (Beck et al., 1985), cognitive therapy emphasizes identification and testing of beliefs maintaining PTSD, particularly beliefs regarding continued overestimation of threat and underestimation of one's ability to cope. Cognitive restructuring helps identify and revise PTSD-related negative automatic thoughts that stem from these dysfunctional beliefs, and in doing so, it reduces negative emotions and behaviors.

The overall goal is to help patients move from being passive victims to active survivors. Specifically, automatic thoughts about the implications of the disaster, such as overestimations of the possibility of experiencing future disasters ("A terrorist attack may happen again"), assumptions that the disaster has made an indelible, global, and permanent change in their lives ("I will never be the same again"), overgeneralizations of the fear to normal life events (e.g., riding the subway), and personalizations of the event ("Bad luck follows me") are modified to reduce the sense of continued threat from the traumatic event.

Interpretations made by individuals regarding their behavior during the disaster ("I should have stayed behind to help my friend"), regarding their initial PTSD symptoms ("I mentally snapped when the earth began to move"), regarding the behavior of others in the aftermath of events ("No one appreciates what I have gone through"), and regarding the consequences of the trauma ("I can no longer be effective as a mother") are also modified.

In a consecutive case series, 20 patients treated with cognitive therapy showed highly significant improvement in symptoms of PTSD, depression, and anxiety (Ehlers, Clark, Hackmann, McManus, & Fennel, 2005). A subsequent randomized controlled trial comparing cognitive therapy to a 3-month wait-list condition for survivors of a variety of traumatic experiences found that cognitive therapy led to greater reduction in symptoms and disability (Ehlers et al., 2005). Treatment gains were well maintained at 6-month follow-up and good treatment outcome was related to greater changes in dysfunctional posttraumatic cognitions.

The benefits of cognitive therapy have been confirmed in disaster survivors (Clark, 2000; Ehlers et al., 2003) and appear to be generalizable to community-based clinics (Clark, 2000). For example, a consecutive series of 91 patients with PTSD resulting from a car bomb that exploded in the center of Omagh, Northern Ireland, in 1998, were treated 10 months after the event, for an average of eight cognitive therapy sessions. Clinically significant improvements were observed, with the degree of improvement being comparable to that reported in prior research trials (Clark, 2000).

Overall, although cognitive restructuring appears to be effective (Foa et al., 2000; Marks et al., 1998), some studies have found that cognitive restructuring in addition to exposure therapy may be no more effective than exposure alone (Foa & Rauch, 2004; Marks et al., 1998).

STRESS INOCULATION TRAINING

Stress inoculation training (SIT; Meichenbaum, 1985) is a multicomponent intervention that teaches patients effective coping skills; relaxation, guided self-dialogue, covert modeling (successful confrontation of an anxiety-provoking situation in imagination), role playing, and thought stopping (e.g., subvocally saying the word "stop!" to interrupt intrusive thoughts). Evidence suggests that SIT is effective but may not be as effective as prolonged exposure and that it may not add anything above and beyond prolonged exposure alone (Foa et al., 1991; Foa et al., 1999). Moreover, research suggests that attempting to suppress trauma-related cognitions may, in fact, paradoxically increase the frequency and intensity of the thoughts (Harvey & Bryant, 1998).

In summary, CBT is considered to be the first-line treatment option for individuals diagnosed with PTSD, with a special emphasis on exposure therapy to trauma memories and current feared but objectively safe situations. Cognitive therapy is also recommended to modify dysfunctional cognitions that maintain a sense of current and future threat. Expert consensus guidelines recommend that medications be considered only in combination with CBT and as viable alternatives to CBT alone in adults when the course is chronic or severe, and in children only when symptoms are severe. A combination of medications and CBT is recommended over CBT alone only when comorbidity is present.

SEPTEMBER 11, 2001: A CASE STUDY

T. F. is a single, 35-year-old banker who was at work in his office directly opposite the World Trade Center on September 11, 2001. T. F. described 9/11 as the "day that changed my life forever." He recalled stepping over body parts as he fled the building and being "swallowed up" by billowing smoke. He described feeling completely suffocated and sure that he would never resurface.

In the days following the attack, T. F. reported disjointed memories of the day's events: how he had learned that the North Tower had been struck; how he had fled down the stairwell and out into the street; and how he had walked 3 miles to a friend's home in Chelsea. He described blurred memories combined with vivid snapshots of events that terrorized him on a daily basis. Particularly vivid snapshots included the view of the World Trade Center from his office, the south tower being hit, office workers leaping to their deaths, and the utter darkness and heat in the stairwell as he descended to the lobby. He was unable to shake these images and often awoke in a cold sweat after nightmares featuring these and other events.

Immediately after the disaster, all residents of T. F.'s apartment complex in Battery Park City (adjacent to the World Trade Center site) were barred from returning to their homes. He described feeling desolate, overwhelmed, and out of control over the next few days as he arranged temporary housing, contacted family and friends, and purchased amenities for his day-to-day needs.

T. F. attended a group therapy session arranged by his bank a week later and remembered "spinning out of control" as he heard other survivors describe their experiences. He experienced a panic attack in the room and began to feel as if he were suffocating. He left the group therapy session after an hour and did not return.

T. F. presented for treatment 9 months later, at the suggestion of his mother, who felt that his evaluation of his recovery was inaccurate. He described feeling better but not "back to the way [he] was." He said he was seeking treatment because his bank was planning to relocate his department back to its quarters downtown and he felt unable to make the move.

When he presented for treatment, T. F. reported symptoms of heightened anxiety, increased muscle tension, irritability, nightmares, and intrusive thoughts about the events surrounding 9/11. He reported feeling jumpy and watchful at all times and stated that he could not tolerate loud noises. T. F. also described a sense of dread on encountering reminders of the attack (e.g., smells associated with the day, traveling to the general area of the disaster, and the drone of a jet engine). He intentionally attempted to avoid anything that evoked memories of 9/11 for him.

T. F. recalled his former excitement about living in a city that was always in motion, and felt that he had "fit in well" with the city's rhythm. Now, T. F. felt his pulse quicken with each stranger who walked by, grew irritable when fighting his way through throngs of tourists, and could not wait to reach home. He fantasized about moving to a small town far away from the dangers that he sensed lurked everywhere in Manhattan.

T. F. also reported a substantial decline in social support following 9/11. He was unable to return home immediately following the attack and had to live with a friend until he was able to get insurance to pay for temporary housing. Later, he refused to move back to Battery Park City. Instead, he rented an apartment on Manhattan's Upper East Side, where he had few acquaintances, no friends, and no familiarity with local services and community resources.

In addition, although the bank relocated to temporary quarters in midtown, most of his coworkers were shifted to another branch in Connecticut. By the time T. F. had begun adjusting to his new quarters, he was informed that he would be relocated again, back to refurbished offices near the World Trade Center site. He described this move as "impossible."

T. F. had also been unable to meet with any family members for several weeks following the event. When his mother and sister flew to New York from California, he recalled, he had felt alienated from and disappointed in them. He felt they neither understood what he had experienced nor adequately empathized with his situation. At the time he presented for treatment, T. F. had distanced himself from his parents and sisters, complaining of deep resentment at what he perceived to be their lack of understanding of his ordeal. T. F. had also kept his old friends at a distance, preferring the company of newer friends from his new neighborhood because he felt they understood him.

Although T. F. had no prior history of treatment, the intake evaluation revealed that he had a prior history of undiagnosed unipolar major depressive disorder when he had completed college. The episode had lasted 6 months and had led him to drop out of college for one semester. He had never sought treatment for the episode because he saw it as a weakness and claimed that he had "overcome it by sheer willpower."

A structured diagnostic interview conducted a week after T. F. presented for treatment revealed that T. F. met the criteria in the *Diagnostic and Statistical Manual of Mental Disorders*, fourth edition (DSM-IV; American Psychiatric Association, 1994) for PTSD. His symptom severity score on the Posttraumatic Stress Diagnostic Scale (Foa, Cashman, Jaycox & Perry, 1997) was 34. He scored a total of 24 on the Beck Anxiety Inventory and 15 on the Beck Depression Inventory.

T. F. had the following risk factors for developing PTSD:

Pretrauma (individual) factors: single; male; prior psychiatric history
Trauma factors: proximity to the disaster; intensity of exposure; seeing the attacks in person; disaster characterized by mass violence
Posttrauma factors: relocation; decline in social support; cognitive and behavioral reactions to the trauma

Cognitive Conceptualization

Cognitive models suggest that PTSD occurs when individuals process the event and/or its sequelae in a manner that creates appraisals of either current or impending threat. In keeping with this model, T. F. reported unabated and specific concerns that he would be the victim of another terrorist attack. He felt that he would never be the same, that 9/11 was an instrument of permanent, negative change in his life rather than a time-limited event from which he would recover. He often stated that his old self had "died" and that a different person had emerged from the "ashes of 9/11."

The cognitive model suggests that individuals with PTSD tend to overgeneralize the fear from the trauma to normal life events and thereby perceive normal events as more dangerous than they are in reality. Although T. F. was able to mask his fears publicly, he reported that he felt fearful of being attacked as he walked to work, worked in his office, and rode in cabs, and that he would never be safe again.

The cognitive model also suggests that individuals who experience mental defeat, dissociation, numbness, confusion, and being overwhelmed by sensory impressions during the traumatic event appear to be more likely to develop biased appraisals over time and to develop chronic PTSD (Ehlers & Clark, 1999). T. F. reported several maladaptive interpretations about his behaviors on 9/11, his initial symptoms, and the effects of 9/11 on his life. He agonized about events that he believed he could have handled differently. For example, he remembered feeling frozen, confused, and help-less during the attack; perceived this reaction as having "gone to pieces"; and thus labeled himself a weakling and a coward. He firmly believed that if he had had better command of his senses, he could have helped many of his coworkers. He stated that he had been "tested" and that he had "failed." He now believed that not only had his luck changed but that he had been revealed as a coward who could not face dangerous situations with courage.

T. F. provided several interpretations about how others had behaved or treated him since 9/11. He believed his family did not understand him and were insufficiently supportive of him. He insisted that both his family and his old friends wanted him to put 9/11 behind him and move on, but only because that would be easier for them. Their focus was to make themselves feel better rather than help him, he claimed. He expressed anger and resentment that his family and friends were more focused on alleviating their own pain and anxiety than on his.

Congruent with the cognitive model of PTSD (Ehlers & Clark, 2000), T. F.'s memory for events was blurred and he could not provide a continuous account of his activities on the day of the attack. However, he experienced vivid intrusive thoughts that plagued him throughout the day and at night. These specific memories could be triggered by myriad stimuli, such as smelling smoke or feeling hot, that only further reinforced his belief that he was a coward.

As a result of these negative appraisals, T. F. experienced a number of negative emotions, including anxiety, sadness, guilt, and shame. Although he was able to go to work and appeared superficially to be functioning well, an in-depth assessment revealed that T. F. employed a number of maladaptive strategies to cope with these negative emotions.

By the time he presented for treatment, T. F.'s alcohol consumption had returned to normal after several weeks of excessive alcohol consumption immediately following the disaster. However, he did not travel by subway or bus but instead opted to take cabs or walk but refused cabs with drivers who seemed (to him) to be Muslim. T. F. was always on his guard and often walked out of his office to check that "the outside world" was proceeding as usual. His "emergency backpack," which he kept with him at all times, contained a change of clothes, a toothbrush, a Swiss Army knife, a flash-light, medicines, a vacuum-packed meal, and a bottle of water. He avoided high floors in any building, and other than traveling to work, he rarely moved around Manhattan, especially the area south of Canal Street with its proximity to the World Trade Center site. He escaped settings where he felt hot or smelled or saw smoke (e.g., a barbecue). These coping strategies maintained T. F.'s appraisals of the world as a dangerous place, perpetuating his PTSD symptoms.

T. F.'s symptoms at the time he presented for treatment included the following:

- Cognitive:
  - Intrusive phenomena: intrusive thoughts, flashbacks, nightmares.
  - Automatic thoughts: "I will never be the same again"; "I reacted badly to 9/11."

- Cognitive processes: overestimating danger, catastrophizing, underestimating own ability to cope, "should" statements, self-focused attention, personalization, overresponsibility.
- Assumptions: "I'm always in danger and so must take extraordinary precautions."
- Schemata: "I am weak and vulnerable to danger"; "People are threatening and may harm me"; "The world is a dangerous place."
- Affective: anxiety, irritability, sadness, guilt, shame.
- Physiological: muscle tension, difficulty staying asleep, fatigue, exaggerated startle response, hypervigilance, restlessness.
- Behavioral coping strategies:
  - Avoidance behaviors: inability to travel on public transportation, travel in general vicinity of disaster site, go to high floors, move around Manhattan.
  - Safety behaviors: carrying emergency equipment constantly, monitoring news reports or leaving office regularly to check on occurrence of further disasters.
  - Escape behaviors: shying away from contact with individuals of Middle Eastern descent, retreat from smoke and perceived heat.

Treatment

The goal of acute crisis intervention is to provide "psychological first aid" in order to reduce initial distress and foster both short- and long-term adaptive functioning through natural emotional processing (National Child Traumatic Stress Network and National Center for PTSD, 2004; Padesky et al., 2002). In the acute aftermath of 9/11, T. F. promptly received support through FEMA (Federal Emergency Management Administration) and other agencies to address his urgent needs for safety and physical shelter. He expressed profound gratitude that he did not encounter into bureaucratic obstacles and believed that his postdisaster physical assistance went as well as he could have imagined.

T. F.'s need for psychological sustenance, however, was not addressed as well. About 10 days after 9/11, he was referred to a group therapy session that he recalled as an extremely negative experience. He reported that he was not in the "correct frame of mind" to attend therapy because he was not sleeping and was extremely tired. He recalled listening with a heavy heart to other people's reactions and particularly remembers one of his coworkers crying, a fact that had both embarrassed and troubled him. T. F. described feelings of being suffocated and trapped as he heard seemingly endless stories about 9/11. He described being told in the session that he might have PTSD and might need treatment, which had triggered his premature departure from the session because, he said, he became fearful that he would go insane and never recover.

When he presented for treatment, T. F. was educated about CBT and antidepressant medications as effective treatments for PTSD (Ballenger et al., 2000). Based on Expert Consensus Guidelines (Foa et al., 1999), a multicomponent CBT treatment was initiated, offering education about common trauma reactions; breathing and relaxation training; prolonged imaginal exposure to the assault; *in vivo* exposure to feared, but safe, situations; and cognitive restructuring to feared beliefs. Prolonged imaginal exposure to trauma memories plus cognitive restructuring comprised the bulk of treatment sessions.

In contrast to the messages he had received during his group therapy session, T. F. was educated about normal and expected responses to trauma, such as anxiety, nightmares, and irritability, including that these effects were transient for the vast majority of individuals. His symptoms and reactions on 9/11 were normalized and validated as real yet temporary. Using the cognitive-behavioral model of PTSD and evolutionary models of anxiety, T. F. was helped to understand why his symptoms were adaptive in the presence of danger but had not abated over time. The goals and treatment rationale were outlined and linked to specific components of treatment. T. F. exhibited significant relief combined with some initial skepticism on hearing optimistic messages about his recovery.

T. F.'s generalized hyperarousal and difficulty staying asleep also became an immediate target of treatment. Following basic sleep hygiene training, T. F. learned deep, diaphragmatic breathing and muscle relaxation exercises early in treatment to help him sleep and to reduce his level of physiological arousal. He experienced immediate relief, which resulted in his increased optimism and commitment to therapy.

In light of findings that the size, vitality, and closeness of social networks are strongly related to positive mental health outcomes (Norris, 2001), support networks of friends, family, and other individuals suffering from PTSD were created to facilitate T. F.'s therapeutic improvement. Although T. F. was unable to immediately bridge the distance with his family and close friends, he gradually reconnected with these networks as his symptoms abated over the course of treatment. He was able to accept the support offered by others instead of drawing away from them as he became aware that his sense of resentment had partially grown out of his misperceptions of how others had behaved toward him.

An assessment of daily living revealed that on weekday evenings and weekends, T. F. typically stayed home or left the city. Through a discussion of prior interests and hobbies, T. F. was encouraged to pursue past hobbies such as jogging in the park and visiting with friends.

Cognitive Therapy

Following Beck's original cognitive-behavioral model of anxiety (Beck et al., 1985), cognitive restructuring was employed to help T. F. accept that he had experienced a tragic, catastrophic event that had affected him significantly but not permanently.

T. F. slowly accepted that his reactions during 9/11 and the days following were normal and expected. He was helped to see that recovery was possible even in the wake of a catastrophic event such as 9/11 and that his symptoms had persisted because he had used avoidance as a way of coping with his anxiety. T. F. was also helped to identify, test, and revise his tendency to overestimate the likelihood of his falling victim to future terrorist attacks.

His assumptions and beliefs that the attack had permanently disabled him, rendering him weak and vulnerable, had supported his sense of acute distress and thus were repeatedly modified. He started to understand that his initial paralysis and subsequent urge to escape were instinctive and adaptive reactions to danger. This helped reduce his guilt and anxiety about his inability to help others and his urge to flee.

T. F. also recognized that his coping methods were perpetuating his sense of danger and the resulting anxiety. This provided immense relief for him because it challenged prior assumptions that he was intrinsically weak. As his optimism about his inherent resilience increased, T. F. also examined and modified his earlier harsh judgments regarding the behavior of others and slowly repaired his fractured relationships with friends and family. His tendency to issue global judgments and labels, toward both himself and persons of Middle Eastern descent, was also modified.

Exposure Therapy

To prepare for future exposure sessions, T. F. was asked at the outset of treatment to keep a journal of all his intrusive phenomena. Initially, the journal contained a jumble of thoughts, memories, and images that spontaneously intruded on his consciousness. As his hyperarousal and general anxiety lessened via relaxation and restructuring exercises, T. F. was encouraged to piece the scenes together sequentially and develop a narrative of the day. T. F. systematically confronted memories of the disaster during and between sessions, using the script he developed and other aids to recreate the event such as videotaped footage, photos, and newspaper articles. Detailed and painful images, such as his initial paralysis and confusion, his slow descent down the dark stairwell, his horror at encountering body parts as he fled the disaster site, were added in over the course of later sessions as T. F. habituated to initial exposure sessions.

Once T. F. habituated to the memories of 9/11, imaginal and *in vivo* exposure were conducted to target present-day situations that he continued to avoid, endured with distress, or endured with the aid of safety behaviors. Although the ultimate goal of exposure was to increase his overall range of movement throughout Manhattan and his overall hierarchy contained a wide range of situations creating tremendous anxiety, a working hierarchy was created to help T. F. reach his specific goal of relocating back to his downtown branch. Initial items required T. F. to travel south of Canal Street, first by car and then by public transportation. These were followed by items requiring more proximal exposure to the disaster site. Because T. F. was unable to discard all safety behaviors at the outset, safety behaviors such as carrying his emergency backpack were built into his exposure hierarchy and shed as he moved upward.

Imaginal exposure sessions were also conducted in preparation for *in vivo* exposure to situations creating more severe anxiety (e.g., standing near the disaster site and walking down the stairwell in his office). Finally, T. F. was gradually exposed to both interoceptive symptoms (e.g., heat and increased heartbeat) and external cues triggering continued anxiety (e.g., smoke and sound of jet engines).

Within 4 months of beginning treatment, T. F. exhibited a significant decline in overall anxiety and irritability, reported minimal flashbacks and nightmares, significantly reduced hyperarousal, and improved sleep. After 8 months, T. F. had achieved his goal of successfully relocating back to his office. Once the majority of his acute symptoms declined, sessions were reduced to every other week and became focused on maintaining gains and preventing relapse.

CONCLUSION

Research shows that the majority of disaster survivors experience common reactions that abate over time, suggesting that resilience is the most common outcome. Based on the available evidence, crisis interventions in the acute aftermath should attend to basic safety and physical needs, foster social support, educate survivors about normal, transient responses to trauma, and prevent pathological beliefs about the possibility of permanent damage.

An essential aspect of crisis intervention is identifying the subgroup of individuals who face increased risk of psychological impairment and developing targeted interventions to address their needs. Several risk factors, including gender, age, prior psychiatric illness, degree of exposure, a loss of resources, and specific cognitive styles, appear to be related to the development of PTSD. CBT prevention programs emphasizing exposure and cognitive restructuring have demonstrated efficacy by reducing the development of PTSD in at-risk individuals. Clinicians must balance the necessity of intervening early for at-risk individuals against the danger of intervening unnecessarily in cases in which individuals may recover on their own, with enough time and support.

Substantial research points to CBT as the first-line treatment for individuals who develop PTSD. Exposure-based strategies, emphasizing habituation to the memory of the event, and exposure to continued fear and avoidance of objectively safe events, appear to be the most effective. Cognitive therapy to modify dysfunctional cognitions that maintain a sense of current and future threat is also recommended. Recent developments in new generations of CBT emphasizing acceptance and mindfulness also offer future promise as emerging treatments for PTSD (Orsillo & Batten, 2005).

REFERENCES

Abenhaim L., Dab, W., & Salmi, L. R. (1992). Study of civilian victims of terrorist attacks. *Journal of Clinical Epidemiology, 45,* 103–109.

Ali, T., Dunmore, E., Clark, D., & Ehlers, A. (2002). The role of negative beliefs in posttraumatic stress disorder: A comparison of assault victims and non-victims. *Behavioural and Cognitive Psychotherapy, 30,* 249–257.

American Psychiatric Association. (1994). *Diagnostic and statistical manual of mental disorders* (4th ed.). Washington, DC: Author.

American Psychiatric Association. (2000). *Diagnostic and statistical manual of mental disorders* (4th ed., text rev.). Washington, DC: Author.

Ballenger, J. C., Davidson, J., Lecrubier, Y., Nutt, D. J., Foa, E. B., Kessler, R. C., et al. (2000). Consensus statement on posttraumatic stress disorder from the International Consensus Group on depression and anxiety. *Journal of Clinical Psychiatry, 61*(Suppl. 5), 60–65.

Beck, A. T., Emery, G., & Greenberg, R. (1985). *Anxiety disorders and phobias: A cognitive perspective*. New York: Basic Books.

Bisson, J. I., & Deahl, M. P. (1994). Psychological debriefing and prevention of post-traumatic stress. *British Journal of Psychiatry, 165*, 717–720.

Blanchard, E. B., Hickling, E. J., Devineni, T., Veazey, C. H., Galovski, T. E., Mundy, E., et al. (2003). A controlled evaluation of cognitive behavioral therapy for posttraumatic stress in motor vehicle accident survivors. *Behaviour Research and Therapy, 421*, 79–96.

Breslau, N., Davis, G. C., Andreski, P., & Peterson, E. (1991). Traumatic events and posttraumatic stress disorder in an urban population of young adults. *Archives of General Psychiatry, 48*, 216–222.

Breslau, N., Kessler, R., Chilcoat, H., Schultz, L., Davis, G., & Andreski, P. (1998). Trauma and posttraumatic stress disorder in the community. *Archives of General Psychiatry, 55*, 626–632.

Bryant, R. A., Harvey, A. G., Dang, S. T., Sackville, T., & Basten, C. (1998). Treatment of acute stress disorder: A comparison of cognitive-behavioral therapy and supportive counseling. *Journal of Consulting and Clinical Psychology, 66*, 862–866.

Bryant, R. A., Moulds, M. L., & Nixon, R. V. D. (2003). Cognitive behaviour therapy of acute stress disorder: A four-year follow-up. *Behaviour Research and Therapy, 41*, 489–494.

Bryant, R. A., Sackville, T., Dang, S. T., Moulds, M., & Guthrie, R. (1999). Treating acute stress disorder: An evaluation of cognitive behavior therapy and supportive counseling techniques. *American Journal of Psychiatry, 156*, 1780–1786.

Cancro, R. (2004). Mental health impact of September 11. *Molecular Psychiatry, 9*, 1055–1056

Canino, G. J., Bravo, M., Rubio-Stipec, M., & Woodbury, M. (1990). The impact of disaster on mental health: Prospective and retrospective analyses. *International Journal of Mental Health, 19*, 51–69.

Clark, D. M. (2000, June). *A community survey of the psychological consequences of the Omagh bomb and predictors of PTSD*. Paper presented as part of a symposium on the effects of the Omagh bombing presented at the International Congress of Cognitive Therapy, Catania, Italy.

Curran, P., Bell, P., Murray, A., Loughrey, G., Roddy, R., & Rocke, L. (1990). Psychological consequences of the Enniskillen bombing. *British Journal of Psychiatry, 156*, 479–482.

Devilly, G. J., & Cotton, P. (2003). Psychological debriefing and the workplace: Defining a concept, controversies and guidelines for intervention. *Australian Psychologist, 38*, 144–150.

Devilly, G. J., & Cotton, P. (2004). Caveat emptor, caveat venditor, and critical incident stress de-briefing/management (CISD/M). *Australian Psychologist, 39*(1), 35–40.

Disaster Mental Health Response Handbook. (2000). Retrieved January 11, 2006, from *www.nswiop.nsw.edu.au/ Resources/Disaster_Handbook.pdf*

Dunmore, E., Clark, D. M., & Ehlers, A. (1999). Cognitive factors involved in the onset and maintenance of posttraumatic stress disorder (PTSD) after physical or sexual assault. *Behaviour Research and Therapy, 37*(9), 809–829.

Dunmore, E., Clark, D. M., & Ehlers, A. (2001). A prospective investigation of the role of cognitive factors in persistent posttraumatic stress disorder (PTSD) after physical or sexual assault. *Behaviour Research and Therapy, 39*(9), 1063–1084.

Ehlers, A., & Clark, D. M. (2000). A cognitive model of posttraumatic stress disorder. *Behaviour Research and Therapy, 38*, 319–345.

Ehlers, A., Clark, D. M., Hackmann, A., McManus, F., & Fennell, M. (2005). Cognitive therapy for post-traumatic stress disorder: Development and evaluation. *Behaviour Research and Therapy, 43*(4), 413–431.

Ehlers, A., Clark, D. M., Hackmann, A., McManus, F., Fennell, M., Herbert, C., et al. (2003). A randomized controlled trial of cognitive therapy, a self-help booklet, and repeated assessments as early interventions for posttraumatic stress disorder. *Archives of General Psychiatry, 60*, 1024–1032.

Ericsson (n.d.). *Disaster statistics: What is a "disaster"?* Retrieved January 21, 2006, from *www.ericsson.com/ericsson/corporate_responsibility/ericssonresponse/awareness/statistics.shtml*

Foa, E. B. (2000). Psychosocial treatment of posttraumatic stress disorder. *Journal of Clinical Psychiatry, 61*(Suppl. 5), 43–48.

Foa, E. B., Cashman, L., Jaycox, L., & Perry, K. (1997). The validation of a self-report measure of PTSD: The Posttraumatic Diagnostic Scale-TM (PDSTM). *Psychological Assessment, 9*(4), 445–451.

Foa, E. B., Davidson, J. R. T., & Frances, A. (1999). The Expert consensus guide series: Treatment of PTSD. *Journal of Clinical Psychiatry, 60*(16), 10–33.

Foa, E. B., Hearst-Ikeda, D., & Perry, K. J. (1995). Evaluation of a brief cognitive-behavioral program for the prevention of chronic PTSD in recent assault victims. *Journal of Consulting and Clinical Psychology, 63*(6), 948–955.

Foa, E. B., Keane, T. M., & Friedman, M. J. (2000). Guidelines for treatment of PTSD. *Journal of Traumatic Stress, 13*(4), 539–588.

Foa, E. B., & Rauch, S. A. M. (2004). Cognitive changes during prolonged exposure versus prolonged exposure plus cognitive restructuring in female assault survivors with posttraumatic stress disorder. *Journal of Consulting and Clinical Psychology, 72*, 879–884.

Foa, E. B., & Rothbaum, B. O. (1998). *Treating the trauma of rape: Cognitive behavioral therapy for PTSD.* New York: Guilford Press.

Foa, E. B., Rothbaum, B. O., Riggs, D. S., & Murdoch, T. B. (1991). Treatment of posttraumatic stress disorder in rape victims: A comparison between cognitive-behavioral procedures and counseling. *Journal of Consulting and Clinical Psychology, 59*, 715–723.

Fullerton, C. S., Ursano, R. J., Norwood, A. E., & Halloway, H. H. (2003). Terrorism and disaster. In R. J. Ursano, C. S. Fullerton, & A. E. Norwood (Eds.), *Terrorism and disaster: Individual and community mental health interventions.* Cambridge, UK: Cambridge University Press.

Galea, S., Ahern, J., Resnick, H., Kilpatrick, D., Bucuvalas, M., Gold, J., et al. (2002). Psychological sequelae of the September 11 terrorist attacks in New York City. *New England Journal of Medicine, 346*, 982–987.

Galea, S., Vlahov, D., Resnick, H., Ahern, J., Susser, E., Gold, J., et al. (2003). Trends of probable post-traumatic stress disorder in New York City after the September 11 terrorist attacks. *American Journal of Epidemiology, 158*(6), 514–524.

Gerrity, E. T., & Steinglass, P. (2003). Relocation stress following catastrophic events. In R. J. Ursano, C. S. Fullerton, & A. E. Norwood (Eds.), *Terrorism and disaster: Individual and community mental health interventions.* Cambridge, UK: Cambridge University Press.

Gidron, Y. (2002). Posttraumatic stress disorder after terrorist attacks: A review. *Journal of Nervous and Mental Disease, 190*(2), 118–121.

Hamblen, J. (2005, September). *Terrorist attacks and children—A National Center for PTSD fact sheet.* Retrieved December 11, 2005, from *www.ncptsd.va.gov/facts/ disasters/fs_children_disaster.html*

Harvey, A., & Bryant, R. (1998). The relationship between acute stress disorder and posttraumatic stress disorder: A prospective evaluation of motor vehicle accident survivors. *Journal of Consulting and Clinical Psychology, 66*(3), 507–512.

Herbert, J. D., & Forman, E. M. (2006). Posttraumatic stress disorder. In J. E. Fisher & W. O'Donohue (Eds.), *Practice guidelines for evidence based psychotherapy* (pp. 555–566). New York: Springer.

Herbert, J. D., & Sageman, M. (2004). "First do no harm": Emerging guidelines for the treatment of posttraumatic reactions. In G. M. Rosen (Ed.), *Posttraumatic stress disorder: Issues and controversies* (pp. 213–232). Hoboken, NJ: Wiley.

Hiley-Young, B., & Gerrity, E. T. (1994). Critical incident stress debriefing (CISD): Value and limitations in disaster response. *NCP Clinical Quarterly, 4*(2). Retrieved July 13, 2002, from *www.ncptsd.org/treatment/cq/v4/n2/hiley-yo.html*

Hoven, C. W., Mandell, D. J., & Duarte, C. S. (2003). Mental health of New York City public school children after 9/11: An epidemiologic investigation. In S. Coates, J. L. Rosenthal, & D. S. Schecter (Eds.), *September 11: Trauma and Human Bonds* (pp. 51–74). Hillsdale, NJ: Analytic Press.

Kessler, R., Sonnega, A., Bromet, E., Hughes, M., & Nelson, C. (1995). Posttraumatic stress disorder in the National Comorbidity Survey. *Archives of General Psychiatry, 52*, 1048–1060.

Kilpatrick, D., Saunders, B., Veronen, L., Best, C., & Von, J. (1987). Criminal victimization: Lifetime prevalence, reporting to police, and psychological impact. *Crime and Delinquency, 33*(4), 479–489.

Litz, B. T., Gray, M. J., Bryant, R. A., & Adler, A. B. (2002). Early intervention for trauma: Current status and future directions. *Clinical Psychology: Science and Practice, 9*(2), 112–134.

Marks, I. M., Lovell, K., Noshirvani, H., Livanou, M., & Thrasher, S. (1998). Treatment of post-traumatic stress disorder by exposure and/or cognitive restructuring. A controlled study. *Archives of General Psychiatry, 55*, 317–325

McFarlane, A. C. (1986). Posttraumatic morbidity of a disaster: A study of cases presenting for psychiatric treatment. *Journal of Nervous and Mental Disease, 147*(1), 4–13.

McGinn, L. K., & Massey, K. (2004, November). *The relationship between cognitive factors and coping styles and comorbid symptoms of PTSD, worry, and depression in the NYC Metropolitan area two years after the attack on the world trade center.* Paper presented at the annual convention of the Association for the Advancement of Behavior Therapy, New Orleans.

McNally, R. J. (2004). Conceptual problems with the DSM-IV criteria for posttraumatic stress disorder. In G. M. Rosen (Ed.), *Posttraumatic stress disorder: Issues and controversies* (pp. 1–14). Chichester, UK: Wiley.

Mitchell, J. (1983). When disaster strikes . . . : The critical incident stress debriefing process. *Journal of Emergency Medical Services, 8*, 36–38.

National Child Traumatic Stress Network and National Center for PTSD. (2004, September). *Psychological first aid: Field operations guide.* Retrieved June 2006 from *www.ncptsd.va.gov/pfa/PFA_9_6_05_Final.pdf*

Norris, F. H. (2001, September). *50,000 disaster victims speak: An empirical review of the empirical literature, 1981–2001.* Retrieved December 11, 2005, from *obssr.od.nih.gov/Activities/911/disaster-impact.pdf*

Norris, F. H. (2002). Disasters in urban context. *Journal of Urban Health, 79*(3), 308–314.

Norris, F. H., Byrne, C. M., Diaz, E., & Kaniasty, K. (2005, May). *Psychosocial resources in the aftermath of natural and human-caused disasters: A review of the empirical literature, with implications for intervention—A National Center for PTSD fact sheet.* Retrieved December 11, 2005, from *www.ncptsd.va.gov/facts/disasters/fs_resources.html*

Norris, F. H., Friedman, M. J., Watson, P. J., Byrne, C. M., Diaz, E., & Kaniasty, K. (2002). 60,000 disaster victims speak: Part I. An empirical review of the empirical literature, 1981–2001. *Psychiatry, 65*(3), 207–239.

North, C. S., Nixon, S. J., Shariat, S., Mallonee, S., McMillen, J. C., Sptiznagel, E. L., et al. (1999). Psychiatric disorders among survivors of the Oklahoma City bombing. *Journal of the American Medical Association, 282*(8), 755–762.

Norwood, A. E., Ursano, R. J., & Fullerton, C. S. (2000). Disaster psychiatry: Principles and practice. *Psychiatric Quarterly, 71*(3), 207–226.

Orsillo, S. M., & Batten, S. V. (2005). Acceptance and commitment therapy in the treatment of posttraumatic stress disorder. *Behavior Modification, 29*, 95–129.

Padesky, C. A., Candido, D., Cohen, A., Gluhoski, V., McGinn, L.K., Sisti, M., et al. (2002). *Academy of Cognitive Therapy's Trauma Task Force Report.* Retrieved January, 2002,

from *academyofct.org/Info/Zoom.asp?InfoID=150&szparent=252&szPath=Add&InfoGroup=
General&InfoType=Article&SessionID=gugukqweq*

Perkonigg, A., Kessler, R., Storz, S., & Wittchen, H. (2000). Traumatic events and post-traumatic stress disorder in the community: Prevalence, risk factors and comorbidity. *Acta Psychiatrica Scandinavica, 101,* 46–59.

Raphael, B., & Meldrum, L. (1995). Does debriefing after psychological trauma work? *British Medical Journal, 310,* 1479–1480.

Resick, P. A. (2004, November). *Beyond cognitive processing: A reconceptualization of post-trauma pathology.* Presidential address conducted at the Association for the Advancement of Behavior Therapy Annual Convention, New Orleans.

Resick, P. A., Nishith, P., Weaver, T. L., Astin, M. C., & Feuer, C. A. (2002). A comparison of cognitive processing therapy with prolonged exposure and a waiting condition for the treatment of posttraumatic stress disorder in female rape victims. *Journal of Consulting and Clinical Psychology, 70,* 867–879

Resick, P. A., & Schnicke, M. K. (1992). Cognitive processing therapy for rape victims. *Journal of Consulting and Clinical Psychology, 60,* 748–756.

Resick, P. A., & Schnicke, M. K. (1993). *Cognitive processing therapy for rape victims.* Newbury Park, CA: Sage.

Rubonis, A. V., & Bickman, L. (1991). Psychological impairment in the wake of disaster: The disaster-psychopathology relationship. *Psychological Bulletin, 109*(3), 384–399.

Schlenger, W. E., Caddell, J. M., Ebert, L., Jordan, B. K., Rourke, K. M., Wilson, D., et al. (2002). Psychological reactions to terrorist attacks: Findings from the National Study of Americans' Reactions to September 11. *Journal of the American Medical Association, 288*(5), 581–588.

Shalev, A. Y., Adessky, R., Boker, R., Bargai, N., Cooper, R., Freedman, S., et al. (2003). Clinical intervention for survivors of prolonged adversities. In R. J. Ursano, C. S. Fullerton, & A. E. Norwood (Eds.), *Terrorism and disaster: Individual and community mental health interventions* (pp. 162–188). Cambridge, UK: Cambridge University Press.

Shore, J. H., Tatum, E. L., & Vollmer, W. M. (1986). Psychiatric reactions to disaster: The Mount St. Helens experience. *American Journal of Psychiatry, 143*(5), 590–595.

Silove, D., & Bryant, R. (2006). Rapid assessment of mental health needs after disasters. *Journal of the American Medical Association, 296*(5), 576–578.

Smith, E. M., North, C. S., McCool, R. E., & Shea, J. M. (1990). Acute postdisaster psychiatric disorders: Identification of persons at risk. *American Journal of Psychiatry, 147*(2), 202–206.

Solomon, S. D., & Green, B. L. (1992). Mental health effects of natural and human-made disasters. *PTSD Research Quarterly, 3*(1), 1–8.

Thailand Center of Excellence for Life Sciences. (2006). *TCELS Projects: Tsunami PTSD Genomics Center.* Retrieved March 13, 2006, from *www.tcels.or.th/project/* TSUNAMI%20PTSD%20GENOMICS%20CENTER_en.pdf

Udwin, O., Boyle, S., Yule, W., Bolton, D., & O'Ryan, D. (2000). Risk factors for long-term psychological effects of a disaster experienced in adolescence: Predictors of post traumatic stress disorder. *Journal of Child Psychology and Psychiatry, 41*(8), 969–979.

van der Kolk, B. A., McFarlane, A. C., & Weisaeth, L. (Eds.). (1996). *Traumatic stress: The effects of overwhelming experiences on mind, body, and society.* New York: Guilford Press.

van Etten, M. L., & Taylor, S. (1998). Comparative efficacy of treatments for post-traumatic stress disorder: A meta-analysis. *Clinical Psychology and Psychotherapy, 5,* 126–144.

Voelker, R. (2006). Post-Katrina mental health needs prompt group to compile disaster medical guide. *Journal of the American Medical Association, 295,* 259–260.

Werner, E., & Smith, R. (1982). *Vulnerable but invincible: A longitudinal study of resilient children and youth.* New York: McGraw-Hill.

Yehuda, R. (1999). *Risk factors for posttraumatic stress disorder.* Washington, DC: American Psychiatric Press.

Yehuda, R., & McFarlane, A. C. (1995). Conflict between current knowledge about posttraumatic stress disorder and its original conceptual basis. *American Journal of Psychiatry, 152,* 1705–1713.

Yehuda, R., & McFarlane, A. C. (1997). Introduction. In R. Yehuda & A. C. McFarlane (Eds.), *Psychobiology of posttraumatic stress disorder* (pp. 11–15). New York: New York Academy of Sciences.

Yeomans, P., Herbert, J. D., & Forman, E. (in press). Western trauma discourse exposure and posttraumatic symptoms among Burundians with traumatic event histories. *Journal of Traumatic Stress.*

Young, A. (2004). When traumatic memory was a problem: On the historical antecedents of PTSD. In G. M. Rosen (Ed.), *Posttraumatic stress disorder: Issues and controversies* (pp. 127–146). New York: Wiley.

Young, B. H., Ford, J. D., & Watson, P. J. (2005, July). *Survivors of natural disasters and mass violence—A National Center for PTSD fact sheet.* Retrieved December 11, 2005, from *www.ncptsd.va.gov/facts/disasters/fs_survivors_disaster.html*

Yule, W. (2001). Posttraumatic stress disorder in the general population and in children. *Journal of Clinical Psychiatry, 62*(Suppl. 17), 23–28.

SUGGESTED READINGS

Ehlers, A. & Clark, D. (2000). A cognitive model of posttraumatic stress disorder. *Behaviour Research and Therapy, 38,* 319–345.

Ehlers, A., Clark, D.C., Hackmann, A., McManus, F., & Fennell, M. (2005). Cognitive therapy for post-traumatic stress disorder: Development and evaluation. *Behaviour Research and Therapy, 43*(4), 413–431.

Foa, E. B., Davidson, J. R. T., & Frances, A. (Eds.). (1999). The expert consensus guideline series: Treatment of posttraumatic stress disorder. *Journal of Clinical Psychiatry, 60*(Suppl. 16).

National Child Traumatic Stress Network and National Center for PTSD. (2004, September). *Psychological first aid: Field operations guide.* Retrieved April 4, 2006, from *www.ncptsd.va.gov/pfa/PFA_9_6_05_Final.pdf*

Rosen, G. M. (Ed.). (2004). *Posttraumatic stress disorder: Issues and controversies.* New York: Wiley.

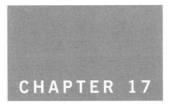

CHAPTER 17

Terrorism

Stevan E. Hobfoll
Tamar Galai-Gat
Dawn M. Johnson
Patricia J. Watson

*T*he restoration of the social and behavioral functioning of survivors of terrorism and mass casualty trauma is critical. At this time, however, there is no evidence-based consensus as to which interventions are effective (Gersons & Olf, 2005). Critical incidence debriefing has been the most well-researched intervention after such events, but the evidence suggests that it either is not effective or has a somewhat negative impact (for recent reviews, see Carlier, Lamberts, van Uchelen, & Gersons, 1998; Litz & Gray, 2002; McNally, Bryant, & Ehlers, 2003). This has led clinicians and researchers to examine other potential interventions based on more indirect evidence that they are likely to be effective. Here we consider evidence-informed interventions, because we believe that they are the most scientifically valid at this time. However, it is also possible to argue that given the variety of types of attacks and mass casualty events, there will never be a clear, evidence-based array of interventions to cover the multitude of situations and populations that may be affected. Many of the ideas we present in this chapter were first put forward in a working panel on disaster and mass casualty treatment organized by the National Center for PTSD and the Substance Abuse and Mental Health Services Administration (SAMSHA) in the fall of 2004 (Hobfoll et al., in press), and that panel deserves much of the credit for our summary in this chapter.

In this chapter, we consider two families of interventions—broad-based public mental health and more individual and small-group clinical interventions. The former are different from what most clinicians are used to and likely to be out of many clinicians' comfort range. However, when terrorism or disaster strikes, clinicians are often called on to stretch their repertoire to meet the broader public health needs of communities. We saw this after the hurricane and flooding of New Orleans and neighboring areas in 2005's Hurricane Katrina, where clinicians from across the country came to aid in these more public mental health kinds of efforts. Second, we consider more individual and small-group interventions for those who are showing earlier signs of traumatic stress, often called *acute stress reactions*. Again, clinicians may be less well versed in these interventions because they are more likely to have experience with trauma after the dust has settled. Indeed, many interventions for traumatic stress (Foa & Meadows, 1997; Foa & Rothbaum, 1998; Resick & Schnicke, 1992) have instructed that clinicians must wait until the causes of the trauma (e.g., violence in women's lives) have subsided and until the survivors are free of substance use. It is the precise nature of intervention with survivors of terrorism and mass casualty that the source of the threat may still be active. Survivors may still be in war zones or zones of political instability and follow-up attacks are often salient aspects of the environment. Hence, what is different about the clinical interventions we outline in this chapter is that they are designed to be used when life is still chaotic and when relative safety has to be considered a goal of treatment and not an already achieved state (Bryant, Harvey, Dang, Sackville, & Basten, 1998).

Terrorism and mass trauma are among the most frightening and emotionally devastating events that can occur (Norris, Friedman, & Watson, 2002; Shalev & Freedman, 2005). Therefore, it is critical that clinicians recognize that people's reactions should not be regarded as necessarily pathological responses or as precursors of subsequent disorder. What is often the case, nevertheless, is that these traumas are experienced with extreme distress and require community and at times clinical intervention (Bleich, Gelkopf, & Solomon, 2003; Galea et al., 2002). Many individuals will have transient stress reactions in the aftermath of terrorism and mass casualty and these reactions may recur occasionally, even years after the precipitating events. This means that many people will require interventions that provide support and resources that maximize opportunities for their transition to normalcy, rather than traditional diagnosis and clinical treatment. Thus, we outline interventions in their broad sense, ranging from provision of community support and public health messaging to clinical assessment and intensive intervention.

Although obvious on some levels, it is important that we contextualize what is occurring in situations of terrorism and mass trauma and why they are so traumatic. First, the extreme physical, social, and psychological demands of such situations range from manageable fear to terror, depending on people's extent of exposure (Bleich et al., 2003; Galea et al., 2002; Hobfoll et al., 2006; Rubin, Brewin, Greenberg, Simpson, & Wessely, 2005). Such situations include severe physical injury, witnessing of horrific violence and devastation, and witnessing of events that challenge the basic sense of the way the world works (e.g., beheadings of innocent individuals, bodies floating in flooded areas, a kindly appearing woman exploding a bomb on a bus, buildings that were symbols of strength and wealth collapsing in fire, and change from safety to extreme terror in a moment without warning). Such events are often outside the repertoire of personal, familial, organizational, and communal resources and coping repertoires, leaving people feeling helpless to respond. In countries where terrorism is more common, such as Israel, there is, conversely, a familiar ritual involving the media, the public, and the municipal workers, but given that being involved in an attack is still a rare event for any individual, this sense of helplessness may still be omnipresent. The loss of loved ones may be as extreme an experience or worse than injury or threat of death to the self. Hence, such experiences as looking in rubble for lost relatives or searching hospitals for dead and wounded are experienced with agony and extreme distress. Mass casualty also means that many family members may have been injured or killed, with all the attendant social, personal, and economic consequences. Just waiting to hear about the safety of loved ones can be a devastating time of deep anguish. Because terrorism is often a continued threat, these wounds cannot easily heal and are evoked each time a new threat occurs.

What also differentiates terrorism and mass casualty from many other types of trauma is a loss of territory, or the loss of territory that is considered safe. What was once a secure base—home, work, playgrounds, public transportation, the vegetable market—becomes a place of threat and future horror. Survivors of rape or violent crime experience such a loss too, but the difference is that the future threat is often imagined as survivors overgeneralize. In the case of terrorism and mass casualty, the continued threat may actually be increasingly likely in the future and not a matter of overgeneralization and exaggerated appraisal.

Finally, what distinguishes terrorism and mass casualty from other types of trauma is that clinicians are often themselves under threat or survivors at the same time that they are offering intervention. First, they may have themselves been involved or threatened by virtue of being in the area at the time of the original event. Even if they are offering their services after coming from afar, they are open to the same threat of follow-up attack or disaster and may often witness the traumatic aftermaths of scenes of mass casualty where bodies are still being removed from rubble, where their own loved ones may be missing or be under continued threat, or where they must live under difficult conditions in tent cities where people are daily receiving death notification. They lose the same sleep; often lack proper clothing, blankets, food or water; and may even feel targeted by other survivors because they represent the "system" that may be seen as having failed to protect or appropriately respond. This is an extreme version of secondary exposure because they are both participant-survivors and witnesses. In Jerusalem, for example, therapists travel on the same buses, sit in the same cafes, and shop in the same market as others.

When people are confronted with such extreme threat they naturally respond psychologically, psychophysiologically, and neurologically in ways that signal the body's confrontation, distress, and adaptation to the environment (McFarlane & van der Kolk, 1996). Biological and psychological adaptation to such extreme events is required for survival and is wired within us in a Darwinian sense (Hobfoll, 1998; van der Kolk & McFarlane, 1996). This means that people's reactivity is deeply embedded in the brain and in psychophysiology (Friedman, Charney, & Deutsch, 1995;

Panksepp, 1998; Yehuda, 1998; Yehuda, McFarlane, & Shalev, 1998). Restoring people to a sense of safety and calm is essential in both animals and humans in order to reduce the psychobiological responses that accompany extreme fear and anxiety (Bryant, 2006).

PUBLIC MENTAL HEALTH INTERVENTIONS

Public mental health intervention (PMH) includes an array of strategies rather than any specific treatment protocols. In general, PMH intervention should (1) promote safety, (2) return people to a sense of calm and control over hyperarousal and numbing reactions, (3) increase sense of self-efficacy and communal efficacy, (4) facilitate social connections to loved ones and significant others, and (5) restore and maintain hope. As all those these goals are interconnected, we use this sequencing as a framework for our presentation.

Promotion of Safety

The goal of terrorism is the disruption of the social order, a breakdown of the public's feeling of safety—so that the impact of the terrorist act is way beyond the sphere of those directly affected. It is the nature of terrorism and mass casualty trauma that people are exposed to events that threaten them, their loved ones, and things they most deeply value (Basoglu et al., 2005; Briere & Elliot, 2000; de Jong, 2002a, 2002b; Hobfoll et al., 1991; Shalev, Tuval-Mashiach, & Hadar, 2004; Ursano, McCaughey, & Fullerton, 1994). With this threat comes an appraised sense and a reality of being unsafe and at continued risk, sometimes referred to as loss of the "protective shield" (Bell, Flay, & Paikoff, 2002; Pynoos, Goenjian, & Steinberg, 1995). It may actually be more common for clinicians to consider sense of psychological safety, as in the case of rape survivors. However, in situations of terrorism and mass casualty, clinicians must also consider the actual safety of individuals and aid in their making safety plans, even if absolute safety may not be realistic. A central goal of intervention therefore is to restore the protective shield, aiding appraised sense of safety and fostering decisions and actions that will promote safety (see Table 17.1).

First, clinicians must aid the orderly movement of people into safer circumstances. This is best accomplished using principles psychologists have considered in fear messaging (Rogers & Mewborn, 1976; Rogers, 1983). These principles include providing accurate information; avoiding exaggeration of the fear message; recommending concrete, clear steps (e.g., orange alerts are dysfunctional if not paired with clear, recommended, achievable action); and providing accurate, real-time feedback as people respond and circumstances change. This may be more difficult than it seems, as people will risk their lives and interfere with aid and rescue efforts to find a lost relative even if their actions objectively hamper first responders' efforts to save that relative.

TABLE 17.1. Safety: Goals and Suggested Strategies

Goals	Suggested strategies
Physical safety • Medical evaluation (some traumatized individuals are not even aware that they have been injured) • Encouraging realistic appraisal of traumatic event and future threats • Identifying real threats to safety • Developing crisis plan to manage ongoing threats Emotional safety • Restoring a sense of power and control • Normalizing acute trauma reactions • Teaching adaptive coping strategies and self-regulation techniques (breathing, etc.)	• Provision of safe environments • Challenge exaggerated appraisals of danger • Safety planning • Problem solving • Psychoeducation on acute stress reactions • Redirecting clients' focus from those aspects that are out of their control to those that are within their control • Providing accurate information regarding future risks

Second, clinicians should aid, design, and facilitate efforts to work with media on messaging. This is important because several studies have found that exposure to televised images of traumatic events are related to greater psychological distress (Ahern et al., 2002; Pfefferbaum et al., 2002; Schlenger et al., 2002; Silver, Holman, McIntosh, Poulin, & Gil-Rivas, 2002). Young children and those already experiencing psychological distress are especially vulnerable (Fremont, 2004; Pfefferbaum et al., 2002). Although the intent of media and government messaging is to inform and instruct, other factors in the real world often impede these goals. Media know that sensational news sells. This is especially problematic in the world of 24-hour-a-day news, as each hour must appear to bring something new. Further, graphic displays may be seen as attracting viewers. This means that news exaggerates, sensationalizes stories, and rehashes old news in ways that portray loss, destruction, death, and damage as worse than they are. If the choice is one story stating that accurate estimates are that 1,000 people have died and another stating that the figure may climb as high as 5,000 deaths, it is the latter story that will be the focus of the news leader and the feature story.

Politicians also may use situations of trauma and mass casualty to promote their political agendas. If the government wishes to increase support for retaliation it might exaggerate the nature and extent of an attack or the possibility of future attacks. Mental health professionals should be voices of reason in such instances, acting as consultants to the media and the political process. Consultation will be facilitated if they have had prior relationships with the media or been part of the political process, but it is also possible in real-time situations. These principles can also be translated to smaller-scale tragedies such as school shootings, where they can be used by school leadership, local politicians, and local media.

Principles of modeling apply to safety on a public health level too. A lesson can be learned here from what the army teaches military officers in combat: specifically, display reasonable, calm actions. As a metaphor, there is nothing to be gained by acting nervous under fire or even ducking when an incoming missile approaches. Thus, mental health professionals can promote a sense of safety by going about their work and taking reasonable, but not unreasonable, precautions. Just being at school on time the day after a tragedy or setting up an aid area within a hurricane- or tsunami-devastated area sends an important message about safety. Instructing other personnel in the importance of their behavioral display extends this principle.

One tool that can be used to increase this sense of safety is the display of accurate odds of further threat occurring—for example, the odds of being killed in an airline flight prior to September 11 were 1:7 million and the odds of being killed in a flight after September 11 (1:1.4 million). Even the odds of being in a building that was tragically hit on September 11, 2001, was about 2 in 10,000 for New Yorkers on that day. In Israel, during the entire period of the Al Aqsa Intifada from September 2000 to the time of the writing of this chapter, the odds of being killed in a terrorist attack were about 1 in 8,000 over a 5-year period. Compare this to the odds of dying in a coast-to-coast car trip (1:14,000), or cardiovascular disease (1:4), cancer (1:4), stroke (7:100), homicide (7:1,000). Such messaging helps people understand the nature of the new threat. This does not mean that people are advised to take risks, but it does mean that if people want to do something about their safety they should limit driving under the influence of alcohol, fatty foods, and smoking, not overreacting to attack. The goal of terrorism is to disrupt people's lives and make them feel unsafe everywhere. This technique helps people react in a more proportional way.

Intervention postterrorism and mass casualty should seek to interrupt the posttraumatic stimulus generalization, which causes people to link posttraumatic stimuli to aspects of the original event (Bryant et al., 1998; Foa & Rothbaum, 1998; Gersons, Carlier, Lamberts, & Van der Kolk, 2000; Resick, Nishith, Weaver, Astin, & Feuer, 2002). Exposure therapy accomplishes this through a combination of imaginal exposure and real-world, *in vivo* exposure. Both techniques are designed to relink associated images, people, and events with safety ("The building that was bombed was unsafe, all buildings are not unsafe," "Going to work that day was dangerous, but going to work other days is safe"). Their efficacy and efficiency are evidence based. Although originally designed for rape survivors, the seeking-safety approach can be applied to post-mass casualty treatment (Najavits, 2002). This approach focuses on teaching contextual discrimination in the face of trauma and loss triggers, develops more adaptive cognitions and coping skills, and utilizes grounding techniques to enhance people's sense of safety (Najavits, Weiss, Shaw, & Muenz, 1998). Mental health professionals need to adapt these treatments to the safety requirements and cognitions associated with the specific circumstances their population is confronted with, recognizing that danger in terms of continued terrorism, further flooding, or other threats may or may not be realistic.

Evidence from the front-line treatment of combatants also supports the centrality of bringing individuals to safety, even if that safety is relative. Hence, if intervention considers safety a relative state, bringing survivors or those threatened to a place of relative safety will help restore their sense of calm and control. Thus in Israel, bringing combatants who are experiencing acute distress disorder to safe zones is a key principle of immediate treatment (Solomon & Benbenishty, 1986; Solomon, Shklar, & Mikulincer, 2005). This breaks both the cognitive and physiological cycles associated with the threat–survival connection.

Calming

Anxiety, depression, and other displays of emotionality are normal following terrorist attacks and mass casualty events. Some anxiety is not only normal but aids vigilance. A case in point is the avoidance that many Jerusalemites developed of traveling by bus during the periods of frequent suicide bombings on buses. Clearly, this is a realistic precaution, but it should also be emphasized that many cannot afford this luxury.

This suggests that intervention should let this be known so that people do not interpret their emotional upheaval as pathological. Similarly, it should be communicated to people that some level of denial can be healthy as it allows individuals to titrate the amount of news of harm little by little, letting in what they can cope with at that time (Breznitz, 1983). It becomes problematic, however, if levels of distress heighten to the extent that they interfere with sleep, eating, self-care, decision making, and performance of critical life tasks. Moreover, if allowed to continue unabated, these levels of distress may become chronic and more intractable with time. Extreme emotions that continue may also diminish individuals' sense of control, and when they feel out of control, their anxiety, depression, and fear may be furthered. Extreme emotionality during the posttrauma period may also be associated with panic attacks, dissociation, and later posttraumatic stress disorder (PTSD) (Harvey & Bryant, 2002; Shalev et al., 1998). Finally, physiological and cognitive demands associated with heightened arousal may compete with other physiological and psychological resources that are necessary for attention and action, causing functional decrements precisely when optimal functioning is required.

There is convincing evidence that these early interventions are not effective in preventing subsequent psychological disorder (see McNally et al., 2003). A major reason why psychological debriefing (such as critical incident stress debriefing) has been criticized in recent years is that it may exacerbate arousal. For example, requiring people to ventilate feelings in the immediate aftermath of trauma can increase arousal at a time when they need to calm down and restore equilibrium. It is possible that this increase in arousal may be the reason that debriefing exacerbates some people's stress reactions after trauma (Bisson, Jenkins, Alexander, & Bannister, 1997; Hobbs, Mayou, Harrison, & Worlock, 1996). Furthermore, because first responders are told not to debrief about "operational complaints" (officers did not send enough or the correct equipment; government officials held them back) (clearly a political decision), they are prevented from offering the kind of problem solving and venting that might be helpful.

Most successful psychological and pharmacological treatments for trauma target restoration of self-regulation and calming of extreme emotions that are out of individuals' control or chronic (Davidson, Landerman, Farfel, & Clary, 2002; Follette, & Ruzek, 2006; Foa, Keane, & Friedman, 2000; Friedman, Davidson, Mellman, & Southwick, 2000). Again, considering the example of combatants who are experiencing acute stress disorder, restoring a sense of calm is seen as critical to their immediate care and to reducing the future risk of PTSD (Solomon, 2003). Even exposure-based therapies that act to temporarily heighten emotionality through exposure do so with the goal of decreasing this emotionality in the face of imagined and *in vivo* fear-producing stimuli (Foa & Rothbaum, 1998; Resick & Schnicke, 1992).

Clinicians have a number of therapeutic tools that can be applied to decreasing hyperarousal (see Table 17.2). Individuals with severe agitation may be aided by grounding techniques that remind them that they are no longer in the threat–trauma condition and that their thoughts and feelings cannot harm them the way the original event could. In this way, grounding counteracts dissociative tendencies. Breathing retraining, deep muscle relaxation, yoga, mindfulness, and meditation techniques have all been used to limit hyperarousal and give individuals a restored sense of control as they can use these techniques on their own once learned (Carlson, Speca, Patel, & Goodey, 2003; Cohen Warneke, Fouladi, Rodriguez, & Chaoul-Reich, 2004; van de Put & Eisenbruch, 2002). We still require systematic research on pharmacological approaches to induce calming, but several medications hold promise, including antiadrenergic agents, antidepressants and conventional anxiolytics (Friedman & Davidson, 2007; Pitman et al., 2002).

One of the more comprehensive treatments that can be applied post-mass casualty is Meichenbaum's (1974) stress inoculation training (SIT). This is a general set of cognitive-behavioral techniques that can be combined to aid stress resistance. SIT includes muscle relaxation training, breathing control, assertiveness training, role playing, modeling, thought stopping, positive reframing, and self-talk. SIT has been successfully applied to treatment of sexual assault and accident survivors (Foa et al., 1991; Kilpatrick et al., 1982). It has also been applied effectively to combatants in Israel, which suggests that it might generalize well to survivors of terrorism and mass casualty (Solomon, 2003).

TABLE 17.2. Calming: Goals and Suggested Strategies

Goals	Suggested strategies
• Reducing levels of anxiety • Restoring physical self-regulation • Reducing numbing reactions • Approaching safe triggers • Improving self-care • Limiting unnecessary exposure to triggers • Reducing risk of future PTSD	• Psychoeducation on acute stress reactions • Self-soothing • Sleep hygiene • Grounding techniques • Relaxation training • Stress inoculation training • Cognitive restructuring • *In vivo* exposure • Imaginal exposure/recapitulation • Medications

A brief version of exposure therapy has also been adapted to secondary prevention of PTSD with survivors of accident and assault. Studies of this adaptation have found it to be successful (Bryant et al., 1998; Bryant, Haney, Guthrie, & Moulds, 2003; Bryant, Sackville, Dang, Moulds, & Guthrie, 1999; Foa, Hearst-Ikeda, & Perry, 1995). A recent study by Foa, Zoellner, and Feeny (2006) compared exposure therapy with more supportive counseling with those suffering acute stress reactions and found both treatments to be effective but that exposure therapy more quickly relieved symptoms. Such efficiency should not be undervalued, as acute stress reactions are experienced painfully and limit functioning that is critical in the posttrauma period.

On a more public health level, most people will benefit from several messages that promote calming. In particular, research suggests that normalization of the posttrauma experience is key. Solomon (2003), discussing intervention with combatants with acute stress disorder, noted that a key element of intervention is communicating to them that their "extreme" reactions are quite normal and in most cases will subside in a matter of days or weeks. People are calmed by hearing that they are not "going crazy" or "weak" because they are experiencing fear-induced anxiety, depression, numbness, or bouts of anger—that they are having normal reactions to an abnormal situation—and the calming techniques further enhance their sense of control, which in turn further enhances emotional stability.

Cognitive-behavioral problem-solving techniques can be taught on individual, group, organizational, and even media levels. The fact that the problems in such situations are largely shared can be turned to an advantage as many problem-solving techniques and strategies can be offered for what people might typically be confronting. These strategies can be tailored to make them appropriate for different age groups, settings, or cultural subgroups. Some of the tasks that require problem solving are instrumental, such as applying for federal aid or getting a roof repaired. Others are more interpersonal, such as how much to explain circumstances to children or being emotionally labile and irritable with loved ones. Still other tasks are emotional, such as promoting sleep hygiene and dealing with increased alcohol use or problems in concentration due to anxiety or intrusive images.

Monitoring reexposure can also be integrated into individual, group, organizational and media-based treatments, which is important in diminishing hyperarousal and panic attacks. People naturally seek information postterrorism and mass casualty, but rather than decreasing their fears, the opposite often occurs. In general, continuous news viewing should be avoided. Those with normal levels of anxiety would still do well to limit exposure to once in the morning, afternoon, and evening for, say, half an hour. Those experiencing more significant hyperarousal or panic reactions might be advised to limit their exposure to print news or even the half-hour report on radio, which is less graphic than television news. Those who are having difficulty with this level of exposure may be willing to rely on a trusted other for important updates that are stripped of descriptions of fear-inducing stimuli (politicians warning of exaggerated threats, descriptions of dead bodies, etc.). This might be better than complete detachment from the news, as lack of information can itself provoke anxiety.

Promoting Sense of Self- and Communal Efficacy

One of the first casualties of severe traumas is people's sense of competency (Benight, 2004; Benight, Freyaldenhoven, Hughes, Ruiz, & Zoschke, 2000; Foa & Meadows, 1997; Resick & Schnicke, 1992). Therefore, intervention on all levels must work to reverse this negative view of the self and group from a sense of helplessness to a sense of competency. Benight and Harper's (2002) work suggests that intervention is most efficient if based on the specific competencies people need in the posttrauma period, as opposed to more generalized life competencies. Such intervention is also an aid to efficient treatment, because once again the pathways to efficacy are to a great extent common for people experiencing a common trauma (de Jong, 1995; de Jong, Komproe, & van Ommeren, 2003; Sampson, Raudenbush, & Earls, 1997). Treatment can therefore translate intervention to specific skills that people require during this period.

Indeed, many of the interventions discussed under restoring safety and calming have a simultaneous impact on sense of self and communal efficacy (see Table 17.3). As people feel that they can restore their safety and control their emotions, aid their children, concentrate enough to fulfill life tasks, and make decisions about how much they should expose themselves to news broadcasts they will feel increasingly efficacious (Benight, Swift, Sanger, Smith, & Zeppelin, 1999; Ginzburg, Solomon, Dekel, & Neria, 2003). A key intervention principle here is not doing "for them" but "with them." Many cognitive-behavioral interventions lend themselves to these feelings as therapists are sharing expertise and helping to make clients more capable through skill building, homework, tapes, and worksheets.

Expanding this principle of self-help, clinicians should seek to learn from survivors what they need and encourage them to provide ideas for what they think can work. Bringing parents into the school to help design effective treatment for their children will not only increase their involvement but also offer them a sense that they are still in the critical parental role. When the larger community is impacted by the trauma circumstances, it is critical to involve the natural leaders, spiritual leaders, and intact organizations and groups in the "therapeutic" process. The expert serves as consultant rather than "savior."

Those working in economically disadvantaged regions need to promote self-government, integrate culturally consonant processes with treatment, and rely on sur-

TABLE 17.3. Self-Efficacy/Communal Efficacy: Goals and Suggested Strategies

Goals	Suggested strategies
• Restoring a sense of power and control • Empowerment • Reducing feelings of helplessness • Instilling a sense of competence • Enhancing group cohesion	• Case management • Community interventions with local agencies that provide material and financial resources • Skill building • Problem solving • Advocacy • Participation in resource building

vivors to become vehicles to restore safety, provide resources, and as active as possible (de Jong & Clarke, 1996). This may appear less efficient than bringing in armies of volunteers and experts from the outside. However, it will ultimately be more efficient and has the added benefit of instilling communities with many of the skills they will need in the midterm and long-term aftermath, when all the volunteers have gone home.

This approach also extends to authority figures at schools and in other agencies. People in authority, feeling helpless, often ask professionals to come and "do something," but the greatest benefit such professionals can provide is to consult with these people and empower them to assist those under their care. Consultation is more effective, in the long run, than direct intervention, and it may be the only reasonable way to impact a community, given that the number of experienced mental professionals is necessarily limited.

Two elements are critical to treatment postterrorism and mass casualty that may be overlooked by mental health professionals if they focus on cognitive and emotional aspects alone. Specifically, people require certain skills and behaviors in such an environment. Many of their perceptions and emotions are actually well founded and accurate. Thus, changing the emotion or cognition may undermine treatment, as these are natural responses to the adaptation process. Hence, it is critical that interventions focus on new, adaptive behaviors and skills to increase sense of efficacy (Bandura, 1997; Benight, Ironson, et al., 1999; Hobfoll, 2002; Ozer & Bandura, 1990). This, in turn, will aid cognitive and emotional adjustment. Using soldiers and first responders as models, it can be seen that the emphasis is on training them in adaptive skills and behaviors that suit the challenges they face (Keinan, Friedland, & Sarignaor, 1990; Solomon, 2003). This includes relying on the unit, which may be more natural in collectivist societies but counter to some of the natural tendencies in individualistic cultures. A key principle of such treatment is achieving "small wins" as people succeed in practicing increasingly difficult skills and behaviors (Hobfoll et al., 1991; Meichenbaum, 1974).

The second aspect of self- and communal efficacy that mental health professionals might ignore is that empowerment relies on access to material and financial resources (Rappaport, 1981). Resource loss has been shown to be one of the strongest predictors of PTSD and psychological distress following trauma, and in many cases it is the critical predictor of well-being and functioning (Benight, Ironson, Benight, Swift, et al., 1999; Freedy, Shaw, Jarrell, & Masters, 1992; Galea et al., 2002; Hobfoll et al., 2006), yet it is actually ignored in most predictive models and clinical treatises on trauma. The most vulnerable segments of the population postterrorism and disaster are the poor, children, elderly, and ethnic minority groups (Galea et al., 2002; Hobfoll et al., in press; Ironson et al., 1997; Norris & Kaniasty, 1996). Thus, it is critical, though not typical, mental health services to integrate with social services, financial aid, and provision of shelter, food, and opportunities for protection, rebuilding, or relocating. Such linkage is paramount given the extent of damage to infrastructure, loss of jobs, loss of home, and loss of income that may occur following terrorism or mass casualty. It is psychologically critical because otherwise survivors will increase their self-blaming as they fail to recover without access to necessary material and financial resources.

Fostering Connections to Others

Social support and fostering social interactions are invaluable in many stressor situations. It is both critical and a dynamic difficult process following terrorism and mass casualty because events often threaten or result in the loss of multiple family members, disrupt support systems, and may make interpersonal communication impossible due to moving people to temporary shelter, disruption of phone service, failure to make e-mail connection, and often fear of venturing out to make social contact.

Those who can sustain social support following terrorism and mass casualty are better able to cope, adapt better to the posttrauma environment, and have better mental health outcomes in the short-term, midterm, and even many years later (Galea et al., 2003; Green et al., 1990; Norris, Baker, Murphy, & Kaniasty, 2005; Solomon et al., 2005). The first priority in postterrorism and mass casualty settings is reconnecting people with their loved ones, reestablishing community ties, and re-creating the "village" of social interconnections that existed prior to the trauma (de Jong, 2002a, 2002b; Litz & Gray, 2002; Shalev, Tuval-Mashiach, & Hadar, 2004; Ursano, Fullerton, Norwood, & Weiseth, 1995). As the temporary communities may or may not actually be temporary, it may have long-term impact as well. Postdisaster temporary settings can be sources of support and succor or places of competition, violence, and even posttrauma retribution.

Clinicians will be aided in their intervention design by the social support deterioration, deterrence (SSDD) model of Kaniasty and Norris (1993; Norris & Kaniasty, 1996). The SSDD model suggests that people are certainly aided by the provision of social support following disaster and this model fits what we have learned about postterrorism environments (Hobfoll, Canetti-Nisim, & Johnson, 2006). However, two other aspects of the process must be highlighted. First, those who lack social support resources require more active assistance, either professional support or help in activating their support systems. Second, at the same time that social support is active and helpful, it is not an endless resource. Hence, although initial periods are characterized by a high degree of support, support systems quickly deteriorate under the pressure of overuse and the need of individuals to get on with their own lives. This suggests not only that those who begin with low levels of social support are vulnerable but also that chronic and ongoing demands will drain even rather robust support systems. Intervention should educate survivors regarding this problem, as support processes can be modified when people are made aware of such problems and are taught how best to activate and moderate the support they both give and receive (Freedy & Hobfoll, 1994). This means that intervention in these cases should be a priority as natural support networks may have disintegrated or been disrupted (de Jong, 2002a; Sattler et al., 2002) (see Figure 17.1).

Freedy and Hobfoll (1994) outlined several steps in the support process. These are depicted in Figure 17.1. This tool helps people understand that social support often

Process	Time Frame 1	Time Frame 2	Time Frame 3 thru *n*
Identify support needs and sources (yours and theirs)			
Ask for aid—specifics			
Use aid/advise/support			
Offer feedback Check feelings			
Note how things are helping you; people need to hear that the support they give is worthwhile			
Ask for and offer further assistance			

FIGURE 17.1. Building social support: A worksheet and strategy.

does not occur spontaneously, especially when there are major protuberances in the environment, such as those that occur following situations of mass casualty. It is important to underscore that social support requires nurturance. A number of interfering assumptions are also common and should be underscored, as depicted in Table 17.4.

Although social support aids people's coping, emotional reactions, and efforts, not all social processes are supportive. Therefore, interventionists must help people modify negative social interactions, even those that are not intended to be negative (see Table 17.5). Potential supporters might overburden individuals and sharing bad news without respite wears people down (Andrews, Brewin, & Rose, 2003; Hobfoll & Lon-

TABLE 17.4. Mistaken Support Assumptions and Corrective Cognitions and Actions

Mistaken assumption	Corrective assumption or action
"Only spontaneous support is valid."	"People may not be aware of our needs, but may still very much care about us."
"I don't want to burden others."	"What would you want your family or best friends to do if they needed support?" (Answer: "Let me know. I want to help.")
"Asking for support means I'm weak."	"Would you see a friend or family member as weak if they needed you to talk to, help with childcare, help fix a roof?"
"Others have their own problems."	"True, so sharing support is often the key. Even if you have difficulties there are things you can do for others. Be a good listener, watch their kids, pick up groceries for them when you go to the store."
"I'll just feel worse if I share my feelings."	"Actually, research shows that people feel better when they share their feelings. It's often hard to start."
"Now that support has started, everything should just go smoothly."	"No, support is like a back itch. It moves and changes over time. So, you have to update and check in whether you're the support provider or the support recipient."

TABLE 17.5. Connections/Relationships: Goals and Suggested Strategies

Goals	Suggested strategies
• Encouraging use of existing sources of social support • Connecting with new sources of social support • Reducing further deterioration of social support • Limiting access to negative sources of social support and undermining	• Support groups/supportive milieu • Case management • Religion/spirituality • Psychoeducation on the importance of social support • Challenging mistaken assumptions that interfere with asking for help • Communication strategies • Establishing boundaries • Diversifying support resources so as not to overburden specific sources of support

don, 1986). People may minimize problems, provide unrealistic expectations for quick return to full functioning, and provide invalidating messages. Even messages with positive intent, such as "You just need to rely on God," may have a negative impact, as God may appear to be quite absent during such periods and prayers may have appeared to have gone unanswered (Wortman & Lehman, 1985). Relationships may also be historically characterized by undermining, and these negative social interactions can be especially devastating (Rook, 1984). This can become exacerbated due to the competition for limited resources that may occur following mass casualty (Giel, 1990).

These principles can also be applied in large-scale interventions in majority world countries. Hence, efforts to promote social support networks in temporary refugee camps are effective (de Jong, 2002a, 2002b). De Jong (2002b) suggests adopting the concept of treating temporary sites as villages rather than camps. Camps are temporary sites for displaced persons who are at risk of becoming quickly helpless and invalidated. Villages, in contrast, have leadership structures, places of worship, places for entertainment and congregation of women's and men's activities, and places for children to play under supervision. Further, this strategy increases the likelihood that intervention will be consonant with the cultural values of the community. This relates back to the need to intervene in ways that enhance self- and collective efficacy as noted earlier. It also acts to preserve social structures that help keep communities intact and to preserve rules, order, and social supervision (i.e., the rule of law). However, communities may still need help policing, as chaos is fertile ground for violent and criminal activity. Even in the resource-rich United States, after Hurricane Andrew hit south Florida in 1992, motorcycle gangs extorted money as sham roofing crews. Government may likewise still need to aid residents postdisaster against powerful others (e.g., state governments sued insurance companies on behalf of residents for their failure to follow their contractual obligations after Hurricane Katrina in 2005 in Louisiana and Mississippi).

Raising Positive Expectancies

A basic principle of self-regulation theory is that people are aided by positive expectancies that their behavior will lead to their achieving their goals (Carver & Scheier, 1998). Antonovsky (1979) broadened this principle, which he believed overemphasized "rugged individualism." Instead, he argued that people who have a sense of coherence are better able to cope with major stressors, basing his work on his study of Holocaust survivors. He defined sense of coherence as a "global orientation that expresses the extent to which one has a pervasive, enduring though dynamic feeling of confidence that one's internal and external environments are predictable and that there is a high probability that things will work out as well as can reasonable be expected" (p. 123). He went on to state that "a sense of coherence . . . does not at all imply that one is in control. It does involve one as a participant in the processes shaping one's destiny as well as one's daily experiences. . . . The crucial issue is not whether power to determine such outcomes lies in our own hands or elsewhere. What is important is that the location of power is where it is legitimately supposed to be" (p. 128).

One of the first casualties of terrorism and mass casualty is the sense of hope and positive expectations. The world appears to be turned "topsy-turvy." Restoring hope becomes critical and demands attention to both overt occurrences and deep-seated values because such traumas often shatter people's world view (Janoff-Bulman, 1992). PTSD is often accompanied by the difficulty of imagining a positive future and is likely to be accompanied by catastrophizing that undermines hope and encourages a sense of despair, fatalism, and resignation. This loss of hope and sense of helplessness are not inevitable by any means, as studies also indicate that many survivors of major trauma are resilient (Antonovsky, 1979; Lomranz, 1990; Shmotkin, Blumstein, & Modan, 2003).

There is danger of hingeing hope on personal efficacy (Hobfoll, Briggs-Phillips, & Stines, 2003). This overly Western view can be seen as having been applied to the survivors of Hurricane Katrina in New Orleans in 2005. Survivors were blamed for not evacuating, for looting, and for criminal activity. Later it became known that the poor had few resources to aid their evacuation, had nowhere to go, and were unlikely to be looting despite the government's failure to deliver basic water and food supplies, and that criminal activity was mainly perpetrated by known criminals who received carte blanche when police deserted flooded areas.

There are several avenues for enhancing hope following terrorism and mass casualty (see Table 17.6). Studies suggest that those showing acute stress reactions respond well to supportive counseling and exposure therapies, but that exposure therapies may be more efficient in achieving positive results (Foa et al., 2006). This preliminary research, demonstrating the therapeutic efficacy and cost-effectiveness of early and appropriate identification and treatment of trauma-related disorders itself, can enhance hope among both professionals and survivors. Cognitive-behavioral treatments might need to increase their focus on people's tendencies to take personal responsibility for their emotional upheaval or experience self-blame and guilt over events that

TABLE 17.6. Positive Expectancies: Goals and Suggested Strategies

Goals	Suggested strategies
• Fostering a sense of coherence • Identifying positive goals • Challenging fatalistic cognitions • Encouraging positive coping • Encouraging a sense of community resiliency	• Provision of accurate assessments of damage and recovery efforts • Focusing on positives • Redirecting clients' focus from those aspects which are out of their control to those that are within their control • Cognitive restructuring • Pleasant activity planning • Use of clear, achievable goals or "small wins"

occurred during the trauma sequence, such as failure to save loved ones, not being where they "should" have been, and magical ideas about this being punishment for some past transgression (Bryant et al., 1998; Foa et al., 1995). Seligman and Peterson's (1995) learned optimism and positive psychology model is also relevant. They focus on identifying positive goals, amplifying healthy cognitions and emotions, and building people's strengths. This can be paired simultaneously with disputing catastrophic thinking that undermines hope. Other useful techniques include guided self-dialogue (Foa & Rothbaum, 1998; Meichenbaum, 1974) to restructure irrational fears, control self-defeating overgeneralizations regarding inevitable failure, and encourage positive coping. These, in turn, raise sense of self- and communal efficacy, as we detailed earlier.

Related to enhancing hope is research on benefit finding after trauma. In this regard, some research shows that traumatic growth enhances well-being. Some studies indicate that benefit finding is associated with increased hope and better psychological adaptation months and even years after trauma (Antoni et al., 2001; King & Miner, 2000; Stanton et al., 2001). Other research, however, found quite the opposite. Hobfoll et al. (2006), studying terrorism in Israel, found that those who experienced traumatic growth had higher levels of PTSD. This might, however, indicate that those who were having greater difficulty increased their search for meaning and closeness to others. Another aspect of the findings of this study makes this second interpretation circumspect, because traumatic growth was also related to greater hatred and distrust of other ethnic groups and greater support for violent retaliation. Another study of the forced evacuation of Jewish settlers from Gaza by this same research group found the same measure of traumatic growth to be related to better mental health outcomes (Hall et al., in press). A major difference in the two circumstances was that in the case of terrorism, traumatic growth was cognitive, whereas in the case of the Gaza evacuation, these individuals were actively involved in behaviors aimed at realizing their dreams. This suggests the possibility that if people turn traumatic growth to action, such active coping may prove beneficial. Clearly, work on traumatic growth is in its infancy and caution should be exercised in translating it to treatment.

Hope is raised when communities show that they can work together. This includes returning to life tasks, addressing the psychological and physical harm done by the trauma, and attending to rituals that memorialize the community's strengths. Adger, Hughes, Folke, Carpenter, and Rockstrom (2005) point out that community resiliency emerges when communities work to mobilize assets, expand and repair social networks, and invest social capital in recovery. Community leaders, organizations, and religious leaders can enhance positive expectancy by helping people make accurate assessments of the extent of damage, proposing and setting in motion positive goals, and building new strengths and community apparatuses that will be required in the posttrauma period of rebuilding. There is often a fine line between correcting weaknesses in warning and response systems and becoming so involved in blame that rebuilding efforts are paralyzed.

CASE STUDIES: APPLYING THE PRINCIPLES
TO THE INDIVIDUAL LEVEL

The following case examples may help readers appreciate the focus on connections, hope, sense of self- and collective efficacy, and positive expectations as applied to individual treatment.[1]

Case 1: Lily

Note the key nature of connections in this woman's life.

Lily, a woman in her 50s, was brought to the crisis center by her family the morning after the suicide bombing of a café. She had been sitting with two of her children inside the cafe late at night, after having had a friendly conversation with the security guard who was killed minutes later while trying to block the terrorist. This was Lily's second experience with a terrorist attack. A few years previously she was injured in a terrorist attack at a family celebration, when incendiary bombs were thrown on the dance floor. Her clothes caught fire and she suffered burns. As a result, she spent 3 months in the hospital and 2 years in rehabilitation. This second bombing reactivated memories and fears from the previous event, and Lily was overwhelmed by the conviction that there was no safe place for her or her children: "How can I be certain this won't happen a third time?" she kept saying. She arrived at the crisis center hyperventilating, distraught, overwhelmed, and crying incessantly, after a sleepless night. The image of the dead security guard tormented her. She couldn't bring herself to eat, and felt choked. She kept reliving moments and was concerned with what would have happened. She felt guilty for having initiated the outing.

The first meeting was held with the mother and her family. At first, the therapist normalized Lily's reaction and helped manage the anxiety using breathing regulation. This proved effective. Once Lily was calmer, they began spontaneously reconstructing the event from their different perspectives, and with the help of some reframing, a narrative emerged of mutual concern and assistance in the immediate aftermath of the bombing, of active coping and survival: The family members had sought each other out and assisted one another out of the devastated café. The children had physically supported the mother, and the youngest had retrieved her cellular phone and called a relative to inform him they had survived. This emerging narrative had a calming effect on Lily, as she began to take stock of the situation and find meaning in the chaos and terror she had experienced. Over the next 6 weeks there were another seven sessions, in which Lily processed her trauma and reaffirmed her belief in the importance of her family in her life. She struggled with her fears and avoidance, forcing herself to go to cafes and the supermarket through *in vivo* exposure techniques.

---

[1] We have received permission from all individuals to write about their trauma experiences and have also changed certain key details to limit possible identification. We are thankful to the Metiv Crisis Center at Herzog Hospital in Israel, where one of us (T. G. G.) is employed.

Two months later, at a follow-up meeting, Lily reported a feeling of well-being. She still experienced dreams in which she heard explosions and people shouting, but she considered this normal.

She had changed her priorities: "I have no control over certain things, and I might be in another bombing, but I want to influence what I *do* have control over. I want to live my life as best I can," she said to the therapist.

The therapist maintains follow-up with Lily, who calls the therapist before every Jewish holiday. Lily reports feeling well and gives details of her family's concerns. She was considering early retirement, and looked forward to developing her interest in studying art. Among her other plans is volunteer work, helping others who have gone through similar experiences. Recently Lily invited her therapist to her son's wedding. The therapist went—a very moving experience for both the therapist and her client.

Case 2: Uri

Note the focus on self-efficacy in particular for this former soldier, as well as the failure of his superiors to offer appropriate support.

Uri, a first responder in his late 30s, came to the crisis center seeking help following a suicide bombing on a bus the previous month. He had arrived first on the scene and witnessed a second bus exploding before his eyes. He rushed to the first bus and tried to enter it, but the smoke prevented his doing so. He then tried to resuscitate an elderly woman outside until the paramedics arrived. He suffered burns but was only treated hours later, as he was busy assisting the survivors.

This was not Uri's first traumatic event. As part of his job he had been involved in many rescue operations and had been decorated for his valor. But he felt that there was something different about this event. Uri found it very difficult to return to his routine; he suffered from lack of sleep, physical tension and hypervigilance, sore muscles, depression, and reliving of the terrible scenes that revisited him "like movies"— especially of a woman he could not save. He was distressed because he had always perceived himself as strong and had never reacted in this way in the past.

He was also troubled by the reactions of his superiors, who told him that he should just "forget about it" and return to normal. Uri was diagnosed with PTSD and started immediately on a treatment course of exposure therapy (trauma-focused cognitive-behavioral treatment), aimed at confronting the traumatic situations in a safe and systematic way in order to change his perception about the traumatic event and regulate his tension and anxiety. Uri was encouraged to return to the active sports he loved so well as part of the effort to regulate his physiological arousal. He found the strength to continue with his treatment despite lack of support from his commanders and his worry that this would adversely affect his promotion.

Following the treatment, which Uri undertook like a true soldier, overcoming his fears and pain, he was able to return to work in a different position. The flashbacks dissipated, and Uri was able to participate in family events and visit public places again. He was still grappling with issues of self-image and the need to redefine his idea of resilience. His wife, who was very appreciative of the progress he made, sent the trauma center staff homemade cake and a symbolic gift.

On follow-up 1 year later, Uri reported further improvement. He is still suffering from high arousal and is being treated with antidepressant medication. He is, however, functioning well in a different job within the service and has withstood the pressure to take early retirement. Uri feels that although he hasn't returned to his previous level of functioning, he has stabilized. He is now able to cope with day-to-day life and has reconnected to his resilience and vitality. He sees it as his mission to help raise awareness for the distress experienced by first responders and for the lack of support for them in the culture of these organizations.

Case 3: Joel

Joel was a bystander in one instance of a terrorist attack and later he was directly caught in one. Note the mixed use of exposure therapy and grief counseling and a focus on connections (as both sources of trauma exposure and support).

Joel, a single man in his 20s, had a steady job, was socially active, and had a warm, supportive relationship with his family. He came to the crisis center asking for help just a few hours after a suicide bombing on a bus below his flat. It was early morning, and a first blast woke him. He went to the window and opened it to see what had caused the noise. Then he said, "The blast burst into my home through the window." He first heard the quiet, and then the sounds of injured people and shouting erupted. He saw the smoke and the scattered bodies and smelled the burned flesh. Joel immediately phoned for help, and after the first responders arrived, he went to work, but found that he could not concentrate. The sights and smells kept intruding. A fellow worker referred him to the crisis center, and he came in 5 hours after the bombing.

It transpired that due to the location of his flat—over a busy, much-targeted intersection—he had witnessed a number of terrorist attacks prior to the one that brought him to seek help. In the past Joel had always mobilized, called 911 and the media, been interviewed, and returned to his daily routine very quickly. This time, something different was happening. He felt very anxious and jumpy, could not concentrate, felt nauseous, and was overwhelmed with doubts and questions: "Why did I choose to live here?"; "Perhaps I should leave"; "Why is death pursuing me?"

He responded well to the intervention, which served to calm him down, reduce anxiety over his reactions by normalizing them, structure his experience, and validate his questions and his concerns for his safety. This was a single-session intervention—Joel reported on follow-up that he had resolved some of the questions that had bothered him, was calmer, had returned to work, and had made the decision to relocate to a quieter neighborhood.

Two years later, Joel walked through the door again, this time bringing members of his extended family with him. He asked for his therapist, and there, in the waiting room, told her in a rush that he had been through another terrorist attack 3 days previously. This time he had been staying with his family and a few friends in a resort hotel. Terrorists had planted a bomb, and most of the hotel was devastated. Joel was able to escape the building with a relative—a small child—in his arms. He was extremely active in assisting other victims and survivors. After fretful hours following the bombing, he learned that the rest of his family and friends had been in another part of the building, farther from the explosion, and were physically unharmed. The young woman he had just started dating, however, was among those killed.

Beginning a day after the attack, Joel experienced severe emotional stress. He had flashbacks and experienced fear of another terrorist attack. He oscillated between the intrusive memories and avoidance of all reminders of the event. He reported hypervigilance and trouble sleeping. Joel also had outbursts of weeping and blamed himself for not being able to save the young woman as well.

Although Joel returned to work, he was not able to function at his previous level. The therapy, which lasted 2 months, focused first on the traumatic images through use of exposure. Only after the posttraumatic symptoms subsided was Joel able to mourn and begin working through his traumatic loss. He gradually returned to functioning, and his sense of competence and vitality was restored.

On follow-up, Joel reported having "bounced back," and was functioning well in the work, social, and family spheres. He had just returned from a vacation, with some of the same friends, at a resort hotel close to the one that had been bombed, and he reported having had a good time.

CONCLUSION

We have identified five principles of intervention following the important work of the panel sponsored by the National Center for PTSD and SAMSHA (Hobfoll et al., 2006). These principles do not provide a specific set of interventions that have stood the test of controlled clinical trials, and it is our contention that such a set of interventions may elude us for many years, and may indeed be impossible to achieve. These five principles, however, guide priorities for intervention following terrorism and mass casualty events. They can guide intervention in two ways. First, intervention should use them as yardsticks and guides to develop intervention. Second, interventions that do not focus on these five principles should be viewed circumspectly. We cannot a priori say that all such interventions would not prove successful, but there would be increased need to justify investing resources in them over alternative interventions that do focus on one or more of these five principles.

Looking across these principles, one of the key elements of intervention is pairing psychological and pharmacological intervention with an understanding that terrorism and mass casualty often result in a drastic diminishment of personal, social, and condition resources that individuals, families, and groups require to recover or maintain their well-being following trauma (Hobfoll, 1991, 1998). This massive decline in resources must be attended to or treatment will enter a victim-blaming mode because people will be unable to respond to efforts to provide aid. This means that psychosocial intervention must be tied to financial, material, social, and community resources in an integrated, interwoven manner. Normally, the mental health professional refers clients for such needs, but such referral would lead to likely failure in the post-mass casualty environment. Rather than refer for services, the watchword must be partnering with other services and even offering services in an integrated, one-stop package.

As a final caution, we must emphasize that many of the individuals and communities that are most devastated by mass trauma were not in a healthy, resource-endowed state prior to trauma. Hence, the idea of returning them to normalcy is a mistaken concept as they as individuals, groups, families, and communities that are at most trauma risk are often already not doing well and receiving an unfair slice of society's riches (Fullilove, 2005; Galea et al., 2002). This offers an opportunity for intervention that might address these imbalances and offer such individuals, groups, and communities an opportunity to participate in not just rebuilding but achieving a better future.

REFERENCES

Adger, W. N., Hughes, T. P., Folke, C., Carpenter, S. R., & Rockstrom, J. (2005). Social-ecological resilience to coastal disasters. *Science, 309*, 1036–1039.

Ahern, J., Galea, S., Resnick, H., Kilpatrick, D., Bucuvalas, M., Gold, J., et al. (2002). Television images and psychological symptoms after the September 11 terrorist attacks. *Psychiatry, Interpersonal and Biological Processes, 65*(4), 289–300.

Andrews, B., Brewin, C. R., & Rose, S. (2003). Gender, social support, and PTSD in victims of violent crime. *Journal of Traumatic Stress, 16*(4), 421–427.

Antoni, M H., Lehman, J. M., Kilbourn, K. M., Boyers, A. E., Culver, J. L., Alferi, S. M., et al. (2001). Cognitive-behavioral stress management intervention decreases the prevalence of depression and enhances benefit finding among women under treatment for early-stage breast cancer. *Health Psychology, 20*, 20–32.

Antonovsky, A. (1979). *Health, stress, and coping.* San Francisco: Jossey-Bass.

Bandura, A. (1997). *Self efficacy: The exercise of control.* New York: Freeman.

Basoglu, M., Livanou, M., Crnobaric, C., Franciskovic, T., Suljic, E., Duric, D., et al. (2005). Psychiatric and cognitive effects of war on former Yugoslavia. *Journal of the American Medical Association, 294*(5), 580–590.

Baum, A., Cohen, L., & Hall, M. (1993). Control and intrusive memories as possible determinants of chronic stress. *Psychosomatic Medicine, 55*, 274–286.

Bell, C. C., Flay, B., & Paikoff, R. (2002). Strategies for health behavioral change. In J. Chunn (Ed.), *The health behavioral change Imperative: Theory, education, and practice in diverse populations* (pp. 17–40). New York: Kluwer Academic/Plenum Press.

Benight, C. C. (2004). Collective efficacy following a series of natural disasters. *Anxiety, Stress, and Coping, 17*(4), 401–420.

Benight, C. C., Freyaldenhoven, R. W., Hughes, J., Ruiz, J. M., & Zoschke, T. A. (2000). Coping self-efficacy and psychological distress following the Oklahoma City bombing. *Journal of Applied Social Psychology, 30*, 1331–1344.

Benight, C. C., & Harper, M. L. (2002). Coping self-efficacy perceptions as a mediator between acute stress response and long-term distress following natural disasters. *Journal of Traumatic Stress, 15*(3), 177–186.

Benight, C. C., Ironson, G., Klebe, K., Carver, C. S., Wynings, C., Burnett, K., et al. (1999). Conservation of resources and coping self-efficacy predicting distress following a natural disaster: A causal model analysis where the environment meets the mind. *Anxiety, Stress and Coping, 12*(2), 107–126.

Benight, C. C., Swift, E., Sanger, J., Smith, A., & Zeppelin, D. (1999). Coping self-efficacy as a mediator of distress following a natural disaster. *Journal of Applied Social Psychology, 29,* 2443–2464.

Bisson, J. I., Jenkins, P. L., Alexander, J., & Bannister, C. (1997). Randomized controlled trial of psychological debriefing for victims of acute burn trauma. *British Journal of Psychiatry, 171,* 78–81.

Bleich, A., Gelkopf, M., & Solomon, Z. (2003). Exposure to terrorism, stress-related mental health symptoms, and coping behaviors among a nationally representative sample in Israel. *Journal of the American Medical Association, 290*(5), 612–620.

Breznitz, S. (1983). Anticipatory stress reactions. In S. Breznitz (Ed.), *The denial of stress* (pp. 225–255). New York: International Universities Press.

Briere, J., & Elliott, D. (2000). Prevalence, characteristics, and long-term sequelae of natural disaster exposure in the general population. *Journal of Traumatic Stress, 13,* 661–679.

Bryant, R. A. (2006). Cognitive behavior therapy: Implications from advances in neuroscience. In N. Kato, M. Kawata, & R. K. Pitman (Eds.), *PTSD: Brain mechanisms and clinical implications* (pp. 255–270). Tokyo: Springer-Verlag.

Bryant, R. A., Harvey, A. G., Dang, S. T., Sackville, T., & Basten, C. (1998). Treatment of Acute Stress Disorder: A comparison of cognitive-behavioral therapy and supportive counseling. *Journal of Consulting and Clinical Psychology, 66*(5), 862–866.

Bryant, R. A., Harvey, A. G., Guthrie, R. M., & Moulds, M. L. (2003). Acute psychophysiological arousal and posttraumatic stress disorder: A two-year prospective study. *Journal of Traumatic Stress, 16*(5), 439–443.

Bryant, R. A., Sackville, T., Dang, S. T., Moulds, M., & Guthrie, R. (1999). Treating acute stress disorder: An evaluation of cognitive behavior therapy and supportive counseling. *American Journal of Psychiatry, 156,* 1780–1786.

Carlier, I. V., Lamberts, R. D., van Uchelen, A. J., & Gersons, B. P. (1998). Disaster-related posttraumatic stress in police officers: A field study of the impact of debriefing, *Stress Medicine, 14,* 143–148.

Carlson, L. E., Speca, M., Patel, K. D., & Goodey, E. (2003). Mindfulness-based stress reduction in relation to quality of life, mood, symptoms of stress, and immune parameters in breast and prostate cancer outpatients. *Psychosomatic Medicine, 65*(4), 571–581.

Carver, C. S., & Scheier, M. R. (1998). *On the self-regulation of behavior.* New York: Cambridge University Press.

Cohen, L., Warneke, C., Fouladi, R. T., Rodriguez, M. A., & Chaoul-Reich, A. (2004). Psychological adjustment and sleep quality in a randomized trial of the effects of a Tibetan yoga intervention in patients with Lymphoma. *Cancer, 100*(10), 2253–2260.

Davidson, J. R. T., Landerman, L. R., Farfel, G. M., & Clary, C. M. (2002). Characterizing the effects of Sertratine in post-traumatic stress disorder. *Psychological Medicine, 32*(4), 661–670.

de Jong, J. T. V. M. (1995). Prevention of the consequences of man-made or natural disaster at the (inter)national, the community, the family and the individual level. In S. E. Hobfoll, & M. W. de Vries (Eds.), *Extreme stress and communities: Impact and intervention* (pp. 207–229). Boston: Kluwer.

de Jong, J. T. V. M. (Ed.). (2002a). *Trauma, war and violence: Public mental health in sociocultural context.* New York: Plenum-Kluwer.

de Jong, J. T. V. M. (2002b). Public mental health, traumatic stress and human rights violations in low-income countries: A culturally appropriate model in times of conflict, disaster and peace. In J. de Jong (Ed.), *Trauma, war and violence: Public mental health in sociocultural context* (pp. 1–91). New York: Plenum-Kluwer.

de Jong, J. T. V. M., & Clarke, L. (Eds.). (1996). *Mental health of refugees* [online]. Geneva, Switzerland: World Health Organization. Available at *whqlibdoc.who.int/hq/1996/a49374.pdf* de Jong, J. T. V .M., Komproe, I. H., & van Ommeren, M. (2003). Common mental disorders in post-conflict settings. *Lancet, 361*(6), 2128–2130.

Foa, E. B., Hearst-Ikeda, D., & Perry, K. J. (1995). Evaluation of a brief cognitive-behavioral program for the prevention of chronic PTSD in recent assault victims. *Journal of Consulting and Clinical Psychology, 63*(6), 948–955.

Foa, E. B., Keane, T. M., & Friedman, M. J. (Eds.). (2000). *Effective treatments for PTSD: Practice guidelines from the International Society for Traumatic Stress Studies.* New York: Guilford Press.

Foa, E. B., & Meadows, E. A. (1997). Psychosocial treatment for posttraumatic stress disorder: A critical review. *Annual Review of Psychology, 48,* 449–480.

Foa, E. B., & Rothbaum, B. O. (1998). *Treating the trauma of rape: Cognitive-behavioral therapy for PTSD.* New York: Guilford Press.

Foa, E. B., Rothbaum, B. O., Riggs, D., & Murdock, T. (1991). Treatment of posttraumatic stress disorder in rape victims: A comparison between cognitive-behavioral procedures and counseling. *Journal of Consulting and Clinical Psychology, 59,* 715–723.

Foa, E. B., Zoellner, L. A., & Feeny, N. C. (2006). An evaluation of three brief programs for facilitating recovery after assault. *Journal of Traumatic Stress, 19,* 29–43.

Follette, V. F., & Ruzek, J. I. (2006). *Cognitive-behavioral therapies for trauma* (2nd ed.). New York: Guilford Press.

Freedy, J. R., & Hobfoll, S. E. (1994). Stress inoculation for reduction of burnout: A Conservation of Resources approach. *Anxiety, Stress, and Coping, 6,* 311–325.

Freedy, J. R., Shaw, D. L., Jarrell, M. P., & Masters, C. R. (1992). Towards an understanding of the psychological impact of natural disasters: An application of the conservation of resources stress model. *Journal of Traumatic Stress, 5*(3), 441–454.

Fremont, W. P. (2004). Childhood reactions to terrorism-induced trauma: A review of the past 10 years. *Journal of the American Academy of Child and Adolescent Psychiatry, 43*(4), 381–392.

Friedman, M. J., Charney, D. S., & Deutsch, A.Y. (Eds.). (1995). *Neurobiological and clinical consequences of stress: From normal adaptation to post-traumatic stress disorder.* Philadelphia: Lippincott-Raven.

Friedman, M. J., & Davidson, J. R. T. (2007). Pharmacotherapy for PTSD. In M. J. Friedman, T. M. Keane, & P. A. Resick (Eds.) *Handbook of PTSD: Science and practice* (pp. 376–405). New York: Guilford Press.

Friedman, M. J., Davidson, J. R. T., Mellman, T. A., & Southwick, S. M. (2000). Pharmacotherapy. In E. B. Foa, T. M. Keane, & M. J. Friedman (Eds.), *Effective treatments for PTSD: Practice guidelines from the International Society for Traumatic Stress Studies* (pp. 326–329). New York: Guilford Press.

Fullilove, M. (2005). *Root shock: How tearing up city neighborhoods hurts America, and what we can do about it.* New York: Random House.

Galea, S., Ahern, J., Resnick, H., Kilpatrick, D., Bucuvalas, M., Gold, J., et al. (2002). Psychological sequelae of the September 11 terrorist attacks in New York City. *New England Journal of Medicine, 346,* 982–987.

Galea, S., Vlahov, D., Resnick, H., Ahern, J., Susser, E., Gold, J., et al. (2003). Trends of probable post-traumatic stress disorder in New York City after the September 11 terrorist attacks. *American Journal of Epidemiology, 158*(6), 514–524.

Gersons, B. P., Carlier, I. V., Lamberts, R. D., & van der Kolk, B. (2000). A randomized clinical trial of brief eclectic psychotherapy in police officers with posttraumatic stress disorder. *Journal of Traumatic Stress, 13*(2), 333–347.

Gersons, B. P., & Olff, M. (2005). Coping with the aftermath of trauma. *British Medical Journal, 330*(7499), 1038–1039.

Giel, R. (1990). Psychosocial processes in disasters. *International Journal of Mental Health, 19*(1), 7–20.

Ginzburg, K., Solomon, Z., Dekel, R., & Neria, Y. (2003). Battlefield functioning and chronic PTSD: Associations with perceived self-efficacy and causal attribution. *Personality and Individual Differences, 34*(3), 463–476.

Green, B. L., Lindy, J. D., Grace, M. C., Gleser, G. C., Leonard, A. C., Korol, M., et al. (1990). Buffalo Creek survivors in the second decade: Stability of stress symptoms. *American Journal of Orthopsychiatry, 60*(1), 43–54.

Hall, B. J., Hobfoll, S. E., Palmieri, P, Johnson, R., Shapira, O., & Galea, S. (in press). The psychological impact of forced settler disengagement in Gaza: Trauma and posttraumatic growth. *Journal of Traumatic Stress.*

Harvey, A. G., & Bryant, R. A. (2002). Acute stress disorder: A synthesis and critique. *Psychological Bulletin, 128,* 886–902.

Hickling, E. J., & Blanchard, E. B. (1997). The private practice psychologist and manual-based treatments: Posttraumatic stress disorder secondary to motor vehicle accidents. *Behavior Research and Therapy, 35*(3), 191–203.

Hobbs, M., & Mayou, R., Harrison, B., & Worlock, P. (1996). A randomized controlled trial of psychological debriefing for victims of road traffic accidents. *British Medical Journal, 313,* 1438–1439.

Hobfoll, S. E. (1991). Traumatic stress: A theory based on rapid loss of resources. *Anxiety Research: An International Journal, 4,* 187–197.

Hobfoll, S. E. (1998). *Stress, culture, and community: The psychology and philosophy of stress.* New York: Plenum Press.

Hobfoll, S. E. (2002). Social and psychological resources and adaptation. *Review of General Psychology, 6,* 307–324.

Hobfoll, S. E., Briggs-Phillips, M., & Stines, L. R. (2003). Fact or artifact: The relationship of hope to a caravan of resources. In R. Jacoby & G. Keinan (Eds.), *Between stress and hope: From a disease-centered to a health-centered perspective* (pp. 81–104). Westport, CT: Praeger.

Hobfoll, S. E., Canetti-Nisim, D., & Johnson, R. J. (2006). Exposure to terrorism, stress-related mental health symptoms, and defensive coping among Jews and Arabs in Israel. *Journal of Consulting and Clinical Psychology, 74,* 207–218.

Hobfoll, S. E., & London, P. (1986). The relationship of self-concept and social support to emotional distress among women during war. *Journal of Social and Clinical Psychology, 4,* 189–203.

Hobfoll, S. E., Spielberger, C. D., Breznitz, S., Figley, C., Folkman, S., Green, B. L., et al. (1991). War-related stress: Addressing the stress of war and other traumatic events. *American Psychologist, 46,* 848–855.

Hobfoll, S. E., Watson, P., Bells, C. C., Bryant, R. A., Brymer, M. J., Friedman, M. J., et al. (in press). Five essential elements of immediate and mid-term mass trauma intervention: Empirical evidence. *Journal of Psychiatry: Interpersonal and Biological Processes.*

Ironson, G., Wynings, C., Schneiderman, N., Baum, A., Rodriguez, M., Greenwood, D., et al. (1997). Posttraumatic stress symptoms, intrusive thoughts, loss, and immune function after Hurricane Andrew. *Psychosomatic Medicine, 59,* 128–141.

Janoff-Bulman, R. (1992). *Shattered assumptions: Toward a new psychology of trauma.* New York: The Free Press.

Kaniasty, K., & Norris, F. H. (1993). A test of the social support deterioration model in the context of natural disaster. *Journal of Personality and Social Psychology, 64*(3), 395–408.

Keinan, G., Friedland, N., & Sarignaor, V. (1990). Training for task-performance under stress: The effectiveness of phased training methods, part 2. *Journal of Applied Social Psychology, 20*(18), 1514–1529.

Kilpatrick, D. G., Veronen, L. J., & Resick, P. A. (1982). Psychological sequelae to rape: Assessment and treatment strategies. In D. M. Dolays & R. L. Meredith (Eds.), *Behavioral medicine: Assessment and treatment strategies* (pp. 473–497). New York: Plenum Press.

King, L. A., & Miner, K. N. (2000). Writing about the perceived benefits of traumatic events: Implications for physical health. *Personality and Social Psychology Bulletin, 26,* 220–230.

Litz, B. T., & Gray, M. J. (2002). Early intervention for mass violence: What is the evidence? What should be done? *Cognitive and Behavioral Practice, 9*(4), 266–272.

Lomranz, J. (1990). Long-term adaptation to traumatic stress in light of adult development and aging perspectives. In M. A. Stephens, J. H. Crowther, S. E. Hobfoll, & D. L. Tennenbaum (Eds.), *Stress and coping in later-life families* (pp. 221–235). New York: Hemisphere.

McFarlane, A. C., & van der Kolk, B. A. (1996). Trauma and its challenge to society. In B. A. van der Kolk & A. C. McFarlane (Eds.), *Traumatic stress: The effects of overwhelming experience on mind, body, and society* (pp. 24–46). New York: Guilford Press.

McNally, R. J., Bryant, R. A., & Ehlers, A. (2003). Does early psychological intervention promote recovery from posttraumatic stress? *Psychological Science in the Public Interest, 4*(2), 45–79.

Meichenbaum, D. (1974). *Cognitive behavior modification.* Morristown, NJ: General Learning Press.

Najavits, L. M. (2002). *Seeking safety: A treatment manual for PTSD and substance abuse.* New York: Guilford Press.

Najavits, L. M., Weiss, R. D., Shaw, S. R., & Muenz, L. R. (1998). Seeking safety: Outcome of a new cognitive-behavioral psychotherapy for women with posttraumatic stress disorder and substance dependence. *Journal of Traumatic Stress, 11*(3), 437–456.

Norris, F. H., Baker, C. K., Murphy, A. D., & Kaniasty, K. (2005). Social support mobilization and deterioration after Mexico's 1999 flood: Effects of context, gender, and time. *American Journal of Community Psychology, 36*(1–2), 15–28.

Norris, F. H., Friedman, M. J., & Watson, P. J. (2002). 60,000 disaster victims speak, part II: Summary and implications of the disaster mental health research. *Psychiatry: Interpersonal and Biological Processes, 65*(3), 240–260.

Norris, F. H., & Kaniasty, K. (1996). Received and perceived social support in times of stress: A test of the social support deterioration deterrence model. *Journal of Personality and Social Psychology, 71,* 498–511.

Ozer, E. M., & Bandura, A. (1990). Mechanisms governing empowerment effects: A self-efficacy analysis. *Journal of Personality and Social Psychology, 58*(3), 472–486.

Panksepp, J. (1998). *Affective neuroscience: The foundations of human and animal emotions.* New York: Oxford University Press.

Pfefferbaum, B., Doughty, D. E., Reddy, C., Patel, N., Gurwitch, R. H., Nixon, S. J., et al. (2002). Exposure and peritraumatic response as predictors of posttraumatic stress in children following the 1995 Oklahoma City bombing. *Journal of Urban Health—Bulletin of The New York Academy of Medicine, 79*(3), 354–363.

Pitman, R. K., Sanders, K. M., Zusman, R. M., Healy, A. R., Cheema, F., Lasko, N. B., et al. (2002). Pilot study of secondary prevention of posttraumatic stress disorder with propranolol. *Biological Psychiatry, 51*(2), 189–192.

Pynoos, R. S., Goenjian, A., & Steinberg, A. M. (1995). Strategies of disaster intervention for children and adolescents. In S. E. Hobfoll & M. de Vries (Eds.), *Extreme stress and communities: Impact and intervention* (pp. 445–471). Dordrecht, Netherlands: Kluwer.

Rappaport, J. (1981). In praise of paradox: A social policy of empowerment over prevention. *American Journal of Community Psychology, 9,* 1–25.

Resick, P. A., Nishith, P., Weaver, T. L., Astin, M. C., & Feuer, C. A. (2002). A comparison of cognitive-processing therapy with prolonged exposure and a waiting condition for the treatment of chronic posttraumatic stress disorder in female rape victims. *Journal Of Consulting and Clinical Psychology, 70*(4), 867–879.

Resick, P. A., & Schnicke, M. K. (1992). Cognitive processing therapy for sexual assault victims. *Journal of Consulting and Clinical Psychology, 60*(5), 748–756.

Rogers, R. W. (1983). Cognitive and physiological processes in fear appeals and attitude change:

A revised theory of protection motivation. In J. Cacioppo & R. Petty (Eds.), *Social psychophysiology* (pp. 153–176). New York: Guilford Press.

Rogers, R. W., & Mewborn, C. R. (1976). Fear appeals and attitude change: Effects of a threat's noxiousness, probability of occurrence, and the efficacy of the coping responses. *Journal of Personality and Social Psychology, 34,* 54–61.

Rook, K. S. (1984). The negative side of social interaction: Impact on psychological well-being. *Journal of Personality and Social Psychology, 46,* 1097–1108.

Rubin, G. J., Brewin, C. R., Greenberg, N., Simpson, J., & Wessely, S. (2005). Psychological and behavioural reactions to the bombings in London on 7 July 2005: Cross sectional survey of a representative sample of Londoners. *British Medical Journal, 331*(7517), 606–611.

Sampson, R. J., Raudenbush, S. W., & Earls, F. (1997). Neighborhoods and violent crime: A multilevel study of collective efficacy. *Science, 277,* 918–924.

Sattler, D. N., Preston, A. J., Kaiser, C. F., Olivera, V. E., Valdez, J., & Schlueter, S. (2002). Hurricane Georges: A cross-national study examining preparedness, resource loss, and psychological distress in the U.S. Virgin Islands, Puerto Rico, Dominican Republic, and the United States. *Journal of Traumatic Stress, 15*(5), 339–350.

Schlenger, W., Cadell, J., Ebert, L., Jordan, B., Rourke, K., Wilson, D., et al. (2002). Psychological reactions to terrorist attacks: Findings from the National Study of Americans' Reactions to September 11. *Journal of the American Medical Association, 288,* 581–588.

Shalev, A. Y., & Freedman, S. (2005). PTSD following terrorist attacks: A prospective evaluation. *American Journal of Psychiatry, 162*(6), 1188–1191.

Shalev, A. Y., Sahar, T., Freedman, S., Peri, T., Glick, N., Brandes, D., et al. (1998). A prospective study of heart rate response following trauma and the subsequent development of posttraumatic stress disorder. *Archives of General Psychiatry, 55,* 553–559.

Shalev, A. Y., Tuval-Mashiach, R., & Hadar, H. (2004). Posttraumatic stress disorder as a result of mass trauma. *Journal of Clinical Psychiatry, 65*(1), 4–10.

Shmotkin, D., Blumstein, T., & Modan, B. (2003). Tracing long-term effects of early trauma: A broad-scope view of Holocaust survivors in late life. *Journal of Consulting and Clinical Psychology, 71*(2), 223–234.

Silver, R. C., Holman, E. A., McIntosh, D. N., Poulin, M., & Gil-Rivas, V. (2002). Nationwide longitudinal study of psychological responses to September 11. *Journal of the American Medical Association, 288,* 1235–1244.

Solomon, Z. (2003). *Coping with war-induced stress: The Gulf war and the Israeli response.* New York: Plenum Press.

Solomon, Z., & Benbenishty, R. (1986). The role of proximity, immediacy, and expectancy in frontline treatment of combat stress reaction among Israelis in the Lebanon war. *American Journal of Psychiatry, 143,* 613–617.

Solomon, Z., Shklar, R., & Mikulincer, M. (2005). Front line treatment of combat stress reaction: A 20 year longitudinal evaluation study. *American Journal of Psychiatry, 162,* 2309–2314.

Stanton, A. L., Danoff-Burg, S., Sworowsky, L., & Collins, C. (2001). Randomized, controlled trial of written emotional disclosure and benefit finding in breast cancer patients. *Psychosomatic Medicine, 63,* 122–122.

Ursano, R. J., Fullerton, C. S., & Norwood, A. E. (1995). Psychiatric dimensions of disaster: Patient care, community consultation, and preventive medicine. *Harvard Review of Psychiatry, 3*(4), 196–209.

Ursano, R. J., McCaughey, B. G., & Fullerton, C. S. (1994). Trauma and disaster. In R. J. Ursano, B. G. McCaughey, & C. S. Fullerton (Eds.), *Individual and community responses to trauma and disaster* (pp. 3–28). Cambridge, UK: Cambridge University Press.

van de Put, W. A. C. M., & Eisenbruch, I. M. (2002). The Cambodian experience. In J. T. V. M. de Jong (Ed.), *Trauma, war and violence: Public mental health in sociocultural context* (pp. 93–155). New York: Plenum-Kluwer.

van der Kolk, B. A., & McFarlane, A. C. (1996). The black hole of trauma. In B. A. van der Kolk & A. C. McFarlane (Eds.), *Traumatic stress: The effects of overwhelming experience on mind, body, and society* (pp. 3–23). New York: Guilford Press.

Yehuda, R. (1998). Psychoneuroendocrinology of post-traumatic stress disorder. *Psychiatric Clinics of North America, 21,* 359.

Yehuda, R., McFarlane, A., & Shalev, A. (1998). Predicting the development of posttraumatic stress disorder from the acute response to a traumatic event. *Biological Psychiatry, 44,* 1305–1313.

SUGGESTED READINGS

Bryant, R. A., Harvey, A. G., Dang, S. T., Sackville, T., & Basten, C. (1998). Treatment of Acute Stress Disorder: A comparison of cognitive-behavioral therapy and supportive counseling. *Journal of Consulting and Clinical Psychology, 66*(5), 862–866.

de Jong, J. T. V. M. (Ed.). (2002a). *Trauma, war and violence: Public mental health in sociocultural context.* New York: Plenum-Kluwer.

Foa, E. B., & Rothbaum, B. O. (1998). *Treating the trauma of rape: Cognitive-behavioral therapy for PTSD.* New York: Guilford Press.

Hobfoll, S. E. (1998). *Stress, culture, and community: The psychology and philosophy of stress.* New York: Plenum Press.

Najavits, L. M. (2002). *Seeking safety: A treatment manual for PTSD and substance abuse.* New York: Guilford Press.

Resick, P. A., Nishith, P., Weaver, T. L., Astin, M. C., & Feuer, C. A. (2002). A comparison of cognitive-processing therapy with prolonged exposure and a waiting condition for the treatment of chronic posttraumatic stress disorder in female rape victims. *Journal of Consulting and Clinical Psychology, 70*(4), 867–879.

Solomon, Z. (2003). *Coping with war-induced stress: The Gulf war and the Israeli response.* New York: Plenum Press.

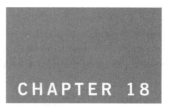

CHAPTER 18

Problem Solving and Crisis Intervention

Joop J. Meijers

*H*ebrew is a 2,000-year-old language that was revived in the late 19th and early 20th centuries. The word that denotes *crisis* in Hebrew has an interesting and intriguing history. The modern word used for crisis is *mashber*. The core meaning of this word is "to break." The related word *shewer* refers to "that which is broken." It can also mean "solution.". Interestingly, in the book of Isaiah (Chapter 37), the term *mashber* refers to "the exit of the uterus" (i.e., the point at which a newborn exits the womb during childbirth). The *mashber*, or crisis, that the prophet is referring to is a situation in which a woman who, under duress, has no strength left to endure childbirth. From this concept, the Talmud derives another meaning from the term *mashber*. In the Talmud (circa 200 C.E.), *mashber* stands for the bed or chair on which the mother gives birth. In essence, the child's birth is the problem and, at the same time, the solution.

The original Greek term *crisis*, which derives from the term *klinein*, means "to judge" or "to decide." The Hebrew term refers to an existential moment in which something is ruptured, broken, or destroyed in order to make room for something new or different. Crisis is like a birth, in that the infant breaks through, out of the womb, and into the outside world. In this way, a crisis is a "critical," decisive situation in which a problem is forcefully broken up and solved. In other words, crisis is an opportunity for growth and development. The famous expression "strike while the iron is hot" refers to the same concept: that sometimes the best opportunity to change an existing situation is when the situation becomes malleable. Only then is change a possible solution.

In this chapter, the concept of "problem solving" is derived from the original cognitive-behavioral model of interpersonal problem solving (IPS), developed in the early 1970s by D'Zurilla and Goldfried (1971) and further developed and elaborated on by Nezu (2004), Spivack and Shure (1974), and others. The main thesis of this chapter is that IPS offers a fruitful and worthwhile model for the development of strategies in coping with a variety of crisis situations.

We understand that crisis situations are those in which an individual is confronted by a real or perceived need to find a rather quick solution to a circumstance that is real or is perceived as demanding. The IPS model guides an individual facing a crisis through a series of cognitive and behavioral steps that increase the chances of finding a solution to the crisis. Often, but not always, the solution presents in the form of a new behavioral response that changes the situation. Sometimes the solution response is a cognitive-emotional response that changes the person's feelings about and attitude toward the crisis situation so that it becomes easier to accept or live with. Thanks to the solution response, the situation loses its crisis character and becomes more tolerable.

It is well known that the emotional impact of a crisis situation impairs cognitive functioning. Once we are faced with a crisis, it is very difficult to "problem solve." Therefore, it is posited that IPS training, in which a series of steps is needed to solve problems, can become part of an individual's personal skills. A metaphor might be best to illustrate this point: In many monsoon countries, people learn how to cope with wet roads on rainy days by learning how to skid in a productive fashion. Most drivers train until they reach a level of proficiency at which they can react automatically by applying the brakes of their motor vehicle at a moment's notice. In the same vein, training in IPS can benefit individuals in crisis situations where they have to make crucial decisions—sometimes in split seconds—that allow little time for them to engage their cognitive functions.

The model proposed in this chapter was initially developed from work with parents, children, and teachers who, on a daily basis, face one crisis after the other. IPS is a general skill, or a form of metacognition, that can easily be generalized to other situations. Consequently, it may be considered a general skill used to cope with crisis situations in different settings with various populations under different circumstances.

PROBLEMS AS CRISES AND CRISES AS PROBLEMS

An underlying assumption of this chapter is the link between problems and crises. Not all problems evolve into crises. Some problems are simply situations that require a solution. So, when does a problem actually evolve into a crisis? The answer depends on how one defines a crisis, as well as on how a particular individual (not the researcher or clinician) defines his/her crises.

The *Merriam-Webster Online Dictionary* offers the following definitions of a "crisis":

> **a:** the turning point for better or worse in an acute disease or fever **b:** a paroxysmal attack of pain, distress, or disordered function **c:** an emotionally significant event or radical change of status in a person's life <a midlife crisis> **2:** the decisive moment (as in a literary plot) **3a:** an unstable or crucial time or state of affairs in which a decisive change is impending; especially : one with the distinct possibility of a highly undesirable outcome <a financial crisis> **b:** a situation that has reached a critical phase <the environmental crisis>

D'Zurilla and Nezu (1999) define a problem as

> any life situation or task (present or anticipated) that demands a response for adaptive functioning but no apparent response is immediately apparent or available to the person due to the presence of some obstacle or obstacles. (p. 11)

Comparing D'Zurilla and Nezu's (1999) definition of a problem using the previous definition of crisis, one notices the overlap of basic characteristics: Both definitions imply a turning point, a situation that demands a decision that can change the situation for better or worse. With both definitions, the individual must make a choice. In both circumstances, the situation is significant enough that the individual cannot ignore it. He/she *must* make a decision. An important difference, however, seems to exist as well: In a crisis the individual seems not to have the luxury of delaying his/her response. The situation is critical in the respect that it forces the individual to respond immediately, which is not the case in problem solving in general. The aforementioned definitions lack the urgency of what would be considered a crisis situation.

In the inverse, a crisis is *always* a problem that needs to be solved. From this perspective, all IPS models that have been described and subjected to experimental and empirical research form an important part of the tools available to cope with crises.

However, for IPS to be a useful coping tool in crisis situations, two questions must be answered:

1. Is there any evidence that in the emotionally arousing situation of a crisis, enough "cognitive space" is left to at least remember the main IPS steps one has to follow in order to cope with a crisis?
2. Can IPS indeed lead to a significant reduction in stress and arousal so that one can effectively cope with the crisis situation?

In his book *The Explosive Child*, Ross Greene (2001) describes explosive children's tendency to "melt down" in crisis situations. Once they are in such a state of emotional disarray, their ability to think the problem through rationally deteriorates.

Before answering these two questions, it might be prudent to describe the main problem-solving models available to us. After describing the models and their practical applications, I address the two aforementioned questions.

INTERPERSONAL PROBLEM-SOLVING MODELS

The main impetus to the more recent work on IPS reverts to an early article by D'Zurilla and Goldfried (1971). The authors articulated "interpersonal problem solving" as an important cognitive-behavioral skill that could be essential in maintaining one's mental health. Behaviorists in general contended that the skill consisted of a chain of cognitive and behavioral responses that, when available, increased the probability that one could respond to a problematic situation in such a way that the aversive aspects of the situation were reduced or eliminated while the positive consequences increased. Their definitions of *problem*, *problem solving*, and *solution* have been adopted by more recent researchers and clinicians—for example, D'Zurilla and Nezu (1999):

> Problem: "any life situation or task (present or anticipated) that demands a response for adaptive functioning but no apparent response is immediately apparent or available to the person due to the presence of some obstacle or obstacles" (D'Zurilla & Nezu, 1999, p. 11).
>
> Problem solving: "the self-directed cognitive-behavioral process by which a person attempts to identify or discover effective or adaptive solutions for specific problems encountered in everyday living" (D'Zurilla & Nezu, 1999, p. 10).
>
> Solution: "a situation-specific coping response or response pattern (cognitive and/ or behavioral) that is the product or outcome of the problem-solving process when it is applied to a specific problematic situation" (D'Zurilla & Nezu, 1999, p. 12).

Based on an extensive review of the literature the authors present a prescriptive working model of steps that, if taken sequentially, would improve the chances of finding and applying new solutions to existing problems. They specify a number of different "stages" through which the individual would have to pass to arrive from the earlier perception of a problem to the later solution. Their so-called prescriptive problem-solving model consists of two parts:

1. *Problem orientation*: the motivational base of problem solving which, in crisis situations, is almost always a given, considering the urgency of the crisis situation that leaves an individual little choice.
2. *Problem-solving proper*: the process by which an individual attempts to find an effective or adaptive solution to the crisis through the rational application of problem-solving strategies and techniques.

DIFFERENT PROBLEM-SOLVING MODELS
AND THEIR RELEVANCE FOR CRISIS INTERVENTION

After D'Zurilla and Goldfried's (1971) pioneering model was developed, a variety of other IPS models were developed. Two of the more influential models with implication for IPS as a crisis intervention are those introduced by Spivack and Shure (1974) and their team at Hahnemann University in Philadelphia, as well as Elias's (2006) work on problem-solving skill training in the schools. An additional model worth mentioning is the application of IPS developed by Alan Kazdin (2005) as an integral part of his parent management training protocol for work with parents of conduct-disordered children. In addition to the traditional learning principles of operant conditioning, reinforcement, and modeling, Kazdin ascribes importance to problem-solving skills for a variety of situations in which parents and children are uncertain as to what to do or how to behave in order to cope well in a problematic situation. In his earlier work, Kazdin used IPS principles to help conduct-disordered children in institutional settings (e.g., Kazdin, Siegel, & Bass, 1992; Kazdin, 2005). Although Kazdin's work is impressive and effective, it is not expounded here because, basically, he applied existing notions of IPS to conduct disorder problems without offering a new conception of IPS.

Spivack and Shure's Model

The main problem-solving skill emphasized by Spivack and Shure (1976) is known as MEPS (means–ends problem solving). There is an overlap between this skill and the third stage in the D'Zurilla and Goldfried (1971) model. Based on their extensive research with different populations (aggressive and normal children, psychiatric populations) Spivack, Platts, and Shure (1976) found that the (learned and learnable) skill of cognitively generating different means to problem situations greatly increased the chance that the individual who was trained in MEPS, in the real-life problem situation, while confronted with the immediate need to act, would execute the appropriate response and solve the problem situation. According to the authors, MEPS is a separate identifiable skill that can be taught independently and generalized to real-life problems and, consequently, to crisis situations.

In crisis situations, there may be a natural and spontaneous tendency to do the first thing that comes to mind. In some cases, this may be doing nothing at all. Individuals previously trained in MEPS skills might be in a better position to quickly think of the most appropriate response. Spivack and Shure (1974) found evidence for a correlation between MEPS skills and a decrease in aggressive behavior in children confronted with provocative and threatening situations. To the degree that one can conceptualize those situations as a kind of crisis situation for those children, having experienced MEPS training was helpful in finding alternative, constructive solutions to some of the problems the children often face.

One of the attractive aspects of Shure and Spivack's work is the applicability of the model to young, kindergarten children, 5 years of age (Spivack & Shure, 1974). Most other models of crisis intervention are not applicable to such young populations.

In later work, Shure (1994) extended the model to work with mothers of young children. In a clear and instructive book, written specifically for parents, she demonstrates how mothers (or fathers) can integrate problem-solving skills in dealing with educational crises and problems, if and when they occur. Here, also, preventive training is purported to provide parents with tools that they can use later in real-life crisis situations.

Elias's Model

In 1992 Elias and Clabby described a so-called social problem-solving curriculum, specifically designed for coping with problems and crises in school situations. Their original aim was to develop an approach that would help at-risk children "to think carefully and independently through decisions and problems." "We will help them to see that they have choices and some control over their lives" (Elias & Clabby, 1992). In developing their problem-solving model, the authors refer to Bronowski's) *The Ascent of Man*. Elias and Clabby (1992) cite Bronowski's belief that human beings have core skills that allow the potential for human survival and development:

> These qualities include the ability to think of several ways to reach a goal; forethought, analysis and planning; . . . the ability to recognize and use feelings as information with which to guide decision making, problem solving and action. (p. 12)

The authors list a number of social decision-making and problem-solving skills that, in their view, are essential. They translated the skills into specific steps that a schoolchild (or whoever faces a crisis situation) can use in coping with the problem:

1. Look for signs of different feelings.
2. Define the problem (crisis) for yourself.
3. Decide on your goal.
4. Stop and think of as many solutions to the problem or crisis as you can.
5. For each solution think of all the things that might happen next.
6. Choose your best solution.
7. Plan it and make a final check.
8. Try it and rethink it.

Elias developed his model over a period of 20 years in which he demonstrated the effectiveness of the model as applied to schoolchildren's coping with problem and crisis situations (Elias, 2006). Implicit in Elias's model is the distinction between the motivational part of IPS (e.g., feelings) and IPS proper (skills) like thinking of many different solutions.

Goldfried, D'Zurilla, and Nezu's Model

Of all the different problem-solving models, the one initiated by Goldfried and D'Zurilla and further developed by D'Zurilla and Nezu is no doubt the more influential model, on both a theoretical and an empirical level. Their prescriptive model (i.e., what people *should* do to better solve problems and cope with crisis situations) offers the most comprehensive and integrative model available for coping with crises.

For the aforementioned reason, in the section that follow we discuss their model in more detail and offer an illustration of the application of the model itself.

CRISES COPING THROUGH PROBLEM SOLVING: THE PROCESS

The general prescriptive problem-solving process consists of two parts:

1. *Problem-solving orientation*: motivational steps and stages that set the tone and conditions for effective problem solving. This relates to all the beliefs, attitudes, feelings a person has about problems in life—that is, his/her general ideas about how normal or abnormal it is to have problems at all or face crises and his/her beliefs in his/her ability to deal with crises and problems or the belief that crises are life situations that can be dealt with effectively.
2. *Problem solving proper*: all the activities an individual can generate to actually solve his/her problems and cope successfully with crises.

Problem-Solving Orientation

One never enters a crisis in a state of *tabula rasa*. Many factors determine how one responds to crisis. Because the defining characteristics of a crisis are its urgency and immediacy, there is no need for prior training in labeling feelings as signs of a problem or crisis. Most individuals are clearly able to determine when they are in the midst of a crisis. In this respect crisis coping is different from traditional problem solving where individuals do not always realize they have a problem. Once in crisis, orientation is an important factor that will influence the outcome of the coping process.

An important focus is the preexisting attitudes and schemata that influence one's perception of a crisis, the personal beliefs about one's general potential to solve difficulties in life. Two concepts are relevant to the preexisting attitudes: self-efficacy and outcome expectancy (see Bandura, 1997). As Bandura purported, the general belief in one's ability to solve problems in general, formed over years of positive or negative experience, would clearly influence the degree to which one is motivated to spend the time and energy to initiate the steps needed to face a crisis or solve a problem. Bandura's experimental work demonstrates that it is possible to change self- and outcome expectancy. But the change is often slow. Clinically this means that preventive work on self- and outcome expectancy should be an important element of any school or parent training program where there is a high probability of crises. Once an individual finds him/herself in a crisis situation, there is not always enough time to work on the motivational component of IPS models. And, as some research shows, unless the motivational element is present, IPS programs are much less effective (Nezu, 2004).

It should be part of every person's real-life curriculum to accept the possibility that he/she will be forced to face one or more crises in his/her lifetime. Such crises may include death, chronic illness, divorce, natural disasters, war, terror, chronic unemployment, and so on. Such situations are unavoidable in a world where many forces are beyond one's control. The same applies to "day-to-day crises" that although not as existential as the aforementioned are nevertheless stressful enough to qualify as crises. Such instances include having children with severe emotional or behavioral problems, robbery, theft, sudden illness, a fire, and so on. How to prepare individuals for the inevitable crisis situation during their life is the issue. Preventive crisis-coping programs as part of ongoing curricula in schools may be a major step in addressing this issue.

Hayes, Follette, and Linehan (2004), in the mindfulness tradition, talk about the important role of so-called acceptance skills: the ability to accept a given situation for what it truly is, as long as the situation does indeed exist. This means that one neither identifies fully with the situation nor rejects or escapes it but faces the situation as it presents itself in reality. In a way, this is quite similar to the well-known exposure principle of traditional behavior therapy. The proposal of acceptance skills is an important part of the orientation stage in IPS. This concept agrees with the notion of IPS style as mentioned by Nezu (2004). Nezu makes a distinction between three different styles of IPS: impulsive IPS, avoidance IPS, and rational IPS. In the first two instances, individuals also try to cope with problems and crises by either impulsively acting on the first thing that comes to mind or passively waiting to see what will happen next. Those are considered to be inadequate crises-coping mechanisms. A so-called rational coping style, based on the prescriptive IPS model, is considered to be a better alternative.

Two other orientation elements should also be mentioned here:

1. The willingness to view crises as challenges instead of as threats
2. The realization of and willingness to accept the fact that time and effort are needed in order to deal with a crisis.

Is it possible to instill these attitudes as part of a "program"? Or are these attitudes such an integral part of cultural training that it is impossible to teach them as one is able teach IPS skills?

Although IPS research demonstrates that one can be trained in IPS skills, there is no evidence (yet) that the above-mentioned attitudes can be instilled within a reasonable period of time. What does this mean for intervention? Perhaps one has to assess to what degree these attitudes already exist in order to be able to estimate the chances of successfully running an IPS program in the context of crisis intervention. As Nezu (2004) indicates, although an individual can be trained in IPS in the absence of these attitudes, it will work less effectively without them.

Problem Solving Proper

The core of any IPS program consists of seven clearly defined steps or stages that, when learned and applied consecutively, increase the probability of solving a problem or coping with a crisis constructively. The steps were originally conceptualized and developed by D'Zurilla and Goldfried (1971) but eventually evolved over the years. The following is a more recent version of the original model, as applied to crisis coping. The model offered is based on the version developed by D'Zurilla and Nezu (1999). (For an extended discussion of the stages we refer the interested reader to the manual published in their 1999 book.)

1. Attempting to identify and "accept" a crisis when it occurs.
2. Defining the crisis by formulating in your own words what the crisis is about.
3. Attempting to understand the crisis.
4. Setting reasonable goals (behavioral or emotional).
5. Generating alternative behavioral and/or emotional coping with crisis situations.
6. Evaluating and subsequently choosing the more promising of the alternatives.
7. Implementing the chosen alternatives.
8. Evaluating the efficacy of the total process and—if needed—taking corrective action at one of the previous stages.

Some Critical Remarks Concerning the Different Stages of Crisis Coping

Because excellent texts exist that describe extensively the different stages of the IPS model, this chapter offers only a few critical remarks about each of the steps.

STAGE 1: IDENTIFYING AND ACCEPTING A CRISIS WHEN IT OCCURS

Compared with a typical, day-to-day problem, it can be assumed that in crisis situations the phenomenological experience is always one of crises. If in a regular problem situation it is not always clear to the individual that he/she "has a problem, in a crisis the urgency and intensity of the situation are such that most people have an immediate and unavoidable experience of stress, tension that cannot be escaped. One could almost say that instead of the individual having a problem "the problem has the individual." Therefore, the major problem in this stage is not the identification of the situation as a crisis but the acceptance that this is a crisis situation. According to Hayes, Strosahl, and Wilson (1999), acceptance is the opposite of avoidance and suggests that one is prepared to recognize and "take in" the fact that a crisis does exist (p. 77). At its highest level, *acceptance* means "abandonment of dysfunctional change agendas and an active process of experiencing feelings as feelings, processing thoughts as thoughts, recalling memories as memories." Germer, Siegel, and Fulton (2005) define acceptance as "means to accept our experience without judgment or preference, with curiosity and kindness" (p. 118). Crisis intervention at this stage is designed to help the individual accept the crisis in the aforementioned sense, not acceptance as "resignation" but acceptance as a springboard and necessary condition for any future coping. Linehan's (1993) notion of the dialectical relationship between an acceptance and change agenda is particularly relevant to this stage.

STAGE 2: DEFINING THE CRISIS AND FORMULATING IN YOUR OWN WORDS

The transition between vague, amorphous feelings and fuzzy, unarticulated thoughts, images, and memories floating around in the free-association preverbal space to the stage of verbalizing is crucial. D'Zurilla and Goldfried's original statement that a "problem well defined is a problem half-solved" has merit. Although a crisis may be the outcome of an objective situation (death, illness), the impact is always mediated by the perception and following definition of the objective situation. To use a modern term, the *narrative* or *cognitive construction* of the crisis situation will determine any following crisis-solving operations. The IPS model offers useful guidelines to optimalize this stage of the process:

- Gather as much factual information about the crisis as possible.
- Define the crisis in your own words.
- Be concrete and specific in your formulation.
- Define the here and now and the desired end in concrete terms.
- Choose realistic goals.

Lazarus and Folkman (1984) distinguish between two sets of goals: problem-focused coping and emotion-focused coping. In *problem-focused coping* the emphasis is on attempts to change the external situation so that the crisis is solved or made less acute. In *emotion-focused coping* the emphasis is on attempts to make the situation bearable enough by influencing the emotional reaction to the crisis so that one can live with the situation even when it cannot be changed. The latter is relevant when one has no control over the situation while the former is useful when one has some control over the factors that determine the outcome of the crisis situation. Based on Lazarus, D'Zurilla and Nezu (1999) write: "the optimal set of goals for any particular problematic situation would be a set that aims to: (1) change the negative aspects of the situation that can be changed and (2) reduce, minimalize, or tolerate the distress caused by the negative conditions that cannot be changed" (p. 25).

There is one issue in all IPS models that often is not mentioned explicitly: In itself, the act of verbalizing vague, unstructured thoughts may well be a necessary and sometimes sufficient condition that enables the person to move to the next stage of the problem-solving process. This transformation of free-floating thoughts into a narrative, story, or any other verbal product (diary, letter, report, homework assignment) is crucial.

STAGE 3: UNDERSTANDING THE CRISIS

Although given a separate place in the chain of steps and stages, understanding is an elaboration of one of the principles that constitutes the second stage. Understanding relates to the "gestalt" of the crisis with special emphasis on three elements:

- The situation as it is in the *here and now*—the present—is experienced as aversive and undesirable.
- The situation as it—preferably—*should be*: the desired situation that is strived for.
- The stumbling blocks, barriers, and obstacles that constitute a very difficult path to get from the situation as it is to the situation as desired (the obstacles may relate both to those that are inherent in the person's abilities, capacities, limitations etc., as well as to external constraints not under the person's control).

Closely related to this is the next stage.

STAGE 4: SETTING REASONABLE GOALS (BEHAVIORAL OR EMOTIONAL)

The goals that are set depend on others to the degree that the crisis is a function of factors under one's control or beyond one's control and also—correlated with the degree of control—on the emphasis to be placed on problem-focused or emotion-focused coping. By way of illustration, an individual who faces a crisis due to the death of a beloved spouse is faced by a situation caused by factors beyond his/her control. In all probability a reasonable goal for the outcome of the crisis is related to emotion-focused problem solving. The individual may well define the possible outcome of the crisis as "being able to accept the finality of the death of a spouse and being able to live one's life to the fullest with and in that awareness." Here the desirable goal ("situation as desired") is foremost the reduction of negative emotions in order to make room for "living to the fullest" under the new circumstances.

An example of setting reasonable goals would be if an able and healthy young adult were suddenly confronted with a crisis after being dismissed from employment. In all probability he would choose "seeking new employment" as a reasonable and possible goal. Although not totally under his control, he might have some control over the situation because he could apply for a number of available positions listed in the newspapers.

In the literature two strategies are mentioned as important during this stage:

- State your goals in concrete and specific terms.
- Avoid stating goals that are unrealistic or unlikely to be attained.

It is obvious that applying these strategies, especially the second one, is easier said than done. Factors to consider when working on the second strategy are preexisting levels of aspiration, general reality testing, self-image, and factual knowledge about existing conditions.

STAGE 5: GENERATING ALTERNATIVES

Once having chosen one's goals in concrete and specific terms, how does one get through the crisis situation? The basic assumption of IPS models is that the more alternative pathways one can think of to accomplish one's goal, the better the chances are to identify the most promising means to the end. Four rules are being proposed:

1. The more alternatives, the better ("quantity breeds quality").
2. While generating alternative ideas do not judge or scrutinize the ideas. Doing so prematurely only blocks the creative process of "brainstorming."
3. Generate as many alternatives as possible but also think of a *variety* of different means.
4. Combine and synthesize different pathways.

Most IPS theoreticians assume that this stage is the most important. If one had time to learn only one stage of the model, this would be the step to master. The underlying assumption is that people are so fixed and rigidly set in their ways of thinking that—especially when under heavy emotional pressure and stress—they fall back on well-known patterns that are ingrained and overused. Sometimes it is necessary to "think outside of the box." Training in alternative solutions may well be one of the more promising methods to do so. Thus from a preventive standpoint, it is desirable to include this step in regular curricula taught in normal school situations or parenting programs in the community.

STAGE 6: EVALUATING ALTERNATIVES AND DECIDING
ON A COURSE OF ACTION

This part of the model is also known as "decision making." Contrary to rational decision making under normal problematic conditions, here we are dealing with the difficult topic of decision making under stress, when the cognitive apparatus is constrained and restrained by emotional factors. The literature is divided about the effects of stress on decision making. Many authors refer to the well-known Yerkes–Dodson law, which assumes an inverted U relationship between emotional arousal and performance efficiency: When arousal is too low or high the performance is impaired. Only with moderate levels of arousal will the performance be optimal (Yerkes & Dodson, 1908). But not everyone agrees, and there is some evidence that sometimes performance improves thanks to the effects of stress (Easterbrook, 1959). Janis, as cited in D'Zurilla and Nezu (1999), mentions the negative consequences of stress as related to problem solving and decision making: "narrowing the range of perceived alternatives, overlooking long-term consequences, inefficient information-seeking, erroneously evaluating expected outcomes and using oversimplified decision rules" (p. 62). Janis and Mann (1977) identified two maladaptive decision-making patterns that result from high emotional stress:

- Defensive avoidance
- Hypervigilance

In defensive avoidance a person tends to procrastinate and/or to shift the decision making to someone else. This is similar to the previously mentioned "passive" problem-solving style. In hypervigilance the person impulsively jumps between alternatives and without thinking much seizes on the first solution that comes to mind without considering pros and cons, or long-term consequences. Because these two patterns threaten to overshadow the otherwise useful rules about decision making in normal problem situations, the first and most important rule for IPS in crisis situations would be to become aware that the existing stress in the background is going to exert its strong influence on the decision-making process. Therefore, the individual in a crisis is advised to go through the decision-making rules of the D'Zurilla and Nezu (1999) model supervised or assisted by another person he/she trusts (whether it is a relative, teacher, counselor, or therapist) who can point out the traps that he/she might fall in when engaged in decision making. If, while getting feedback from a trusted source, the individual in a crisis goes through the regular decision-making rules, the individual still improves his/her chances to successfully cope.

STAGE 7: IMPLEMENTING THE CHOSEN ALTERNATIVE

After having decided on a viable alternative, one has to put it into practice. The silent assumption is that the response or actions needed to do so are in the individual's existing repertoire. Ideally, in the previous stage, the individual decided on an alternative that he/she thought could be executed. Otherwise, he/she would first have to learn the new response or skill needed to perform the solution response. For example, an individual decided that the best way to cope with the situation was to wait until the crisis itself had passed, or ceased, while remaining as relaxed as possible. If the individual had no relaxation skills, this solution would not be feasible. The individual would first have to learn relaxation skills. If another individual decided that the best way to cope with the crisis of a divorce was to start looking for another spouse but he lacked assertiveness or other interpersonal skills, the solution would be inadequate. If, however, the individual had the needed emotional and/or behavioral skills in his repertoire, he could then apply the solution.

Four elements are important in this stage of the model:

- Performing the right sequences of responses or actions.
- Self-monitoring the performance while in action.
- Self-evaluation (how well am I doing).
- Self-reinforcement (giving positive feedback when successful).

These four elements are an integral part of Kanfer's (1970) model of self-control that describes and explains how individuals succeed in regulating self-chosen behavior.

One point that has not been stressed enough is underscored by Goldfried and D'Zurilla and mentioned as being very important by Spivack (Spivack & Shure, 1974) and his group: "the awareness that the passage of time is often needed before one can put into practice a solution, or expect the desired outcome." In most of the IPS literature, it is stated that once we put the solution response into practice, the problem is more or less immediately solved. In reality, and especially in crisis situations, this is seldom the case. The element of "time awareness" should be added as an indispensable part of this stage in IPS.

STAGE 8: EVALUATING THE EFFICACY OF THE TOTAL PROCESS
AND—IF NEED BE—TAKING CORRECTIVE ACTION

According to the typical problem-solving model, once the chosen action has been performed, there is a need to compare outcome with the previously stated goal and see if the goal was accomplished. If not, there is a need to return to earlier stages of the model and discover where corrections must be made to reach the goal.

In crisis situations the need may be less pronounced. Often it is the feelings of tension, stress, and arousal that make it quite clear whether the crisis has passed. Because the passage of time plays an important role, it is not always possible to evaluate the coping process immediately after an action has been taken. Especially when the focus is on reducing level of arousal and learning to accept instead of changing a situation, more time is needed before a conclusion can be drawn about the efficacy of the process.

Contrary to normal, day-to-day, and interpersonal problems in living, when coping with a crisis situation, it is not only the last response in the chain that is evaluated but the entire process. Moreso than in cases of regular interpersonal problem solving, in crises the person may conclude that the problem situation cannot be solved by changing it but only by acceptance and a willingness and ability to live with the situation. Sometimes this may take a long time and it happens only after several unsuccessful attempts of "problem-focused" coping. We are reminded of Hayes's idea, derived from Zen Buddhism, of creative hopelessness: A real solution becomes possible only after the person begins to understand and accept that all his/her problem-focused coping was futile because the "solution process" so far was the problem. When clients are prepared to give up their unworkable change agenda they can begin to actually cope with the crisis in their life (Hayes et al., 1999).

AN ILLUSTRATIVE EXAMPLE OF COPING WITH A CRISIS USING THE IPS MODEL

In the following case, first we see what typically occurs, then we apply the IPS model to the crisis situation.

Julia is a 25-year-old school teacher who is new to her profession. Julia's first teaching assignment is with high school students. One of her students, Masha, is very disruptive and has been acting out for quite some time. Masha was warned several times that she could be thrown out of school and prevented from taking part in school activities if her disruptive behaviors were to continue. Masha was vulnerable to her teacher's threats because she had a lot of friends in school and wanted to finish school with good grades. Consequently, being removed form school served as a viable threat. When Masha disturbed the class by her obnoxious and aggressive behaviors one time too many, Julia decided to follow through on her threat.

She sent Masha home. However, as Masha was leaving the classroom, she took a knife out of her pocket and cut herself on the wrists, something that Julia never expected. One of the pupils who passed by saw what happened and called for help. Julia was summoned and, upon arriving at the scene, saw Masha bleeding profusely. Julia started screaming hysterically, took her head in her hands, and began to cry. She was paralyzed by what she saw. She didn't know what to do. It took a minute or so before another more experienced and older teacher arrived on the scene. He took over and managed to deal with the situation effectively.

From Julia's point of view, this was clearly a crisis situation, and she was completely overwhelmed by it. It was completely unexpected and, intuitively, Julia had no idea what to do. Her emotional arousal precluded her from thinking about an appropriate response, and she froze in her tracks.

Had Julia taken part in a specialized training such as the one based on an IPS model, she might have responded very differently. If IPS had been internalized as a cognitive schema triggered in crisis situations, Julia's alternative response would have been more effective.

Any IPS model (stage 1) starts with the notion that strong feelings are a cue that there is a problem—a "crisis to be solved." High levels of arousal function much like a traffic light, which is a clear cue and sign to stop and wait. Ideally speaking, the emotion felt when confronted by a student whose wrists are cut with blood spilling out of the wounds could have become a kind of conditioned stimulus for labeling the situation as a crisis or problem to be solved. If still too overwhelmed, Julia could, ideally, have applied one of the earlier acquired techniques (deep breaths for example) to calm herself enough to be able to think, or to call for help if she felt too overwhelmed to deal with the situation by herself. As a result, Julia would then quickly describe the situation, define the problem, and ask herself the question, "What's going on and how should I respond to this situation?" (stage 2). In a case such as this, there probably are not many alternative formulations or definitions to consider as there was a clear danger to the pupil who cut herself and emergency action was required. Because this is a crisis situation that demands a rather quick solution, it is advisable to skip stages 3 and 4.

Following the stage of defining the problem, it is necessary to generate several alternative courses of action (stage 5). Alternatives for Julia to consider might be to call the nurse, call another person and tell the other person to call the nurse, or call any other person who could be of immediate help; to do something immediately to stop the bleeding (i.e., apply pressure to the wound); or, if she was still too tense, to take some quick deep breaths herself before deciding on an action (such as in-flight instructions that direct a parent to apply the oxygen masks on themselves before applying it to his/her child). We assume that individuals who do not already have the intuitive notion of IPS will, after training have acquired the internal schema "when in crisis there are alternatives to consider." Functionally speaking, such a schema or "script" would make it possible for Julia to think of alternative solutions in the immediate crisis situation. In this respect, Julia would have to decide which of the alternatives to choose.

If Julia possessed the skill to calm herself by taking some deep breaths, she might be able to think more clearly. If she felt the situation with Masha was too dangerous, she might call for help, knowing that Masha might lose too much blood and lose consciousness. Once her decision was made, Julia would take action and follow through on the preferred alternative (stages 6, 7).

The last stage would depend on the outcome of Julia's efforts. If she did not succeed in calming herself down, she probably would call for help. If she felt the Masha's life was in danger, she still might decide to do whatever she could do to stop the bleeding by evaluating the options she had before her (stage 8).

Some crisis situations require a very quick reaction. Although IPS training may take some time, the expectation is that, once the schema of IPS is internalized, it will enable an individual to quickly solve a problem, even when there is little time. Indeed, that is the ultimate aim of any IPS model: Not only will people be able to quickly analyze and solve a crisis situation, but it may not always be necessary to review the different stages.

After receiving enough experience with IPS training, individuals will no doubt skip certain parts of the model to focus on those steps necessary to increase the chance of solving the particular crisis. One may compare the situation with learning to play a musical instrument. Ultimately one is able to improvise. But to reach that point, one needs to master the basic skills. This mastery is essential to be able to refine one's response repertoire in crisis situations. In the same vein, for those who lack the intuitive skills of IPS, it may be helpful first to learn the skills and practice applying them to subsequent real-life crisis situations.

THE ROLE AND IMPACT OF EMOTIONS

One of the working assumptions of the cognitive-behavioral model, of which IPS is a part, is the reciprocal relationship between emotion and cognition. Preexisting emotion can induce certain cognitions (beliefs, attributions), which, in turn, can give rise to further emotions. The IPS model teaches an individual to use emotion as a cue to begin to problem-solve. But, in some crisis situations, the emotion may be so strong that it overwhelms an individual and overrides his/her cognitive process. However, even in highly emotional situations, a fleeting memory associated with the preexisting knowledge of the IPS model may be enough to aid an individual in navigating through a crisis. One is reminded of the famous experiments by the neurologist Delgado (1967) who showed how monkeys whose limbic (anger) system was aroused by electrical stimulation had no control whatsoever over the anger response. The monkeys in the experiment still regulated their actions in accordance with a quick interpretation of the situation (attacking other monkeys lower in the social hierarchy of the colony, but leaving alone those higher up and stronger). This research suggests that even in a heightened state of emotional arousal, an organism can still mediate cognitively.

The emotional aspect of crisis situations creates a special problem for training in IPS. It is very difficult and, in some cases, almost impossible to create training situations that are emotionally comparable to real-life crisis situations. However, if Delgado's experiment can be used as an example, we have reason to assume that even in situations in which it appears as though individuals are out of control, cognitive information processing still occurs. Therefore, in Julia's case, although she felt overwhelmed, one might assume that she would be able to exert some cognitive control that would enable her to cope with the crisis adequately.

"I HAVE MY THEORIES.
DO NOT CONFUSE ME WITH YOUR FACTS."

As has been reviewed thus far, IPS is an elegant and seemingly logical–rational model for teaching individuals how to cope with the stress of crisis situations.

On the basis of a rich theoretical literature and years of clinical experience, one can attest to the usefulness of the IPS model. But a crucial question remains: Does solid research indeed offer enough evidence that the IPS model is effective and efficacious as a helpful intervention for coping with crisis?

To best address this question, the reader is referred to two recent articles that well summarize the research on IPS in relation to coping with stress and crises. In 2007 Malouff, Thorsteinsson, and Schutte published a meta-analysis, based on 31 published studies between 1978 and 2004 with a total of almost 3,000 participants, about the efficacy of problem-solving therapy in reducing mental and physical health problems. Nezu (2004) summarized the overall efficacy of problem-solving therapy but with special emphasis on the effects of IPS on stress reduction.

Nezu reviews a large number of studies that all support the hypothesis that effective problem solving attenuates the negative effects of stress in a variety of subjects with a variety of problems in living. But there is a limitation: Most of the studies are correlational. The strong correlation between problem-solving skills and lower levels of stress in itself does not help us to determine the direction of the relationship.

However, both Nezu and Malouff discuss numerous intervention studies that offer evidence for the efficacy of IPS training and therapy in coping with the stress of various problems. Especially important are the findings about IPS efficacy in dealing with life-threatening illnesses (such as cancer), chronic diseases, and suicidality. Both authors review a number of methodologically sound studies all showing the efficacy of

IPS in reducing stress and improving effective problem solving and quality of life in relation to these crisis situations.

It must be added, however, that the comparisons on which the analyses are based have been used with wait-list control and placebo conditions. Of those studies reviewed, there is little evidence that IPS is superior to other, alternative approaches to crisis intervention and stress reduction. No doubt, IPS offers a rational and systematic model that is effective in crisis intervention; however, if it is no better than other existing models, what is the justification for using it in crisis situations?

The answer might be that as compared with other existing interventions (e.g., Meichenbaum's [2001] stress-reduction programs), IPS offers a metacognitive intervention "par excellence." More than any other existing program, the IPS model teaches individuals how to think, how to analyze problems, how to generate different solutions, and, most important, how to evaluate crisis situations. As a metacognitive skill, it has the added quality that is generalizable to a variety of problem and crisis situations. It is a very "portable" model, that is, once internalized, one easily incorporates it internally to use in future situations. In addition, the IPS model is quite flexible and can be adapted to a variety of circumstances.

It can be applied as a total package or in parts, depending on the need of the individual and the situation. One can build a full-blown intervention along the lines of the IPS model or include elements of IPS in other forms of therapy or interventions. IPS can be applied individually or in a group format. As the research literature shows (Nezu, 2004), IPS can be offered to children, adults, teachers, parents, and caregivers. The training can easily be done by teachers who can help with the generalization by using the IPS model in the natural environment of the classroom.

Because the IPS model is based on metacognitive skills that do not require an average IQ, it can also be applied with populations that are moderately mentally retarded or otherwise challenged (Nezu, 2004, p. 20).

CONCLUSION

IPS based on the original model by D'Zurilla and Goldfried and elaborated by Nezu and others offers a promising and useful framework for crisis intervention.

After more then 30 years of theory development and intervention research, it can be said that IPS is an effective and efficacious intervention, which can be applied to a variety of subject populations with different problems.

Although there is no evidence that IPS works better than other stress-reduction and crisis intervention programs, there are some advantages to IPS over other programs. The format of IPS is flexible and can be constructed and modified in different ways depending on the needs of the clients and the intervention context. IPS teaches clients metacognitive skills for problem solving that can be generalized to different situations and time periods in the life of a person.

IPS offers a model that, following the Hebrew word for crisis—*mashber*—helps with a breakthrough in a crisis situation so that new possibilities can be born.

REFERENCES

Bandura, A. (1997). *Self-efficacy: The exercise of control.* New York: Freeman.

Bronowski, J. (1973). *The ascent of man.* Boston: Little, Brown.

Delgado, J. M. R. (1967). Social rank and radio-stimulated aggressiveness in monkeys. *Journal of Nervous Mental Diseases, 144,* 383–390.

D'Zurilla, T. J., & Goldfried, M. R. (1971). Problem solving and behavior modification. *Journal of Abnormal Psychology, 78*(1), 107–126.

D'Zurilla, T. J., & Nezu, A. M. (1999). *Problem solving therapy. A social competence approach to clinical intervention* (2nd ed.). New York: Springer.

Easterbrook, J. A. (1959). The effect of emotion on cue utilization and the organization of behavior. *Psychological Review, 66,* 183–201.

Elias, M. (2006). The connection between academic and social-emotional learning. In M. Elias & H. Arnold (Eds.), *The educator's guide to emotional intelligence and academic achievement* (pp. 4–11). Thousand Oaks, CA: Corwin Press.

Elias, M. J., & Clabby, J. F. (1992). *Building social problem-solving skills: Guidelines from a school-based program.* San Francisco: Jossey-Bass.

Germer, C. K., Siegel, R. D., & Fulton, P. R. (Eds.). (2005). *Mindfulness and psychotherapy.* New York: Guilford Press.

Greene, R. W. (2001). *The explosive child: A new approach for understanding and parenting easily frustrated, chronically inflexible children.* New York: Quill (HarperCollins).

Hayes, S. H., Follette, V. M., & Linehan, M. M. (2004). *Mindfulness and acceptance: Expanding the cognitive-behavioral tradition.* New York: Guilford Press.

Hayes, S. H., Strosahl, K. D., & Wilson, K. G. (1999). *Acceptance and commitment therapy: An experiential approach to behavior change.* New York: Guilford Press.

Janis, I. L., & Mann, L. (1977). *Decision making: A psychological analysis of conflict, choice, and commitment.* New York: The Free Press.

Kanfer, F. H. (1970). Self-regulation: Research, issues and speculations. In C. Neuringer & J. L. Michael (Eds.), *Behavior modification in clinical psychology* (pp. 178–220). New York: Appleton-Century-Crofts.

Kazdin, A. E. (2005). *Parent management training: Treatment for oppositional, aggressive, and antisocial behavior in children and adolescents.* Oxford, UK: Oxford University Press.

Kazdin, A. E., Siegel, T. C., & Bass, D. (1992). Cognitive problem-solving skills training and parent management training in the treatment of antisocial behavior in children. *Journal of Consulting and Clinical Psychology, 60*(5), 733–747.

Lazarus, R. S., & Folkman, S. (1984). *Stress, appraisal and coping.* New York: Springer.

Linehan, M. M. (1993). *Cognitive-behavioral treatment of borderline personality disorder.* New York: Guilford Press.

Malouff, J., Thorsteinsson, E., & Schutte, N. S. (2007). The efficacy of problem solving therapy in reducing mental and physical health problems: A meta-analysis. *Clinical Psychology Review, 27*(1), 46–57.

Meichenbaum, D. H. (2001). *Treatment of individuals with anger control problems and aggressive behaviors: A clinical handbook.* Clearwater, FL: Institute Press.

Nezu, A. M. (2004). Problem solving and behavior therapy revisited. *Behavior Therapy, 35,* 1–33.

Shure, M. B. (1994). *Raising a thinking child.* New York: Henry Holt.

Spivack, G., Platt, J. J., & Shure, M. B. (1976). *The problem-solving approach to adjustment: A guide to research and intervention.* San Francisco: Jossey-Bass.

Spivack, G., & Shure, M. B. (1974). *Social adjustment of young children: A cognitive approach to solving real-life problems.* San Francisco: Jossey-Bass.

Yerkes, R. M., & Dodson, J. D. (1908). The relation of strength of stimulus to rapidity of habit formation. *Journal of Comparative Neurology and Psychology, 18,* 459–482.

SUGGESTED READINGS

Chang, E. C., D'Zurilla, T. J., & Sanna, L. J. (Eds.). (2004). *Social problem solving: Theory, research and training*. Washington: American Psychiatric Association Press.

D'Zurilla, T. J., & Nezu, A. M. (1999). *Problem solving therapy. A social competence approach to clinical intervention* (2nd ed.). New York: Springer.

Malouff, J., Thorsteinsson, E., & Schutte, N. S. (2007). The efficacy of problem solving therapy in reducing mental and physical health problems: A meta-analysis. *Clinical Psychology Review, 27*(1), 46–57.

Nezu, A. M. (2004). Problem solving and behavior therapy revisited. *Behavior Therapy, 35*, 1–33.

Nezu, A. M., & D'Zurilla, T. J. (in press). Problem-solving therapy. In A. M. Nezu, C. M. Nezu, M. Reinecke, L. C. Sobell & A. Wells (Eds.), *International encyclopedia of cognitive behavior therapy*. New York: Kluwer Academic/Plenum Press.

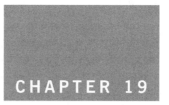

CHAPTER 19

Rape Trauma

Elizabeth Muran

*C*urrent research underscores the imposing effects of experiencing the trauma of rape. The *Diagnostic and Statistical Manual of Mental Disorders*, fourth edition (DSM-IV; American Psychiatric Association, 1994), describes "trauma" as an event that involves perceived or actual threat and elicits an extreme emotional response. The psychological sequelae that are frequently seen in survivors of the trauma of rape is *posttraumatic stress disorder* (PTSD). Traumatic events, especially rape, occur in tremendous numbers, and a significant proportion of survivors will develop PTSD. Moreover, PTSD-like syndromes have been described in the literature for more than 100 years under various labels such as nervous shock, compensation neurosis, hysteria, traumatophobia, and others (Foa, Steketee, & Rothbaum, 1989; Dancu & Foa, 1992). Despite the magnitude and long-standing history of PTSD and rape, the treatment of PTSD is relatively new territory for clinicians. It has only been recognized as a diagnosis since 1980 when it first appeared in DSM-III (American Psychiatric Association, 1980). Subsequently, several cognitive-behavioral treatment programs for PTSD have been developed and studied.

Recent treatment outcome studies have approached better methodological standards (e.g., Rothbaum, Foa, Murdock, Riggs, & Walsh, 1992), bringing important issues and strategies to the foreground and developing an empirical foundation for clinical practice. Cognitive-behavioral treatments have proven to be efficacious, having been the subject of the greatest number of well-controlled outcome studies.

Despite the growing number of rigorous treatment studies, there remains very little information and a serious paucity of empirical findings about crisis intervention strategies with rape survivors (Calhoun & Atkeson, 1991). Crisis intervention counseling is short term, often limited to one or two sessions. It is the earliest and often the only intervention that many rape survivors experience. However, its effects on recovery and the prevention of long-term psychopathology have yet to be well studied. In light of the inherent limitations due to both the brevity of therapeutic contact in crisis intervention and the lack of empirical data, the goal of this chapter is to provide a practical guide for clinicians who are working with rape trauma survivors[1] in crisis.

POSTTRAUMATIC STRESS DISORDER

DSM-III-R (American Psychiatric Association, 1987) described PTSD as an anxiety disorder including a criterion of a precipitating trauma, a stressor that is beyond the range of usual human stressors. Although both acute and chronic reactions following exposure to trauma vary along a continuum of adjustment, some survivors do not recover to their pretrauma level of functioning (Fairbank & Brown, 1987). Only a minority of these survivors seek crisis intervention or longer-term treatment. Within this group, many develop symptoms of PTSD. The hallmark symptoms include persistent, distressing, and intrusive recollections of the trauma; numbing of responsiveness to the environment; avoidance or escape in the presence of trauma-related cues; and a variety of autonomic, dysphoric, or cognitive symptoms that persist longer than 1 month after the trauma (Fairbank & Brown, 1987).

DSM-IV has retained the symptoms of PTSD delineated in DSM-III-R, but it has modified the "trauma" to include characteristics of the actual trauma, as well as the perception of threat to self. Because PTSD cannot be diagnosed until the required symptom constellation has lasted beyond 1 month, DSM-IV has introduced a new disorder called acute stress disorder (ASD), which overlaps PTSD considerably. The differences in criteria between PTSD and ASD are both the duration of symptoms and the emphasis in ASD on dissociative symptoms. ASD can be diagnosed in the immediate aftermath of a trauma, with the disturbance lasting for at least 2 days and less than 1 month. For ASD to be diagnosed, the individual must also experience three of five dissociative symptoms (derealization, depersonalization, dissociative amnesia, subjective sense of numbing, reduction in awareness of surroundings) immediately after the trauma.

In this chapter, rape is addressed as a trauma specifically acknowledged by DSM-IV as a potential precipitant of PTSD. It has been found that shortly after the assault, 94% of rape survivors met criteria for PTSD; 3 months after the assault, 47% of survivors still suffered from PTSD; 17 years later, 16.5% of survivors still experienced PTSD (Rothbaum et al., 1992). This prospective study is indicative of the high prevalence of PTSD following rape. Most relevant to this chapter, almost all the rape survivors seen in the Rothbaum et al. (1992) study initially demonstrated symptoms of PTSD shortly after the assault. Given these findings, we may assume the presence of

---

[1] The term *rape survivor* has been used instead of *rape victim* in order to emphasize the implication of active coping and recovery.

PTSD symptoms (now formally diagnosed as ASD) during initial contact or crisis intervention with these survivors.

GOALS OF CRISIS INTERVENTION WITH RAPE TRAUMA

Recounting the Trauma in a Safe Environment

Although many treatment approaches have been suggested for PTSD, cognitive-behavioral interventions rely primarily on exposure to help PTSD clients. The first step in exposure treatment often entails the verbal revelation of the traumatic event. It is important that this initial stage occur as early as possible. Many psychologists believe that the more successful an individual is at avoiding the stimuli, the more the individual's anxiety will be reinforced. Military psychologists have a long history of treating combat-related PTSD. Their experience indicates that early intervention is crucial to successful treatments. Animal and human learning studies indicate that successful avoidance of a conditioned stimulus results in the strengthening of both the anxiety to that stimuli and the avoidance of that stimuli. Thus, based on well-established learning principles, early intervention is crucial.

Early intervention should focus on providing a sense of safety and support. During the crisis period, most survivors of rape trauma experience high autonomic arousal and are, therefore, more inclined to disclose their traumatic experience to an attentive and supportive listener. The survivor is often driven to repeat descriptions of the assault as a need to retell her[2] experience. The goal is to help the survivor develop a coherent and complete narrative account. The therapist should encourage the recapitulations and the cathartic expressions, sensitively reinforcing the client to continue. It is important at this time that the therapist normalize the intense initial reactions of the survivor while encouraging completion of the story. Of course, complete disclosure will be a difficult process, because many survivors may be unable to recall the entire experience and may also avoid confrontation with the painful memory details.

Many survivors have been inadvertently discouraged by friends and family from sharing their entire experience and their painful emotions. It can be extremely uncomfortable for friends and family members to listen to a recapitulation of the gruesome experience. They may also believe it is in the survivor's best interest to put this negative experience behind, not dwell on it, and carry on with life. Therefore, describing the assault and expressing related cognitions and emotions may be the first complete imaginal exposure for the survivor. Incomplete or spontaneous exposures (e.g., flashbacks, nightmares, and intrusive recollections) can be less therapeutic because they do not include all the conditioned stimuli. As a result, the incompleteness of such recollections may account for the lack of extinction of the PTSD responses. Complete exposure or more conditioned stimuli, on the other hand, may lead to extinction of PTSD responses. Moreover, Keane, Zimmerling, and Caddell (1985) have suggested that

---

[2] Because the majority of rape victims are women, the female pronoun is used throughout this chapter, although we acknowledge that anyone is vulnerable to rape.

providing more cues (conditioned stimuli) during *in vitro* exposure may improve memory and enhance confrontation with the trauma. Furthermore, the subsequent increase in arousal following this memory will lead to better recall and ultimately a better match between the affect at the time of the trauma and the affect at the time of recall; this improved match will facilitate the retrieval of memory details leading to complete exposure.

As the client is relating her experiences, the therapist should assess for PTSD symptoms and the degree to which she has difficulty or avoids recalling and retelling parts of the traumatic event. The therapist should also attend to the maladaptive thoughts and feelings regarding the client's role in the rape and her current perception of herself and her world. A trauma such as rape serves to undo a person's view of herself and the world. Cognitive theorists consider this alteration of fundamental beliefs to be at the core of PTSD (Janoff-Bulman, 1992). Following this assessment, the therapist should reinforce adaptive thoughts and feelings, gently begin challenging inappropriate thoughts and feelings, and finally substitute more adaptive ones.

The rape survivor's appraisal process of the trauma sequelae has been a focus of attention by Ehlers and Clark (2000) as a predictor of the maintenance of PTSD. While observing the wide range of meanings survivors assign to their PTSD symptoms, Ehlers and Steil (1995) suggested that negative appraisals of symptoms predict a maintenance of these symptoms. Other studies have demonstrated that perceived appraisal from others or a perceived inability to relate to others can lead to a sense of alienation, which has been shown to impede recovery in rape survivors. This focus on the survivor's appraisals of symptoms and others' responses to her symptoms needs to be considered by the therapist during this early stage of intervention.

Drawing on cognitive theories, Resick and Schnicke (1992) have suggested an information-processing model whereby the experience of trauma conflicts with preexisting assumptions about the self and the world, and this conflict is manifested in PTSD-like responses. The theory that processing an event requires a modification in existing beliefs is derived from Piaget's (1954) model of cognitive development. He proposed that assimilation and accommodation were two mechanisms used to modify beliefs about an experience. In other words, to reconcile the conflict, the survivor must distort the trauma experience to be more consistent with prior beliefs (assimilation) or alter her beliefs to adjust to this new information (accommodation). In view of this suggestion, the goal of crisis intervention is to help the survivor to neither assimilate (e.g., blaming self for rape) nor overaccommodate (e.g., never feeling safe again). Instead, the therapist's goal is to support the survivor in recalling the trauma, accept that it happened, and begin processing the related emotions.

In the following case vignette, an example of a rape survivor's assimilation and accommodation of being raped is shown.

Caroline, age 19, is in her second year at a small liberal arts college. She shares an apartment with another female and a male college student. The assault occurred when Caroline was alone in her apartment working on a research paper. Her two roommates had gone to a party on campus. When the doorbell rang, a friend of her male roommate was at the door. His name was Peter, and she had remembered him from a class she had taken with her roommate, John, during their freshman year. He had also been at a party at their apartment recently. Peter was asking for John, and Caroline explained that John was at a party on campus. Instead of leaving, Peter asked if he could do some studying at their place while he waited for John to return. Caroline was uncomfortable with this but agreed reluctantly. After a short time, Peter asked that she sit by him to keep him company. Again, she agreed reluctantly. Peter moved closer to her on the couch and ultimately grabbed her. As Caroline protested, he pushed her into her bedroom, threw her on her bed, and raped her with a pillow over her face. Caroline's roommates returned at least an hour after Peter had left, finding Caroline crying uncontrollably on her bed. They insisted on taking her to the college health center, where she was treated medically. She met with a counselor from the center the following day.

During her initial counseling session, Caroline expressed tremendous self-blame (assimilation) for letting Peter in despite her reluctance, and she believed that she could never be trusted to live independently and that her parents would probably want her to go back to living in a dormitory on campus (overaccommodation). While the counselor acknowledged Caroline's feelings as a normal way of assimilating her trauma and overaccommodating for it, she gently challenged her statements and offered more adaptive ones.

Establishing and Maintaining a Therapeutic Alliance

Early intervention should provide a safe environment within which to build an alliance with the survivor. The interpersonal domain is particularly vulnerable, because the trauma of rape is inflicted by another person. Rape trauma, therefore, has a resonating interpersonal valence, underscoring the significance of the therapeutic alliance.

The therapeutic alliance is just as critical to success (and often more difficult to establish) in crisis intervention as it is to any other therapeutic intervention, even though crisis therapy is brief. In fact, this is a limitation that may make the establishment of a therapeutic alliance more difficult, as the therapist, having minimal contact with the client, must be adept at establishing rapport and communicating effectively in a very short time. The therapist should employ both verbal and nonverbal strategies to validate the client's experience and to convey sensitivity, understanding, support, and a positive outlook toward recovery. These strategies, while evoking compassion and acceptance from the therapist, are particularly critical with a survivor of rape. The survivor's trust of self and others has been shaken. Herman (1997) describes core experiences of the rape trauma as powerlessness and distrust. Recovery, therefore, is based on the empowerment of the survivor and establishment of new interpersonal connections. Recovery can take place only within the context of interpersonal relationships. In her renewed connection with others, including the therapist, the survivor recreates psychological faculties previously damaged by trauma (e.g., trust and autonomy).

Another limitation in establishing a therapeutic alliance and inherent in treatment with trauma survivors is their high attrition rate, resulting from their inclination to avoid confrontation with the memory of the trauma and, therefore, the therapy process. Helping the survivor explore and, ultimately, overcome the resistance to confront the painful memories should again be done through a supportive and validating approach.

After normalizing the survivor's experience and defining a course of recovery, it is important here to get a clear agreement on the goals of therapy. Two important aspects of Bordin's (1979) model of the therapeutic alliance are agreement on the goals and agreement on the tasks, which are interdependent with a third aspect, the affective bond between client and therapist. The therapist may see the goals as reducing the anxiety and the avoidance behavior. However, the client may not agree. She may wish to keep the anxiety because it helps motivate avoidance. The client may believe that if she avoids well enough, she can prevent such an event from recurring.

Reaching an agreement on the goals of therapy may not be easy. The client may believe that continued and complete avoidance is achievable and the only reaction likely to bring a sense of safety. The therapist may need to first discuss the appropriateness and achievability of the client's goal. Then the therapist can help the client explore alternative goals. This needs to be done in a sensitive, nonforceful way. The therapist should be checking in regularly with the client for her experience of the therapy process and the therapist (Safran & Muran, 2000), which will serve to give some control to the survivor who has just undergone a trauma that violated her.

Once agreement on the goals is reached, the therapist can work toward achieving agreement on the tasks. This refers to the procedures the therapist will use to help the client reach the agreed-on tasks. The therapist may need to discuss the importance of verbal exposure. Some clients may find the procedure too threatening. Again, it may be necessary for the therapist to stop and address any issue and explore the resistance the client has about the procedures before implementing them. Even though the client may agree to the goals of therapy, as well as to the importance of talking about the rape trauma, she may still be resistant. Talking about the traumatic experience produces a great deal of anxiety. Two possible anxiety reactions that may inhibit the process of therapy at this point are discomfort anxiety and shame.

If a client is resistant to recounting her story, we recommend that the therapist validate the client's experience and report that many survivors of rape have experienced similar difficulty recounting their trauma. Next, the therapist should ask the client how she feels about proceeding with her story. Some clients will have no difficulty reporting that they feel shame, or that the task is too hard for them. If they are able to express these emotions, the therapist can proceed by discussing the importance of targeting these emotions because they block the client's ability to proceed in therapy. However, we find that many clients are unable to acknowledge their emotional blocks. Patiently awaiting the client's insight through reflective or nondirective techniques can be costly. The costs result from the fact that continued avoidance may reinforce the anxiety, and the client may not return for further sessions.

Therefore, an active approach to assessing the resistance by hypothesis drive assessment is recommended (DiGiuseppe, 1991). Using this strategy, the therapist offers hypotheses concerning the emotions or thoughts the client is experiencing. In such a situation, the therapist could say, "Many women who have gone through similar experiences find they are too upset to talk about what happened to them. Does that sound like you?" The therapist waits for the client to respond, and if she affirms the question, the therapist continues, "Some women feel too much shame. They believe others will think badly of them for what happened. Others believe that it is just too hard to discuss these things. After all, the trauma was painful enough. Reliving it is just more painful. Do any of these sound like a reaction you may be having?"

Notice that the client does not have to say much to answer. If she is unwilling to talk about an issue because of an emotional block, a lengthy reply would be unlikely. Providing the possibility for a curt reply makes it easier for her to proceed. Most clients reply honestly, and there seems to be little risk of leading the client.

Restructuring Cognitions Underlying Resistance

Negative, maladaptive appraisals are identified by careful questioning, and cognitive therapeutic strategies are employed to modify negative appraisals. If the client reports that she experiences shame, the therapist would then proceed to uncover the belief that coexists with that shame. Perhaps she believes the therapist will think less of her, or that she was responsible for the rape. It is most important for the therapist to challenge these maladaptive thoughts and to share with the client the fact that he/she does not harbor any such thoughts of the client. Regardless of any poor judgment the client may believe she displayed by putting herself at risk for the rape, it could not have been predicted. The therapist should make clear to the client that she in no way "made" the rapist act as violently as he did. It is also important that the therapist challenge the client's feelings of worthlessness that resulted from the trauma. The experience of the rape in no way undoes all the positive aspects of the client's personality.

The client's discomfort anxiety may be more difficult to change. Ellis (1985) maintains that discomfort anxiety is a frequent cause of resistance in psychotherapy. The recommended therapeutic strategy is to challenge the client's low frustration tolerance (Ellis, 1985, 1986) and replace it with the notion that she can tolerate any level of discomfort that she believes she can handle. We have generally found this strategy to be useful with most clients who resist talking about their emotional upset. However, suggesting to rape survivors (who have experienced an event beyond the range of usual human experiences) that they have a low tolerance for frustration because they resist recounting the trauma may be perceived as an invalidation of the traumatic experience.

Marie Joyce (personal communication, 1992) has proposed a variation on Ellis's (1986) concept of low frustration tolerance. She argues that many clients, blocked by discomfort anxiety from completing a goal, have failed despite levels of frustration and discomfort greater than those of most people in their reference group. The frustration they have tolerated may be average or higher. The problem is that they are just not willing to experience a high enough frustration level that is required to complete the desired task.

Joyce (personal communication, 1992) recommends that we label such cognitive-emotional reactions as frustration intolerance. This frustration intolerance problem seems to arise with most PTSD clients and clients with physical disabilities, chronic illnesses, or other challenging and enduring stressors. Such clients endure greater frustration than the average person. Suggesting that they have low frustration tolerance is inaccurate and invalidating. Joyce recommends that we acknowledge the high degree of frustration they have endured while focusing on the belief that their task is "too difficult" to tolerate. Again, understanding and compassion are critical elements in the therapeutic alliance.

Thus, an important goal is to help survivors of rape develop greater frustration tolerance. Discussing the painful memories of the rape is very difficult, but it is also critical for recovery. It is in their best long-term interest to experience more discomfort temporarily in order to suffer less in the long run.

Gathering and Providing Information

After the client has recounted the trauma experience, it is important to gather information about immediate presenting problems, daily functioning, and available social support. Assessing suicidal risk should be done at this juncture, and steps must be taken as appropriate. Finally, information should be taken about the client's premorbid adjustment, interpersonal relationships, and any previous traumatic experiences.

Following the initial interview, the presence of PTSD symptoms can be efficiently assessed by the PTSD Symptom Scale (PSS; Foa, Riggs, Dancu, & Rodibaum, 1993). Although PTSD cannot be diagnosed before at least 1 month's duration of the symptoms listed here (ASD is the appropriate diagnosis), a preliminary assessment is important for an early measure of the PTSD responses that are present. This can serve as a baseline on which to contrast future changes or treatment gains. Most significantly, such an interview is an important vehicle to normalize the posttrauma experience for the survivor. The client needs to be educated about the most frequently experienced symptoms following a rape. Further, these PTSD responses and the responses specific to rape-related trauma can be normalized by communicating information to the client as follows:

> "Symptoms of posttraumatic stress disorder can develop after a person has experienced a very upsetting event, especially one that is life-threatening, as rape is. These symptoms may affect your normal daily functioning as well as your relationships with others. They can affect you when you reexperience the rape in your thoughts and in your dreams. You may want to avoid activities, situations, feelings, and thoughts that you associate with the rape. You may become easily startled or aroused by anything that reminds you of the rape. You will probably be scared and cry often; you may have difficulty with your appetite and your sleep. You may feel somatic pain or soreness throughout your body, as well as physical symptoms specific to the attack—for example, pain in the anal or vaginal area. Even if you try to block the rape from your mind, there may be a strong desire for you to think about how you could have changed or prevented the rape from happening. After being raped, most women experience diminished self-esteem, degra-

dation, depression, sadness, guilt, shame, embarrassment, self-blame, and anger. Any or all these feelings could affect you intensely and often simultaneously. You could have mood swings, which inhibit social relatedness. If the rapist was someone you knew, your trust in people can be shattered. Whether or not the rapist is someone you knew, the world may no longer feel safe. Sometimes it will seem as though withdrawing is the best way to protect yourself emotionally. Try to remember, though, that it is now more than ever that you need support from your friends and family. Rape can be a very isolating experience, but you are not alone in what you are feeling, and there are people who can help you."

Sharing information about the symptoms that are commonly experienced by other survivors of a rape trauma will normalize the experience, reduce distress over symptoms, and help the client begin to regain a sense of control and normalcy. There is a great deal of information to be provided, and it is understandably difficult for the survivor to concentrate, listen, and assimilate all or even parts of that which has been discussed. Therefore, in addition to the factual information communicated verbally, it may be helpful to provide the client with written handouts concerning rape-related responses as well as common myths about rape.

Coping Strategies

In view of the psychological sequelae of rape, the survivor's daily functioning, interpersonal relationships, and sexual functioning may reflect the negative after-effects of the rape trauma. Therefore, coping strategies should be provided despite the brevity of the crisis intervention phase.

Stress Inoculation Training

Stress inoculation training (SIT) was originally developed by Meichenbaum (1985) in the early 1970s and adapted for use with rape survivors by Kilpatrick, Veronen, and Resick (1982). It is currently the most comprehensive and well-researched program for survivors of sexual assault (Calhoun & Atkeson, 1991). The objective of this program is to provide the survivor with a sense of control over her fears and anxiety by teaching her coping strategies to overcome her fears and improve her functioning in distressing situations.

Although it may not be possible to cover the entire training program within the limited time frame of crisis intervention, the program is well suited for adaptation to various needs and objectives. Ideally, the SIT program is designed to train clients within a course consisting of approximately 12 weekly 90-minute sessions. However, a more realistic goal, depending on the time provided, would be to shorten the educational phase and modify the skills training phase by not teaching all the skills. Possibly, follow-up sessions will be discussed after the initial meeting, and further training can be provided.

SIT is presented in two phases. The first phase is educational, in which learning theory (e.g., principles of stimulus generalization or higher-order conditioning) is presented to the client as it applies to the development of her rape-related responses (i.e., PTSD symptoms). These responses are explained as occurring along three channels (Lang, 1968): (1) physical or autonomic responses, (2) behavioral or motoric responses, and (3) cognitive responses. The interrelationship among these channels can be discussed, using specific examples from the client's experience. The goals of crisis intervention already comprised, in effect, the first phase described earlier in this chapter.

The second phase of SIT is coping skills training, in which a variety of strategies (discussed below) are taught for coping with fear and anxiety.

Breathing Retraining

Breathing affects psychological and physiological states. Teaching slow, rhythmic diaphragmatic breathing is a relaxation tool that can lead to feeling calmer, resulting in long-term changes in anxiety symptoms and the nervous system.

Diaphragmatic breathing is taught and practiced at a rate of approximately 4 seconds each for inhaling and exhaling. Breathing should be through the nose with mouth closed (or lips pursed). Normal breathing should be slow and practiced to attain a smooth and fluid breathing cycle.

Muscle Relaxation

Deeper relaxation can be achieved through Jacobson's (1938) progressive muscle relaxation technique. More recently refined and modified by Bernstein and Borkovec (1973), the technique demonstrates the contrast of tensing and relaxing major muscle groups of the whole body. It should be introduced through simultaneous instruction and demonstration. Typically, a muscle group is tensed for 5 to 10 seconds, attending to the sensation of the tension. Then the muscle is relaxed, and attention is focused on differentiating between the sensation of tensing and that of relaxing. The procedure is practiced in session and taped for daily home practice.

Eye Movement Desensitization and Reprocessing

Eye movement desensitization and reprocessing (EMDR; Shapiro, 2001) is a technique, originally developed for the treatment of PTSD, that uses imaginal exposure and saccadic eye movements in order to jump-start information processing. The treatment has been proven highly effective in most recent outcome studies, particularly in the treatment of rape trauma (Shapiro & Forrest, 2004). EMDR has been shown to deal with the wide range of symptoms often seen in rape survivors, ranging from negative emotions, cognitions, and behaviors to recurring physical disturbances.

This technique involves the survivor imagining a scene from the trauma and focusing on the accompanying cognition and emotion, during which time the therapist moves two fingers across the survivor's visual field repetitively. The survivor must track the therapist's fingers until the anxiety decreases. Each sequence is followed by the survivor reporting her subjective units of distress (SUDs) level and her level of belief in a positive cognition.

The rapid eye movements are meant to stimulate the survivor's information-processing system so that the traumatic experience can be "digested," and the emotional and physical turmoil can be extinguished. During EMDR all pieces of the memory reconnect, allowing the survivor to process the experience fully. The advantage of this treatment in crisis intervention is the quickness and ease of the method. Advocates of EMDR claim that even a single 50-minute session significantly diminishes symptoms.

Covert Modeling

The client is instructed to imagine an anxiety-producing situation and imagine herself confronting it successfully, using the coping strategies she has learned to manage her anxiety. Covert modeling is the imaginal counterpart to role playing. If a client is able to imagine herself getting through a difficult situation successfully, she is more likely to get through it in reality. A non-assault-related situation is chosen first, and the therapist demonstrates overtly how someone else might cope successfully with the situation. Then the client visualizes herself in the situation coping successfully with distress. Finally, an assault-related situation is chosen. The same steps are repeated, in which coping is demonstrated by the therapist, followed by the client imagining herself coping successfully.

Role Playing

The therapist models the desired behavior or communication; then the roles are switched. The client practices a desired response to a rape-related problem. Assertion training can be an important aspect of this skill, as interpersonal situations are often involved. For example, the client may need to communicate her sexual discomfort or fears with her sexual partner. Education and role playing in assertive communication would help to counter-condition the potential anxiety in these situations.

Cognitive Restructuring

Survivors of sexual assault will often endorse maladaptive thoughts of self-blame, future uncontrollability, and the futility of future responses. Cognitive restructuring can help a survivor correct her beliefs that the world is dangerous and that she is incompetent. The goal is to reduce distress by teaching the survivor to identify, evaluate, and change negative and dysfunctional thinking (Foa & Rothbaum, 1998). Cognitive restructuring of her negative self-blaming thoughts should be done in a manner similar to that with other clients (Beck & Emery, 1985; Walen, DiGiuseppe, & Dryden, 1992). Our clinical experience suggests that some areas of traditional cognitive-behavioral therapy may be more helpful than others. Both Beck (1976; Beck & Emery, 1985) and Ellis (1962; Ellis & Dryden, 1987) have identified catastrophizing or "awfulizing" as dysfunctional beliefs leading to anxiety disorders. Challenging this belief has been an important part of therapy for both these pioneers. Rape survivors are likely to report the presence of such beliefs after their trauma and when they experience PTSD symptoms. However, targeting such catastrophizing beliefs in rape survivors and other PTSD clients is not helpful. Regardless of the theory proposed by Beck and Ellis that such beliefs are irrational, are antiempirical, and lead to emotional disturbance, focusing on these beliefs results in a rupture of the therapeutic alliance. Survivors perceive such an intervention as insensitive and invalidating. Given the social context of the prevailing reactions to rape, most people would agree with the following statements: "It is awful to have been raped" and "It would be awful to be raped again." Challenging these specific thoughts is socially unacceptable and will, undoubtedly, result in a broken therapeutic alliance. This suggests that it would be preferable to focus on other dysfunctional beliefs.

Ellis (1994) proposes that dysfunctional beliefs are undergirded by deeper cognitive structures. He suggests that therapists target this "deeper" level, where survivors hold absolutistic shoulds, oughts, and musts that go beyond existent reality (e.g., "Really bad things must never happen to me"), driving them into severe states of panic and depression. When investigating a survivor's attributions and inferences, it may be more thorough to further examine the absolutistic demands underlying the automatic thoughts. Resick and Schnicke (1992) devised an effective procedure, cognitive processing therapy (CPT), for treating PTSD. Ellis (1994) suggests that CPT be coalesced with his rational-emotive behavior therapy (REBT), where core cognitive structures, as well as dysfunctional thoughts, are examined.

Regarding awfulizing beliefs, it is helpful to restructure awfulizing statements in a manner to increase the client's frustration tolerance or self-efficacy. In other words, a revised thought could be, "I lived through an awful experience, and I'm strong enough to survive." This strategy acknowledges the trauma of the rape but redefines the reaction in an adaptive manner. Maladaptive thoughts of self-blame are much more fertile ground for intervention. Given that individuals often derive comfort from the belief that the world is fair and predictable, there is subsequently a search for explanation and meaning. This search predisposes individuals to attribute explanations in the face of trauma, which ultimately may account for responses of self-blame, helplessness, frustration, depression, and anger. Consonant with this theory of causal attribution is one advanced by Janoff-Bulman (1979), who proposes that directing blame for victimization at one's behavior rather than at one's character would result in fewer deficits. In other words, assigning some responsibility for the rape to a changeable behavior (e.g., "I could have walked home with someone from work") may enable the client to regain a sense of control. Assigning blame to one's character (e.g., "I'm a bad person") is maladaptive and has been correlated positively with fear and depression (Meyer & Taylor, 1986). Survivors should be guided toward restructuring their maladaptive thinking accordingly.

Ehlers and Clark (2000) developed a model of PTSD in which key cognitive processes are targeted in treatment. Their model highlights the significance of excessively negative appraisals of the trauma and its sequelae, the disturbance of memory of the trauma, and the role of maladaptive behaviors and cognitions in persistent PTSD. Recent studies of this cognitive model support the effectiveness of cognitive restructuring.

Thought Stopping

The purpose of thought stopping is to end ruminating or obsessive maladaptive self-statements. Despite a lack of empirical support, the advantage of using this technique in crisis intervention is its simplicity and brevity. The client is instructed to think about a feared stimulus, which the therapist interrupts by yelling "Stop!" and clapping simultaneously. The client is instructed to repeat the thought and verbalize "Stop!" first aloud and then subvocally. She learns to use thought stopping covertly. This skill provides a good opportunity to assess the client's maladaptive thoughts, followed by a discussion of why these thoughts are dysfunctional. Some examples of typical maladaptive self-statements following a sexual assault are:

> "I'm damaged goods now."
> "It must have been my fault."
> "Nobody must know that I was raped."
> "I will never be the same again."
> "If I was aroused during the assault, I must be sick."
> "I shouldn't cry this much."
> "I will never trust anyone again."

Guided Self-Dialogue

This technique involves assessing maladaptive cognitions, such as the examples listed above, and substituting them with adaptive ones. (Similar to thought stopping, the advantage of this technique lies in its simplicity and brevity.) Adaptive self-statements are taught in the face of a distressing situation in the following four phases:

1. *Preparation:* Identifying the problem and appraising the negative outcome.
2. *Confrontation:* Breaking down the goal into manageable steps.
3. *Management:* Imagining anxiety as manageable and temporary.
4. *Reinforcement:* Making positive self-statements after taking action.

Social, Medical, and Legal Support

The critical role that family and friends can play in the recovery stage should be emphasized to the survivor. The survivor should be encouraged to depend on the social network she has identified, to confide in others who can provide emotional support. Some survivors may feel safer by moving in with a friend or relative or by having someone move in with them temporarily. Other ways to increase perceptions of safety (e.g., installing a security system) can be explored. It is also important to discuss potential difficulties with intimacy and sexual functioning with the survivor and possibly her sexual partner, facilitating realistic expectations concerning the aftermath of a sexual assault. If possible, any intervention with the survivor's significant others would be helpful.

A rationale for seeking medical treatment should be presented. There may be external and/or internal physical injuries that should receive medical attention immediately. Factual information about potential sexually transmitted diseases and pregnancy should be discussed. Medical intervention may also be necessary (if given immediately following the assault) for forensic evidence. The survivor often experiences the medical intervention received immediately following the assault as extremely invasive, and, therefore, she may react as thought she is reliving the trauma experience. If the survivor is about to confront this situation, potential adverse reactions should be discussed.

Many survivors are as reluctant to seek medical attention as they are to report the assault to the police. Factual information concerning the procedures necessary in reporting a sexual assault, as well possible outcomes, should be discussed (Calhoun & Atkeson, 1991). Criminal reporting (Herman, 1997) is a choice that rests with the survivor. While a decision to report the rape may lead to social restitution, it may realistically engage the survivor with a legal system that may be invalidating or hostile to her. Efforts to establish safety may be undermined. In view of this, the survivor must make an informed decision or she could be retraumatized.

Follow-Up Treatment

During the immediate aftermath of crisis, cognitive-behavioral techniques that include exposure can be dangerous, as exposure procedures create temporarily high levels of arousal. Instead, because crisis intervention is time limited, the focus needs to be on supporting the survivor, helping the survivor stabilize, and developing adaptive coping strategies for the short term. Other cognitive-behavioral treatments that include exposure can, however, be recommended to clients as a follow-up to crisis intervention and for longer-term therapy.

Two cognitive-behavioral therapies, besides SIT, that have been shown to be effective through well-controlled studies are prolonged exposure (PE) and CPT, both of which include an exposure component. In a recent review of the literature on treatment outcome for PTSD, Foa and Meadows (1997) consider PE to be the treatment of choice for long-term gains, having been one of the most rigorously tested procedures to date. SIT is more likely to produce immediate symptom relief; PE has been shown to be the most effective treatment over the long term; CPT shows promising initial findings (Foa & Meadows, 1997).

These traditional, well-researched treatments are undergoing new, promising changes, as they begin to include alternative approaches. More recently developed behavior therapies are emphasizing nontraditional themes such as mindfulness, dialectics, acceptance, spirituality, the therapeutic relationship, and focusing on the present moment. Mindfulness-based therapies integrated with exposure treatment are shown to improve the effectiveness of cognitive-behavioral treatments (Becker & Zayfert,

2001), despite the existing tension between both philosophical positions. A combination of dialectical behavior therapy (DBT; Linehan, 1993), acceptance and commitment therapy (ACT; Hayes, Strosahl, & Wilson, 1999), and functional analytic psychotherapy (FAP; Kohlenberg & Tsai, 1991) is used with traditional exposure treatment, demonstrating the significance of mindfulness and acceptance practices as an enhancement of the cognitive-behavioral model (Hayes, Follette, & Linehan, 2004). Approaching PE and CPT from a mindfulness and acceptance-based perspective offers a more comprehensive approach. While outcome literature indicating the efficacy of mindfulness is promising, further study is needed.

Support without Resistance

Working with rape survivors can be very difficult for the therapist. Therapists' own maladaptive beliefs often get in the way of their helping clients. Working with rape survivors often shatters a therapist's own sense of security or just-world beliefs (Janoff-Bulman, 1992). Anyone (male or female) is a potential target for rape. Working with survivors often reminds therapists of their own vulnerability to danger. Realizing that the survivors cannot bring this on themselves results in the knowledge that anyone could be attacked. Many therapists have difficulty accepting this. Therapists need to be careful not to inadvertently reinforce a survivor's self-blame (e.g., "What were you doing walking alone in the park that late at night?") or the belief that life is fair and we can control our fate. A therapist's verbal or nonverbal reactions can hold a judgment that is subtly conveyed, creating an atmosphere of distrust for the survivor.

Another problem that therapists encounter is their strong empathy with rape survivors. Some therapists do believe that these clients have endured too much suffering and should, therefore, not be asked to reexperience any additional pain by recounting the trauma. Such an empathic attitude may result in supportive therapeutic strategies, but it can also result in protecting the client from exposure interventions, thereby impeding potential therapeutic gains. It is important for therapists to monitor their own beliefs or myths about rape, as these beliefs will undoubtedly be communicated one way or another to the client. If the therapist believes that the traumatic experience is too difficult to face, the client's avoidance will be reinforced.

Working with rape survivors, as with any PTSD client, requires a fine balance between empathy and support on the one hand and encouragement and faith in the survivor's ability on the other.

CONCLUSION

In summary, cognitive-behavioral treatments have been proven effective in reducing PTSD symptoms following rape trauma. Based on established learning principles, early crisis intervention is important for the psychosocial recovery of rape.

Intervention should provide a sense of safety and support for the survivor, as well as a reinforcement of adaptive thinking. The goals of crisis intervention are to help the survivor not blame herself and feel more of a sense of safety and control, while trying to recall, process, and accept the trauma.

The role of intervention immediately following the trauma must be more active, directive than in other therapies, due to the brevity of time. The goals are also limited to what can be accomplished in a very short time. Therefore, it is unreasonable to expect more than some distress reduction, enhancement of coping strategies, and a greater sense of optimism and trust (through a positive connection with the therapist).

Although the most extensively studied psychological treatments for rape trauma are cognitive-behavioral, there remains a lack of outcome studies substantiating the effectiveness of cognitive-behavioral therapy in crisis intervention, as well as a lack of research on the combination of cognitive-behavioral treatments as described in this chapter. Ideally, emerging studies will provide more empirical evidence and a greater understanding of the efficacy of cognitive-behavioral therapy in crisis intervention following rape trauma.

ACKNOWLEDGMENT

I gratefully wish to acknowledge the contribution that the book *Treatment of Rape Victims: Facilitating Psychological Adjustment*, by Karen S. Calhoun and Beverly M. Atkeson (1991), made to the development of this chapter.

REFERENCES

American Psychiatric Association. (1980). *Diagnostic and statistical manual of mental disorders.* (3rd ed.) Washington, DC: Author.

American Psychiatric Association. (1987). *Diagnostic and statistical manual of mental disorders.* (3rd ed., rev.). Washington, DC: Author.

American Psychiatric Association. (1994). *Diagnostic and statistical manual of mental disorders.* (4th ed.). Washington, DC: Author.

Beck, A. T. (1976). *Cognitive therapy and emotional disorders.* New York: International Universities Press.

Beck, A. T., & Emery, G. (1985). *Anxiety disorders and phobias: A cognitive perspective.* New York: Basic Books.

Becker, C. B., & Zayfert, C. (2001). Integrating DBT-based techniques and concepts to facilitate exposure treatment for PTSD. *Cognitive and Behavioral Practice, 8,* 107–122.

Bernstein, D., & Borkovec, T. (1973). *Progressive relaxation training: A manual for the helping professions.* Champaign, IL: Research Press.

Bordin, E. (1979). The generalizability of the psychoanalytic concept of the working alliance. *Psychotherapy, 16,* 252–260.

Calhoun, K. S., & Atkeson, B. M. (1991). *Treatment of rape victims: Facilitating psychosocial adjustment.* New York: Pergamon Press.

Dancu, C. V., & Foa, E. B. (1992). Posttraumatic stress disorder. In A. Freeman & F. M. Dattilio (Eds.), *Comprehensive casebook of cognitive therapy* (pp. 79–88). New York: Plenum Press.

DiGiuseppe, R. (1991). A rational-emotive model of assessment. In M. E. Bernard (Ed.), *Doing rational-emotive therapy effectively* (pp. 88–96). New York: Plenum Press.

Ehlers, A., & Clark, D. M. (2000). A cognitive model of persistent posttraumatic stress disorder. *Behaviour Research and Therapy, 38*, 319–345.

Ehlers, A., & Steil, R. (1995). Maintenance of intrusive memories in posttraumatic stress disorder: A cognitive approach. *Behavioural and Cognitive Psychotherapy, 23*, 217–249.

Ellis, A. (1962). *Reason and emotion in psychotherapy.* New York: Lyle Stuart.

Ellis, A. (1985). *Overcoming resistance: Rational-emotive resistance with difficult clients.* New York: Springer-Verlag.

Ellis, A. (1986). Discomfort anxiety: A cognitive-behavioral construct. In A. Ellis & Grieger (Eds.). *Handbook of rational-emotive therapy* (Vol. 2, pp. 105–120) New York: Springer-Verlag.

Ellis, A. (1994). Post-traumatic stress disorder (PTSD): A rational emotive behavioral theory. *Journal of Rational-Emotive and Cognitive Behavior Therapy, 12*, 3–25.

Ellis, A., & Dryden, W. (1987). *The practice of rational-emotive therapy.* New York: Springer-Verlag.

Fairbank, J. A., & Brown, T. A. (1987). Current behavioral approaches to the treatment of post-traumatic stress disorder. *Behavior Therapist, 3*, 57–64.

Foa, E. B., & Meadows, E. A. (1997). Psychosocial treatments for posttraumatic stress disorder: A critical review. *Annual Review of Psychology, 48*, 449–480.

Foa, E. B., Riggs, D. S., Dancu, C. V, & Rothbaum, B. O. (1993). Reliability and validity of a brief instrument for assessing post-traumatic-stress disorder. *Journal of Traumatic Stress, 6*, 459–473.

Foa, E. B., & Rothbaum, B. O. (1998). *Treating the trauma of rape: Cognitive-behavioral therapy for PTSD.* New York: Guilford Press.

Foa, E. B., Steketee, G., & Rothbaum, B. O. (1989). Behavioral/cognitive conceptualizations of post-traumatic stress disorder. *Behavior Therapy, 20*, 155–176.

Hayes, S. C., Follette, V. M., & Linehan, M. L. R. (2004). *Mindfulness and acceptance.* New York: Guilford Press.

Hayes, S. C., Strosahl, K., & Wilson, K. G. (1999). *Acceptance and commitment therapy: An experiential approach to behavior change.* New York: Guilford Press.

Herman, J. L. (1997). *Trauma and recovery.* New York: Basic Books.

Jacobson, E. (1938). *Progressive relaxation.* Chicago: University of Chicago Press.

Janoff-Bulman, R. (1979). Characterological versus behavioral self-blame: Inquiries into depression and rape. *Journal of Personality and Social Psychology, 37*, 1798–1809.

Janoff-Bulman, R. (1992). *Shattered assumptions: Toward a new psychology of trauma.* New York: The Free Press.

Keane, T. M., Zimmerling, R. T., & Caddell, J. M. (1985). A behavioral formulation of post-traumatic stress disorder in Vietnam veterans. *Behavior Therapist, 8*, 9–12.

Kilpatrick, D. G., Veronen, L. J., & Resick, P. A. (1982). Psychological sequelae to rape: Assessment and treatment strategies. In D. M. Doleys, R. L. Meredith, & A. R. Ciminero (Eds.), *Behavioral medicine: Assessment and treatment strategies* (pp. 473–498). New York: Plenum Press.

Kohlenberg, R. J., & Tsai, M. (1991). *Functional analytic psychotherapy.* New York: Plenum Press.

Lang, P. J. (1968). Fear reduction and fear behavior: Problems in treating a construct. *Research in Psychotherapy, 3*, 90–102.

Linehan, M. M. (1993). *Cognitive-behavioral treatment of borderline personality disorder.* New York: Guilford Press.

Meichenbaum, D. H. (1985). *Stress inoculation training.* Elmsford, NY: Pergamon Press.

Meyer, C. B., & Taylor, S. E. (1986). Adjustment to rape. *Journal of Personality and Social Psychology, 50*, 1226–1234.

Piaget, J. (1954). *The construction of reality in the child.* New York: Basic Books.

Resick, P. A., & Schnicke, M. K. (1992). Cognitive processing therapy for sexual assault victims. *Journal of Consulting and Clinical Psychology, 60,* 748–756.

Rothbaum, B. O., Foa, E. B., Murdock, T., Riggs, D., & Walsh, W. (1992). A prospective examination of post-traumatic stress disorder in rape victims. *Journal of Traumatic Stress, 5,* 445–475.

Safran, J., & Muran, J. C. (2000). *Negotiating the therapy alliance: A relational treatment guide.* New York: Guilford Press.

Shapiro, F. (2001). *Eye movement desensitization and reprocessing: Basic principles, protocols, and procedures* (2nd ed.). New York: Guilford Press.

Shapiro, F., & Forrest, M. (2004). *Eye movement desensitization and reprocessing (EMDR): The breakthrough eye movement therapy for overcoming anxiety, stress, and trauma* (*updated*). New York: Basic Books.

Walen, S. R., DiGiuseppe, R., & Dryden, W. (1992). *The practitioner's guide to rational-emotive therapy* (2nd ed.). New York: Oxford University Press.

SUGGESTED READINGS

Calhoun, K. S., & Atkeson, B. M. (1991). *Treatment of rape victims: Facilitating psychosocial adjustment.* New York: Pergamon Press.

Foa, E. B., & Meadows, E. A. (1997). Psychosocial treatments for posttraumatic stress disorder: A critical review. *Annual Review Psychology, 48,* 449–480.

Foa, E. B., & Rothbaum, B. O. (1998). *Treating the trauma of rape: Cognitive-behavioral therapy for PTSD.* New York: Guilford Press.

Foa, E. B., Steketee, G., & Rothbaum, B. O. (1989). Behavioral/cognitive conceptualizations of post-traumatic stress disorder. *Behavior Therapy, 20,* 155–176.

Resick, P. A., & Mechanic, M. B. (1995). Brief cognitive therapies for rape victims. In A. R. Roberts (Ed.), *Crisis intervention and time-limited cognitive treatment* (pp. 91–126). Newbury Park, CA: Sage.

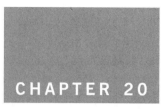

CHAPTER 20

Traumatic Stress Disorders

Laurence Miller

September 11, 2001.

Mention traumatic stress, and almost anyone will invoke that particular national paroxysm. Ironically, however, by the time that tragic event occurred, trauma psychologists and emergency crisis workers already knew a great deal about how to treat traumatic disability syndromes (Miller, 1998e), preventing even greater fear and ignorance from adding to the confusion and horror of that event. This chapter describes the history, phenomenology, symptomatology, and main cognitive-behavioral treatment strategies for traumatic stress syndromes. Reflecting the author's practical experience, the emphasis is on civilian (nonmilitary) traumatic stress, although the principles of evaluation and treatment share more similarities than differences (Miller, 2006a).

HISTORY OF THE TRAUMA CONCEPT

Historically, the pendulum of interest in posttraumatic stress syndromes has swung back and forth between military and civilian traumas (Evans, 1992; Pizarro, Silver, & Prouse, 2006; Rosen, 1975; Trimble, 1981; Wilson, 1994). During warfare, rulers and generals have always had a stake in knowing as much as possible about any factors that might have an adverse effect on their fighting forces. To this end, doctors have been pressed into service to diagnose and treat soldiers with the aim of getting them back to the front lines as quickly as possible. In peacetime, attention turns to the everyday accidents and individual acts of mayhem that can produce stress, pain, and trauma in the lives of civilians.

One of the first modern conceptualizations of posttraumatic stress was put forth by the army surgeon Hoffer who in 1678 developed the concept of *nostalgia*, which he defined as a deterioration in the physical and mental health of homesick soldiers. The cause of this malady was attributed to the formation of abnormally vivid images in the affected soldier's brain by battle-induced overexcitation of the "vital spirits." Here, in effect, was one of the first attempts to explain how a psychological event could affect brain functioning and, in turn, influence health and behavior.

With the 18th and 19th centuries came the mechanized progress of the industrial revolution, bringing with it new and monstrous machines to crush, grind, and flay the scores of workers who tended them too carelessly or toiled too close by. At about the same time, a new form of high-speed transportation, the railroad, began to reveal a disturbing propensity to rattle and strew its passengers about in derailments and collisions. All too often it was noticed, after the physical scars had healed, or even when injury to the body was minor or nonexistent, many accident victims showed lasting disturbances in thought, feeling, and action that could not readily be explained by the conventional medical knowledge of the day. Some patients were afflicted by strange paralyses or neurasthenic fatigues, while others trembled continuously, twitched and postured bizarrely, jumped at the slightest sound, or holed up for weeks or months.

In 1882 Erichson (cited in Wilson, 1994) introduced the concept of *railway spine*, which he believed could be traced to as-yet unobservable perturbations in the structure of the central nervous system caused by blows to the body—never mind that in many cases there was no evidence at all for any such bodily concussions. Others among Erichson's colleagues considered that the strange disorders of sensation and movement might be due to disruptions in the blood flow to the spinal cord, or even to small hemorrhages.

While these organically minded physicians were squinting to discern structural microtraumas in nervous tissue, others expanded their gaze to view the origin of posttraumatic impairment syndromes as a *psychological* phenomenon—albeit straying none too far from the home base of neurophysiology. This was reflected in the theory of *nervous shock*, introduced by Page in 1895 (cited in Wilson, 1994), which posited that a state of overwhelming fright or terror—not physical bangs and jolts—was the primary cause of traumatic impairment syndromes in railway and industrial accidents. Similarly, at around the same time, Oppenheim (1890) theorized that a stimulus perceived through the senses alone, if strong enough, might actually jar the nervous system into a state of disequilibrium.

For his part, the great Charcot (1887) regarded the effects of physical trauma as a form of hysteria, the symptoms arising as a consequence of disordered brain physiology caused by the terrifying memory of the traumatic event. In postulating the impact of a psychological force on the physical functioning of the brain, these late 19th-century theories were reminiscent of Hoffer's conceptualization, two centuries earlier, except that electrophysiological impulses now had replaced vital spirits as the underlying mechanism of the disorder.

Attention, however, soon shifted back to the field of battle. The American Civil War introduced a new level of industrialized killing and with it a dramatic increase in reports of stress-related nervous ailments. Further advances in weapons technology during World War I produced an alarming accumulation of horrid battlefield casualties from machine guns, poison gas, and long-range artillery. This led to the widely applied concept of *shell shock*, a form of psychological incapacitation, at first thought to be produced by the brain-concussive effects of exploding shells. This wartime stress theory was, after all, not too different from the earlier civilian concept of railway spine. In both cases, undocumentable effects on the nervous system were postulated on the basis of observed disorders in behavior.

To this end, physicians continued to marshal new findings about the role of the nervous system in regulating states of arousal and bodily homeostasis. For example, Wilson and his colleagues (Frazier & Wilson, 1918; Mearburg & Wilson, 1918) described a syndrome in traumatized soldiers called *irritable heart*, which they attributed to overstimulation of the sympathetic ("fight-or-flight") branch of the autonomic nervous system.

Even Sigmund Freud got into the act. No stranger to neuroscientific theory and practice himself (Miller, 1984, 1991b), Freud (1920) regarded the tendency to remain "fixated" on traumatic events as having a biological basis. But recurring recollections and nightmares of a frightening nature seemed to fly in the face of Freud's theory of the pleasure principle. Consequently, he was forced to consider a psychogenic cause—that traumatic dreams and other symptoms served the function of helping the traumatized person master the terrifying event by working it over and over in the victim's mind. Unfortunately, this line of theorizing took Freud into some morbid metaphysical speculations about the death instinct and organic dissolution that has had the effect of keeping his ideas on the fringes of trauma theory even to the present day.

Meanwhile, soldiers were still being scared out of their wits on the battlefield and the civilian industrial, railway, and now automobile accident cases continued to pile up. The persistently annoying failure of medical science to discover any definitive organic basis for these debilitating stress syndromes led to a gradual, if grudging, acceptance of psychodynamic explanations, as the Freudian influence began to be felt more generally throughout psychiatry. This contributed to the replacement of shell shock by the more psychological-sounding concept of *war neurosis*.

Apparently making a theoretical virtue of empirical necessity, doctors now no longer felt compelled to tether their diagnoses and treatments to ephemeral defects of nervous tissue. Accordingly, Ferenczi, Abraham, and Simmel (1921) elaborated the basic model of traumatic neurosis that is still largely accepted today among psychodynamic theorists (Horowitz, 1986). Ferenczi's group described the central role of anxiety, the persistence of morbid apprehension, regression of the ego, the attempted reparative function of recurring nightmares, and the therapeutic use of catharsis. For the most part, the patients themselves seemed to do well with the kinds of psychologically cathartic and supportive approaches that were provided by caring counselors, ministers, or nurses.

Continuing research and clinical experience expanded the theoretical base of trauma psychology. After surveying more than 1,000 reports in the international literature published during the World War I, Southard (1919) concluded that shell shock, war neurosis, and similar syndromes were true psychoneuroses. Kardiner (1941) followed a group of patients with war neuroses for more than a decade and concluded that severe war trauma produced a kind of centripetal contraction or collapse of the ego that prevented these patients from adapting to and mastering life's subsequent challenges. Kardiner elaborated a conceptualization of trauma termed *physioneurosis* that is startlingly close to the modern concept of posttraumatic stress disorder. The features of Kardiner's physioneurosis included (1) persistence of a startle response or irritability; (2) a proclivity to explosive behavior; (3) fixation on the trauma; (4) an overall constriction of the personality; and (5) a disturbed dream life, including vivid nightmares.

The experiences of the World War II contributed surprisingly little to the development of new theories and treatments for wartime trauma, now renamed *battle fatigue*. In fact, resistance to the concept of battle fatigue, with its implications of mental weakness and lack of moral resolve, was widespread in both medical and military circles. There was a war on, plenty of good Joes were getting killed and wounded, and the army had little sympathy for the pusillanimous whinings of a few slackers and Nervous Nellies who wouldn't buck up and pull their weight.

But it was becoming apparent that wartime psychological trauma could take place in circumstances other than the actual battlefield. In World War II, then Korea and Vietnam, and most recently in the Persian Gulf wars, clinicians began to learn about disabling stress syndromes associated with large-scale bombings of civilian populations, prisoner of war (POW) and concentration camps, "brainwashing" of POWs, civilian atrocities, and terrorism.

With sad predictability, today's daily media continue to churn out more than ample case material from every imaginable species of human tragedy: war crimes, industrial injuries, plane crashes, auto accidents, rapes, assaults, domestic violence, child abuse, earthquakes, hurricanes, fires, floods, toxic spills, terrorist bombings—the list goes on. In 1980 traumatic stress syndromes were finally codified as an identifiable type of psychopathological syndrome—*posttraumatic stress disorder* (PTSD)—in the American Psychiatric Association's (1980, 1987, 1994, 2000) official *Diagnostic and Statistical Manual of Mental Disorders*.

PTSD: THE SYNDROME

In clinical classification, a *syndrome* is defined as a set of symptoms and signs that occur in a fairly regular pattern from patient to patient, under a given set of circumstances, and with a specific set of causes (even though individual variations may be seen). In this definition, PTSD is a syndrome of emotional and behavioral disturbance that follows exposure to a traumatic stressor or set of traumatically stressful experiences that is typically outside the range of normal, everyday experience for that person. As a result, there develops a characteristic set of symptoms (American Psychiatric Association, 2000; Meek, 1990; Merskey, 1992; Miller, 1994b, 1998e, 1999a; Modlin, 1983; Parker, 1990; Weiner, 1992).

Anxiety

The patient describes a continual state of free-floating anxiety or nervousness. There is a constant gnawing apprehension that something terrible is about to happen. He or she maintains an intensive hypervigilance, scanning the environment for the least hint of impending threat or danger. Panic attacks may be occasional or frequent.

Physiological Arousal

The patient's autonomic nervous system is always on red alert. He/she experiences increased bodily tension in the form of muscle tightness or "knots," tremors or shakiness, restlessness, fatigue, heart palpitations, breathing difficulties, dizziness, headaches, stomach and bowel disturbances, urinary frequency, or menstrual disturbances. About one-half of PTSD patients show a classic startle reaction: surprised by an unexpected door slam, telephone ring, sneeze, or even just hearing their name called, the patient may literally "jump" out of his seat and then spend the next few minutes trembling with fear and anxiety.

Irritability

There is a pervasive chip-on-the-shoulder edginess, impatience, loss of humor, and quick anger over seemingly trivial matters. Friends get annoyed, coworkers shun the patient, and family members may be abused and alienated. A particularly common complaint is the patient's increased sensitivity to children's noisiness or the family's bothering questions.

Avoidance and Denial

The patient tries to blot out the event from his/her mind. He avoids thinking about the traumatic event and shuns news articles, radio programs, or TV shows that remind him of the incident. "I just don't want to talk about it" is the standard response, and the patient may claim to have forgotten important aspects of the event. Some of this is a deliberate, conscious effort to avoid trauma reminders; part of it also involves an involuntary psychic numbing that blunts most incoming threatening stimuli. The emotional coloring of this denial may range from blasé indifference to nail-biting anxiety.

Intrusion

Despite the patient's best efforts to keep the traumatic event out of his/her mind, the horrifying incident pushes its way into consciousness, often rudely and abruptly in the form of intrusive images of the event by day and frightening dreams at night. In the most extreme cases, the patient may experience flashbacks or reliving experiences in which he seems to be mentally transported back to the traumatic scene in all its sensory and emotional vividness, sometimes losing touch with current reality. More commonly, the intrusive recollection is described as a persistent psychological demon that "won't let me forget" the terrifying events surrounding the trauma.

Repetitive Nightmares

Even sleep offers little respite. Sometimes the patient's nightmares replay the actual traumatic event; more commonly, the dreams echo the general theme of the trauma but miss the mark in terms of specific content. For example, a patient traumatized in an auto accident may dream of falling off a cliff of having a wall collapse on him. Or, a sexual assault victim may dream of being attacked by vicious dogs or drowning in a muddy pool. The emotional intensity of the original traumatic experience is retained but the dream partially disguises the event itself. This symbolic reconfiguration of dream material is, of course, one of the main pillars of Freudian psychoanalytic theory.

Impaired Concentration and Memory

The subject complains of having gotten "spacey," "fuzzy," or "ditsy." He/she has trouble remembering names, tends to misplace objects, loses the train of conversations, or cannot keep his/her mind focused on work, reading material, family activities, and so on. The patient may worry that he/she has brain damage or that "I'm losing my mind."

Sexual Inhibition

Over 90% of PTSD subjects report decreased sexual activity and interest; this may further strain an already stressed-out marital relationship. In some cases, complete impotence or frigidity may occur, especially in cases in which the traumatic event involved sexual assault.

Withdrawal and Isolation

The patient shuns friends, neighbors, and family members and just wants to be left alone. He/she has no patience for the petty, trivial concerns of everyday life—bills, gossip, news events—and gets annoyed at being bothered by such things. The hurt feelings this engenders in those he/she rebuffs may spur retaliatory avoidance, leading to a vicious cycle of rejection and recrimination.

Impulsivity and Instability

More rarely, the trauma survivor may take sudden trips; move from place to place; walk off the job; disappear from his/her family for prolonged periods; uncharacteristically engage in drunken binges, gambling sprees, or romantic trysts; make excessive purchases; or take dangerous physical or legal risks. It is as if the trauma has goaded the patient into a "what the hell, life is short" attitude that overcomes his/her usual good judgment and common sense. Obviously, not every instance of irresponsible behavior can be blamed on trauma, but a connection may be suspected when this kind of activity is definitely out of character for that person and follows an identifiable traumatic event. Far from taking such walks on the wild side, however, the majority of trauma survivors continue to suffer in numbed and shattered silence.

ACUTE STRESS DISORDER

Acute stress disorder (ASD) was introduced as a diagnostic category into DSM-IV (American Psychiatric Association, 1994) primarily to help identify those at risk of developing later PTSD. ASD is defined as a reaction to the traumatic stress that occurs within 4 weeks after the index trauma. Although ASD focuses more on dissociative symptoms than does PTSD, it also includes symptoms of reexperiencing, avoidance, and hyperarousal. Preliminary prospective studies suggest that between 60 and 80% of individuals meeting criteria for ASD following a traumatic event will meet criteria for PTSD up to 2 years later.

The ASD diagnosis has been contentious since its inception. It has been criticized on the grounds of being conceptually and empirically redundant with PTSD, as well as pathologizing common symptoms of psychological distress in the immediate aftermath of trauma (Koch, Douglas, Nicholls, & O'Neill, 2006). However, it recognizes that some patients may show traumatic reactions close in time to the injurious event and it reinforces the importance of early treatment where it is clinically indicated.

PARTIAL AND ATYPICAL PTSD SYNDROMES

When fewer than the requisite number of symptoms are tabulated, subsyndromal or partial forms of PTSD may be described (Stein, Walker, Hazen, & Forde, 1997). Thus, one patient may report only traumatic nightmares, while another may experience hyperarousal without numbing/avoidance or reexperiencing symptoms. Note that the actual number of symptoms need not correlate with severity of psychological disability: The subject may be so psychologically disabled by crippling anxiety and sleep loss that he/she may develop secondary cognitive and emotional impairment sufficient to disrupt work and family life.

To account for psychological responses to trauma that do not fit neatly into the DSM diagnostic formulation, Alarcon, Deering, Glover, Ready, and Eddleman (1997) have proposed a PTSD typology to accommodate these unusual variants. Again, clinicians should be careful not to overlook other DSM diagnoses that might fit these patients (Miller, 2002).

The *depressive* subtype presents with psychomotor retardation, social withdrawal, inability to deal with everyday occurrences, loss of interest, low self-esteem, self-criticism, guilt feelings, and suicidality. Differential diagnoses include major depressive disorder and adjustment disorder with depressed mood.

The *dissociative* subtype is characterized by a predominance of flashbacks, hallu-cinatory experiences, depersonalization, derealization, fugue-like amnesic behavior, and symptoms resembling multiple personality disorder. Differential diagnoses include dissociative identity disorder, borderline personality disorder, and temporal lobe epi-lepsy.

The primary manifestation of the *somatomorphic* subtype is chronic pain or some other type of physical symptomatology, typically without clear localization or identifi-able medical cause. Differential diagnoses include the somatoform disorders as well as unrecognized organic injury or illness.

In the *psychotic-like* subtype, the patient shows distortions of consciousness, fan-tasizing, staring, inattentiveness, impaired motivation and volition, paranoia, and behavioral regression. Differential diagnoses include schizophrenia; schizoid, schizo-typal, or paranoid personality disorders; or brain injury effects.

The *organic-like* subtype presents with impaired attention, concentration, learn-ing, memory, and cognition, along with confusion, slowness in thought, speech, and behavior, and in some cases, a dementia-like clinical picture. Differential diagnoses include postconcussion syndrome following brain injury, severe depression, or natu-rally occurring dementias in older patients.

The *neurotic-like* subtype is characterized by anxiety, phobic avoidance, restless-ness, hypersensitivity, obsessionalism, and panic attacks. Differential diagnoses in-clude the anxiety disorders.

EVOLUTION OF THE TRAUMA RESPONSE

But the phenomenology of ASD and PTSD consists of more than a tabulation of index symptoms, and the reaction to a traumatic event can begin within the first few moments of the crisis. Hollywood portrayals to the contrary, during the immediate cri-sis, most people do not become overwhelmed or paralyzed by intense fear or shock; in the breach, many behave quite adaptively (Aldwin, 1994; Weiner, 1992; Miller, 1998e, 2003a, 2004, 2005). Assault victims calculate their avenues of escape; passengers pur-posefully unstrap their seatbelts and climb out of the window of their burning plane or submerging automobile; office workers find the exit and file down the stairwell of the bombed building, even helping others in the process. The entire organism seems to go on automatic and is directed toward survival. A certain degree of adaptive depersonal-ization or dissociation may take place, an unnatural mental detachment from the sur-rounding events that enables the person to deal with the practical survival needs of the situation; this is often described in retrospect as "like being in a dream" or "happening in slow motion." Cinematic wild-eyed panic is extremely rare and disaster manage-ment experts frequently note how difficult it is to get people to move at all during an emergency (Miller, 1998e).

After the event, the numbing depersonalization may continue for some time, the survivor feeling confused and bewildered. It is as if the psychoanesthetic freeze elicited during the trauma incident needs time to thaw out in the more temperate affective climate of real life. Unfortunately, though, "real life" does not last very long, as the intrusive recollective and emotional gale rushes in at the weak chinks that begin to form in the crumbling psychic armor. Thus begins the wrenching emotional seesaw of painful intrusion alternating with numbing denial, along with many of the other post-traumatic stress symptoms described earlier.

In the best cases, the major symptoms and disturbances diminish in the course of weeks to months as the event becomes integrated into the life narrative and personal history of the individual. A more realistic awareness of individual vulnerability is built up, so that basic feelings of security and confidence are restored. However, in some cases, a number of mental roadblocks may stand in the way of the trauma survivor's making peace with him/herself and the world (Everstine & Everstine, 1993; Matsakis, 1994; McCann & Pearlman, 1990; Miller 1994b, 1998e).

One of these involves guilt and stigma. Many trauma survivors believe that they could have somehow prevented the traumatic event from occurring. Others interpret the event as a kind of hard-knocks wakeup call for their poor judgment or as cosmic punishment for past misdeeds. Many survivors feel "marked by fate," especially if this is not their first traumatic experience. Still others experience a violation of their bodily and territorial integrity. They feel fragmented and scattered, and the slightest upset makes them irritable and isolative. They may literally wince when touched or when others encroach upon their personal space, and they become panicky in rooms or in crowds where they are unable to negotiate a clear route of escape.

The traumatic event and its aftermath comprise a shattering existential experience. The trauma survivor is starkly confronted with his/her own vulnerability and mortality in a way that most of us manage to avoid by using the normal, adaptive denials of everyday life, of "business as usual." The victim's existential violation may be all the more painful if the trauma took place at the hands of another person; worse still if the actions of the malfeasor were maliciously intentional or uncaringly negligent. And even more devastating may be traumas perpetrated by a known and heretofore trusted person, such as a family member, friend, workmate, neighbor, doctor, or clergy member.

Being in a trauma mode is difficult to stop and hard to let go of. Many trauma survivors generalize the helplessness of the cognitive survival state to other aspects of their lives, now feeling powerless to control even their own behavior or to influence the actions of others. Or, they may impute domineering or retaliatory motives to anyone who tries to exert even the normal, socially appropriate influence or control over them (e.g., bosses, doctors, parents, or spouses). In some cases, outright paranoia and hostility may develop.

Even after things seem to have calmed down, when the trauma survivor has achieved some measure of delicate equilibrium, the stresses or returning to the normal routines of work and family life may trigger PTSD reactions. Also, delayed PTSD reactions may crop up years or even decades after the event as illness or the aging process begins to deplete the individual's adaptive reserves.

In general, the more severe the trauma and the longer the trauma response persists, the more pessimistic the outcome. That is why it is important for all traumatic disability patients to receive quick, effective treatment (Miller, 1998e). And even after a delay, or when the trauma syndrome takes time to surface, proper treatment can still have a significant impact, so no situation should ever be considered categorically hopeless.

TYPES OF CIVILIAN TRAUMATIC STRESS SYNDROMES

As noted in the historical section, much of the initial interest in traumatic stress reactions came from the field of military psychology and psychiatry. However, most of the PTSD cases that are seen by practitioners in routine mental health practice involve civilian instances of ASD and PTSD.

Medical Procedures

Emergency medical care, lifesaving though it may be, often employs procedures for which the patient has little or no preparation (Shalev, Schreiber, Galai, & Melmed, 1993). The emotional impact of serious illness or injury may be compounded by these invasive, painful, and frightening medical procedures, such as those that occur in emergency treatment for a heart attack, motor vehicle accident, or workplace injury. Intrusive recollection and avoidance of stimuli are frequently observed among hospitalized survivors of trauma but tend to be time limited and self-remitting. However, medical conditions or procedures themselves may constitute possible traumatic stressors, as they are often associated with sudden onset, a feeling of helplessness, or lack of control by the patient and a perceived or actual threat to life (Miller, 1994b, 1998e).

Pain

In addition to fear and threat to life, one of the most traumatically stressful aspects of injuries, or the treatment of them, may be the unavoidable physical pain that is sometimes involved (Miller, 1993a, 1994b, 1998e, 2002). Research shows that the prevalence of PTSD among physically injured survivors of stressful events is higher than that of survivors without physical injury in both war and civilian trauma and that pain can be the most stressful aspect of injury trauma (Helzer, Robins, & McEnvoi, 1987; Pitman, Orr, Forgue, de Jong, & Claiborn, 1989; Schreiber & Galai-Gat, 1993), although, in some cases, physical injury may actually defuse and limit the stress response by giving the patient something "real" on which to focus his/her concern (Modlin, 1983).

Traumatic Brain Injury

Injuries that produce pain syndromes also often produce traumatic brain injuries that may result in a *postconcussion syndrome* (PCS). Although this is usually conceptualized by neuropsychologists in terms of the cognitive impairment involved, the emotional and psychodynamic effects may be even more traumatizing (Miller, 1991a, 1993c, 1993d, 1998e, 2001b; Parker, 1990, 2001; Small, 1980). Brain injury is a distinctive form of stressor because the person's very organ of coping has been damaged. Thus, the individual's ability to maintain vocational, domestic, or academic responsibilities—one's normal hold on reality—is impaired. Significant features of PCS stress reactions include anxiety, depression, anger, intrusive thoughts, preoccupation with the trauma, self-deprecation, social withdrawal, disintegration of selfhood, and behavioral regression. Impulsivity, egocentricity, and lack of insight into deficits and behavior may cause further alienation from family and care providers.

Toxic Trauma and the Toxic Stress Syndrome

Exposure to toxic substances in the home or workplace may produce a variety of neurological, cognitive, and emotional disturbances that are typically attributed to the direct physical effects of toxic materials on the nervous system (Eskanazi & Maizlish, 1988; Hartman, 1995). In addition, however, the experience of a potentially life-threatening or health-impairing chemical poisoning episode can be overwhelmingly frightening, leading to the development of a PTSD-like *toxic stress syndrome* (Miller, 1993b, 1995b, 1998e; Morrow, Ryan, Goldstein, & Hodgoon, 1989; Morrow, Ryan, Hodgoon, & Robin, 1991, Schottenfield & Cullen, 1985). Symptoms include anxiety, depression, impaired concentration, somatic preoccupation, intrusive recollections, and traumatic dreams. Often, symptoms are triggered by trauma reminders, especially by exposure to odors. Emotional disturbance and psychological and behavioral impairment are often uncorrelated with level and duration of toxic exposure.

Motor Vehicle Accidents

We live in a car culture, and motor vehicle accidents (MVA) are a major cause of injury and death in people under 30 (Blanchard & Hickling, 2003). A wide variety of post-MVA traumatic psychological symptoms have been described, including anxiety, panic attacks, intrusive recollections (e.g., flashbacks), driving and riding phobias, traumatic nightmares, and disruption of work and family life (Blanchard, Hickling, Taylor, Loos, & Gerardi, 1994; Brom, Kleber, & Defares, 1989; Foeckler, Garrard, Williams, Thomas, & Jones, 1978; Hodge, 1971; Kuch, 1987; Kuch & Swinson, 1985; Malt, Hoivik, & Blikra, 1993; Munjack, 1984; Parker, 1996). Because MVA can result in a number of injuries, an "unholy trinity" often occurs consisting of (1) PCS due to closed-head injury, (2) chronic pain due to low back or cervical whiplash injury, and (3) PTSD, which exacerbate one another in a vicious cycle (Miller, 1998a).

Disasters

Although the posttraumatic reactions to natural and man-made disasters in many ways resemble those to other traumatic stressors, several features make the disaster experience unique (Abueg, Woods, & Watson, 2000; Aldwin, 1994; Freedy,

Shaw, Jarrell, & Masters, 1992; Green 1991; Raphael, 1986; Ursano, Fullerton, & Norwood, 1995; Weiner, 1992). First, there is often little or no warning, such as in an earthquake or building collapse. Even when advance warning is available, as with a hurricane that is tracked for days, people often display a stupefying capacity for denial and minimization until it is too late. Second, most disasters—chemical spills, earthquakes, tsunamis, nuclear power plant meltdowns, terrorist attacks—generally occur in a relatively short time frame. By the time the full extent of the threat is realized, the worst may be over and the aftermath must be dealt with. Third, disasters typically involve extreme danger, including loss of life. At the very least, people lose something of value, often in both material and human terms. Fourth, both natural and technological disasters provide very little chance for people to exert any kind of meaningful human control; helplessness magnifies the traumatic effect of disasters. Finally, disasters happen to many people simultaneously, often causing victims to feel that the whole world is coming to an end, or that the larger world has abandoned them. On the positive side, a sense of communal purpose can be important in mitigating the effects of traumatic stress.

Crime Victim Trauma

The effects of trauma are often magnified when the harm comes through intentional human malevolence. These psychic injuries violate our sense of security, stability, and community. The suddenness, randomness, and fundamental unfairness of criminal assaults can overwhelm victims with helplessness and despair. As difficult as it may be to bear the traumas of injury and loss that occur in accidents and mishaps of nature, far more wrenching are the wounds that occur as the result of the callous and malicious depredations of others. Trauma due to interpersonal violence can thus be among the most severe and long lasting (Falsetti & Resnick, 1995; Foa & Riggs, 1993; Freedy, Resnick, Kilpatrick, Dansky, & Tidwell, 1994; Hough, 1985; Miller, 1998c, 2001a; Rothbaum, Foa, Riggs, Murdock, & Walsh, 1992; Spungen, 1998).

Workplace Violence

Many people spend most of their waking hours at work, so not feeling safe on the job can produce both chronic stress and acute trauma. The National Institute of Occupational Safety and Health reports that homicide is the second leading cause of death in the workplace. Murder is the number-one workplace killer of women and the third leading cause of death for men, after MVA and machine-related fatalities (Kinney, 1995; Labig, 1995; Mantell & Albrecht, 1994). Annually, robberies account for the greatest number of deaths, followed by business disputes, personal disputes, and law enforcement line-of-duty deaths. The majority of workplace homicides are committed by firearms. For every actual killing, there are anywhere from 10 to 100 sublethal acts of violence committed at work (Flannery, 1995; Labig, 1995). Workplace violence combines crime victimization with a violation of the expectations of safety and security we come to expect at a familiar jobsite, similar to violence that occurs at home (Blythe, 2002; Dennenberg & Braverman, 1999; Miller, 1999b).

Terrorism

The word *terrorism* derives from the Latin, *terrere*, which means "to frighten," and the first recorded use of the term as it is currently understood derives from the 18th-century Reign of Terror associated with the French Revolution. Although we may think of it as a recent crisis in this country, terrorism is as old as civilization, as timeless as human conflict, and it has existed ever since people discovered that they could intimidate the many by targeting the few. However, terrorism has achieved special prominence in the modern technological era, beginning in the 1970s as international terrorism, continuing in the 1980s and 1990s as American domestic terrorism, and apparently coming full circle in the 21st century with mass terror attacks on U.S. soil by foreign nationals. Arguably, the two culmination points of domestic and international terrorism in the past decade have been Oklahoma City and the World Trade Center. Many experts believe that the worst is yet to come (Bolz, Dudonis, & Schultz, 1996; Kuzma, 2000; Savitch, 2003), although others believe the threat has been overblown (Mueller, 2005).

Essentially, terrorism is the "perfect" traumatic stressor, because it combines the elements of malevolent intent, actual or threatened extreme harm, and fear of the future. Terrorist attacks combine features of criminal assaults, disasters, and acts of war. Accordingly, much of our clinical knowledge in treating terror victims is adapted from experiences in treating these other kinds of cases, and terrorism will be an important part of trauma psychology in the 21st century (Kratcoski, Edelbacher, & Das, 2001; Miller, 2006b; Strebnicki, 2001).

It might be assumed that the enormity of a nationwide trauma like 9/11 might provide a kind of reality check, help some patients put their own idiosyncratic crises and preoccupations into perspective, and actually aid them in coping—a kind of "there but for the grace of God go I" reaction. Instead, it has been my clinical experience that if anything, many people's personal tragedies have been magnified by the national trauma: "Here I am, struggling with my alcohol abuse, or my social phobia, or my dysfunctional work behavior, or my chronic pain syndrome, or my lousy marriage, or my rotten kids—and now I have to deal with *this, too?*" Thus, for many people, the effect of a generalized trauma seems to be summative with, not ameliorative to, their more personal traumas and tribulations (Miller, 2003a, 2003b, 2004, 2005).

Critical Incident Stress

Special challenges are faced by the men and women in law enforcement, firefighting, paramedic, and other emergency services who regularly have to deal with the most violent, impulsive, and predatory members of society, to display professionalism in the face of citizens undergoing the most emotional events of their lives, and to frequently confront cruelties and horrors that most civilians only view from the sanitized distance of their newspapers and TV screens. Handling the combination of both routine stresses and episodic crises requires a certain adaptively defensive toughness of attitude, temperament, and training. Without this resolve, these crisis workers could not do their jobs effectively. Sometimes, however, the stress is just too much, and the very toughness that facilitates smooth functioning in their daily duties now becomes an impediment to these helpers seeking help for themselves. Accordingly, specialized forms of treatment are required (Blau, 1994; Bohl, 1995; Dunning, 1999; Henry, 2004; McMains, 1991; Miller, 1995a, 1998e, 1999c, 2000a, 2006a; Mitchell & Everly, 1996; Paton & Smith, 1999; Reese, 1987; Sheehan, Everly, & Langlieb, 2004; Silva, 1991; Solomon, 1995; Toch, 2002; Williams, 1991).

THEORIES OF PTSD AND THE TRAUMA RESPONSE

As noted earlier in the historical introduction, theorizing about traumatic disability syndromes has always swung between mentalistic and physicalistic accounts. Kretschmer (1926) originally described two classes of naturalistic behavioral responses that organisms use to ward off threats. The first he characterized as the *violent motor reaction* which involves active attempts to attack or escape from the source of the danger. The second was called the *sham death* or *immobilization reflex*, in which inaction and seemingly stuporous features predominate.

Ludwig (1972) revised and expanded Kretschmer's (1926) formulation by positing a pervasive natural tendency for animals and humans to react in progressively more primitive ways when confronted with potentially dangerous and inescapable situations. Under such conditions, organisms readily and automatically resort to behaviors appropriate at earlier stages of development, behaviors that appear regressive or "immature." These include babbling, rocking, crying, vivid fantasizing, mute withdrawal, incontinence, and so on—the kinds of reaction often associated with "shell shock" or other kinds of acute traumatic states.

Psychodynamic theories of the trauma response (Brom & Kleber, 1989; Horowitz, 1986; Modlin, 1983) generally focus on the self-protective mechanisms used by the ego to deal with overwhelming stimulation. These include fight-or-flight responses, numbing and dissociation, displacement of anxiety onto external objects or situations, behavioral regression, and cognitive or interpretive control mechanisms (Thompson, 1981). In this way, the victim tries to preserve at least the illusion of control and thereby diminish the threat of recurrence. Many people would rather blame themselves than feel helpless.

Neuropsychological theories of PTSD (Charney, Deutsch, Krystal, Southwick, & Davis, 1993; Dietz, 1992; Kolb, 1987; Miller, 1997, 2000b; Sapolsky, Krey, & McEwen, 1984) tend to invoke interactions between the emotional processing mechanisms of the brain's limbic system and the cognitive-interpretive mechanisms of the cerebral cortex (Miller, 1990)—a concept that actually goes back to Freud (1920) and Pavlov (1927). In this framework, perturbations in corticolimbic functioning induced by trauma prevent the assimilation and dissipation of the psychophysiological crisis response, thus inhibiting resolution of the traumatic memory. This theory especially focuses on the neurosensitizing effect of stress-induced glucocorticoid hormones on the *hippocampus*, the brain's system for storing emotionally relevant memories.

PSYCHOTHERAPY OF THE TRAUMATIZED PATIENT

The variety of PTSD syndromes described earlier and the complex neuropsycho-dynamics that contribute to the unique clinical expression in individual cases necessarily demand that psychotherapists show some degree of clinical flexibility in their treatment of traumatized patients. In the present context, it may require some latitude in what are considered cognitive-behavioral forms of therapy.

General Therapeutic Considerations

Several authorities (Brom & Kleber, 1989; Everstine & Everstine, 1993; Shalev et al., 1993) have stressed the need to consider the trauma response and its corresponding treatment in terms of a series of stages that may vary in length and intensity from patient to patient, depending on such factors as premorbid personality, past experience, prior trauma, and the patient's interpersonal support systems. A conceptualization that takes into account the neuropsychobiological bases of PTSD is Everly's (1990, 1993, 1995) two-factor model of PTSD treatment, consisting of (1) a *neurobiological hypersensitivity* involving heightened nervous system and endocrine responsivity, and (2) a *psychological hypersensitivity* involving disruptions and transfigurations in the individual's world view and self-concept. Accordingly, the following is an outline of therapeutic procedures for treating traumatic disability syndromes of many types (Miller, 1998e).

Educative and Supportive Measures

Although physical trauma is almost always treated solicitously by medical professionals, psychological trauma is frequently disregarded or dismissed. Such disenfranchised suffering only serves to entrench disability and impede recovery. Thus, the first step is to treat traumatic stress syndromes with the respect they deserve. Indeed, research and clinical experience show that early, intensive, and appropriate treatment within the first weeks and months of any physically or psychologically traumatic event improves the prognosis for all kinds of traumatic disability syndromes (Miller, 1998e). Accordingly, Modlin (1983) recommends that far from coddling patients into permanent invalidism, appropriately solicitous clinical attention and a reasonable interval of convalescence can actually prevent the development of subsequent persistent traumatic disability.

This approach involves the therapist first demonstrating his/her understanding by asking questions that elicit the nature of the common PTSD symptoms, then offering a comprehensible explanatory model that emphasizes the universality and normality of the stress response and its manifestations. This process is replicated in each session. The patient may not completely grasp the psychological explanation, but what he/she does hear is that the therapist understands what he/she has gone through, believes the patient has a legitimate clinical syndrome that has a name and a causal explanation, and that the clinician knows what to do about it.

The importance of providing concrete, practical help to patients is often over-looked (Brom & Kleber, 1989; Werman, 1984), such as referrals to law enforcement, legal, and social service agencies. Patients at first may refuse these measures, and unless medically necessary, therapists should refrain from forcing the issue, in order to give the patient some sense of autonomy and control over what happens to him, all the while continuing to provide realistic reassurance (Matsakis, 1994).

In the acute trauma stage, the patient's concept of reality is profoundly altered. Accordingly, in the first phase of contact, the therapist should try to bring structure to the experiences of the trauma patient in an adaptive, reality-oriented manner. This is done by first following the narrative of the patient and then identifying the emotions as they are expressed. During this initial stage, the therapist encourages the patient in only a limited way to explore his/her feelings further or deeper, as a prematurely intense discussion of emotions may increase confusion and evoke an atmosphere of crisis. As time passes and the patient begins to recapture a sense of fundamental safety and control, he/she will need this structuring form of support less and less. The therapist can then adopt a more probing and challenging approach that incorporates con-frontation and reality testing, although the atmosphere of understanding and trust remains the most important basis of the therapeutic relationship (Brom & Kleber, 1989; Everstine & Everstine, 1993; Shalev et al., 1993).

Treating Posttraumatic Symptoms

For many patients, the frightening and disorienting symptoms of PTSD are the most disabling part of the syndrome. For some, achieving some measure of control over symptoms is the first step in allowing themselves to believe they can recover from the trauma. For others, even the attempt to deal with symptoms must await the achieve-ment of some degree of confidence and stability. For some patients, it is a reciprocal cycle, with small increments in equanimity allowing small steps toward symptom con-trol, which in turn produce greater confidence and further attempts at mastery, and so on. In still other cases, patients may come to understand that, while symptoms may be managed and controlled, they may never completely disappear but can be relegated to the background of consciousness, like "mental shrapnel" that only aches on occasion (Everstine & Everstine, 1993; Matsakis, 1994; Miller, 1994b, 1998e).

Exposure and Desensitization

Most symptom-oriented treatments for posttraumatic disturbances employ a behav-ioral or cognitive-behavioral approach. Thompson (1992) points out that posttrau-matic stress symptoms may be particularly appropriate for graded exposure thera-pies in which patients gradually learn to confront the stimuli they would otherwise avoid. These kinds of therapies are derived from *systematic desensitization*, origi-nally used to treat phobias and now well integrated into behavioral medicine (Miller, 1994a). In the cognitive-behavioral treatment of PTSD, the aim is to reduce posttraumatic reactions such as flashbacks, intrusive memories, and startle responses through habituation, thereby bringing about the extinction of the conditioned aver-sive response.

Exposure therapy for desensitization is typically conducted through imagination during a relaxation exercise or in real-life (*in vivo*) situations. Both methods may be used in combination, the imagination exercise paving the way for the *in vivo* training. In general, such strategies have been found useful in mitigating posttraumatic anxiety, intrusive memories, nightmares, hyperarousal, and hypersensitivity to sounds (Cooper & Clum, 1989; Keane, Fairbank, Caddell, & Zimmerling, 1989; Thompson, 1992).

My own experience in applying this type of approach has been mixed. Many patients seem to "get with the program," learn the relaxation technique, and desensi-tize themselves effectively to the traumatic situation. However, the most successful cases are typically the ones with the least distressing traumatic experiences. A few of the more severely traumatized patients resist all attempts at desensitization, fearing that "letting down their guard" during relaxation will render them vulnerable to over-whelming emotional arousal, a problem that has been noted for relaxation therapies in general (Lazarus & Mayne, 1990; Miller, 1994a). In such cases, a supportive-expressive cognitive therapy approach is often successful in helping patients work through the traumatic fear and pain of the injuring event in a more "rational" manner—trying, in effect, to turn the posttraumatic vigilance and rumination to con-structive therapeutic advantage. In other cases, a version of the *mental toughness training* I teach to law enforcement and emergency services personnel (Miller, 2006a, 2007) is useful for many kinds of patients to achieve interim cognitive and emotional control—a form of "splinting the psyche" to allow other forms of therapy and healing to take place.

Posttraumatic Flashbacks

Waking flashbacks may occur in any sensory modality, and often in multiple senses simultaneously; these symptoms are what make many patients fear they are "going crazy." As noted previously, the therapist should normalize the processes as much as possible, helping the patient to understand that this a natural and expectable part of the recovery process, that the flashbacks will eventually fade, and that there are learnable ways to manage intrusive symptoms (Everstine & Everstine, 1993; Matsakis, 1994; Modlin, 1983). The patient does not have to fight the flashback; it is possible to ride out many episodes without being overwhelmed, once he/she understands the nature and self-limiting quality of these symptoms—similar to the cognitive-behavioral approach taken with panic attacks and chronic pain flare-ups (Miller, 1993a, 1998e).

Many flashbacks and other PTSD symptoms are triggered by stimuli in the envi-ronment; others may be triggered by internal stimuli and sometimes these may not be conscious. Anniversary dates, people, places, objects, and certain emotional states can serve as triggers. The first step in helping patients cope with trauma triggers is to help them identify those triggers (Mataskis, 1994). Other times, patients will come to ther-apy all too painfully aware of what stimuli trigger their posttraumatic symptoms; if anything, they are paralyzed into avoidance, withdrawal, and inactivity by the con-stant vigilance against exposing themselves to trigger situations.

In either case, once triggers have been identified, the full range of relaxation and behavioral desensitization techniques may be applied. However, as noted earlier, for many patients, this may be threatening in itself, so for these patients, a more cognitively based approach involves planning ahead for anticipated trigger situations. Matsakis (1994) recommends training the patient to ask him/herself certain questions when faced with potential trigger situations; these may be individualized for each patient:

"How have I reacted to similar situations in the past?"
"Did anything terrible happen?"
"What are the chances of something bad happening again?"
"If the worst happens, what can I do to help myself?"
"Whom can I ask for help and how can they help me?"

Just the act of going through this kind of list often helps build a cognitive firewall between the spark of the triggering stimulus and the tinderbox of traumatic memories that can flare into a full-scale emotional conflagration. In addition, taking time to "think it through" gives the patient experience in using his/her own brain to solve problems—the epitome of the cognitive therapy approach—thus increasing the sense of control. Similar Socratic questioning techniques may be used by therapists themselves in crisis intervention with suicidal or decompensating patients (Gilliland & James, 1993; Miller, 1998e, 2005, 2006a). With symptomatic PTSD patients, the therapist may first model these adaptive coping questions and self-statements and then teach the patient to utilize them in trigger situations.

Dreams and Nightmares

Traumatic dreams are seldom rote replications of the traumatic incident itself. Instead, they tend to recapitulate the emotional terror of the event and/or symbolically represent important issues related to the event, such as survival, betrayal, and loss. Matsakis (1994) recommends the technique of having the patient "rewrite" the nightmares, incorporating empowering themes and outcomes into the revised narratives—a version of cognitive restructuring familiar to cognitive-behavioral therapists. However, some patients may view this as trivializing their dream experiences and the trauma itself. I have found that incorporating such revisioning into the waking therapeutic imagery exercises is generally more acceptable to patients because it suggests a reinterpretation of alternatives rather than "changing the script" of their dreams, which many patients find difficult or impossible to do, especially in the beginning stages of treatment.

Matsakis (1994) also recommends "beating the dreams to death" through repeated exposure and reiteration, thereby stripping them of their intimidating power. This is actually an extension of the technique of repeated ventilation, exploration, and working through of traumatic material in general. Again, my only caveat here is that the reexposure be truly dissipative and stress innoculative, not retraumatizing. This requires the therapist to know when the patient is ready to handle the traumatic dream material and perhaps combining the repetition with other therapeutic techniques, such as relaxation or cognitive restructuring.

Numbing, Dissociation, and Self-Harm

In posttraumatic therapy, intrusive symptomatology constitutes the proverbial "squeaky wheel that gets the grease" because it draws the most attention and seems to cause the most distress. For some patients, however, equal or greater disturbance is produced by the "zoning-out" numbing response of the posttraumatic syndrome. These may not be observed unless specifically asked for (Matsakis, 1994).

Some patients, especially those who have been multiply traumatized from an early age and who may have received diagnoses of borderline personality disorder, respond to numbing by dissociation and self-mutilating behavior. In such cases, Matsakis (1994) recommends teaching the patient less harmful and more reality-grounding forms of self-stimulation, such as taking a cold shower, drinking a carbonated beverage, using a wrist-snapping rubberband, doing some form of vigorous exercise, or handling a "safe object" such as a teddy bear. Several of my patients have learned to substitute the application of ice or the teeth of a comb to their skin in place of self-mutilating with a cigarette or knife blade (Miller, 1998e).

Posttraumatic Psychotherapy

As effective as they are, therapeutic symptom-reduction strategies have their limitations in dealing with the full cognitive and emotional range of posttraumatic stress reactions and bringing about a reintegrative healing of the personality. Eventually, most authorities agree, some form of constructive confrontation with the traumatic experience has to take place.

General Posttraumatic Therapy Guidelines

At some point in treatment, the therapist takes the trauma patient back to the event and has him/her discuss it in progressive degrees of detail. The goal is to counteract maladaptive avoidance tendencies and to diminish the chance that they will congeal into long-standing patterns of behavioral constriction. In the case of the avoidant victim who has been coping with trauma by downplaying its importance, the moment of graphic recapitulation may occur much later in the course of therapy and its onset may catch the therapist by surprise. This late outpouring of emotion should not necessarily be confused with "regression" but may in fact represent a sign of progress. Sometimes sufficient therapeutic trust, ego bolstering, and working through of peripheral issues must take place to lay the groundwork for direct exploration of the traumatic event itself (Brom et al., 1989; Everstine & Everstine, 1993; McCann & Pearlman, 1990).

In this framework, then, posttraumatic treatment should facilitate the repair of the patient's adaptive defense mechanisms, at the same time assisting the patient to reenter family, work, community, and other social roles. With these parallel therapeutic activities, both internal and external psychological integration can proceed. Bringing repressed thoughts to the surface or confronting disturbing or distorted memories should be handled with extreme care and sensitivity to ensure that the experience is one of corrective mastery, not retraumatization.

Mood Swings

Emotional lability is a frequent posttraumatic symptom and such mood swings can be confusing and disorienting, especially if they occur or recur late in the treatment process. The patient by this time has gotten a taste of psychological stability and may think that the worst of the ordeal is finally over. Then he/she hits some snag of frustration, stress, or disappointment and is yanked back into a state of anxiety and depression. During this unsettling process, patients will probably require even more therapeutic support than usual because they may feel they are backsliding and "losing it." These episodes should be viewed as an expectable response to these jarring bumps in the road to recovery and the patient should be reassured that this is not necessarily a sign of regression. A temporarily increased amount of therapeutic contact may be necessary at these times (Everstine & Everstine, 1993; McCann & Pearlman, 1990).

Anger

At some phase in the therapeutic process, mood swings may portend a phase of emerging anger, as the patient begins to get in touch with the fact that malignant or neglectful actions of others may have caused his/her trauma. Patients may be angry that the trauma occurred at all; that it happened to them when it did; that they were injured; that their loved ones died; that they have had to suffer secondary wounding and residual physical, psychological, and financial scars; that they have been mistreated by the medical and legal systems; that they have forever been banished from a sense of rightness and goodness in the world; and that they are now forced to engage in a therapeutic process that is effortful, expensive, and emotionally painful and draining (Everstine & Everstine, 1993; Matsakis, 1994; Miller, 1998e).

While this anger must eventually be faced and dealt with, pushing the emotion to the surface too quickly may impel the patient to act out in a dangerous way, to become paralyzed with helpless rage leading to depression, to develop a masochistic countertransference with the therapist and symbolically recreate the traumatic experience, or to flee the therapeutic setting entirely. Therefore, it is important that the therapist first help the patient to regain the requisite level of ego strength that will enable him/her to eventually express anger appropriately and constructively, in a manner that will not alienate those around her (Everstine & Everstine, 1993).

Matsakis (1994) has developed an effective program of posttraumatic anger management, the main components of which I have found useful with many types of PTSD patients (Miller, 1994b, 1995a, 1995b, 1998b, 1998c, 1998e, 1999a, 1999b, 2000c, 2003a, 2004, 2005). This begins with validating the anger because, especially where the trauma occurred at the malicious hands of others, patients may have very good reason to be angry. But angry feelings need not be expressed as angry acts, because the latter are often ultimately self-defeating, and good judgment in the service of avoiding further self-harm is always an important goal. However, where appropriate, patients can be supported or encouraged to take constructive action (e.g., within the judicial system, in support group work, and in political involvement). Indeed, a number of post-9/11 family survivors have turned their grief and anger into constructive action in just this manner (Miller, 2003a, 2003b, 2004, 2005).

In the clinical setting, much controversy surrounds whether overtly and forcefully venting anger is a legitimate therapeutic means of "letting off steam" or whether such emotional displays only serve to reinforce and further entrench the rageful feelings. As in most areas of clinical judgment, the therapist must know his/her patient well enough to determine whether or not angry expressions will be productive and to be able to tell how much is too much. Certainly, there should be nothing in terms of content that is categorically off limits for discussion. But unproductive spewing for spewing's sake should not be encouraged. Even here, there are exceptions because sometimes the pain of recollection gets too great and the patient really does just have to scream. The key is to allow such venting at an appropriate time and place and to follow it up with constructive therapeutic processing.

There are other, less dramatic, but often equally effective ways for patients to vent, such as talking to another person about their anger (obviously, much of this will occur in the therapeutic sessions), writing about their anger, speaking the anger into a tape recorder, drawing a picture about their anger, or telling God about their anger. Other techniques for managing anger include taking time outs, keeping an "anger diary" and discussing the entries during therapy, and, most important, encouraging the patient to behave in self-empowering ways that give him/her a feeling of greater control (Matsakis, 1994). Anger feeds on helplessness, so any way that a patient's sense of control can be legitimately increased—getting a better handle on emotions, improving relationships with supportive friends or family members, taking productive action—will go a long way toward reducing the need for defensive, reflexive action.

As noted earlier, constructive legal, social, or political activities are often perfect outlets of this type. It is important to remember, however, that a socially directed action must be valid for its own sake, not just be an egocentric healing project; otherwise, the activity risks turning into an irrational and compulsively driven crusade that ultimately harms both the patient and the people he/she works with. Here is another area in which therapeutic and commonsense guidance are crucial. In this vein, therapists must also be careful not to impose their own philosophical or political agendas on patients but to guide them to find their own direction and voice.

Existential Issues and Therapeutic Closure

Taking action in the real world raises another important issue. In virtually every case of significant trauma, the patient struggles with shattered assumptions and fantasies about fairness, justice, security, and the meaning of life. It is part of the essential task of psychotherapy to help the trauma patient come to terms with these existential issues. Some patients obsess over what they did or should have done to avoid or escape more serious harm or to help other people, and with these individuals, the therapeutic task becomes one of reorienting these individuals to a more realistic state of self-acceptance. Many patients need to pass the anniversary date of the traumatic event, especially if their trauma was severe, before they can begin to bring the trauma response to closure. The process of simultaneously externalizing and integrating the trauma event allows the last stages of recovery to take place. As the trauma patient approaches closure, the therapist can help him/her form a newly realistic and adaptive self-image, which becomes the foundation for a healthy future (Calhoun & Tedeschi, 1999; Everstine & Everstine, 1993; Miller, 1998d; Tedeschi & Calhoun, 2004; Tedeschi & Kilmer, 2005).

Everly (1994, 1995) emphasizes the need to help traumatized patients reintegrate their sense of self as well as their shattered world view in order to regain a feeling of existential safety. This necessitates carefully paying attention to what the patient tells the therapist in order for the clinician to discern what specific aspects of the patient's self-schema and worldview have been most affected. Then, posttraumatic reintegration can be approached from one or more of three main perspectives, as follows.

First, the trauma can be *integrated into the patient's existing worldview*: these things happen, cars do get into accidents on the highway, people do get mugged, but there are certain precautions one can take to minimize the risk of this happening in the future so that the patient can feel safe again.

Second, the trauma can be alternatively *understood as a parallel aspect of the existing worldview*, that is, an "exception to the rule": buildings are almost always safe and structural collapses almost never happen, so this tragedy, while certainly awful, is a one-shot deal that will most likely never happen to the same person again. Interestingly, for all the media attention concerning terrorism, such acts are still so rare that the chance of any one person being affected even once, much less repeatedly, are vanishingly small (Miller, 2005; Mueller, 2005).

Third, the trauma can be used to demonstrate the invalidity of the patient's existing perspective and the *need to create a new and modified worldview* in which the trauma more readily fits: your mugging shows that the world is not all filled with good people, that justice does not always work out, that sometimes the innocent suffer and the guilty go free. But you can fashion a new way of looking at things that allows both realism and cautious optimism; you can learn to be realistic, even skeptical about human nature and motives, but without allowing yourself to turn into a soul-shriveled cynic.

Everly (1995) believes that each of these approaches is successively less ego syntonic and therefore successively more difficult to apply in therapeutic practice. However, I have found that much depends on the nature of the traumatic event and the type of patient. Predominantly externalizing patients seem to cleave to the once-in-a-lifetime, "lightning doesn't strike twice" type of explanation, putting their trust in fate or God or sheer statistical improbability. The "what can I personally do to keep this from happening again" type of reframe appeals more to patients who already possessed a degree of self-efficacy before the trauma and are therefore willing and able to try to solve problems by their own efforts once the therapist shows them the way.

Hanscom (2001) describes a treatment model that emerged from her work with survivors of torture, and that may be applied more broadly to victims of trauma of many types, especially incidents involving interpersonal violence. In this model, an essential condition of healing is the reestablishment of the experience of trust, safety, and the ability to have an effect on the world. This relearning relies less on particular therapeutic techniques and procedures than on the compassionate human interaction and therapeutic alliance between the survivor and a counselor who is willing and able to listen effectively.

Hanscom (2001) describes what she calls the *HEARTS model*, which is an acronym for the following:

- *H = Listening to the HISTORY.* This includes providing a gentle environment, listening with body language, attending the flow of speech; hearing the voice and tone of the speaker, observing the speaker's movements and reactions, looking at facial expressions, remaining quietly patient, and listening compassionately. Clinicians will recognize this as a basic description of "active listening."
- *E = Focusing on EMOTIONS and reactions.* This involves using reflective listening, asking gentle questions, and naming the emotions.
- *A = ASKING about symptoms.* This involves using your own personal and therapeutic style to investigate current physical symptoms, current psychological symptoms, and suicidality.
- *R = Explaining the REASON for symptoms.* This includes showing how the symptoms fit together, describing how the body reacts to stress and trauma, explaining the interaction between the body and mind, and emphasizing that these are normal symptoms that normal people have to a very abnormal event.
- *T = TEACHING relaxation and coping skills.* This involves instructing the patient in relaxation skills, such as abdominal breathing, meditation, prayer, imagery, visualization, and others, and discussing coping strategies (e.g., recognizing how they have coped in the past, reinforcing old and healthy strategies, and teaching new coping skills).
- *S = Helping with SELF-CHANGE.* This involves discussing the person's world view—the original view, any changes, adaptations, or similarities—and recognizing the positive changes in the self.

In general, existential treatment strategies that focus on a quest for meaning, rather than just alleviation of symptoms, may productively channel the worldview conflicts generated by the trauma event, such as helping the patient to formulate an acceptable "survivor mission" (Shalev et al., 1993). Indeed, in the best cases, the rift and subsequent reintegration of the personality leads to an expanded self-concept and even a new level of psychological and spiritual growth (Bonanno, 2005; Calhoun & Tedeschi, 1999; Tedeschi & Calhoun, 1995, 2004; Tedeschi & Kilmer, 2005). Some trauma survivors are thus able to make positive personal or career changes out of a renewed sense of purpose and value in their lives. Of course, not all trauma victims are able to achieve this successful reintegration of the ordeal and many struggle with at

least some vestige of emotional damage for a long time, perhaps for life (Everstine &
Everstine, 1993; Matsakis, 1994; McCann & Pearlman, 1990).

Therefore, my main caution about these transformational therapeutic conceptualizations is that they be presented as an opportunity, not an obligation. The extraction of
meaning from adversity is something that must ultimately come from the patient him/
herself, not be foisted on the patient by the therapist. Such existential conversions by the
sword are usually motivated by a need to reinforce the therapist's own meaning system,
or they may be part of what I call a therapeutic "Clarence-the-Angel fantasy" (Miller,
1998e), wherein the enlightened therapist swoops down and, by dint of the clinician's
brilliantly insightful ministrations, rescues the patient from his/her darkest hour.

Realistically, we can hardly expect all or even most of our traumatized patients to
miraculously transform their tragedy and thereby acquire a fresh, revitalized, George
Baileyan outlook on life—how many *therapists* would respond this well? But human
beings do crave meaning (Yalom, 1980) and if a philosophical or religious orientation
can nourish the patient in his/her journey back to the land of the living, then our therapeutic role must sometimes stretch to include some measure of guidance in affairs of
the spirit.

CASE STUDY

Ivan, an émigré from the former Soviet Union and proud recent U.S. citizen, was driving home on the highway from a pleasant evening spent with out-out-town relatives
who had been visiting for the Christmas holiday. Some of these relatives had recently
been reunited after a long separation in various locations in North America and Eastern Europe and a number of them were in the car on their way back to the hotel. At
one point, Ivan's back started to ache from the uncomfortable seat of the rental car, so
he pulled over and asked his brother to drive. His brother joked about how "you
always make me do the dirty work," as he goodnaturedly took over the wheel.

They continued on their road trip when, suddenly, seemingly out of nowhere, a
huge, off-duty charter bus careened into their lane, forcing the car up against a concrete retaining wall. The combination of friction and gas spill from the ruptured chas-
sis caused the car to erupt in flames. The panicked occupants poured from the burning
vehicle and clambered to safety.

Or so they thought. Relief at their narrow escape soon turned to horror when a
head count revealed that one of their number was missing. Several male members of
the group ran back to the car to find Ivan's teenage nephew pinned in the back seat,
surrounded by flames. The fire was too hot for the men to get at the trapped youth and
a few of them suffered burns on their hands and faces while struggling to reach
through the flames. Ivan's last clear image was of his nephew crying out to him for
help. In the next hellish moments, Ivan could hear the boy screaming until smoke and
flames engulfed him and the anguished voice was stilled.

For several months afterward, friends and relatives described Ivan as a "human
vegetable." The burn injuries on his hands and a wrenched hip required a short period

of hospitalization and a few weeks of rehab, but otherwise his physical injuries were mostly minor cuts and bruises. Because of his general lack of responsiveness in the hospital, doctors at first feared that Ivan had sustained brain damage in the accident or perhaps an allergic reaction from the morphine used for his burn pain. But all the medical tests were normal. A psychiatric consult was called in, a tentative diagnosis of "posttraumatic depression" was made, and medication was prescribed. Physically healed, he was discharged a few days later.

When I first met Ivan, he was curled up in a chair in my office at the clinic where I worked, as I arrived for the first appointment of the day. His wife had driven him to the appointment and the reception staff had let him into the office because he could not tolerate being with the other people in the waiting room. The initial clinical interview with Ivan made it clear that he was suffering the classic PTSD symptoms of intrusive recollection, frightening dreams, emotional numbing alternating with panic and depression, phobic avoidance of car-related activities, and, above all, a crippling depression that no amount of medication could dent.

Because of his withdrawn clinical presentation and because he reported having banged his head while trying to get his nephew out of the car, I administered a standard neuropsychological test battery. Ivan's intellectual and cognitive functioning were surprisingly intact—above average, in fact, on most of the measures. This further confirmed the impression that Ivan's mortal wound was not in his brain but in his soul. Over the course of our subsequent psychotherapy sessions, it became clear how the effects of this traumatic event were inextricably tied in with the complex interpersonal dynamics of Ivan's extended family. Virtually all the common themes of psychotherapy were played out in this case: love, hate, loyalty, jealousy, rivalry, religion, politics, money, and the legal aspects of the case. However, there was one salient issue that seemed to define Ivan's reaction to his trauma and his steps toward recovery.

Ivan could not get off the idea that his nephew's death was his "fault" because he stopped to change drivers to ease his aching back. As an initial therapeutic approach, we discussed the important differentiations between temporal causation and volitional causation: Ivan did not make the bus veer out of its lane; there was no way to anticipate the event; millions of people change drivers and nothing happens; if there is any fault to be had, it is with the driver or the bus's maintenance crew, and so on. But Ivan, for all his innate intelligence, seemed fixated on blaming himself for the accident. More than simple logic was obviously at play. The following is a condensation of the therapeutic dialogue that took place over several sessions.

IVAN: If I hadn't pulled over, we would have been in a different spot when that bus came by.

THERAPIST: Did you have control over the bus's actions?

IVAN: No, but we would have been someplace else.

THERAPIST: So any time that any good or bad thing ever happens, it's always because of a specific, conscious choice a person makes? We have total control over everything that happens to us?

IVAN: No, some of it is in God's hands.

At this point, the therapist may be tempted to say something like, "Well, how do you know *this* wasn't in God's hands?" But that type of response usually leads to an irresolvable theological debate that places the therapist in the uncomfortable position of challenging the patient's religious doctrines. Instead, I chose to guide the discussion back to a realm that was more psychological in nature and probably more to the crux of the problem: the patient's motivations.

THERAPIST: Why did you pull the car over?

IVAN: I told you, my back hurt.

THERAPIST: If somebody else told you that they changed drivers because their back hurt, would you think there was something wrong with that?

IVAN: But with that other person, nobody died.

THERAPIST: What would have changed the outcome of your accident?

IVAN: If I kept driving.

THERAPIST: Why should you—or anyone—have kept driving with an aching back?

IVAN: I shouldn't have been concerned with my own pain. I should have been concerned about my nephew, about the people in the car.

THERAPIST: At that point, you had no idea that a bus was coming down the road, so how was continuing to suffer with back pain going to help your passengers?

IVAN: (*Becomes tearful.*) I should have taken better care of my family, not worry about my own comfort.

With this admission, Ivan was able to tell me about the family dynamics that appeared to underlie his seemingly irrational guilt. It turned out that there was some bad blood involving part of his family accusing him of having abandoned his kin by getting out of the then-repressive regime of his Eastern European country. These family members' plaint was summed up along the lines of: "How can you think only of your own comfort by going to America? What about the rest of us stuck here in our home country? How can you be so selfish?" Ivan had also recently married an American woman of a different religion, and his family accused him of doing so only to establish residency, and this was seen as a further abandonment of both faith and family. When the marriage began to sour, Ivan felt the need for greater support from his family of origin, many of whose members were now castigating him for his betrayal.

Working through some of these family issues helped Ivan become more at ease with his choices in life and their resulting impact on his extended family. But the idea that his actions had "caused" the accident stubbornly persisted. It emerged that this had to do precisely with the existential, religious, and cosmic issues that I had sidestepped at the beginning of the treatment process: In addition to family psychodynamics, psychotherapy was going to have to deal with the existential aspects of this case. This was because without this emotional assumption of personal responsibility—illogical as he and I intellectually knew it to be—Ivan's philosophical world would fall apart. Again, the following is a condensation of a therapeutic dialogue that took place over several sessions.

IVAN: If it's not my fault, then it's God's fault, and then there's no God because how could God do such a terrible thing, and then there's no reason for anything.

THERAPIST: How do you figure that?

IVAN: This man [the bus driver] falls asleep or doesn't pay attention for a few seconds and my "little brother" [a cultural term of endearment for the nephew] dies like that, an innocent boy dies like that. There has to be some explanation.

THERAPIST: And you're it?

IVAN: Look, I'm not crazy and I'm not a bad person. I know I didn't deliberately wish harm on my nephew. But I was the weak link in the chain that made all this happen.

THERAPIST: What could you have done differently?

IVAN: Not get out of the car. Next time, I don't get out of the car.

THERAPIST: Next time?

IVAN: There's no next time, my nephew's dead.

What became clear in this case, as with many others, is that taking blame for something that happened *this time* at least provided Ivan with the illusion of control that, if he were ever again in a position to do something different *next time*, a horrible tragedy like this would not recur—that there might be some imagined time in the future that he could change, atone, and undo this kind of horrible event by taking some different action. More broadly and symbolically, maybe sometime, somewhere Ivan could be in a position to help his family, to undo or mitigate the abandonment and betrayal that they had accused him of and that he had internalized. It would thus have been countertherapeutic—indeed, cruel—to try to rip away this vestige of control. Instead, we chose to focus on what practical steps Ivan could take to repair the relationship with his extended family, to help them and protect them in the real world.

As cognitive-behavioral therapists, then, we must not lose sight of the fact that being *too* cognitive, *too* rational, may deprive our patients of the critical dose of meaning their psychic wounds need to heal. If the ostensibly illusionary belief system constitutes a somewhat philosophically disfiguring scar, then this is what the patient may need to move on at this point in time. Someday, this blemish might be further reduced by cosmetic therapy, but for right now, we must squelch our Clarence-the-Angel fantasy to make it all come out right.

This does not mean that we peddle fairytales or abet the conjuring of fanciful correlations but only that we respect our patients' meaning systems as long as they do not dysfunctionally impede recovery and adaptation to real life. Most treatments for overwhelming traumas—physical or psychological—are necessarily incomplete and if our patient can learn to ambulate again with a psychic limp, then he/she is still walking. By acknowledging the limitations in what we can realistically accomplish, we gain a greater respect and appreciation of the real good that we do.

CONCLUSION

The field of psychotraumatology has expanded to the point where no single clinician can be an expert in every syndrome. But the basic principles of effective crisis intervention and psychotherapy with trauma survivors are remarkably consistent and generalizable. Thus, the clinician who acquires expertise in trauma intervention will be an invaluable asset is dealing with the challenges of our new century.

REFERENCES

Abueg, F. R., Woods, G. W., & Watson, D.S. (2000). Disaster trauma. In F. M. Dattilio & A. Freeman (Eds.), *Cognitive-behavioral strategies in crisis intervention* (2nd ed., pp. 243–272). New York: Guilford Press.

Alarcon, R. D., Deering, C. G., Glover, S. G., Ready, D. J., & Eddleman, H. C. (1997). Should there be a clinical typology of posttraumatic stress disorder? *Australian and New Zealand Journal of Psychiatry, 31,* 159–167.

Aldwin, C. M. (2007). *Stress, coping, and development: An integrative perspective* (2nd ed.). New York: Guilford Press.

American Psychiatric Association. (1980). *Diagnostic and statistical manual of mental disorders* (3rd ed.). Washington, DC: Author.

American Psychiatric Association. (1987). *Diagnostic and statistical manual of mental disorders* (3rd ed., rev.). Washington, DC: Author.

American Psychiatric Association. (1994). *Diagnostic and statistical manual of mental disorders* (4th ed.). Washington, DC: Author.

American Psychiatric Association. (2000). *Diagnostic and statistical manual of mental disorders* (4th ed., text rev.). Washington, DC: Author.

Blanchard, E. B., & Hickling, E. J. (2003). *After the crash: Psychological assessment and treatment of survivors of motor vehicle accidents.* Washington, DC: American Psychological Association.

Blanchard, E. B., Hickling, E. J., Taylor, A. E., Loos, W. R., & Gerardi, R. J. (1994). Psychological morbidity associated with motor vehicle accidents. *Behavior Research and Therapy, 3,* 283–290.

Blau, T. H. (1994). *Psychological services for law enforcement.* New York: Wiley.

Blythe, B. T. (2002). *Blindsided: A manager's guide to catastrophic incidents in the workplace.* New York: Penguin.

Bohl, N. (1995). Professionally administered critical incident debriefing for police officers. In M. I. Kunke & E. M. Scrivner (Eds.), *Police psychology into the 21st century* (pp. 169–188). Hillsdale, NJ: Erlbaum.

Bolz, F., Dudonis, K. J., & Schultz, D. P. (1996). *The counter-terrorism handbook: Tactics, procedures, and techniques.* Boca Raton: CRC Press.

Bonanno, G. A. (2005). Resilience in the face of potential trauma. *Current Directions in Psychological Science, 14,* 135–138.

Brom, D., & Kleber, R. J. (1989). Prevention of posttraumatic stress disorders. *Journal of Traumatic Stress, 2,* 335–351.

Brom, D., Kleber, R. J., & Defares, P. B. (1989). Brief psychotherapy for posttraumatic stress disorder. *Journal of Consulting and Clinical Psychology, 57,* 607–612.

Calhoun, L. G., & Tedeschi, R. G. (1999). *Facilitating posttraumatic growth.* Mahwah, NJ: Erlbaum.

Charcot, J. M. (1887). *Lecons sur les maladies du system nerveux* (Vol. 3). Paris: Progress Medical.

Charney, D. S., Deutsch, A. Y., Krystal, J. H., Southwick, S. M., & Davis, M. (1993). Psychobiologic mechanisms of posttraumatic stress disorder. *Archives of General Psychiatry, 50,* 294–305.

Cooper, N. A., & Clum, G. A. (1989). Imaginal flooding as a supplementary treatment for PTSD in combat veterans: A controlled study. *Behavior Therapy, 20,* 381–391.

Dennenberg, R. V., & Braverman, M. (1999). *The violence-prone workplace: A new approach to dealing with hostile, threatening, and uncivil behavior.* Ithaca, NY: Cornell University Press.

Dietz, J. (1992). Self-psychological approach to posttraumatic stress disorder: Neurobiological aspects of transmuting internalization. *Journal of the American Academy of Psychoanalysis, 20,* 277–293.

Dunning, C. (1999). Postintervention strategies to reduce police trauma: A paradigm shift. In J. M. Violanti & D. Paton (Eds.), *Police trauma: Psychological aftermath of civilian combat* (pp. 269–289). Springfield, IL: Thomas.

Eskenazi, B., & Maizlish, N. A. (1988). Effects of occupational exposure to chemicals on neurobehavioral functioning. In R. E. Tarter, D. H. Van Thiel, & K. L. Edwards (Eds.), *Medical neuropsychology: The impact of disease on behavior* (pp. 223–264). New York: Plenum Press.

Evans, R. W. (1992). The postconcussion syndrome and the sequelae of mild head injury. *Neurologic Clinics, 10,* 815–847.

Everly, G. S. (1990). PTSD as a disorder of arousal. *Psychology and Health: An International Journal, 4,* 135–145.

Everly, G. S. (1993). Psychotraumatology: A two-factor formulation of posttraumatic stress. *Integrative Physiological and Behavioral Science, 28,* 270–278.

Everly, G. S. (1994). Short-term psychotherapy of acute adult-onset posttraumatic stress. *Stress Medicine, 10,* 191–196.

Everly, G. S. (1995). The neurocognitive therapy of posttraumatic stress: A strategic meta-therapeutic approach. In G. S. Everly & J. M. Lating (Eds.), *Psychotraumatology: Key papers and core concepts in post-traumatic stress* (pp. 159–169). New York: Plenum Press.

Everstine, D. S., & Everstine, L. (1993). *The trauma response: Treatment for emotional injury.* New York: Norton.

Falsetti, S. A., & Resnick, H. S. (1995). Helping the victims of violent crime. In J. R. Freedy & S. E. Hobfoll (Eds.), *Traumatic stress: From theory to practice* (pp. 263–285). New York: Plenum Press.

Ferenczi, S., Abraham, K., & Simmel, E. (1921). *Psychoanalysis and the war neuroses.* Vienna: International Psycho-Analysis Press.

Flannery, R. B. (1995). *Violence in the workplace.* New York: Crossroad.

Foa, E. B., & Riggs, D. S. (1993). Posttraumatic stress disorder and rape. In J. Oldham, M. B. Riba, & A. Tasman (Eds.), *American Psychiatric Press review of psychiatry* (Vol. 12, pp. 273–303). Washington, DC: American Psychiatric Press.

Foeckler, M. M., Garrard, F. H., Williams, C. C., Thomas, A. M., & Jones, T. J. (1978). Vehicle drivers and fatal accidents. *Suicide and Life-Threatening Behavior, 8,* 174–182.

Frazier, F., & Wilson, R. M. (1918). The sympathetic nervous system and the "irritable heart of soldiers." *British Medical Journal, 2,* 27–29.

Freedy, J. R., Resnick, H. S., Kilpatrick, D. G., Dansky, B. S., & Tidwell, R. P. (1994). The psychological adjustment of recent crime victims in the criminal justice system. *Journal of Interpersonal Violence, 9,* 450–468.

Freedy, J. R., Shaw, D., Jarrell, M. P., & Masters, C. (1992). Towards an understanding of the psychological impact of natural disaster: An application of the conservation resources stress model. *Journal of Traumatic Stress, 5,* 441–454.

Freud, S. (1920). Beyond the pleasure principle. In J. Strachey (Ed. & Trans.), *The standard edition of the complete psychological works of Sigmund Freud* (Vol. 18, pp. 7–64). New York: Norton.

Gilliland, B. E., & James, R. K. (1993). *Crisis intervention strategies* (2nd ed.). Pacific Grove, CA: Brooks/Cole.

Green, B. L. (1991). Evaluating the effects of disasters. *Psychological Assessment, 3*, 538–546.

Hanscom, K. L. (2001). Creating survivors from trauma and torture. *American Psychologist, 56*, 1032–1039.

Hartman, D. E. (1995). *Neuropsychological toxicology: Identification and assessment of human neurotoxic syndromes* (2nd ed.). New York: Plenum Press.

Helzer, J. E., Robins, L. N., & McEnvoi, L. (1987). Post-traumatic stress disorder in the general population. *New England Journal of Medicine, 317*, 1630–1634.

Henry, V. E. (2004). *Death work: Police, trauma, and the psychology of survival.* New York: Oxford University Press.

Hodge, J. R. (1971). The whiplash neurosis. *Psychosomatics, 12*, 245–249.

Horowitz, M. J. (1986). *Stress response syndromes* (2nd ed.). New York: Aronson.

Hough, M. (1985). The impact of victimization: Findings from the British Crime Survey. *Victimology, 10*, 498–511.

Kardiner, A. (1941). *The traumatic neuroses of war.* Washington, DC: National Research Council.

Keane, T. M., Fairbank, J. A., Caddell, J. M., & Zimmerling, R. T. (1989). Implosive (flooding) therapy reduces symptoms of PTSD in Vietnam combat veterans: A controlled study. *Behavior Therapy, 20*, 245–260.

Kinney, J. A. (1995). *Violence at work: How to make your company safer for employees and customers.* Englewood Cliffs, NJ: Prentice Hall.

Koch, W. J., Douglas, K. S., Nicholls, T. L., & O'Neill, M. L. (2006). *Psychological injuries: Forensic assessment, treatment, and the law.* New York: Oxford University Press.

Kolb, L. C. (1987). A neuropsychological hypothesis explaining posttraumatic stress disorders. *American Journal of Psychiatry, 144*, 989–995.

Kratcoski, P. C., Edelbacher, M., & Das, D. K. (2001). Terrorist victimization: Prevention, control, and recovery. *International Review of Victimology, 8*, 257–268.

Kretschmer, E. (1926). *Hysteria.* New York: Basic Books.

Kuch, K. (1987). Treatment of posttraumatic stress disorder following automobile accidents. *Behavior Therapy, 10*, 224–225.

Kuch, K., & Swinson, R. P. (1985). Posttraumatic stress disorder after car accidents. *Canadian Journal of Psychiatry, 30*, 426–427.

Kuzma, L. (2000). Trends: Terrorism in the United States. *Public Opinion Quarterly, 64*, 90–105.

Labig, C. E. (1995). *Preventing violence in the workplace.* New York: Amacom.

Lazarus, A. A., & Mayne, T. J. (1990). Relaxation: Some limitations, side effects, and proposed solutions. *Psychotherapy, 27*, 261–266.

Ludwig, A. M. (1972). Hysteria: A neurobiological theory. *Archives of General Psychiatry, 27*, 771–777.

Malt, U. F., Hoivik, B., & Blikra, G. (1993). Psychosocial consequences of road accidents. *European Psychiatry, 8*, 227–228.

Mantell, M., & Albrecht, S. (1994). *Ticking bombs: Defusing violence in the workplace.* New York: Irwin.

Matsakis, A. (1994). *Post-traumatic stress disorder: A complete treatment guide.* Oakland, CA: New Harbinger.

McCann, I. L., & Pearlman, L. A. (1990). *Psychological trauma and the adult survivor: Theory, therapy, and transformation.* New York: Brunner/Mazel.

McMains, M. J. (1991). The management and treatment of postshooting trauma. In J. T. Horn & C. Dunning (Eds.), *Critical incidents in policing* (rev ed., pp. 191–198). Washington, DC: Federal Bureau of Investigation.

Mearburg, J. C., & Wilson, R. M. (1918). The effect of certain sensory stimulations on respiratory and heart rate in cases of so-called "irritable heart." *Heart, 7*, 17–22.

Meek, C. L. (1990). Evaluation and assessment of post-traumatic and other stress-related disorders. In C. L. Meek (Ed.), *Post-traumatic stress disorder: Assessment, differential diagnosis, and forensic evaluation* (pp. 9–61). Sarasota, FL: Professional Resource Exchange.

Merskey, H. (1992). Psychiatric aspects of the neurology of trauma. *Neurologic Clinics, 10,* 895–905.

Miller, L. (1984). Neuropsychological concepts of somatoform disorders. *International Journal of Psychiatry in Medicine, 14,* 31–46.

Miller, L. (1990). *Inner natures: Brain, self, and personality.* New York: St. Martin.

Miller, L. (1991a). Psychotherapy of the brain-injured patient: Principles and practices. *Journal of Cognitive Rehabilitation, 9*(2), 24–30.

Miller, L. (1991b). *Freud's brain: Neuropsychodynamic foundations of psychoanalysis.* New York: Guilford Press.

Miller, L. (1993a). Psychotherapeutic approaches to chronic pain. *Psychotherapy, 30,* 115–124.

Miller, L. (1993b). Toxic torts: Clinical, neuropsychological, and forensic aspects of chemical and electrical injuries. *Journal of Cognitive Rehabilitation, 11*(1), 6–20.

Miller, L. (1993c). The "trauma" of head trauma: Clinical, neuropsychological, and forensic aspects of posttraumatic stress syndromes in brain injury. *Journal of Cognitive Rehabilitation, 11*(4), 18–29.

Miller, L. (1993d). *Psychotherapy of the brain-injured patient: Reclaiming the Shattered Self.* New York: Norton.

Miller, L. (1994a). Biofeedback and behavioral medicine: Treating the symptom, the syndrome, or the person? *Psychotherapy, 31,* 161–169.

Miller, L. (1994b). Civilian posttraumatic stress disorder: Clinical syndromes and psychotherapeutic strategies. *Psychotherapy, 31,* 655–664.

Miller, L. (1995a). Tough guys: Psychotherapeutic strategies with law enforcement and emergency services personnel. *Psychotherapy, 32,* 592–600.

Miller, L. (1995b). Toxic trauma and chemical sensitivity: Clinical syndromes and psychotherapeutic strategies. *Psychotherapy, 32,* 648–656.

Miller, L. (1997). Neurosensitization: A pathophysiological model for traumatic disability syndromes. *Journal of Cognitive Rehabilitation, 15*(6), 12–23.

Miller, L. (1998a). Motor vehicle accidents: Clinical, neuropsychological, and forensic aspects. *Journal of Cognitive Rehabilitation, 16*(4), 10–23.

Miller, L. (1998b). Our own medicine: Traumatized psychotherapists and the stresses of doing therapy. *Psychotherapy, 35,* 137–146.

Miller, L. (1998c). Psychotherapy of crime victims: Treating the aftermath of interpersonal violence. *Psychotherapy, 35,* 336–345.

Miller, L. (1998d). Ego autonomy and the healthy personality: Psychodynamics, cognitive style, and clinical applications. *Psychoanalytic Review, 85,* 423–448.

Miller, L. (1998e). *Shocks to the system: Psychotherapy of traumatic disability syndromes.* New York: Norton.

Miller, L. (1999a). Treating posttraumatic stress disorder in children and families: Basic principles and clinical applications. *American Journal of Family Therapy, 27,* 21–34.

Miller, L. (1999b). Workplace violence: Prevention, response, and recovery. *Psychotherapy, 36,* 160–169.

Miller, L. (1999c). Critical incident stress debriefing: Clinical applications and new directions. *International Journal of Emergency Mental Health, 1,* 253–265.

Miller, L. (2000a). Law enforcement traumatic stress: Clinical syndromes and intervention strategies. *Trauma Response, 6*(1), 15–20.

Miller, L. (2000b). Neurosensitization: A model for persistent disability in chronic pain, depression, and posttraumatic stress disorder following injury. *Neurorehabilitation, 14,* 25–32.

Miller, L. (2000c). Traumatized psychotherapists. In F. M. Dattilio & A. Freeman (Eds.), *Cognitive-behavioral strategies in crisis intervention* (2nd ed., pp. 429–445). New York: Guilford Press.

Miller, L. (2001a). Crime victim trauma and psychological injury: Clinical and forensic guide-lines. In E. Pierson (Ed.), *2001 Wiley expert witness update: New developments in personal injury litigation* (pp. 171–205). New York: Aspen.

Miller, L. (2001b). Family therapy of traumatic brain injury: Basic principles and innovative strategies. In M. M. MacFarlane (Ed.), *Family therapy and mental health: Innovations in theory and practice* (pp. 311–330). New York: Haworth.

Miller, L. (2002). What is the true spectrum of functional disorders in rehabilitation? *Physical Medicine and Rehabilitation: State of the Art Reviews, 16*, 1–20.

Miller, L. (2003a). Psychological interventions for terroristic trauma: Symptoms, syndromes, and treatment strategies. *Psychotherapy, 39*, 283–296.

Miller, L. (2003b). Family therapy of terroristic trauma: Psychological syndromes and treatment strategies. *American Journal of Family Therapy, 31*, 257–280.

Miller, L. (2004). Psychotherapeutic interventions for survivors of terrorism. *American Journal of Psychotherapy, 58*, 1–16.

Miller, L. (2005). Psychotherapy for terrorism survivors: New directions in evaluation and treat-ment. *Directions in Clinical and Counseling Psychology, 17*, 59–74.

Miller, L. (2006a). *Practical police psychology: Stress management and crisis intervention for law enforcement.* Springfield, IL: Thomas.

Miller, L. (2006b). The terrorist mind: I. A psychological and political analysis. *International Journal of Offender Rehabilitation and Comparative Criminology, 50*, 121–138.

Miller, L. (2006c). The terrorist mind: II. Typologies, psychopathologies, and practical guide-lines for investigation. *International Journal of Offender Rehabilitation and Comparative Criminology, 50*, 255–268.

Miller, L. (2007). *METTLE: Mental toughness training for law enforcement.* Flushing, NY: Looseleaf Law Press.

Mitchell, J. T., & Everly, G. S. (1996). *Critical incident stress debriefing: Operations manual* (rev. ed.). Ellicott City, MD: Chevron.

Modlin, H. C. (1983). Traumatic neurosis and other injuries. *Psychiatric Clinics of North Amer-ica, 6*, 661–682.

Morrow, L. A., Ryan, C. M., Goldstein, G., & Hodgson, M. J. (1989). A distinct pattern of per-sonality disturbance following exposure to mixtures of organic solvents. *Journal of Occu-pational Medicine, 32*, 743–746.

Morrow, L. A., Ryan, C. M., Hodgson, M. J., & Robin, N. (1991). Risk factors associated with persistence of neuropsychological deficits in persons with organic solvent exposure. *Jour-nal of Nervous and Mental Disease, 179*, 540–545.

Mueller, J. (2005). Six rather unusual propositions about terrorism. *Terrorism and Political Vio-lence, 17*, 487–505.

Munjack, D. J. (1984). The onset of driving phobias. *Journal of Behavior Therapy and Experi-mental Psychiatry, 15*, 305–308.

Oppenheim, H. (1890). Tatsachliches und hypthothetisches uber das wesen der hysterie. *Berlin Klinik Wschr, 27*, 553.

Parker, R. S. (1990). *Traumatic brain injury and neuropsychological impairment: Sensorimotor, cognitive, emotional, and adaptive problems in children and adults.* New York: Springer-Verlag.

Parker, R. S. (1996). The spectrum of emotional distress and personality changes after minor head injury incurred in a motor vehicle accident. *Brain Injury, 10*, 287–302.

Parker, R. S. (2001). *Concussive brain trauma: Neurobehavioral impairment and maladap-tation.* Boca Raton: CRC Press.

Paton, D., & Smith, L. (1999). Assessment, conceptual and methodological issues in researching traumatic stress in police officers. In J. M. Violanti & D. Paton (Eds.), *Police trauma: Psy-chological aftermath of civilian combat* (pp. 13–24). Springfield, IL: Thomas.

Pavlov, I. P. (1927). *Conditioned reflexes: An investigation of the physiological activity of the cerebral cortex.* New York: Oxford University Press.

Pitman, R. K., Orr, S. P., Forgue, D. F., de Jong, J. B., & Claiborn, J. M. (1989). Prevalence of posttraumatic stress disorder in wounded Vietnam veterans. *American Journal of Psychiatry, 146*, 667–669.

Pizarro, J., Silver, R. C., & Prouse, J. (2006). Physical and mental health costs of traumatic experiences among Civil War veterans. *Archives of General Psychiatry, 63*, 193–200.

Raphael, B. (1986). *When disaster strikes: How individuals and communities cope with catastrophe.* New York: Basic Books.

Reese, J. T. (1987). Coping with stress: It's your job. In J. T. Reese (Ed.), *Behavioral science in law enforcement* (pp. 75–79). Washington, DC: Federal Bureau of Investigation.

Rosen, G. (1975). Nostalgia: A forgotten psychological disorder. *Psychosomatic Medicine, 5*, 342–347.

Rothbaum, B. O., Foa, E. B., Riggs, D. S., Murdock, T., & Walsh, W. (1992). A prospective examination of posttraumatic stress disorder in rape victims. *Journal of Traumatic Stress, 5*, 455–475.

Sapolsky, R. M., Krey, L. C., & McEwen, B. S. (1984). Glucocorticoid-sensitive hippocampal neurons are involved in terminating the adrenocortical stress response. *Proceedings of the National Academy of Sciences, 81*, 6174–6177.

Savitch, H. V. (2003). Does 9-11 portend a new paradigm for cities? *Urban Affairs Review, 39*, 103–127.

Schottenfield, R. S., & Cullen, M. R. (1985). Occupation-induced posttraumatic stress disorders. *American Journal of Psychiatry, 142*, 198–202.

Schreiber, S., & Galai-Gat, T. (1993). Uncontrolled pain following physical injury as the core trauma in post-traumatic stress disorder. *Pain, 54*, 107–110.

Shalev, A. Y., Schreiber, S., Galai, T., & Melmed, R. N. (1993). Post-traumatic stress disorder following medical events. *British Journal of Clinical Psychology, 32*, 247–253.

Sheehan, D. C., Everly, G. S., & Langlieb, A. (2004, September). Current best practices: Coping with major critical incidents. *FBI Law Enforcement Bulletin*, pp. 1–13.

Silva, M. N. (1991). The delivery of mental health services to law enforcement officers. In J. T. Reese, J. M. Horn & C. Dunning (Eds.), *Critical incidents in policing* (rev ed., pp. 335–341). Washington, DC: Federal Bureau of Investigation.

Small, L. (1980). *Neuropsychodiagnosis in psychotherapy* (rev. ed.). New York: Brunner/Mazel.

Solomon, R. M. (1995). Critical incident stress management in law enforcement. In G. S. Everly (Ed.), *Innovations in disaster and trauma psychology: Applications in emergency services and disaster response* (pp. 123–157). Ellicott City, MD: Chevron.

Southard, E. (1919). *Shell-shock and other neuropsychiatric problems.* Boston: Leonard.

Spungen, D. (1998). *Homicide: The hidden victims. A guide for professional.* Thousand Oaks, CA: Sage.

Stein, M. B., Walker, J. R., Hazen, A. L., & Forde, D. R. (1997). Full and partial posttraumatic stress disorder: Findings from a community survey. *American Journal of Psychiatry, 154*, 1114–1119.

Strebnicki, M. A. (2001). The psychosocial impact on survivors of extraordinary, stressful, and traumatic events: Principles and practices in critical incident response for rehabilitation counselors. *Directions in Rehabilitation Counseling, 12*, 57–72.

Tedeschi, R. G., & Calhoun, L. G. (1995). *Trauma and transformation: Growing in the aftermath of suffering.* Thousand Oaks, CA: Sage.

Tedeschi, R. G., & Calhoun, L. G. (2004). Posttraumatic growth: Conceptual foundations and empirical evidence. *Psychological Inquiry, 15*, 1–18.

Tedeschi, R. G., & Kilmer, R. P. (2005). Assessing strengths, resilience, and growth to guide clinical interventions. *Professional Psychology: Research and Practice, 36*, 230–237.

Thompson, J. (1992). Stress theory and therapeutic practice. *Stress Medicine, 8*, 147–150.

Thompson, S. C. (1981). Will it hurt less if I can control it? A complex answer to a simple question. *Psychological Bulletin, 90*, 89–101.

Toch, H. (2002). *Stress in policing*. Washington, DC: American Psychological Association.

Trimble, M. R. (1981). *Post-traumatic neurosis: From railway spine to whiplash*. New York: Wiley.

Ursano, R. J., Fullerton, C. S., & Norwood, A. E. (1995). Psychiatric dimensions of disaster: Patient care, community consultation, and preventive medicine. *Harvard Review of Psychiatry, 3*, 196–209.

Weiner, H. (1992). *Perturbing the organism: The biology of stressful experience*. Chicago: University of Chicago Press.

Werman, D. S. (1984). *The practice of supportive psychotherapy*. New York: Brunner/Mazel.

Williams, T. (1991). Counseling disabled law enforcement officers. In J. T. Reese, J. M. Horn & C. Dunning (Eds.), *Critical incidents in policing* (pp. 377–386). Washington, DC: Federal Bureau of Investigation.

Wilson, J. P. (1994). The historical evolution of PTSD diagnostic criteria: From Freud to DSM-IV. *Journal of Traumatic Stress, 7*, 681–698.

Yalom, I. D. (1980). *Existential psychotherapy*. New York: Basic Books.

SUGGESTED READINGS

Everstine, D. S., & Everstine, L. (1993). *The trauma response: Treatment for emotional injury*. New York: Norton.

Gilliland, B. E., & James, R. K. (1993). *Crisis intervention strategies* (2nd ed.). Pacific Grove: Brooks/Cole.

Miller, L. (1998). *Shocks to the system: Psychotherapy of traumatic disability syndromes*. New York: Norton.

Miller, L. (2006). *Practical police psychology: Stress management and crisis intervention for law enforcement officers*. Springfield, IL: Thomas.

Weiner, H. (1992). *Perturbing the organism: The biology of stressful experience*. Chicago: University of Chicago Press.

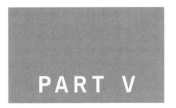

PART V

General Issues in Crisis Work

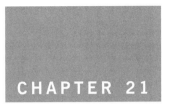

CHAPTER 21

Legal and Ethical Issues in Crisis Intervention

Leon VandeCreek
Samuel Knapp

*C*risis intervention is an important service that mental health professionals perform. As with any other professional service, the practitioner is required to adhere to certain legal and ethical standards of behavior. Failure to do so can place the professional at risk for a malpractice suit, charges of ethical misconduct, investigation by a licensure board, and other forms of civil liability. Although crisis intervention services pose a higher risk of liability than most other professional services, these risks must be placed in perspective. The risks are relatively small, the legal requirements are generally consistent with good quality care, and the fear of disciplinary actions should not detract practitioners from delivering high-quality care.

Of course, mental health professionals are motivated by more than just the desire to avoid being disciplined. Even if the risk of professional liability is low, practitioners want to do more than merely adhere to basic ethical standards (Knapp & VandeCreek, 2006).

Unfortunately, the very nature of crises may place a significant emotional burden on practitioners. Requests for emergency services may come late at night or from persons who walk into the office without an appointment. Often the individuals are accompanied by police or relatives who have been under stress themselves and may present themselves in a demanding, pushy, or rude manner. Practitioners may not have time to consult with colleagues.

In one sense, the most severely disturbed patients may be the easiest to evaluate. The danger of their behaviors and the intensity of their distress may leave no doubt that hospitalization or referral is the proper course of action. When the danger is more remote or when the distress is less severe, however, the decisions become more difficult. At what point does a person's refusal to eat constitute neglect of self? When is a suicidal gesture severe enough to be considered a suicidal act? When does a person's behavior cross the line to posing imminent danger to self or others? And what is the prevailing standard of care that must be followed in crisis situations?

No mental health professional can make these decisions with complete accuracy. Despite our extensive study of human behavior, we are limited in our ability to predict dangerousness or to anticipate the course of a disorder. Furthermore, the stakes are often high in crisis situations. Recommending patients for involuntary hospitalization may lead to a deprivation of their civil liberties and may make some patients more resistant to seeking treatment voluntarily in the future. On the other hand, failure to hospitalize a person may mean that a life is endangered. Reporting a family to a child welfare agency because of suspected child abuse may result in substantial intrusions into their privacy, yet the failure to make such a report may seriously jeopardize the welfare of the child.

This chapter reviews several of the areas in which professionals may face ethical and legal challenges in managing patients in crisis situations. Suggestions for conducting a risk-managed practice are offered.

LEGAL AND ETHICAL REGULATION OF PRACTICE

Crisis intervention, like other forms of professional practice, is regulated by a variety of mechanisms, such as malpractice law, other tort remedies, the codes of ethics of professional associations and licensing boards, and other laws.

Four criteria must be met to sustain a malpractice charge. First, the practitioner must have a professional relationship with the patient. This criterion is usually met when the practitioner accepts the patient's request for care. If a crisis occurs in the midst of ongoing therapy, then this criterion clearly has already been met. There is some ambiguity with this criterion, however, when practitioners receive contacts from potentially new patients who are in crisis. Does a crisis telephone call establish a therapist–patient relationship? Courts have suggested that it does if the practitioner offers advice or agrees to see the patient for treatment.

Second, it must be proven that the practitioner's behavior deviated from the accepted standard of care used by similar practitioners of similar orientation and in similar circumstances. Typically courts rely on expert testimony to determine the appropriate standard of care. Practitioners who claim to be specialists are expected to adhere to the standards of their specialty. The trend in health care litigation is also to rely on a national standard of care rather than on a local standard of care.

Third, it must be shown that the practitioner's negligent care was the proximate cause of an injury to the patient. Traditionally, proximate cause is defined as a cause that produces an injury in a natural and continuous sequence, unbroken by any other intervening causes. The breach must be the sole cause of the injury. Today, a more liberal definition of proximate cause has become increasingly common. Now, the "but-for" and the "substantial-factor" tests have been allowed by some courts. The but-for test requires that the patient establish that it was more probably true that the injury would not have happened but for the practitioner's acts; the substantial-factor test requires that the acts of the defendant be just that, a substantial factor.

Finally, the patient must prove that an injury resulted from the proximate cause. Claims of injury in mental health have taken many forms, including emotional distress, divorce, harm to self or others, and appearance of new symptoms or an exacerbated state of an already existing condition. Patients may claim any form of injury, although the patient must prove that the injury exists and was caused by the practitioner's conduct.

The courts recognize that mental health treatment is not an exact science and that bad outcomes may occur even when appropriate care has been provided. An unwelcome outcome in treatment, therefore, is not necessarily evidence of negligence. The question is whether the practitioner followed accepted procedures in assessing and treating the patient.

In addition to charges of malpractice, crisis intervention workers may also be liable for other torts (or wrongdoings) such as malicious prosecution, abuse of process, or false imprisonment. Each of these torts has its own specific criteria and is usually invoked in the context of involuntary civil commitments. (They will be discussed later.)

Furthermore, practitioners are regulated by ethics codes. If the practitioner is licensed, then it is likely that the licensing law has incorporated an ethics code into its regulations and violations could result in a disciplinary action, including, in extreme cases, losing one's license. Practitioners who are members of professional associations have ethics codes binding on them by virtue of their membership. In contrast to malpractice claims where patients must prove they were harmed, patients do not have to prove they were harmed when they charge the practitioner under ethics codes and licensure laws.

Finally, miscellaneous laws, such as child protective service laws, also regulate practitioners' behaviors. Although the exact wording of child protective service laws varies from state to state, typically the laws include the provision of a penalty (usually a misdemeanor) for practitioners who are mandated to report child abuse but fail to do so.

These disciplinary mechanisms overlap and interact with each other, such that a practitioner could be fined for failing to report suspected child abuse, be disciplined by a licensing board for failing to follow a law regulating professional practice, and, if a child were harmed as a result of the failure to report, be liable for a civil suit.

ACCEPTING AND REFERRING PATIENTS

Depending on the setting, practitioners may or may not have the right to refuse to accept particular patients who require crisis intervention care. In private settings, practitioners may decline to accept patients who appear to require crisis intervention care. Public settings and managed care settings often do not allow such refusals. Regardless of the setting, once a patient has been accepted into care, the practitioner must provide the necessary care or refer the patient. Practitioners may not refuse to provide crisis care to their ongoing patients just because they do not prefer to work under crisis conditions or because their busy schedules do not lend themselves to crisis care.

Practitioners or settings that advertise crisis intervention services and telephone crisis centers may be held to higher standards of care (a standard of specialists) for crisis contacts than are general practitioners. It is a good practice when referring crisis patients to ensure that they have in fact availed themselves of alternative services.

Practitioners have a responsibility to convey relevant information when making a referral. For example, in *Greenburg v. Barbour* (1971), a physician had allegedly failed to inform the admitting physician at a hospital of the dangerousness of a man seeking treatment at the hospital. The patient was not admitted and subsequently became assaultive. The court held that the failure to transmit this important information concerning violent behavior was contrary to acceptable medical practice.

Practitioners must also be alert to the potential for charges of abandonment if patients are not provided adequate care when in crisis. De facto abandonment could occur if practitioners, while on vacation, do not provide adequate coverage for patients, if the practitioners' schedules are so overloaded that they cannot accommodate the needs of their existing patients, or they fail to provide 24-hour crisis services to patients in need of immediate care.

DANGEROUS PATIENTS

Although patient homicides and suicides are rare, they do occur. Suicide is a leading cause of death in the United States and all mental health practitioners can expect to treat a suicidal patient sometime in their career. The lifetime rate of death by suicide is reported to be 0.72% with an adult annual incidence rate of approximately 10.7 per 100,000 people (National Institute of Mental Health, 2002). Few things are as stressful to a practitioner as managing a patient who poses a danger to self or others.

Danger to Others

The California court case of *Tarasoff v. Regents of the University of California* (1976) established a duty to protect identifiable victims from the foreseeable acts of dangerous patients (see details of the case in VandeCreek & Knapp, 2001). The *Tarasoff* decision was binding only in California, but since then most other states have produced case law or statutory law that outlines practitioners' responsibilities when patients present an imminent danger to harm others. Most, but not all, require or permit some kind of intervention on the part of practitioners even if it means breaking confidentiality.

Practitioners should follow three important steps when confronted with patients who threaten to harm others: (1) determine the foreseeability of harm, (2) develop an appropriate therapeutic intervention, and (3) implement that intervention (Appelbaum, 1985). Substantial data exist on assessing dangerousness that is not reviewed here (see, e.g., Borum, 2000). If a practitioner determines that a third party, or a class or group of parties, is in imminent danger, then the practitioner needs to develop an intervention plan that is designed to reduce the danger. In many states, the law provides an option of warning the identifiable third party. However, even in those cases, practitioners need to consider other ways to diffuse the danger besides breaking confidentiality. These options may include a referral for medication, increased frequency of therapy sessions, monitoring the patient between sessions, and involving family members in monitoring the patient (if clinically indicated). In some instances, the patient's threats are aimed at a spouse or partner, and couple or marital therapy may be beneficial (Harway & Hanson, 2004).

Finally, the practitioner needs to ensure that the treatment plan is implemented as intended or modified as needed. For example, it does little good to refer a patient for a psychiatric evaluation and then do nothing if the patient fails to keep the appointment.

As with other treatment planning, it is desirable to involve the patient in the treatment planning as much as possible. If a patient makes a credible threat to a third party, it is best to involve the patient in the formulation of the plan to reduce the risk even when the plan calls for alerting the potential victim.

Generally, it is wise to adhere to certain moral principles such as respect for patient autonomy, but when it is essential to break that moral principle, the goal is to do so with as little violation to the principle of autonomy as possible. If the danger is imminent and the patient continues to issue threats, then practitioners may still involve the patient in the decision making as much as clinically possible. It may mean, for example, that the practitioner can ask the patient if the warning should be made by phone with the patient present or if the patient would prefer not to be in the room when the call is made.

Maximizing Patient Autonomy

Dr. Aruba became convinced that a patient she had seen for seven sessions was an imminent threat to his ex-girlfriend. The patient shared a plan to shoot her, and Dr. Aruba believed that he intended to carry out the plan. At the outset of therapy Dr. Aruba had shared with the patient the limits to confidentiality, including the provision that she could break confidentiality if she became convinced that the patient was an imminent threat to another person. She believed that at this moment she was permitted, and indeed required, to break confidentiality by contacting the potential victim. Nonetheless, she also believed that therapy was still a powerful factor in changing the patient's approaches to anger management and she wanted to minimize the negative effects on the patient and their therapeutic alliance when she notified the ex-girlfriend. To minimize the violation to the principle of patient autonomy, she discussed with the patient her intention to notify the potential victim and she offered to assist the patient in making the call from the office. While the patient refused to make the call himself, he did agree that she was in danger at the moment and he did acknowledge that killing her would provide only momentary satisfaction followed by a lifetime of regret. Dr. Aruba contacted the ex-girlfriend and the patient was impressed with the therapist's allegiance to him and stayed in therapy.

A few courts have expanded the duty to protect when there is no identifiable victim but, rather, when the victim falls within "a zone of danger." In *Lipari v. Sears* (1980), a court found liability to the public at large. A patient discontinued day treatment, purchased a shotgun, and shot several people at a nightclub. The federal court ruled that the psychotherapists had a responsibility to protect the public even though no specific victim was identifiable. It is not necessary that the psychotherapist "knew the identity of the injured party, but only that therapist could have reasonably foreseen unreasonable risk of harm to injured party or a class of persons of which injured party was a member" (p. 186). The case was settled out of court for $200,000 (Beck, 1987).

Courts in at least two states have ruled that the duty to protect does not apply to them. In *Boynton v. Burglass* (1991), the Third District Court of Appeals of Florida declined to adopt the *Tarasoff* standards for Florida. In *Nasser v. Parker* (1995), the Virginia Supreme Court ruled that psychotherapists have no duty to control the behavior of outpatients. This is an area of law that is continually evolving and practitioners should be aware of the standard their state has adopted.

Duty to Protect and HIV Infection

In recent years, practitioners have experienced a unique twist to the duty to protect as some patients may pose a risk to infect others with HIV/AIDS. The question arises whether the duty to protect applies to persons who threaten others by their sexual behavior or through sharing intravenous needles. Practitioners need to consult their state laws for guidance.

We have learned of no cases in which health care practitioners have been sued for failing to warn identifiable third parties of the potential harm from a patient who is engaging in such high-risk behavior. In fact, some state statutes specifically prohibit such disclosures. For the most part, practitioners should rely on their psychotherapeutic skills to diffuse danger to the public or to identifiable third parties.

Mental health practitioners should not force themselves into dichotomous thinking (warn or not warn) when treating patients who are infected with HIV or other infectious diseases. Fortunately, a body of literature is developing on ways to interview HIV-infected persons and encourage voluntary disclosure (e.g., Anderson & Barret, 2001). For example, we know that HIV-positive patients often do not share their serostatus with partners because of fear of domestic abuse or other forms of retaliation. The failure to disclose may be less a function of sociopathy on the part of the patient than a function of the pathology in the relationship. Even when permitted by law, warning should only be considered as an absolute last resort after attempts at voluntary disclosure or habit change have failed.

Child Abuse

Child abuse is a generic term that refers to nonaccidental physical injury, neglect, sexual abuse, and emotional abuse of a child. Different states have different specific definitions and inclusions, but all states include at least nonaccidental injury and neglect within their definitions of child abuse. All states require professionals who are treating abused children to make reports when appropriate, but the criteria of "appropriateness" differ. Some states require practitioners to report child abuse when they come across it in the course of their professional activities. This would mean, for example, reporting child abuse even if it occurred several years before. Other states do not require the reporting of abuse unless it is uncovered as part of the child's therapy. The threshold for reporting is low to ensure the reporting of all potential cases and to leave the final determination in the hands of the child welfare agency.

Child abuse reporting laws include incentives to report in the form of immunity for reports made in good faith and penalties for mandated reporters who fail to make appropriate reports. For bad faith to be proven, it must be determined that the reporter knew that no abuse had occurred but made the report anyway.

Critics contend that mandatory reporting laws create more problems than they solve. For example, adults who seek treatment to improve their childrearing skills and who admit to abuse may find that their family structure is threatened when a report is made. The process of reporting and the subsequent investigation may create a crisis within the family, and the family may feel betrayed and refuse to continue in treatment if the report was made by the therapist.

Practitioners are placed in a difficult position with regard to abuse reporting. On the one hand, therapists encourage patients to be candid and to share even their best kept secrets, and patients expect these communications to be held confidential. When practitioners must then report a suspicion of abuse, both parties rightfully feel violated. The sense of betrayal can be greatly minimized if practitioners inform patients at the outset of treatment, and throughout treatment as needed, about the limits to confidentiality. Practitioners who work with children and with families with whom issues of abuse are to be expected can make special efforts to develop collegial relationships with staff members of child welfare agencies. Thus, when abuse reports must be made, the practitioner can accurately inform the patient about what to expect. Further, if a cooperative relationship is in place, child welfare agencies may also be willing to let the practitioner play a primary role in addressing an abuse problem.

Elder Abuse

Almost all states have laws that permit, but do not necessarily require, practitioners to report the abuse of older adults. Often the definition of older adults is broad (as young as age 55) and the definition of abuse is broad and includes physical abuse and financial exploitation. A few states permit the reporting of abuse of vulnerable persons (e.g., developmentally disabled adults), or of spousal abuse.

Suicide

Most practitioners become involved in at least some suicide crises. The literature suggests that 10–15% of patients with major psychiatric disorders will die by suicide (Brent, Kupfer, Bromet, & Dew, 1988) and 20% of psychologists and 50% of psychiatrists will lose a patient to suicide during their career (Chemtob, Hamada, Bauer, Kinney, & Torigoe, 1988; Chemtob, Hamada, Bauer, Torigoe, & Kinney, 1988). Inpatient units and their employees, which have greater control over the behavior of their patients, are more vulnerable to lawsuits following the suicide of a patient than are those practitioners who treat outpatients.

Courts have typically followed three criteria when assessing professional liability in cases of suicide: the foreseeability of the suicide attempt, the reasonableness of the practitioner's judgment in developing an appropriate treatment plan, and the thoroughness with which the treatment plan was implemented. These are identical to the three criteria we recommended for assessing and treating patients who threaten harm to others.

Practitioners must use reasonable judgment in determining the foreseeability of a suicide attempt. That is, they must use acceptable professional procedures to assess the total clinical picture of the patient, the intent for suicide, the potential means for accomplishing the suicide, and other factors relevant to treatment. Practitioners should have a good understanding of suicide assessment and intervention. Good sources of information include Bongar (2002), the *Air Force Guide for Managing Suicidal Behavior* (*www.suicidology.org*; Oordt et al., 2005), and the *Practice Guidelines for the Assessment and Treatment of Patients with Suicidal Behavior* (American Psychiatric Association, 2003). As with patients who are dangerous to others, it is important for practitioners to develop a treatment plan that addresses the specific risk of suicide as well as the underlying diagnosis and to implement (or modify) that treatment plan. Liability has not been found when patients have unexpectedly attempted suicide (*Dalton v. State*, 1970; *Paradies v. Benedictine Hospital*, 1980). However, when the treatment plan has overlooked, ignored, or neglected evidence of suicidal tendencies, then courts have found liability (*Dinnerstein v. United States*, 1973; *Eady v. Salter*, 1976).

When suicidal tendencies are uncovered, the practitioner must address suicidality in the treatment plan. The failure to take reasonable precautions when suicidal intent is recognized would be grounds for liability. For example, in *Texarkana Memorial Hospital, Inc. v. Firth* (1988), a woman was admitted for suicidal risk and psychosis. When she was admitted, the locked ward of the hospital had no open beds. Consequently, she was sedated and placed in an open ward with no special suicide precautions. When she awakened, she jumped to her death. Her estate was awarded $950,000 for gross negligence by the hospital.

The third criterion addresses the thoroughness with which the treatment plans are implemented. In *Abille v. United States* (1980), the government was judged to be liable when a nurse ignored the physician's instructions and allowed a depressed patient (who later committed suicide) to leave the ward without an escort. In *Cominsky v. New York* (1979), a hospital was found at fault for failure to observe closely a patient as the physician had ordered; however, the physician was not found at fault. In contrast, the failure of a psychotherapist to inform other staff members about an increase in suicidal potential might leave the therapist liable but absolve the uninformed staff.

Patients with diagnoses such as borderline personality disorder present a special problem for crisis intervention workers. Sometimes these patients cut or mutilate themselves by burning themselves with cigarettes, banging their arms and/or heads, or dripping acid on themselves. Self-mutilation is typically a severe event for the average depressed person, but some patients with borderline personality disorder are chronic parasuicides. They may engage in these behaviors for secondary gain, such as revenge against another person, or the pain may temporarily distract them from their emotional pain. Furthermore, hospitalization may be therapeutically contraindicated for some of these patients. Yet, suicidal gestures should not be dismissed automatically because some such patients die from them.

Crisis workers need to evaluate such situations carefully. A major determinant is whether to recommend hospitalization in the presence of severe depression. If the patient with borderline personality disorder is experiencing severe depression, including life-threatening ideation and other factors indicating lethal intent, then it is important to consider hospitalization. On the other hand, practitioners should not be stampeded into recommending hospitalization for all such cases. Often hospitalizations are contraindicated (Paris, 2002).

There is no duty to warn relatives of potential suicides. Of course, practitioners have the responsibility to take reasonable steps to prevent suicides and may, if their discretion leads them, take unusual steps, including notifying friends or relatives. To our knowledge, no court has found liability when practitioners have enlisted the aid of others to protect a patient from suicide. Likewise, ethics codes of mental health professions permit disclosure of confidential information in order to protect patients from harm.

In all cases of suicidal patients, it is important for practitioners to carefully document their decisions and actions. Practitioners are not liable for mistakes in judgment but for failure to use acceptable clinical care in assessing and treating patients.

CIVIL COMMITMENTS

The grounds for liability in cases of involuntary civil commitments have broadened in recent years. A variety of tort remedies are available in lawsuits surrounding involuntary civil commitments that are not found in other tort situations. These include malicious prosecution (for inappropriately participating in a commitment proceeding), abuse of process (using the commitment proceedings for personal ends rather than care of the patient), and false imprisonment (confinement outside the purview of the law). Furthermore, government employees can be held liable under section 1983 of the Civil Rights Act which prohibits them from depriving citizens of their civil liberties (Knapp & VandeCreek, 1987).

On the other hand, practitioners who are involved in involuntary commitments are usually granted broad immunity protections by their states. The purpose of these laws is to reduce the fear of lawsuits for practitioners who must make difficult decisions under trying circumstances. Although these laws do not provide complete immunity, practitioners can greatly reduce their legal risks by following the legal procedures carefully, being thorough in their evaluations of patients, and documenting their findings conscientiously.

THE SAFETY NET: RISK MANAGEMENT STRATEGIES AND THE "CULTURE OF SAFETY"

Although practitioners must always be aware of the possibility of disciplinary actions, for the most part, good risk management principles are consistent with good clinical care and respect for overarching moral principles (Bennett, Bricklin, Harris, Knapp, & VandeCreek, in press). On the whole, practitioners perform their duties in a legal and ethical manner when they adhere to the laws of their state and licensing board and to the overarching ethical principles such as beneficence (promoting patient welfare), nonmaleficence (avoiding harm to patients), and respect for patient autonomy. Practitioners will find that when they are faced with life-endangering patients, the state laws and ethics codes provide only general standards but do not provide clear directions for how to handle specific patients. Consequently, practitioners need to look to these overarching moral principles for guidance.

Some practitioners have found it helpful to have their behavior guided by a "culture of safety" (Bennett et al., in press; Knapp & VandeCreek, 2006), in which they create a safety net when working in high-risk situations. Some common risk management strategies provide the foundation for that safety net, as do some specific redundant systems of information and data. We describe below the application of such a safety net to clinical emergencies.

When faced with high-risk situations, professionals are wise to give special attention to risk management strategies designed to enhance patient welfare and, at the same time, ensure that acceptable standards of care are delivered and documented. The three most common and effective types of risk management strategies that can be implemented in a culture of safety are consultation, documentation, and informed consent (Bennett et al., in press).

A culture of safety is a practice environment that recognizes that sometimes "the perfect storm" can occur. Sometimes the confluence of patient characteristics and external events is such that a tragedy is likely to occur. Just as every airplane has backup systems in the event the first one fails, every practitioner working in crisis situations needs to have a second set of eyes looking at a case. For example, when working with suicidal patients, one psychotherapist routinely gave her patients a brief screening inventory before every session, as a second source of data to supplement the self-report of the patient in her session. At times, patients deny suicide intent when asked directly in session but report high suicidal ideation on brief written measures. Other family members and friends can also serve as redundant sources of data for dangerous patients.

Consultation is another component of the safety net. Legally speaking, consultation is an activity that occurs between legal peers, and the person receiving the consultation has the authority to reject or accept the recommendations of the consultant. Consequently, those providing consultation have very low legal liability. When crises occur, however, professionals often do not have the opportunity to consult with others; they are faced with an immediate problem and must respond based on the information they have at the moment. On the other hand, practitioners often address chronic crises that go on over days or weeks, or they may sense that certain patients are doing poorly and are at risk of entering a crisis. Consultation helps ensure that an adequate standard of care is being delivered. Furthermore, the mere act of obtaining a consultation may have emotional benefits and just talking out the case or preparing for the consultation can help the practitioner develop a better understanding of how the case should be conceptualized.

Documentation should be increased with crisis cases. The general rule in risk management is "if it isn't written down, it didn't happen." In the event of a tragedy and a lawsuit, courts will give very high deference to records. The general assumption by courts is that the records are accurate and there is a very high threshold for a plaintiff to successfully challenge what is written in the record. The documentation should follow the "ninth-grade algebra teacher" model (Bennett et al., in press), in which the practitioner records the steps that he/she followed and the reasoning behind the final decision. In the worst-case scenario, if a tragedy were to occur and the practitioner were to be sued, the notes would document the thoroughness of the treatment plan and intervention.

Informed consent becomes especially important when treating patients who are at high risk for emergencies. Of course, in the first meeting, the practitioner needs to review basic information, including office or agency policies on after-hours coverage, confidentiality and its limitations, and other issues. Informed consent is best conceived as an ongoing process, not a one-time event. Consequently, the practitioner may need to review these issues periodically during the course of therapy. For example, if the practitioner is treating a patient who presents a risk of harming others, the practitioner can remind the patient of the ethical or legal obligation to break confidentiality to protect the life of an identifiable third party or a class of third parties, depending on the state law.

These risk management strategies are best operationalized when the ethical obligations of practitioners are kept in mind. For example, consultation should not be undertaken as a pro forma activity to give an appearance of competence but as a sincere effort undertaken to improve the quality of care, and informed consent should be completed to engage the patient in clinical decision making as much as possible.

CONCLUSION

Many scholars agree that mental health practitioners will continue to face ethics and malpractice complaints as laws become more complex. As mental health practices become more sophisticated and effective and thereby more standardized, it will become easier to establish standards of care. This increased precision will reduce the difficulty for practitioners to determine what is appropriate care and ironically may make it easier for patients to demonstrate malpractice when standards are not met.

Practitioners and agencies can take several steps to minimize the risks of malpractice. They should (1) maintain accurate records of patient care, (2) engage patients in the process of informed consent, (3) consult with colleagues to ensure that assessments and interventions meet standards of care, (4) strive to honor patients' rights to confidentiality, (5) accept only as many patients as can be carefully treated, (6) know state laws regarding duty to protect and warn and abuse reporting, (7) keep up to date in training on assessment and intervention with crisis patients, (8) establish a redundant system of protection for emergencies, and (9) exercise caution with new modalities of health care.

REFERENCES

Abile v. United States, 482 F. Supp. 703 (N.D. Cal. 1980).

American Psychiatric Association. (2003). *Practice guidelines for the assessment and treatment of patients with suicidal behaviors*. Available at *www.psych.org/psych_prac/treatg/pg/pg_suicidalbehavior.pdf*.

Anderson, J., & Barret, R. (2001). *Ethics in HIV-related psychotherapy*. Washington, DC: American Psychological Association.

Appelbaum, P. (1985). *Tarasoff* and the clinician: Problems in fulfilling the duty to protect. *American Journal of Psychiatry, 142*, 429.

Beck, J. (1987). The psychotherapists' duty to protect third parties from harm. *Mental Disability Law Reporter, 11*, 141–148.

Bennett, B., Bricklin, P., Harris, E., Knapp, S., & VandeCreek, L. (in press). *Risk management: A patient focused approach*. Washington, DC: American Psychological Association Insurance Trust.

Bongar, B. (2002). *The suicidal patient: Clinical and legal standards of care* (2nd ed.). Washington, DC: American Psychological Association.

Borum, R. (2000). Assessing violence risk among youths. *Journal of Clinical Psychology, 56*, 1263–1288.

Boynton v. Burglass, 590 So. 2d 446 Fla. Ct. App., 3d Dist., 1991).

Brent, D. A., Kupfer, D. J., Bromet, E. J., & Dew, M. A. (1988). The assessment and treatment of patients at risk for suicide. In A. J. Frances & R. E. Hales (Eds.), *American Psychiatric Press review of psychiatry* (Vol. 7, pp. 353–385). Washington, DC: American Psychiatric Press.

Chemtob, C. M., Hamada, R. S., Bauer, G. B., Kinney, B., & Torigoe, R. Y. (1988). Patient suicide: Frequency and impact on psychiatrists. *American Journal of Psychiatry, 145*, 224–228.

Chemtob, C. M., Hamada, R. S., Bauer, G. B., Torigoe, R. Y., & Kinney, B. (1988). Patient suicide: Frequency and impact on psychologists. *Professional Psychology: Research and Practice, 19*, 416–420.

Cominsky v. New York, 71 A.D.2d 699, 418 N.Y.S.2d 233 (1979).

Dalton v. State, 308 N.Y.S.2d 441 (1970).

Dinnerstein v. United States, 486 F.2d 34 (2nd Cir. 1973).

Eady v. Salter, 380 N.Y.S.2d 737 (App. Div. 1976).

Greenberg v. Barbour, 322 F. Supp. 745 (1971).

Harway, M., & Hanson, M. (2004). *Spouse abuse* (2nd ed.). Sarasota, FL: Professional Resource Press.

Knapp, S., & VandeCreek, L. (1987). A review of tort liability in involuntary civil commitment. *Hospital and Community Psychiatry, 38,* 648–651.

Knapp, S., & VandeCreek, L. (2006). *Practical ethics: A positive approach.* Washington, DC: American Psychological Association.

Lipari v. Sears, 497 F. Supp. 185 (D. Neb. 1980).

Nasser v. Parker, 455 S.E.2d 502 (Va. 1995).

National Institute of Mental Health. (2002). *Suicide facts.* Available at *www.nimh.nih.gov/research/suifact.htm*

Oordt, M., Jobes, D., Rudd, M. D., Fonseca, V., Runyan, C., Stea, J., et al. (2005). Development of a clinical guide to enhance care for suicidal patients. *Professional Psychology: Research and Practice, 36,* 208–218.

Paradies v. Benedictine Hospital, 431 N.Y.S.2d 175 (App. Div. 1980).

Paris, J. (2002). Chronic suicidality among patients with borderline personality disorder. *Psychiatric Services, 53,* 738–742.

Tarasoff v. Regents of the University of California, 551 P.2d 334 (1976).

Texarkana Memorial Hospital, Inc. v. Firth, 746 S.W.2d 494 (1988).

VandeCreek, L., & Knapp, S. (2001). Tarasoff *and beyond* (3rd ed.). Sarasota, FL: Professional Resource Press.

SUGGESTED READINGS

Bongar, B. (2002). *The suicidal patient: Clinical and legal standards of care* (2nd ed.). Washington, DC: American Psychological Association.

Borum, R. (2000). Assessing violence risk among youth. *Journal of Clinical Psychology, 56,* 1263–1288.

Borun, R., & Verhaagen, D. (2006). *Assessing and managing violence risk in juveniles.* New York: Guilford Press.

Monahan, J., & Steadman, H. (1996). Violent storms and violent people: How meteorology can inform risk communication in mental health law. *American Psychologists, 51,* 931–938.

Norko, M., & Baranoski, M. (2005). The state of contemporary risk assessment research. *Canadian Journal of Psychiatry, 50,* 18–26.

VandeCreek, L., & Knapp, S. (2001). Tarasoff *and beyond* (3rd ed.). Sarasota, FL: Professional Resource Press.

Index